Stevens & Lowe's
Human Histology
FOURTH EDITION

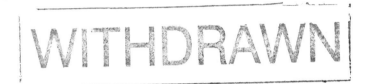

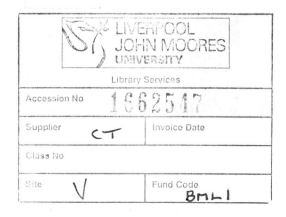

Stevens & Lowe's
Human Histology

FOURTH EDITION

James S. Lowe

BMedSci, BMBS, DM, FRCPath
Professor of Neuropathology
University of Nottingham Medical School
Nottingham, UK

Peter G. Anderson

DVM, PhD
Professor of Molecular and Cellular Pathology
Director of Pathology Undergraduate Education
Department of Pathology
The University of Alabama at Birmingham
Birmingham, Alabama, USA

ELSEVIER
MOSBY

ELSEVIER
MOSBY

1600 John F. Kennedy Blvd.
Ste 1800
Philadelphia, PA 19103-2899

STEVENS & LOWE'S HUMAN HISTOLOGY, FOURTH EDITION   ISBN: 978-0-723435020

Library of Congress Cataloging-in-Publication Data

Lowe, J. S. (James Steven), author. Stevens & Lowe's human histology / James S. Lowe, Peter G. Anderson.—Fourth edition.
     p. ; cm.
   Stevens and Lowe's human histology
   Human histology
   Includes index.
   Preceded by Human histology / Alan Stevens, James Steven Lowe. 3rd ed. 2005.
   ISBN 978-0-7234-3502-0 (pbk.)
   I. Anderson, Peter G. (Pathologist), author.   II. Stevens, Alan (Pathologist).
Human histology. Preceded by (work):   III. Title.   IV. Title: Stevens and Lowe's human histology.   V. Title: Human histology.
   [DNLM: 1. Histology—Atlases.   2. Histology—Examination Questions. QS 504]
QM551
611'.018—dc23
                                                                    2014016496

Content Strategist: Meghan Ziegler
Content Development Specialist: Stacy Matusik
Publishing Services Manager: Hemamalini Rajendrababu
Project Manager: Nisha Selvaraj
Design Direction: Ellen Zanolle/Ryan Cook

Printed in China
Last digit is the print number: 9 8 7 6 5 4 3 2

About This Book

Considerable thought has gone into designing this book to meet the requirements of students who have a limited time in which to assimilate information, yet need to take in maximum detail without re-reading portions of text or becoming fatigued. Many features of this book have been designed to ease reading and assimilation and to highlight clinical relevance, which hopefully will facilitate understanding and thus make it easier to remember details. There is a saying that goes: 'Memorization is what we do when what we are trying to learn makes no sense' (anonymous). Our goal with this revised textbook is to make it easier for students to understand histology in a relevant context so you do not have to resort to rote memorization.

Summary Headings

These headings (bold-faced declarative sentences scattered throughout) provide a summary of the forthcoming text, giving a quick overview of the whole section. These have proven to be popular with students as a high yield overview of each section.

Figure Legends

The figure legends are, in general, not repetitive of the main text and are designed to be read when referenced from the main text. This serves two purposes: first, it maintains the flow of information and, second, it provides a refreshing break from reading the main text. For this reason, many of the captions are used as the vehicle to explain complex pieces of information, particularly those relating to three-dimensional structure.

Clinical Example Boxes

 We have chosen many clinical examples to illustrate the vital role that an understanding of histological structure will play in subsequent studies of human biology, disease and clinical practice.

Practical Histology Boxes

 Many students give up microscopy because they feel that they cannot see what they have just read about. The practical histology sections are designed to put histology into a classroom teaching perspective and hopefully lessen the anxiety of the students who feel that they cannot use a microscope.

Advanced Concept Boxes

 In these sections, we supply more advanced knowledge than is strictly necessary for an understanding of the basic principles. These sections often contain the results of up-to-date research, including some of the most important elements of progress in cell biology.

Key Facts Boxes

 These provide a number of the most important Key Facts relating to the subject just covered. They are ideal for pre-examination panic states to get a student's thoughts in-line and focused on the most important concepts.

Throughout the book, you will see that small sections of text have been emboldened. These are problem-based 'hooks' – text that will be of particular use to readers using the book as a reference for problem-based or case-based study.

End of Chapter Review Questions

 These simple questions in true/false format allow a student to assess both memory and comprehension.

We have also added some problem-based learning exercises in the form of brief clinical histories, followed by simple, fairly broad questions aimed to get the student to think about histology in relation to clinical problems.

The answers to both the true/false and case-based questions can be found in the appendix at the back of the book.

Online Review Questions

Laura F. Cotlin, PhD, Associate Professor, Dept of Cell, Developmental and Integrative Biology, University of Alabama at Birmingham, has written online review questions for this edition of *Human Histology*. These questions are available online at https://studentconsult.inkling.com.

Feedback

Many of the changes in the presentation of this book have been stimulated by comments about previous editions made by teachers and students who used the book for their courses and personal study. This has proved so successful that we again wish to canvas the comments of the users of the fourth edition in the hopes of further improving it in subsequent editions. We hope that teachers and students will again take this opportunity to have an input into the creation of this valuable teaching resource, and are happy to receive suggestions about any new material and illustrations which could be included.

We can be contacted by letter at the address given but are also happy to receive comments by e-mail at: pga@uab.edu.

Preface to the Fourth Edition

Changes in medical education have resulted in curricula that emphasize integration and application of relevant knowledge. In this new edition of *Human Histology*, we have endeavoured to highlight the histology that is relevant to disease processes. While providing a thorough traditional overview of histology, we have also attempted to emphasize the structures and the structure–function relationships that are germane to disease pathogenesis. We have tried to highlight histological structures that play key roles in disease pathogenesis in order to help the health professional student learn histology in the context of relevant clinical disease processes. The non-verbose, high yield content, the layout and the add-ons associated with this book are designed to help students learn the histology that informs histopathology and disease pathogenesis.

Preface to the Third Edition

Our philosophy and principles remain as stated at length in the preface to the second edition. We have tried to keep the text and illustrations as user-friendly as possible and have ruthlessly removed padding and verbosity. When faced with a conflict between comprehensiveness and comprehensibility we have chosen comprehensibility every time.

We have also stuck to our principles of only using human material, even though we acknowledge that the ultrastructural illustrations fall short of perfect. You will find no micrographs of the tissues of rodents or charging manta rays in here.

The major educational change since the second edition has been the greater reliance in some courses on problem-based learning. Although this adds an excellent and exciting dimension to student learning, it requires careful organization and close monitoring by a skilled and enthusiastic teacher (or 'facilitator' in current education jargon) if the inexperienced student is to find the clear and correct path through the jungle. We fear it may all end in tears. Nevertheless, we have included some problem-based learning exercises at the end of most chapters, based on brief clinical histories. To be effective, the answers to these problems must be explained at some length, and we have provided these online.

We have also provided a virtual online microscopy lab, comprising histology images which can be wandered over so that many fields of the same image can be examined at different magnifications, accompanied by labels, some explanatory text and feedback questions.

We tiptoe carefully into the 21st Century.

Acknowledgements to the Fourth Edition

It is of course obligatory that we thank all of those who helped in the first three editions of this book, since much of that material still serves as the core of this textbook. In this new edition, the goal is to emphasize clinical relevance and applicability. To this end, every chapter was reviewed by diagnostic pathologists from the Department of Pathology at the University of Alabama at Birmingham. I am indebted to my UAB Pathology colleagues for their time and their helpful suggestions as they reviewed each chapter related to their area of expertise.

All of the new images in this fourth edition were generated from virtual microscopy files. I want to thank Dr Laura Fraser Cotlin from the UAB Department of Cell, Developmental, and Integrative Biology for providing us with the microscopic slide sets used in our UAB histology course. I also want to acknowledge Matthew C. Anderson for his many hours of meticulous work scanning all of the histology and pathology glass slides used to create our extensive UAB Virtual Microscopy library, which served as the resource for the new images in this text.

Acknowledgments to the Third Edition

In addition to all those who helped in the first and second editions of the book, and whose work continues to be a vital part of the project, we are delighted to thank the following: Carol Dunn and Liz Bakowski for producing fantastic histological sections. Irene Smith for patiently typing parts of the manuscript. Anne Kane for her skill and technological ability with Photoshop and patience with our demands. We would also like to extend our sincere thanks to the team from Elsevier who made the parts a whole.

Acknowledgments to the First and Second Editions

We wish to thank the laboratory staff of the University Department of Histopathology, Queen's Medical Centre, Nottingham, for the skill and patience with which they have produced the sections which we have photographed for this book. In particular we are grateful to Ian and Anne Wilson, Angela Crossman, Janet Palmer, Lianne Ward and David McQuire for paraffin sections, Neil Hand for acrylic resin sections and for the immunocyto-chemcial preparations of the pancreatic islets, Ken Morrell and his team for immunocytochemical preparations, and Janet Palmer for enzyme histochemical preparations. We owe a particular vote of thanks to Trevor Gray who has spent many hours searching out suitable material for transmission and scanning electron microscopy, and is responsible for all of the electron micrographs in this book, as well as the thin epoxy resin sections.

Bill Brackenbury photographed all the gross specimens, and also provided us with many of the very low magnification photomicrographs. Isabella Streeter kindly word-processed much of the new textual material and legends for the new illustrations.

Many professional colleagues at Queen's Medical Centre and elsewhere contributed suitable tissue for processing and subsequent photomicrography. Dr J Wendy Blundell provided the arteriograms for Chapter 15 and, with Dr Ian Leach, supplied material and photomicrographs for Chapter 9.

Dr Peter Furness kindly allowed us to use one of his electron micrographs showing the polyanionic sites in the glomerulus. Dr Jane Zuccollo provided us with material relating to human fetal and neonatal histology, and Dr Mark Stephens supplied us with a rare slide of an early human implantation site.

Dr Mark Wilkinson provided material for Chapter 10 and Jocelyn Germaine of the London Hospital kindly made available some of the material used in the section on teeth in Chapter 11. Dr David Clark gave valuable help and advice in the preparation of Chapter 7 and Dr Barbara Bain kindly allowed us to use a transparency of a large granular lymphocyte in Chapter 8. Dr George Lindop some years ago supplied us with a transparency showing the localisation of renin in the human glomerulus; we were unable to find room for it in the first edition, but it is now illustrated as Figure 15.29b. Professor L Michaels generously allowed us to use his transparency of the human organ of Corti (Fig. 19.5b).

We would like to thank all of the staff of Times Mirror International Publishers who have been involved in the preparation of this second edition. Special thanks to Louise Cook, the Development Editor, for keeping us as nearly under control as can be expected, and also for the Belgian beer; to Elaine Graham and Louise Crowe, the Project Managers, for managing to squeeze our quart into a pint pot without getting cross; to Gudrun Hughes, Production Controller, who controlled things; and to Pete Wilder, Lynda Payne, Greg Smith, Richard Prime, Marie McNestry, Mark Willey, Tim Read, Rob Curran and James Lauder who are responsible for all the pretty, arty, illustrational stuff without which this book would be almost drab. Thanks also to Roger Ashton-Griffiths and Ellen Sarewitz who checked our text for idiocies and typographical errors.

Finally, we are grateful to Dianne Zack, our lovely publisher, for her sustained enthusiasm and energy, for the numerous faxes she sent us (when we were flagging) to tell us how brilliant we were, and how scintillating the book was going to be. Not only that, but she also assiduously translated our English writing into American! We still think that 'Oesophagus' looks prettier than 'Esophagus' but are not inclined to argue.

And of course, we still adore Fiona Foley.

Dedication

*We dedicate this book, with love and gratitude
for their patience and tolerance, to our wives,*
Christine Stevens
Pamela Lowe
and
Joan Anderson

And to our children,
Claire Brierley (née Stevens)
Kate Stevens
Nicholas Lowe
William Lowe
Robert Anderson
Matthew Anderson

Table of Contents

Stevens & Lowe's
Human Histology
FOURTH EDITION

Chapter 1

Histology

Introduction

Histology is central to biological and medical science

Histology is the study of the microscopic structure of biological material and the ways in which individual components are structurally and functionally related. It is central to biological and medical science since it stands at the crossroads between biochemistry, molecular biology and physiology on the one side, and disease processes and their effects on the other.

Samples of human biological material can be obtained from many areas of the body by quick, safe techniques (Fig. 1.1), using instruments such as:
- Scalpels for directly accessible tissues such as the skin, mouth, nose, etc.
- Needles into solid organs
- Endoscopic tubes into the alimentary tract or body cavities
- Special flexible cannulae inside blood vessels.

Knowledge of normal histological appearances is essential if abnormal diseased structures are to be recognized, and to comprehend how abnormal biochemical and physiological processes result in disease.

This is an exciting period in histology, for we are now able to explore the physiological and molecular basis of biological structures through the development of techniques that allow us to examine the chemical make-up of living tissues under the microscope. It is now becoming clear why various biological structures are shaped and arranged as they are.

Histology was once an empirical subject

The study of histology began with the development of simple light microscopes and techniques for preparing thin slices of biological material to make them suitable for examination. Despite their simple equipment and somewhat inadequately prepared material, early histologists learned a surprising amount about the structure of biological material. Such studies led Virchow to propound his cellular theory of the structure of living organisms that established the **cell** as the basic building block of most biological material. Each cell was considered as an individual unit surrounded by a wall called the **cell membrane** and containing within it all of the machinery for its function. In those early years a vocabulary of histology was developed, based on light microscopic analysis of cells and accompanied by a limited understanding of cell physiology and function.

Collections of cells having similar morphological characteristics were described as forming **tissues**. These were originally subdivided into four types:
- Epithelial tissues, or cells which cover surfaces, line body cavities or form solid glands such as salivary glands
- Muscular tissues, or cells with contractile properties
- Nervous tissues referred to cells forming the brain, spinal cord and nerves
- Connective tissue, or cells that produce an extracellular matrix and serve to link or support other specialized tissues by forming tendons, bones or fatty tissue.

Modern histology is a precise science

Modern investigative techniques have revolutionized our understanding of cells. The techniques of electron microscopy, cloning of cells in culture, protein sequencing and molecular genetics have also given unprecedented insight into the working of cells.

Although improvements in knowledge and understanding have been matched in other sciences by the rapid emergence of new vocabularies, this has not always been the case in histology. For many years, the terms and classifications that originated from early histological studies were retained. With every new discovery about the structure of living material, attempts were made to force the new information into an old, often inappropriate classification of cells and tissues.

Fortunately, this rigid histological system is now giving way to a more exciting and functional approach, based on our understanding of cell biology.

Cells are Basic Functional Units

Modern knowledge confirms Virchow's correctness in describing the cell as the basic unit of structure of most living organisms.

Cells vary considerably. Although all cells in the human body are ultimately derived from a single fertilized egg, each cell develops structural attributes to suit its function through the process of differentiation, and is a considerably more sophisticated and complex unit than was formerly suspected. Molecular biology has

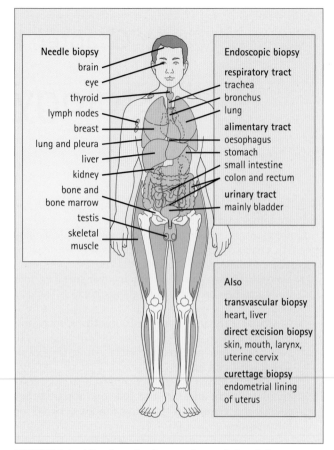

Needle biopsy
brain
eye
thyroid
lymph nodes
breast
lung and pleura
liver
kidney
bone and
bone marrow
testis
skeletal
muscle

Endoscopic biopsy

respiratory tract
trachea
bronchus
lung
alimentary tract
oesophagus
stomach
small intestine
colon and rectum
urinary tract
mainly bladder

Also

transvascular biopsy
heart, liver

direct excision biopsy
skin, mouth, larynx,
uterine cervix

curettage biopsy
endometrial lining
of uterus

FIGURE 1.1 **Histology in diagnostic medicine.** It is now possible to obtain small samples from many areas of the body by various techniques. Histological examination of such samples is an increasingly important and direct way of diagnosing disease.

shown that cells of diverse morphological appearance can be grouped together because of common functional attributes or interactions.

Some cells are adaptable. It has also become apparent that even in the adult, there are populations of highly adaptable, uncommitted cells, which can modify both their structure and their functional activity to adapt to changing environmental demands. This facility is of vital importance in adaptation to internal or external stress, and is commonly seen in disease processes (e.g. replacement of damaged heart muscle by strong fibrous tissue following a heart attack).

The general structural and biological properties of cells are discussed in Chapter 2, and many of their specialized functional attributes in Chapters 3, 4 and 5.

Cells are now classified according to function

It is now possible to classify cells into groups based on their main function. The groupings that will be used in this book are: epithelial cells, supporting cells, contractile cells, nerve cells, germ cells, blood cells, immune cells and hormone-secreting cells (Fig. 1.2). It is important, however, to recognize that a cell may have several functions and be a member of more than one cell group. For example:

- Many of the hormone-producing cells are also epithelial in type, being tightly bound together by specialized junctions to form a gland
- Many immune cells are also blood cells
- Some support cells are also contractile.

The structural and functional specializations delineating each type of cell group are broadly outlined in Chapters 3, 4 and 5, and discussed in more detail throughout the book.

Cell group	Epithelial cells	Support cells	Contractile cells	Nerve cells	Germ cells	Blood cells	Immune cells	Hormone-secreting cells
Example	gut and blood vessel lining, covering skin	fibrous support tissue, cartilage, bone	muscle	brain	spermatozoa	circulating red and white blood cells	lymphoid tissues and white cells (nodes and spleen)	thyroid and adrenal
Function	barrier, absorption, secretion	organize and maintain body structure	movement	direct cell communication	reproduction	oxygen transport, defence	defence	indirect cell communication
Special features	tightly bound together by cell junctions (see Chapter 3)	produce and interact with extracellular matrix material (see Chapter 4)	filamentous proteins cause contraction (see Chapter 5)	release chemical messengers on to surface of other cells (see Chapter 6)	half normal chromosome complement (see Chapters 16 and 17)	proteins bind oxygen, proteins destroy bacteria (see Chapter 7)	recognize and destroy foreign material (see Chapter 8)	secrete chemical messengers (see Chapter 14)

FIGURE 1.2 **Modern functional cell classification.**

Tissues are functional arrangements of cells

A tissue is an assembly of cells arranged in a specific organized fashion. In some cases, the cells are all of the same structure, forming **simple tissues**, for example fat cells forming adipose tissue. However, most apparently distinct tissues contain a mixture of cells with different functions, which may be termed **compound tissues** (Fig. 1.3). For example, 'nervous tissue' contains nerve cells (neurons), support cells (astrocytes), immune cells (microglia) and epithelial cells (ependyma).

The concept of simple and compound tissues is useful in descriptive histology, but for brevity, the unqualified term 'tissue' is used to imply either type.

Connective tissue is a term that underemphasizes its highly specialized role

The one exception to the acceptable use of the term tissue is the old expression 'connective tissue'. This was used to describe a wide range of living material containing cells associated with a dominant extracellular matrix component. In theory, its function was to act as a supporting stroma, serving more highly specialized cell types.

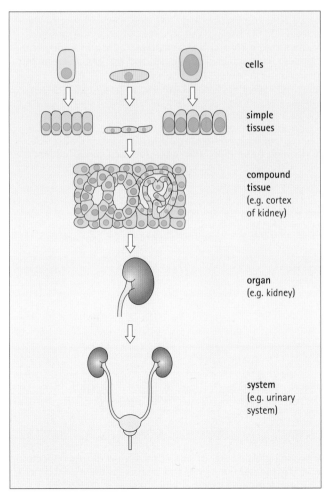

FIGURE 1.3 **Cells, tissues, organs and systems.**

The original group of 'connective tissues' included cell/matrix combinations, such as bone, cartilage, tendon, fibrous tissue, adipose tissue, bone marrow and blood. It has also been traditional to use the term 'loose areolar connective tissue' to describe tissue that is partly made up of support cells that produce an extracellular matrix, but which also contains cells belonging to the immune system (e.g. lymphocytes and macrophages), nerve cells and blood vessels.

In this book, the term 'connective tissue' has been avoided because it underemphasizes the structural organization involved in this group of highly developed tissues. Instead, the concept of support cells is used, which emphasizes the importance of interactions between extracellular matrix and cells.

Support cells and their specializations are discussed in Chapter 4, while bone, tendons and ligaments are discussed in Chapter 13.

Tissues form organs and systems

An organ – for example the heart, liver or kidney – is an anatomically distinct group of tissues, usually of several types, which perform specific functions.

The term 'system' can be used to:
- Describe cells with a similar function but widely distributed in several anatomic sites
- Describe a group of organs which have similar or related functional roles.

The specialized hormone-producing cells scattered in the gut and lung (diffuse endocrine system) cannot be an organ, as they do not form an anatomically distinct mass, whereas the tongue, oesophagus, stomach, intestines, exocrine pancreas and rectum are components of the 'alimentary system', and the kidney, pelvicalyceal system, ureters and bladder are part of the 'urinary system'.

The relationships between cells, tissues, organs and systems are shown in Figure 1.3.

Histology in Other Disciplines

Cell histology is aligned to cell biology

The most common way to study cells is by light microscopy. Tissues are mounted on glass slides as thin preparations, stained with appropriate dyes, illuminated by light and viewed using glass lenses. The analysis of the fine structure of cells by light microscopy is referred to as **cytology**.

There is a limit to the detail that can be resolved using light microscopy, with very small structures within cells being invisible. Until recently, the only way to look at the fine intracellular detail of individual cells was by using electron microscopy, which greatly increases resolution, allowing the subcellular composition of cells to be defined.

These techniques are now complemented by the increasing use of immunohistochemical methods. Antibodies are applied to specific cell constituents to visualize details within cells at the light microscopic level that are not visible by other techniques. For example, the location of specific proteins or subcellular components can now be defined in light microscopic preparations by using immunohistochemical staining techniques.

It is also now possible to demonstrate specific DNA and RNA sequences by the technique of in situ hybridization, thereby gaining fundamental insight into the molecular mechanisms of cells.

A clear understanding of the fine structure and molecular organization of cells greatly improves comprehension of biochemical and physiologic processes. This overlap between structure, physiology, biochemistry and genetics is now embraced by the term 'cell biology'.

Systems histology is aligned to anatomy

Study of the arrangement of different tissues at the microscopic level (systems histology) gives insight into the structure and function of organs and systems. This type of study is an extension of anatomy, and for this reason is often termed 'microscopic anatomy'.

The study of systems histology is an important component of human biology and, in most curricula, is taught alongside normal anatomy.

Histology is essential for understanding pathology

Pathology (understanding disease processes) accounts for a significant portion of most medical curricula. And since most disease processes are associated with histological abnormalities the understanding of systems histology and microanatomy is an important part of the medical student's armamentarium. In modern medicine, despite sophisticated imaging and genetic testing, a histological diagnosis is still the mainstay or the 'gold standard' of clinical practice. This is illustrated in the box below.

 CLINICAL EXAMPLE
HISTOLOGY IN DISEASE DIAGNOSIS

A 20-year-old student develops kidney failure and the cause is not apparent from blood tests or radiology. The renal physician therefore removes a piece of kidney via a needle biopsy so that the diagnosis can be made by histological examination. Special staining methods highlight subtle structural abnormalities by light microscopy (Fig. 1.4), and electron microscopy provides valuable information about abnormalities at a subcellular level. On the basis of the abnormalities that are revealed, an accurate histological diagnosis is made and the renal physician can institute appropriate treatment. Clinical management of this patient requires knowledge of the microanatomy of the kidney. Assessment of progress, and the effectiveness of treatment, are monitored by repeated biopsy.

A 15-year-old girl has swollen lymph nodes in her neck. A surgeon removes one so that it can be examined histologically, and microscopy reveals that the swelling is caused by a form of cancer. The classification of tumours is determined by histology and immunohistochemistry. Accurate histological assessment of tumours is the cornerstone of modern cancer treatment, since the treatment given to this girl depends on the histological type of the tumour (i.e. whether it is derived from muscle, lymphoid cells or endocrine cells). Thus, the pathologist's report, which depends on histological assessment of that specific tumour being accurate, will determine the type of chemotherapy deemed to be most efficacious for each cancer patient's treatment protocol.

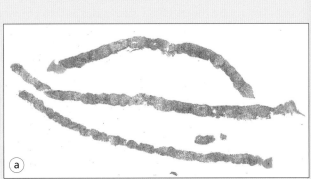

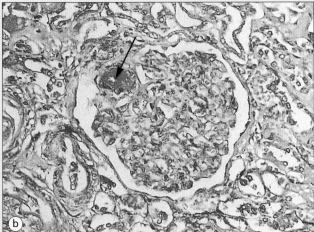

FIGURE 1.4 **Kidney.** (a) Percutaneous needle biopsy sections from a diagnostic case. (b) High-power view of these needle biopsy specimens of kidney (paraffin section, MSB stain). The special stain shows the nature and location of the main abnormality, destruction of the afferent arteriole of the glomerulus by a disease process called 'fibrinoid necrosis' (arrow).

Techniques Used in Histology and Cell Biology

Light Microscopy

Light microscopy using wax-embedded sections is the main technique used in histology

Routine light microscopy uses thin sections of tissue to study cell morphology. Resolution of structures by light microscopy is of the order of $0.2\,\mu m$, but in routine practice with paraffin sections this is seldom better than $0.6\,\mu m$. Sections are usually obtained as follows:
- Tissue is immersed in a preservative solution (fixative), which cross-links or precipitates proteins and prevents degradation
- Tissue is embedded in a firm medium (paraffin wax) for cutting into thin sections
- Tissue is cut into sections (conventionally $5-8\,\mu m$ thick) on a microtome.

The paraffin wax-impregnated thin-sliced sections are mounted on a glass microscope slide and the wax removed with an organic solvent before the section is rehydrated through increasing dilutions of alcohol in water. When fully rehydrated, the sections are stained with any of a number of stains, some of which are outlined below. In routine laboratory practice, it generally takes 24 hours to produce a wax section for histology.

In some cases (for instance surgical biopsies), it is necessary to look at fresh tissues which have not been exposed to protein cross-linking in fixation. In this situation, tissue is made firm enough to cut by freezing; a technique referred to as preparing a frozen section.

Tissue Staining

To see tissue detail, it is necessary to stain the tissue components in a histological section

Cells are virtually colourless and so sections need to be stained for light microscopy. There are four main types of staining:
- Empirical
- Histochemical
- Enzyme histochemical
- Immunohistochemical.

Empirical stains are widely used, and form the basis of most routine stains in histology and histopathology

Many of the stains used have been discovered by trial and error over a period of 100 years or more, and many methods use dyes and principles (e.g. use of mordants) that were developed by the textile industry. In most cases, the precise details of the mechanism of the specific linkage between dye and tissue is not fully understood: sometimes it appears to be related to the sizes of the dye molecules used and sometimes the result of ionic charges on the dye molecules. Empirical stains include van Gieson's and trichrome methods (see 'Advanced Concept' box on p. 6). In some cases, staining is the

ADVANCED CONCEPT
FROZEN SECTIONS

The process of fixation and embedding of biological material in paraffin and other media may destroy certain components, particularly enzymes and some antigenic sites. If frozen water is used as the supporting medium, these are better preserved and can be demonstrated by suitable techniques. Fresh (unfixed) material is rapidly frozen to −150°C to −170°C by immersion in, for example liquid nitrogen, so that it hardens to a solid mass owing to freezing of tissue water. Thin sections ($5-10\,\mu m$) are then cut on a special microtome housed in a refrigerated cabinet (a cryostat), and stained without exposure to alcohol or other organic solvents.

Frozen sections are used to demonstrate the cellular localization of enzymes and soluble lipids, and in the identification of substances using immunofluorescent and immunocytochemical methods.

Further use is made of frozen sections in diagnostic histopathology, when an urgent tissue diagnosis is required of, for example a suspected tumour, while the patient is still on the operating table. In skilled hands, a frozen section of a sample of human tissue stained with haematoxylin and eosin (H&E) can be prepared and examined under the microscope within 5 min of its removal from the body. In this way, a rapid and accurate histological diagnosis can be established while the patient is in the operating theatre, enabling the appropriate surgical room procedure to be performed.

ADVANCED CONCEPT
PARAFFIN EMBEDDING

Paraffin embedding is the standard method of preparing thin sections of biological material for histological examination by light microscopy. It is cheap, comparatively simple and lends itself to automation.

The sample is fixed, usually in an aqueous formalin-based fixative solution, and then progressively dehydrated by passage through a series of alcohol solutions (e.g. 60%, 70%, 90%, 100%) until all water (intrinsic tissue water and fixative water) has been removed and the specimen is thoroughly permeated by absolute alcohol. The alcohol is then replaced by an organic solvent, which is miscible both with alcohol and with molten liquid paraffin wax (alcohol is not miscible with paraffin wax). The resulting specimen is immersed in paraffin wax at a temperature just above the melting point of the wax, which is solid at normal working room temperature. When the biological material is thoroughly permeated by the molten wax, it is allowed to cool so that the wax solidifies. The wax acts as a physical support to the sample, allowing thin sections ($2-7\,\mu m$) to be cut without deformation of the cellular structure and architecture.

ADVANCED CONCEPT
COMMONLY USED HISTOLOGICAL STAINS

Haematoxylin and Eosin (H&E)

The combination of the two dyes, haematoxylin (blue) and eosin (red), is the most useful stain for the examination of biological material; it is simple to perform, reliable, inexpensive and informative. Cell nuclei stain blue (depending on section thickness and the formulation of haematoxylin used), and most components of the cell cytoplasm stain pink/red. Most of the micrographs in this book are stained with H&E, particularly in the Practical Histology sections.

Van Gieson Method

The simple van Gieson method stains collagen pinkish-red and muscle yellow (see Fig. 10.21); it is commonly used in combination with a stain for elastic fibres. The elastic van Gieson (EVG) stain is valuable for demonstrating and differentiating the common support cell fibres, particularly elastic fibres, which stain brown-black, and collagen fibres, which stain pinkish-red; muscle is stained yellow (see Fig. 10.21).

Trichrome Methods

The trichrome methods employ a mixture of three dyes to stain different components in different colours. There are many trichrome methods, and they can be used to demonstrate general architecture, to emphasize support fibres, or to distinguish support fibres from muscle fibres. An important use of a trichrome method is the demonstration of the cellular, osteoid and mineralized components of bone in non-decalcified bone embedded in acrylic resin (see Figs 13.17a, 13.19b).

Silver Methods

Under appropriate conditions, certain biological components, both within cells and in intercellular materials, reduce silver nitrate to form black deposits of metallic silver at the site of chemical reduction. By modifying the conditions of the silver nitrate solution used, these methods can be used to demonstrate a wide range of structures, including reticular fibres (see Fig. 4.5).

Periodic Acid–Schiff (PAS) Method

The widely used PAS method has many applications, particularly in the demonstration of various carbohydrates, either alone (e.g. glycogen; Fig 1.5) or combined with other molecules, such as proteins (e.g. glycoproteins), which are stained magenta. It can therefore be used to delineate basement membranes (see Fig. 4.12a) and some neutral mucins secreted by various secretory epithelial cells. The mucous cells of the stomach are strongly PAS-positive.

Alcian Blue Method

The Alcian blue dye method is used mainly to demonstrate acidic mucins secreted by some epithelial cells (see Fig. 11.44b), and can be combined with the PAS reaction to distinguish between acidic and neutral epithelial mucins. Through control of pH or other variables in the staining solution, the Alcian blue method can be used to demonstrate the extracellular glycosaminoglycan matrix (see Fig. 4.14d) of support cells.

May–Grünwald–Giemsa Method

The use of the May–Grünwald–Giemsa method is confined mainly to the examination of smear preparations of blood and bone marrow cells. Most of the micrographs in Chapter 7 show red and white blood cells stained by this method.

Myelin Methods

Several staining techniques can be used to demonstrate normal myelin. The dye solochrome cyanin is frequently used to demonstrate myelin in paraffin sections (see Fig. 6.24b). Other methods use modified haematoxylin or osmium tetroxide.

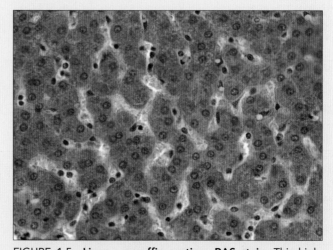

FIGURE 1.5 **Liver – paraffin section: PAS stain.** This high-power photomicrograph shows intense red staining of the liver cell cytoplasm by the PAS stain. It demonstrates the large amounts of glycogen present.

result of a specific chemical reaction between a specific tissue component and a component of the stain solution; these methods are called histochemical methods.

> **In histochemical methods, specific chemical compounds within the tissue can be localized**

A commonly used example of a simple histochemical staining method is the PAS (Periodic Acid–Schiff) reaction, which demonstrates a wide range of tissue carbohydrates, including cytoplasmic glycogen and complex carbohydrate-containing substances, such as epithelial mucins. The rationale of the method is that carbon-to-carbon bonds in 1.2-glycols are cleaved using an oxidative agent, periodic acid. This produces dialdehydes, which then react with the colourless Schiff's reagent (fuchsin–sulfurous acid) to produce a vivid magenta-coloured compound.

Enzyme histochemical techniques identify and localize the sites of activity of particular enzymes

To look at the tissue distribution of specific enzymes, sections of fresh tissue prepared on a cryostat are placed in an incubating solution containing the specific substrate for the enzyme or group of enzymes to be demonstrated, together with any necessary co-factors or inhibitors. The enzyme in the tissue reacts with the substrate to form an insoluble primary reaction product. This is then visualized by its reaction with a visualizing agent, which may be included with the incubating medium or applied as a separate second step.

This technique can be used to show the localization of a vast number of enzymes, including acid and alkaline phosphatases, dehydrogenases and ATPases, and is routinely used to detect abnormalities in certain diseased tissue, particularly muscle (see Fig. 13.4).

As most biological enzyme systems are labile, they may be destroyed by fixation and tissue processing; thus most enzyme histochemical methods are carried out on frozen sections.

Immunocytochemistry uses antibodies to localize specific proteins in tissue sections

Immunocytochemistry is one of the most important innovations in histology. Antibodies to specific cell molecules are used to detect their presence in tissue sections. Polyclonal antibodies to a substance are obtained by inoculating an animal (commonly a rabbit or sheep) with the purified protein and then harvesting serum from which a specific antibody can be extracted. Alternatively, monoclonal antibody may be produced by inoculating a mouse and fusing suitable antibody-producing cells with immortal mouse myeloma cells to continually produce antibodies in tissue culture.

High-resolution light microscopy can be performed with tissue embedded in resin

Resolution of structures by light microscopy using paraffin sections is seldom better than 0.6 μm, the resolution being limited by the thickness of the section, which is rarely thinner than 3 μm. Much better resolution can be obtained by using thinner sections – about 0.5–2 μm – but these cannot be achieved consistently with wax as the embedding medium and using a standard microtome. The use of acrylic and epoxy resins as embedding media allows thinner tissue sections to be cut.

Resin-embedded sections are used increasingly in histology, and examples will be provided in this book where appropriate.

Acrylic resins are a suitable embedding medium for the production of histological sections of non-decalcified bone

Bone, unless severely diseased, is usually too hard to produce thin histological sections using standard paraffin wax as the embedding medium and normal microtome knives. This is because the difference in hardness between the bone and the wax in which it is embedded is too

great, so the bone shatters when the microtome knife blade passes through it, rendering the histology uninterpretable. Bone can be examined histologically in this way only if it is first softened by complete removal of the calcium salts by immersing the fixed bone sample in dilute acid until all the calcium has disappeared; sections can then be produced, but the histology is inevitably modified by the acid treatment. Furthermore, any distinction between mineralized bone and unmineralized osteoid is destroyed by the acid decalcification; this can be important in the diagnosis of some important bone diseases.

ADVANCED CONCEPT
RESINS AND HISTOLOGICAL EMBEDDING MEDIA

Acrylic Resin Embedding

Certain acrylic resins are used in a similar way to paraffin wax as embedding media. When set, they are harder than paraffin wax and offer more support to the tissue than wax. They have two main advantages over paraffin wax for light microscopy:

- With the use of a special microtome, much thinner sections (i.e. 1–2 μm thick) can be obtained than with paraffin wax, giving greater resolution with the light microscope and enabling much more detail to be seen
- They cause very little tissue shrinkage and enable good-quality sections of very hard material to be cut, and are therefore used in the histological examination of mineralized bone (see Figs 13.17a, 13.19b).

Epoxy Resin Embedding

Epoxy resins are the hardest supporting media for biological material. With special sectioning machines, sections as thin as 0.5–1 μm can be cut for high-resolution light microscopy and ultrathin sections can be prepared for transmission electron microscopy.

The transmission electron micrographs in this book were prepared from ultrathin epoxy resin sections. These resins are resistant to the damaging effects of the electron beam in the electron microscope, and continue to support the biological material, whereas other embedding media volatilize in the electron beam.

Most of the staining methods used with paraffin and acrylic resin sections are unable to penetrate epoxy resins. Fortunately, the stain toluidine blue is an exception, and differentially stains biological components in various shades of blue. The greatest cellular detail obtainable by light microscopy is by the use of 0.5–1 μm epoxy resin sections stained with toluidine blue (see Fig. 15.7b,c).

Toluidine Blue Stain

Toluidine blue is used to demonstrate cells and fibres in very thin epoxy resin sections. Toluidine blue is one of the very few dyes that will penetrate the dense epoxy resin to stain the tissue section. It gives considerable cellular detail, staining the various components of the cells and fibres in the shades of blue in a way that represents their relative electron density; hence the resulting blue picture closely resembles a low-power electron micrograph but is blue instead of black.

The problem can be overcome by embedding the bone in an acrylic resin embedding medium (e.g. methylmethacrylate) which, when set (polymerized), has a hardness that is the same as calcified bone, and good sections can be obtained without fragmentation or distortion. Examples are shown in many of the photomicrographs in Chapter 13, e.g. Figures 13.19b and 13.22.

Electron Microscopy

An electron microscope uses parallel beams of electrons instead of light waves

In light microscopy, the degree of magnification and resolution achievable is limited by the wavelength of light. If parallel beams of electrons are used instead of light, much greater magnification can be achieved and allows resolution of structures as small as 1 nm, thus permitting the study of subcellular morphology. There are two main types of electron microscopy used in the study of biological material, **transmission electron microscopy** and **scanning electron microscopy**.

To get the best results in both types of electron microscopy, fixation must be as perfect as can be achieved; this means that the fixative solution (glutaraldehyde) must act on the tissues as soon as possible after the tissue sample has been obtained. The best results are obtained by perfusing the tissues of an anaesthetized animal prior to sacrifice, since its organs are still being oxygenated by an intact and functioning blood circulatory system, as subcellular structures can be structurally altered as soon as they become anoxic. This technique obviously cannot be applied to human histology, so electron microscopy of human tissues is never as good as that obtained from experimental animals. In this book, we have stuck to the principle of illustrating only human tissues, as there are often marked species differences in subcellular organelles (see Fig. 10.15).

Transmission electron microscopy allows resolution of subcellular structures in very thin tissue sections

In transmission electron microscopy, the electrons in a vacuum chamber pass through a very thin section of fixed tissue, some components of which absorb all the electrons ('electron dense'), whereas others allow the passage of all electrons through the other side of the tissue sections ('electron lucent'). Some tissue elements allow only a percentage of electrons through, the remainder being absorbed by the tissue. The electrons that pass through strike a phosphorescent screen, allowing direct vision of the image, or a photographic plate, which renders the image as a permanent record in black, white and various shades of grey. The natural variations of electron density and electron lucency of the tissue components are emphasized by the use of 'stains', such as osmium tetroxide, which has an affinity for lipid components and renders them more electron dense, and other solutions of heavy metal salts.

Tissue preparation for transmission electron microscopy demands the use of very small tissue fragments ($<2\,mm^3$) to allow the fixative to penetrate all parts of the tissue as quickly as possible; the tissue sample must be placed in the fixative as soon as possible after removal and separation from the oxygen supply.

The fixed fragment is embedded in an epoxy resin (see 'Advanced Concepts', p. 7) and very thin sections (of the order of $0.1\,\mu m$, in contrast with paraffin sections, usually in the order of $3.0\,\mu m$ at best) are cut on a special machine, an 'ultramicrotome', using either diamond knives or special glass knives. These ultrathin epoxy resin sections are then placed in the electron microscope on a supporting copper mesh grid.

Scanning electron microscopy allows resolution of three-dimensional subcellular structures

Scanning electron microscopy uses solid pieces of tissue rather than ultrathin tissue sections, and allows perception of three-dimensional views of the surface of cells, tissues and subcellular structures.

A small piece of fixed tissue is dried and coated in gold. An electron beam then scans the specimen and electrons produced from the surface are used to reconstruct a fine three-dimensional representation of the surface (see Figs 7.2b, 7.14b, 11.11, 11.12b, 11.39d).

If living cells are frozen and then fractured, there is a tendency for the fractures to open cells along membranes and distinct planes, which can then be studied using the electron microscope. This technique of 'cryo-fracture' provides information about the surface features of cell membranes.

Light and electron microscopes have similar components, with similar functions

Both have four major systems:
- An **illuminating system**, which includes a source of radiation
- A system to hold the specimen in the radiation beam
- An **imaging system**, which consists of a number of lenses to produce the final magnified image of the specimen
- An **image translating system**, which allows the magnified image to be visualized and recorded.

Figure 1.6 illustrates the similarities between the two microscopes.

In the **light microscope**, the illuminating system comprises a low-voltage electric lamp, with an adjustable **condenser lens** which focuses and concentrates the light into the plane of the object. After passing through the specimen, the light passes into the **objective lens**, the function of which is to collect the light rays and form a magnified intermediate image within the body tube above the objective lens. The **projector lens** in the microscope eyepiece further magnifies the intermediate image and presents the retina of the eye with a magnified virtual image, which appears to the microscopist to be in the plane of the tissue specimen.

In the **electron microscope**, the 'illuminating' system comprises the source of radiation (an electron gun) and a condenser lens system, which focuses the electrons on to the specimen. Like all lenses in an electron

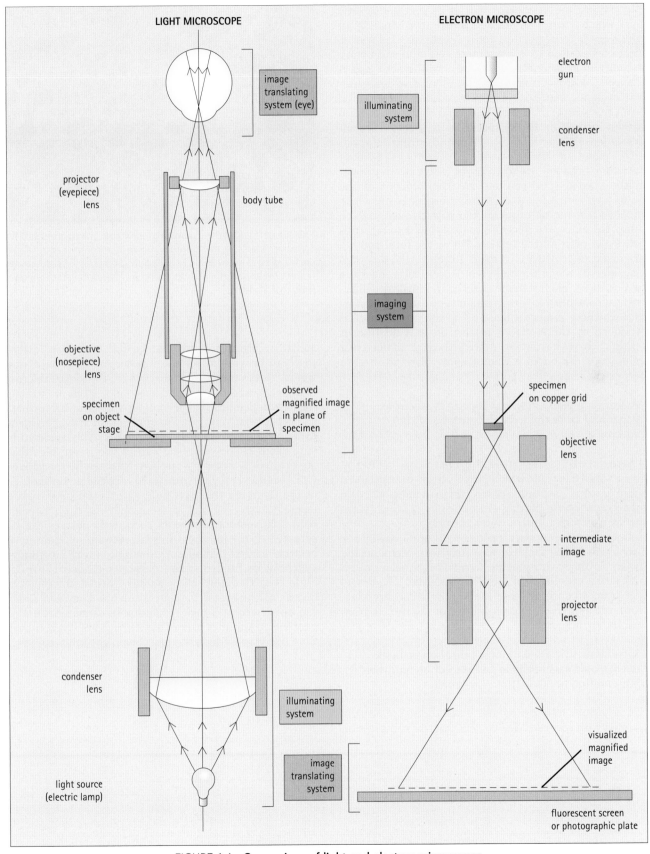

FIGURE 1.6 **Comparison of light and electron microscopes.**

microscope, the condenser lens is an electromagnetic coil, which creates a magnetic field, the strength of which can be controlled to deflect electrons. To focus an electron beam on to a given plane (e.g. the specimen), the current passing through the electromagnetic coil is changed. Most electron microscopes have two condenser lens systems, the first of which reduces the electron beam from about $50\,\mu m$ to $1\,\mu m$, and this narrow beam is then focused on to the specimen by the second condenser lens. When the focused electrons strike the specimen, many of the electrons pass through without deviation, but some are scattered by heavy atoms present in the stained specimen and are knocked out of the beam. This forms a pattern in the emergent beam, which is converted into an image by the objective lens, which brings the emergent electrons to focus a few millimetres below the plane of the section. Below the focal point, a magnified intermediate image is formed, which is then magnified by the projector lens or lenses (there are often two or three, one after the other). The final magnification is controlled by the amount of current passing through these projector lenses. The magnified image is produced by the electrons passing on to a fluorescent screen, where it can be viewed through a binocular microscope, or on to a photographic plate to make a permanent image (Fig. 1.7).

A scanning electron microscope uses electrons generated from the irregular surface of the specimen

Whereas the transmission electron microscope creates an image using electrons which pass through the specimen from a static electron source, the scanning electron microscope uses a moving electron source, which scans the specimen in a square raster pattern.

Low-energy secondary electrons are produced by the interaction of the incident electrons with atoms in the surface layer of the specimen, which has been coated with a thin even layer of metal such as gold. The detection system converts these low-energy secondary electrons into a three-dimensional image of the surface from which they originated.

Virtual microscopy is the digitalization of light microscopic specimens in full resolution and their presentation on a computer or tablet.

For virtual microscopy the glass slides are usually scanned with special slide scanners that use compression

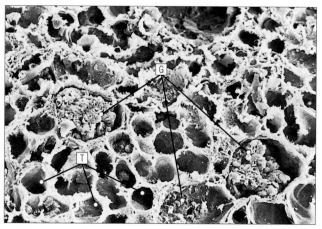

FIGURE 1.7 **Kidney (scanning electron micrograph).** This scanning electron micrograph shows the components of the cortex of the kidney, which are largely glomeruli (G) and tubules (T). At higher magnification more surface details are evident (see Fig. 15.11).

and tiling algorithms to produce full resolution images that can be viewed on a computer or tablet in a way similar to the traditional microscope. For virtual microscopy, glass slides are digitalized and saved in various formats depending on the scanner software. All formats allow for relatively fast visualization of the specimens using software specifically designed for this application (the client or viewer). The size of the image files that are created by scanning can vary between 50 megabytes (MB) and several gigabytes (GB), depending on the size of the tissue on the glass slide and the maximum slide magnification. The images are usually saved on a server with a large storage capacity so that the images can be accessed via the internet. Special software solutions have been developed that allows visualization with a common web browser. Students can access the plethora of "Virtual Slide boxes" online and examine virtual microscopic images of the tissue they are studying. Digitized slides can be viewed at a high resolution by large numbers of people and the files cannot be damaged or broken over time like glass slides and traditional light microscopes.

Chapter 2

The Cell

Introduction

Living cells of all types have certain defining attributes in common. They are composed of smaller elements, termed 'subcellular structures', which provide the framework for cellular activities.

An important component of the cell is its surrounding wall, which consists of a cell membrane. Specialized adaptations of cell membrane surround small elements inside cells termed **organelles**. The fluid inside the cell, the cytosol, is a dense proteinaceous liquid which contains many of the essential enzymes and metabolites. The genetic material, in the form of chromosomes, is contained in the nucleus, and energy for cellular activity is largely generated by mitochondria. There is a constant generation of new structural elements within the cell, and this takes place in the membrane systems of the endoplasmic reticulum (ER) and Golgi. Equally, cells have to take in substances from outside and break them down using a system of small organelles called **lysosomes** that contain powerful digestive enzymes. The shape of cells and much of the movement that takes place within cells is organized by an internal scaffolding of proteins known as the cytoskeleton.

The cell cycle of coordinated cell division and growth is achieved by duplication of genetic material (mitosis) and cell contents (cytokinesis).

This chapter describes the main building blocks of cells and the functional relationships that exist between them.

Cells have a common basic structure

Cells have many common features which are independent of any specialized function (Fig. 2.1):
- An outer membrane surrounds each cell and separates it from its environment and from other cells
- They are composed of a solution of proteins, electrolytes and carbohydrates (cytosol), divided up into specialized functional compartments (organelles) by inner membrane systems
- Their shape and fluidity are partly determined by the arrangement of internal filamentous proteins (intermediate filaments, actin and microtubules) which form the cytoskeleton.

Cell membranes delineate several compartments within cells, each with a specialized function.

The main membrane-bound compartments are:
- The nucleus, which contains the cellular DNA
- Mitochondria, which provide energy
- Endoplasmic reticulum (ER), which is involved in biosynthesis of protein and some lipids
- Golgi, which is involved in processing biosynthetic products for incorporation into the cell or for secretion
- Vesicles, which act as temporary packages of material undergoing transport around the cell
- Lysosomes, which contain hydrolytic enzymes to digest macromolecules within the cell
- Peroxisomes, which contain enzymes involved in fatty acid metabolism.

Cell Membranes

Cell membrane structure is based on a lipid bilayer

The outer membrane surrounding each cell and the membranes surrounding internal cellular organelles have a common basic structure of a lipid bilayer containing specialized proteins in association with surface carbohydrates.

The most important determinant of membrane structure is the lipid component. Each type of membrane lipid molecule has one hydrophilic end and one hydrophobic end (Fig. 2.2); thus they are amphipathic. Such lipids spontaneously form a bilayer in water, with the hydrophobic ends forming an inner layer between the outwardly directed hydrophilic groups.

This basic cell membrane structure, into which membrane proteins are inserted (Fig. 2.3), confers important functional attributes:
- The membrane is a fluid, allowing lateral diffusion of membrane proteins and facilitating cell mobility
- The polar lipid composition leads to a variable permeability to different substances, it being highly permeable to water, oxygen and small hydrophobic molecules such as ethanol, but virtually impermeable to charged ions, such as Na^+ and K^+
- Breaks and tears are sealed spontaneously as the polar nature of lipids eliminates free edges where hydrophobic groups would come into contact with the aqueous environment
- Membrane proteins are placed to perform functional roles in processes such as transport,

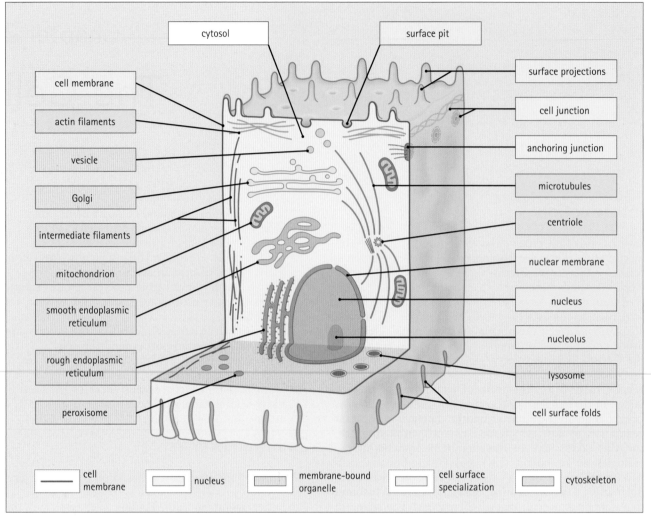

cytosol		surface pit

cell membrane

actin filaments

vesicle

Golgi

intermediate filaments

mitochondrion

smooth endoplasmic reticulum

rough endoplasmic reticulum

peroxisome

surface projections

cell junction

anchoring junction

microtubules

centriole

nuclear membrane

nucleus

nucleolus

lysosome

cell surface folds

| —— | cell membrane | | nucleus | | membrane-bound organelle | | cell surface specialization | | cytoskeleton |

FIGURE 2.1 **Cell structure.** The main constituents of a cell and their distribution.

enzymatic activity, cell attachment and cell communication.

There are three major types of membrane lipid: phosphoglycerides, cholesterol and glycolipids

Lipid forms 50% of the mass of cell membranes.

Phosphoglycerides (phospholipids) make up about 50% of the lipid component and tend to surround membrane proteins, often specifically anchoring proteins with enzyme or transport functions. There are three major phosphoglycerides in the cell membrane:

- Phosphatidylcholine
- Phosphatidylserine
- Phosphatidylethanolamine.

Cholesterol in the cell membrane limits the movement of adjacent phospholipids and makes the membrane less fluid and more mechanically stable.

Glycolipids are found in the outer face of cell membranes with their associated sugars exposed to the extracellular space, where they may be involved in intercellular communication.

The sphingolipids are the main type of glycolipid in cell membranes. An important membrane glycolipid is galactocerebroside, which is a major component of myelin, the fatty insulation layer around nerves (see Chapter 6). Another group of important glycolipids is the gangliosides, which constitute up to 10% of the lipid in nerve cell membranes.

The composition of inner and outer lipid layers is not the same. For example, high concentrations of certain phospholipids in the inner face may be needed to complement the presence of an inner membrane protein because certain proteins need to be linked with specific phospholipids. Islands of high concentration of sphingolipids and cholesterol can form in the membrane to produce **lipid rafts**. These rafts are typically 50 nm in size and can carry specific proteins or cell-signalling molecules. In this way, a lipid raft acts as a specialized membrane domain able to associate or segregate different proteins or signalling molecules.

Membrane proteins carry out most of the specialized functions of cell membranes

The types of membrane protein encountered vary according to cell type. Integral membrane proteins are those that span the lipid bilayer of the cell membrane,

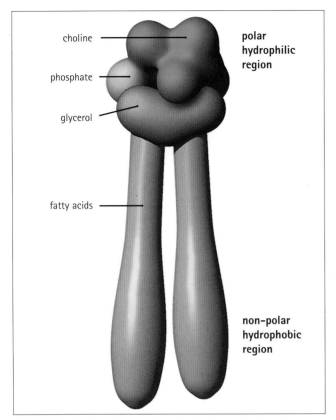

choline

polar
hydrophilic
region

phosphate

glycerol

fatty acids

non–polar
hydrophobic
region

FIGURE 2.2 **Membrane phospholipid molecule.** A membrane phospholipid molecule, which is the main component of cell membranes and determines the fundamental properties of the cell membrane as a whole.

whereas peripheral membrane proteins are associated with either the inner or the outer half of the lipid bilayer. Membrane proteins have several functions:

- Attach cytoskeletal filaments to cell membrane
- Attach cells to extracellular matrix (e.g. adhesion molecules)
- Transport molecules in or out of cells (e.g. carrier proteins, membrane pump proteins, channel proteins)
- Act as receptors for chemical signalling between cells (e.g. hormone receptors)
- Possess specific enzymatic activity.

Some membrane proteins are able to diffuse laterally over the surface of the cell. Others appear fixed in the cell membrane.

Membrane carbohydrates are mostly present on the membrane surfaces which are not in contact with cytosol

Membranes have associated carbohydrate residues which are mainly confined to the membrane surface that faces away from the cytosol. They are therefore found on the luminal aspect of inner membrane systems as well as on the cell surface, where they have been termed the **glycocalyx**.

Membrane carbohydrates can be demonstrated by staining with lectins, proteins extracted from plants with binding capabilities for specific carbohydrate groups.

Transport In and Out of Cells

Transport of material in or out of a cell takes place by the processes of endocytosis and exocytosis

Substances may diffuse through cell membranes, or they may be transported by special membrane protein transport systems (pumps, carriers or channels). Other material from the extracellular space, as well as the surface membrane, may be incorporated into the cell by invagination of the cell surface in a process termed **endocytosis** (Fig. 2.4a). The invaginated cell membrane fuses to form an **endocytotic vesicle** or **endosome**, which is a small, sealed, spherical membrane-bound body. The membrane and any material incorporated into such a vesicle can then be processed within the cell.

The terms **pinocytosis** (Fig. 2.4b) or **potocytosis** are used when cells take up fluid and small molecules to form small vesicles about 50 nm in diameter. The terms **endocytosis** and **phagocytosis** (Fig. 2.4c) are used when cells ingest large particles to form endosomes more than 250 nm in diameter.

Exocytosis is the reverse of endocytosis, and describes the fusion of a membrane-bound vesicle with the cell surface to discharge its contents into the extracellular space (Fig. 2.4d). This mechanism allows the secretion of products that have been manufactured by the cell. Fusion of vesicles with the cell membrane also allows new membrane to be incorporated into the cell surface.

The two main vesicles involved in transport of substances into cells are derived from surface membrane invaginations called coated pits and caveolae

Small invaginations of membrane constantly form at the surface of most cells to ingest extracellular material, which is then processed by the cell. The invaginations are drawn down to form vesicles; once the contents have been processed, the vesicle membrane returns to the cell surface. Thus, there is a constant shuttle of membrane between cell surface and cell interior (membrane trafficking). These vesicles originate in two main types of specialized area of the cell membrane termed **coated pits** and **caveolae**.

Coated pits are invaginations braced by special membrane-associated proteins and are used to bring material into the cell for further processing (Fig. 2.5). In many instances, special receptor proteins are present in the cell membrane that can bind to specific substances outside the cell and draw them inside in a process termed **receptor-mediated endocytosis**. Coated vesicles may also develop from other internal membrane systems inside cells.

Caveolae are also invaginations of the cell surface membrane but, in contrast to coated pits, are braced by the protein caveolin. Caveolae have three important cellular roles (Fig. 2.6):

- The surface of caveolae may carry receptor proteins which bind to molecules in the extracellular space. They can concentrate substances from the

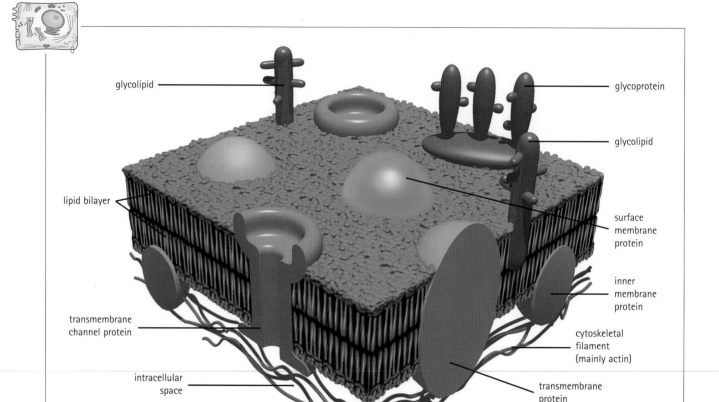

FIGURE 2.3 Cell membrane structure. The cell membrane is composed of a lipid bilayer with phospholipid hydrophobic groups facing inward and hydrophilic groups facing outward. Protein molecules float within this basic structure, with projecting carbohydrate groups being attached to glycolipids or proteins.

extracellular space and transport them into the cell in a process termed **potocytosis**
- They are used to transport material from the extracellular space on one side to the extracellular space on the other in a process termed **transcytosis**. This happens in cells such as the flat cells that line blood vessels (endothelial cells)
- They are also believed to have roles in **intracellular signalling**. The cell membrane associated with caveolae is enriched with many of the cell surface proteins that have function as receptors. Caveolae are believed to allow extracellular events to trigger intracellular secondary cellular messenger systems.

Macropinocytosis and phagocytosis internalize large particles into the cell

Cells internalize material from the extracellular environment by two additional processes:

In **macropinocytosis** the cell extends a crescent-like thin fold of membrane outwards to encapsulate a pool of extracellular fluid, which is then incorporated into the

ADVANCED CONCEPT

There are two types of secretory mechanism. In some cells, secretion occurs by a constant fusion of vesicles with surface membrane, termed the **constitutive secretory pathway**. In other cells, fusion of secretory vesicles with the surface has to be triggered by a signal to the cell, termed the **regulated secretory pathway**.

Several proteins have been defined which mediate the processes of membrane fusion. The Rab family of GTPases controls the specificity of trafficking and docking and recruits tethering factors and fusion factors. So-called 'SNARE' proteins (from SNAp REceptor) are responsible for tethering and docking of the vesicle to the membrane. Different members of the SNARE family are specific to different vesicle systems and cell compartments, allowing specificity of fusion events. A protein called NSF (N-ethylmaleimide-sensitive fusion protein) interacts with proteins called 'SNAPs' (soluble NSF attachment proteins) to mediate membrane fusion.

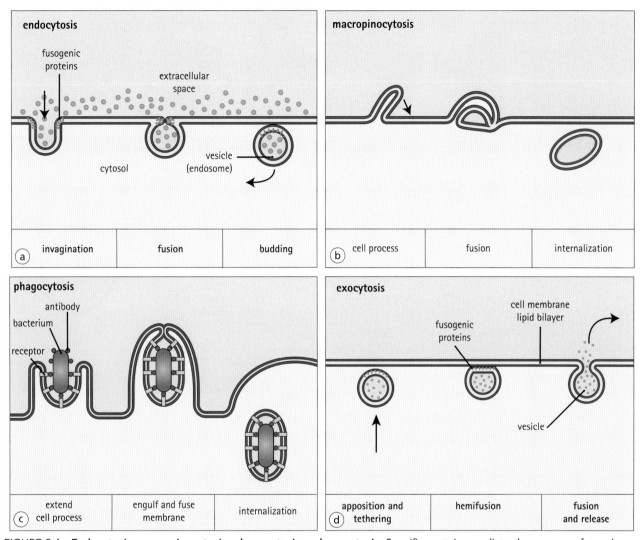

FIGURE 2.4 **Endocytosis, macropinocytosis, phagocytosis and exocytosis.** Specific proteins mediate the process of membrane integration in endocytosis and exocytosis. (a) **Endocytosis.** The invaginated cell membrane fuses to form an endocytotic vesicle (endosome), which is a small, sealed, spherical membrane-bound body. The membrane and any material incorporated into such a vesicle can then be processed within the cell. (b) **Macropinocytosis.** In this process, the cell extends as a sheet to envelop and enclose a large amount of extracellular fluid. Membrane fusion internalizes this within the cell. (c) **Phagocytosis.** In phagocytosis, a particle outside the cell has proteins on its surface that are recognized by receptors on the cell surface. In the case of a foreign particle, such as a bacterium, the protein may be antibody bound to its surface and the receptor recognizes the Fc portion of the antibody. The binding of the receptor leads to activation of cell signalling systems that cause processes to extend from the cell to progressively engulf the particle. Subsequent fusion of the cell membrane leads to internalization of the particle within the cell, contained in a membrane-bound vesicle. (d) **Exocytosis.** This is the fusion of a membrane-bound vesicle with the cell surface to discharge its contents into the extracellular space. This allows the secretion of products manufactured by the cell. Also, fusion of vesicles with the cell membrane allows new membrane to be incorporated into the cell surface.

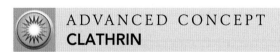

ADVANCED CONCEPT
CLATHRIN

Clathrin is a protein that braces the coated pit membranes. It forms a hexagonal lattice structure that develops as a coat around the outside of the vesicle and accounts for the fuzzy layer seen ultrastructurally.

Assembly of this lattice is believed to drive the invagination of the surface membrane. A protein called 'dynamin' forms a collar around the neck of the invaginating vesicle and is believed to be important in facilitating budding and separation of the formed vesicle from the surface. Several different adapter or assembly proteins are associated with the coat and target the clathrin-coated vesicle to the correct place for docking and transport. The clathrin scaffolding is broken down by a series of proteins in an uncoating reaction once the vesicle is internalized.

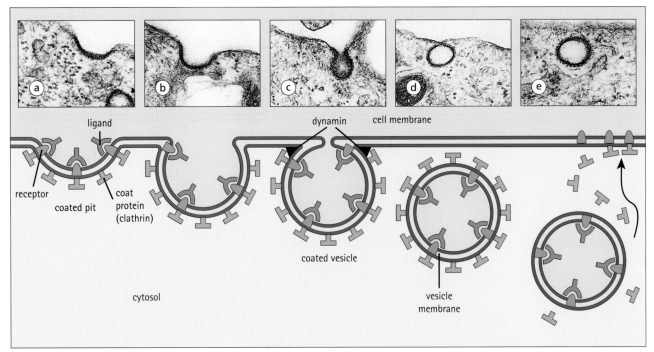

FIGURE 2.5 **Ultrastructure and coated pit formation.** (a) A coated pit is braced by a coat of protein molecules (orange) and bears surface receptors (blue) that bind specific extracellular ligands (red), for example a substance that needs to enter the cell, such as iron. In such cases, the coat protein (visible ultrastructurally as a fuzzy membrane thickening) is clathrin, which forms a hexagonal lattice around the pit membrane. (b,c,d) Assembly of the coat protein lattice drives progressive invagination of the pit to form a coated vesicle. The protein dynamin forms a collar around the neck of the vesicle and assists in budding. (e) Once internalized, the coat protein is shed from the vesicle and returns to the cell surface to form new coated pits. This form of transport into cells is termed receptor-mediated endocytosis and is a feature of the internalization of iron, low-density lipoprotein and some growth factors.

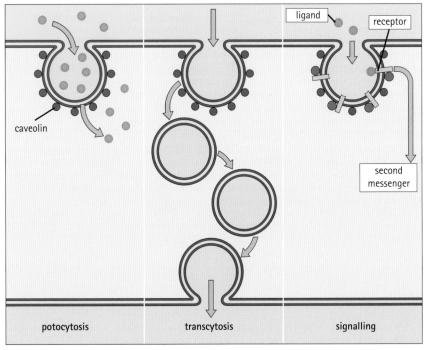

FIGURE 2.6 **Caveolae.** There are three functions of caveolae. First, receptors on caveolae can concentrate substances from the extracellular space and these can then move into the cytosol. This is termed 'potocytosis', and such caveolae remain as invaginations and do not form vesicles. Second, some caveolae form vesicles and internalize material, which is then transported across the cell and released from the other side in a process termed 'transcytosis'. Third, some caveolae are the site of concentration of surface receptors that influence intracellular secondary messenger signal systems, thereby making caveolae an important structure in signal transduction.

cell by invagination of the derived membrane-bound vesicle (see Fig. 2.4b).

In **phagocytosis** an area of the cell surface bears receptors which recognize proteins attached to a – generally – foreign particle in the extracellular space. The proteins that are recognized may be antibodies, for example antibodies bound to a disease-causing bacterium. The binding of receptor and protein triggers extension of the cell membrane to engulf the particle, followed by fusion of the membrane to internalize the particle into the cell, where it then fuses with other vesicles (see Fig. 2.4c).

Cytosol

The cytosol is the fluid matrix of the cell

The cytosol of the cell is a concentrated, dense fluid. This fluid matrix contains the following important components:
- Much of the machinery involved in protein synthesis, protein degradation and carbohydrate metabolism (it is therefore rich in enzyme systems)
- Filamentous proteins that form the cytoskeleton (see p. 26)
- Some products of metabolism, such as glycogen and free lipid, for which it acts as a storage compartment
- Numerous ribosomes, both free in the cytosol and associated with cytosolic surface of rough ER.

Ribosomes are involved in the synthesis of proteins

Ribosomes synchronize the alignment of both messenger RNA and transport RNA in the production of peptide chains during protein synthesis. Ribosomes are small electron-dense particles which impart a blue colour (basophilic) to the cytoplasm of protein-producing cells on light microscopy (Fig. 2.7). Each ribosome is composed of a small subunit which binds RNA, and a large subunit which catalyses the formation of peptide bonds. They are made up of specific ribosomal RNA, as well as specific proteins. Ribosomal RNA is manufactured in the nucleolus (see p. 19).

The Nucleus

The nucleus contains the cellular DNA and the nucleolus

The nucleus is the largest single membrane-bound compartment in the cell and contains the cellular DNA (Fig. 2.8).

In light microscopic preparations, nuclei are spherical or ovoid in shape, generally measuring 5–10 µm in diameter; they stain with basic dyes, such as haematoxylin (i.e. basophilic) and contain a smaller spherical structure, the nucleolus, which synthesizes ribosomal subunits.

Nuclei are bound by two concentric membranes with different functional roles. The inner nuclear membrane contains specific membrane proteins that act as attachment points for filamentous proteins, termed **lamins**, which form a scaffolding to maintain the spherical shape. The outer nuclear membrane binds the perinuclear space, which is continuous with the lumen of the ER; it may be associated with ribosomes in a similar manner to rough ER.

The nuclear membrane is perforated by numerous pores which establish continuity between the cytosol and the nuclear lumen containing the chromatin (Fig. 2.9).

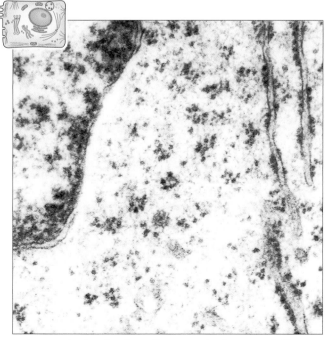

FIGURE 2.7 **Ribosomes.** Electron micrograph showing free ribosomes in the cytosol. They are small electron-dense particles 20–30 nm in diameter, present either singly or in chains called polyribosomes.

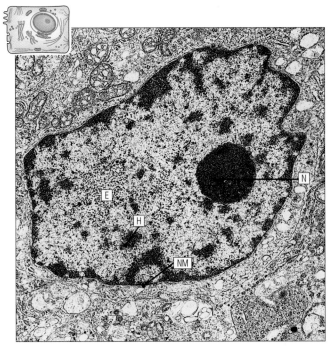

FIGURE 2.8 **Nucleus.** Electron micrograph showing typical cell nucleus. It is bounded by a double nuclear membrane (NM). The nucleolus (N) is clearly visible as an electron-dense circular area. Nucleus chromatin is divided into two types: heterochromatin (H) is dense-staining, whereas euchromatin (E) is light-staining.

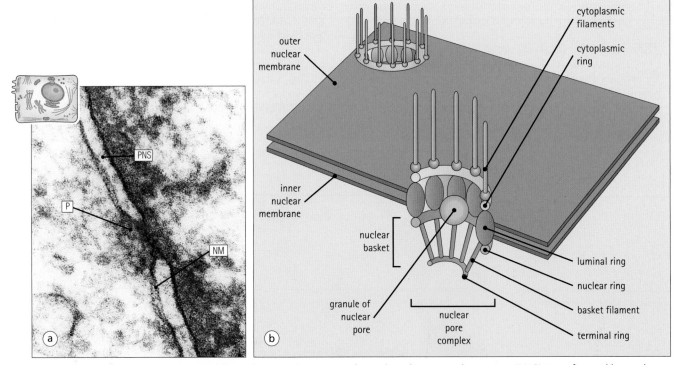

FIGURE 2.9 **Nuclear pore.** (a) The double nuclear membrane (NM) bounding the perinuclear space (PNS) is perforated by nuclear pores (P), which appear as gaps in transmission electron micrographs. (b) Structurally, the pores are formed by concentric rings of eight subunits to form the nuclear pore complex shown in this diagram. Above and below the large protein units are rings from which filaments radiate into nuclear and cytoplasmic spaces. The structure formed by rings and filaments in the nuclear space is termed the 'nuclear basket'. The pores form channels, which allow the transport of small molecules, but restrict the movement of large molecules, between the cytosol and the nucleus. Movement of some proteins into the nucleus is desirable, however, and it is currently thought that the nuclear pore complex recognizes and actively transports specific peptide sequences in proteins destined for the nucleus. In a similar fashion, large ribosomal subunits produced in the nucleus are actively transported into the cytosol. The central granules of the pore complex are believed to be large proteins or components of ribosomes in transit between different cell areas.

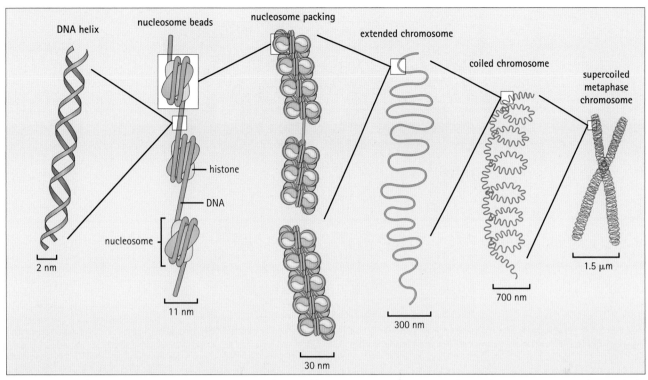

FIGURE 2.10 **Chromatin structure.** DNA is organized around histones into nucleosomes. The nucleosomes are wound into a helix to form chromatin. In chromosomes, this is then wound again into a supercoiled structure.

Nuclear DNA is tightly packed by association with special proteins and forms the chromatin

The nucleus contains DNA wound around proteins called 'histones' to form nucleosomes, which are regular repeating globular structures similar to beads on a string. The nucleosome string is then wound into filaments 30 nm in diameter, which make up the structure of chromatin. Further condensation into distinct chromosomes is possible during cell replication, when chromatin forms large looped domains by attachment to DNA-binding proteins. This relationship is shown in Figure 2.10.

The distribution of chromatin is not uniform, and this reflects varying degrees of unfolding according to whether genes are being transcribed. **Euchromatin** is seen as light-staining electron-lucent areas and represents actively transcribed cellular DNA. **Heterochromatin** is seen as a dense-staining area, often adjacent to the nuclear membrane, and is the highly condensed, transcriptionally inactive form.

The nucleolus is the site of formation of ribosomal RNA in the nucleus

The nucleolus is a spherical area within the nucleus. It measures 1–3 μm in diameter, increasing in size with active gene transcription. Inactive cells have indistinct nucleoli, whereas metabolically active cells have large or multiple nucleoli. In H&E preparations, nucleoli stain blue-pink because of their affinity for both acidophilic and basophilic dyes.

The nucleolus produces ribosomal RNAs, which are packaged with proteins to form ribosomal subunits and exported to the cytosol via the nuclear pore complexes.

Three regions of the nucleolus can be distinguished by electron microscopy (Fig. 2.11):

- **Pars amorpha** (pale areas), so-called 'nuclear organizer regions' with specific RNA-binding proteins, correspond to large loops of transcribing DNA containing the ribosomal RNA genes
- **Pars fibrosa** (dense-staining regions) correspond to transcripts of ribosomal RNA genes beginning to form ribosomes
- **Pars granulosa** (granular regions) correspond to RNA-containing maturing ribosomal subunit particles.

The nuclear lamina is a scaffolding which maintains the shape of the nucleus

The nuclear lamina is a network of protein filaments 20 nm thick that lines the internal nuclear membrane. It is composed of three proteins termed 'nuclear lamins A, B and C', which are organized into filaments and form a regular square lattice as a scaffold beneath the nuclear membrane.

It is thought that this nuclear lamina network interacts with nuclear membrane proteins and acts as a nuclear cytoskeleton, possibly interacting with chromatin in the spatial organization of the nucleus.

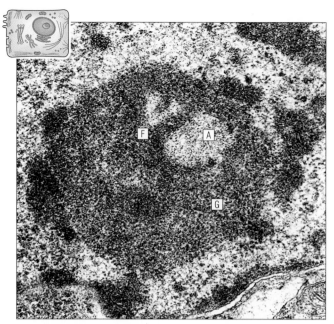

FIGURE 2.11 **Nucleolus.** Electron micrograph showing the nucleolus from a cell actively producing protein. The pars amorpha (A), pars fibrosa (F) and pars granulosa (G) are clearly visible.

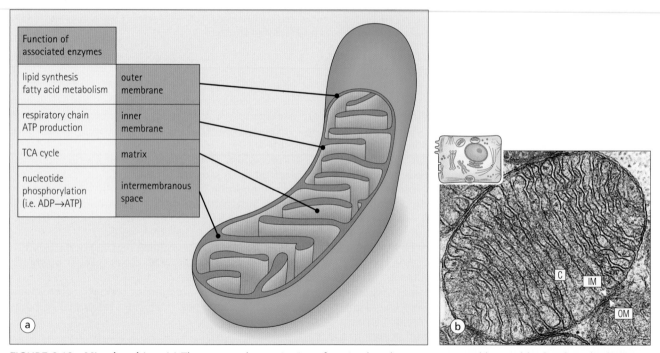

Function of associated enzymes		
lipid synthesis fatty acid metabolism	outer membrane	
respiratory chain ATP production	inner membrane	
TCA cycle	matrix	
nucleotide phosphorylation (i.e. ADP→ATP)	intermembranous space	

FIGURE 2.12 **Mitochondrion.** (a) The structural organization of a mitochondrion accompanied by a table detailing the locations and functions of mitochondrial enzymes. (b) Electron micrograph of a mitochondrion. Note the outer membrane (OM), inner membrane (IM) and cristae (C).

Mitochondria

The mitochondria are the most important sites of ATP production in cells.

Mitochondria are membrane-bound cylindrical organelles (Fig. 2.12), typically measuring 0.5–2 μm in length, which provide energy to cells through oxidative phosphorylation.

Mitochondria are believed to have evolved in human cells as symbiotic prokaryotic organisms similar to bacteria. In support of this hypothesis, each mitochondrion has its own DNA and systems for protein synthesis independent of the cell nucleus.

Each mitochondrion is constructed with two membranes, an outer and an inner, which define two inner mitochondrial spaces, the intermembranous space and the matrix space.

The outer membrane contains specialized transport proteins such as porin, which allow free permeability to molecules up to about 10 kDa molecular weight from the cytosol into the intermembranous space.

The outer mitochondrial membrane also contains transmembrane pores that can assemble and open to release large mitochondrial proteins into the cytosol. This action is triggered by a variety of cell stimuli and leads to activation of cell death mechanisms (apoptosis). In this way, the mitochondrion acts as an important transducer for certain stimuli that lead to cell death.

The inner membrane is highly impermeable to small ions owing to a high content of the phospholipid cardiolipin. This feature is essential to mitochondrial function as it permits the development of electrochemical gradients during the production of high-energy cell metabolites.

The inner membrane is folded into pleats (cristae), thereby increasing its surface area, and is the location of respiratory chain enzymes, as well as ATP synthetase, which is responsible for energy generation.

The intermembranous space contains:

- Metabolic substrates which diffuse through the outer membrane
- ATP generated by the mitochondrion
- Ions pumped out of the matrix space during oxidative phosphorylation. The matrix space contains enzymes to oxidize fatty acids and pyruvate as well as for the citric acid (TCA) cycle. It also contains

mitochondrial DNA and specific mitochondrial enzymes for mitochondrial DNA transcription.

The morphology of mitochondria varies with cell type. In cells with a high oxidative metabolism, mitochondria are commonly large and serpiginous. In steroid hormone-secreting cells, such as those of the adrenal cortex, the cristae are tubular structures rather than flat plates.

Endoplasmic Reticulum (ER) and Golgi

The endoplasmic reticulum and Golgi are involved in protein and lipid biosynthesis

The ER and Golgi are two distinct regions of an inter-communicating membrane-bound compartment involved in the biosynthesis and transport of cellular proteins and lipids (Fig. 2.14). In addition to its functions in biosynthesis, the ER has two other important roles:

- Detoxification or activation of foreign compounds, including several drugs, by ER proteins termed cytochrome P-450 proteins
- Storage of intracellular calcium.

The ER and Golgi are arranged as deeply-folded, flattened membrane sheets or as elongated tubular profiles, their quantity depending on cellular metabolic

---

 CLINICAL EXAMPLE
MITOCHONDRIAL CYTOPATHY SYNDROMES

Mitochondrial DNA is not inherited in the same way as cellular DNA, and in the human, the whole mitochondrial complement of a developing embryo is derived from mitochondria present in the ovum (i.e. maternally derived); there is no paternal contribution.

Abnormal mitochondrial DNA can impair mitochondrial function and lead to defective cell functioning, which mainly results in structural abnormalities of muscle and the nervous system, and metabolic abnormalities derived from failure of oxidative metabolism. Affected individuals can be considered to have mosaics of genetically different mitochondria, a concept termed 'heteroplasmy'. If a large number of abnormal mitochondria are inherited, then it is likely that severe disease will develop. If only a proportion are abnormal, then the resulting disease may be less severe.

The most common patterns of clinical disease are as follows:

- Muscle weakness, particularly affecting the extraocular muscles
- Degenerative disease of the central nervous system (e.g. loss of the optic nerve fibres, loss of cerebellar tissue or degeneration of brain white matter)
- Metabolic disturbances, marked particularly by the development of abnormally high levels of lactic acid.

Such diseases may become manifest at any age from childhood into adult life and diagnosis can be assisted by muscle biopsy (Fig. 2.13), in which abnormal mitochondria can be seen in a proportion of cases. Mutational analysis of mitochondrial DNA is also used in diagnosis.

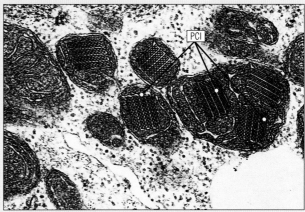

FIGURE 2.13 **Mitochondrial cytopathy.** Electron micrograph of abnormal mitochondria in the muscle cell of a person with muscle weakness. Characteristic paracrystalline inclusions (PCI) are present, and are thought to be composed of excess mitochondrial protein, which accumulates as a result of the genetic abnormality (compare with Fig. 2.12b).

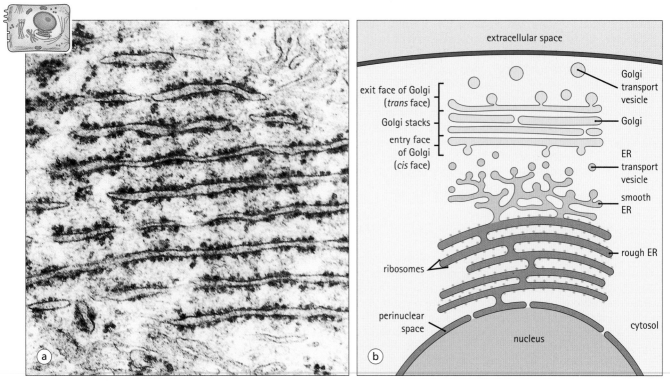

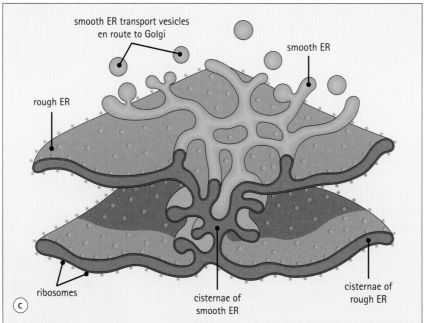

FIGURE 2.14 **Endoplasmic reticulum.** (a) Electron micrograph of rough ER composed of sheets of membrane with ribosomes on the cytosolic surfaces. (b) Relationship between ER and Golgi. The lumen of rough ER (RER) is continuous with the perinuclear space and with the lumen of smooth ER, whereas the Golgi forms a separate membrane system. Communication between ER and Golgi is mediated by small vesicles of ER which break off, move through the cytosol and fuse with Golgi membrane. The vesicles derived from RER are coated with a specific protein, COPII, which targets them for fusion with the Golgi. (c) The spatial relationship between rough ER and smooth ER. Smooth ER cisternae are tubular.

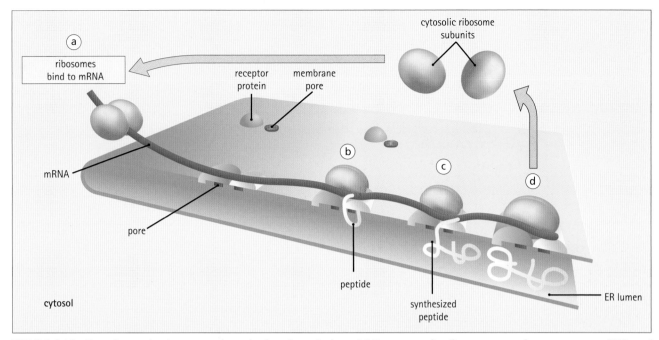

FIGURE 2.15 **Protein synthesis on rough endoplasmic reticulum.** (a) Free cytosolic ribosomes attach to messenger RNA and begin to produce a peptide. (b) The ribosome attaches to a receptor on the ER membrane and the peptide is threaded into the ER lumen via a small protein-lined pore. At any one time, several ribosomes may be transcribing the same messenger RNA strand. (c) The original signal sequence that threads the peptide into the ER lumen is cleaved, and as the peptide is made it forms in the lumen. Some proteins (i.e. those destined to be integral membrane proteins) can also form directly within the ER membrane. (d) After completion of peptide synthesis the ribosome detaches from the receptor protein and returns to the cytosolic free pool.

requirements. Little ER is present in the majority of metabolically inactive cells, but cells that synthesize and secrete protein-containing molecules contain vast amounts. Most cells have only a relatively small quantity of smooth ER, with the exception of cells that secrete or process lipids.

Protein synthesis occurs through interaction of ribosomes, RNA and rough endoplasmic reticulum

Protein synthesis begins in the cytosol, where messenger RNA attaches to free ribosomes and translation produces the new peptide. The first portion of the RNA forms a signal sequence. Proteins destined to remain in the cytosol have a different signal sequence from those destined for entry into membranes or for secretion.

Ribosomes producing peptides with the signal sequence for a membrane or secreted protein become attached to the surface of the ER where the rest of the peptide is translated (Fig. 2.15). The attachment of ribosomes to the ER gives it a studded appearance, hence this portion is called 'rough ER'.

Protein synthesis by rough ER results in either the attachment of membrane proteins to ER membrane or retention of proteins destined for secretion or retention within the ER lumen. These newly made proteins then enter the smooth ER for transport to the Golgi.

The smooth endoplasmic reticulum is the site of membrane lipid synthesis and protein processing

Smooth ER is a vital cell membrane system. As well as processing synthesized proteins, it is the site of cell lipid synthesis, particularly membrane phospholipids. The lipid synthetic enzymes are located on its outer (cytosolic) face with ready access to lipid precursors.

Once synthesized and incorporated into the outer part of the smooth ER membrane lipid bilayer, phospholipids are flipped over into the inner part by specific transport proteins colloquially termed 'flipases'.

The Golgi is a membrane system involved in the sorting, packaging and transporting of cell products

From the smooth ER, further processing of synthesized macromolecules takes place in the Golgi. To reach the Golgi, vesicles bud from the smooth ER and travel in cytosol to fuse with its inner face. Membrane proteins are incorporated into the Golgi membrane, whereas luminal proteins enter the Golgi space (Fig. 2.16a).

The Golgi membrane system has three important roles:
- **Modification** of macromolecules by the addition of sugars to form oligosaccharides
- **Proteolysis** of peptides into active forms
- **Sorting** of different macromolecules into specific membrane-bound vesicles for subsequent incorporation into a membrane, transport into the lumen of a specific membrane-bound organelle, or extracellular secretion.

To facilitate the roles of modification, proteolysis and sorting, the Golgi is divided into three functional components (see Fig. 2.16): the **cis face**, the **medial Golgi** and the **trans-Golgi network**.

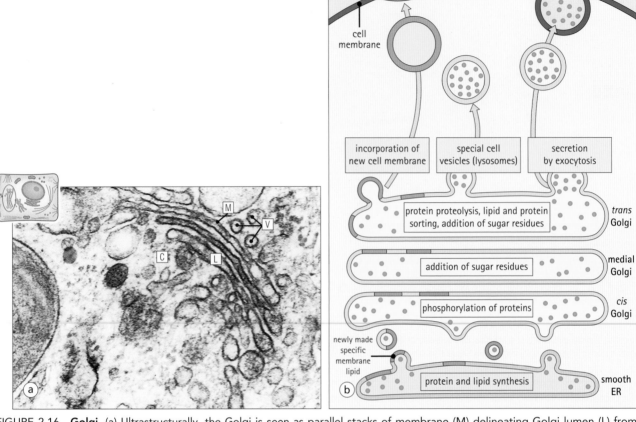

FIGURE 2.16 **Golgi.** (a) Ultrastructurally, the Golgi is seen as parallel stacks of membrane (M) delineating Golgi lumen (L) from the cytosol (C). Transport vesicles (V) can be seen en route from the ER. (b) Golgi has three functional parts: the nuclear-facing cis face receives transport vesicles from smooth ER and phosphorylates certain proteins; the central medial Golgi adds sugar residues to both lipids and peptides to form complex oligosaccharides; the trans Golgi network performs proteolytic steps, adds sugar residues and sorts different macromolecules into specific vesicles which bud off the trans face. Golgi vesicles have a specific coat protein that targets vesicles to the correct compartment. Coat protein complexes (COPI) coat vesicles moving between Golgi compartments. Sorting is performed by specific membrane receptor proteins, which recognize signal groups on macromolecules and direct them into correct vesicles. New membrane lipid synthesized in the smooth ER makes its way into the cell membrane via the Golgi.

Vesicles

Very small membrane-bound bodies are called vesicles and are derived from several compartments

Vesicles are small spherical membrane-bound organelles. They are formed by the budding off of existing areas of membrane and have two main functions. They:
- Transport or store material within their lumina
- Allow the exchange of cell membrane between different cell compartments.

The main types of vesicle are:
- Cell surface-derived endocytotic (i.e. pino- or phagocytotic) vesicles
- Golgi-derived transport and secretory vesicles
- ER-derived transport vesicles
- Lysosomes (see below)
- Peroxisomes (see p. 25).

The cellular distribution of these vesicles can be determined by immunohistochemical staining for specific vesicle-associated proteins or specific vesicle contents.

Lysosomes are part of the acid vesicle system, which is involved in degradation of proteins

A lysosome is a membrane-bound organelle with a high content of hydrolytic enzymes operating in an acid pH. It thus functions as an intracellular digestion system, processing either material ingested by the cell or effete cellular components. This definition encompasses a variety of membrane-bound organelles derived from slightly different sources and with different functional roles.

Lysosomes are now considered to be only one part of the acid vesicle system, a group of vesicles so named

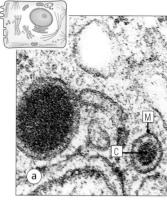

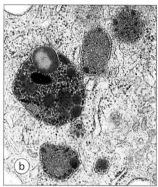

FIGURE 2.17 **Lysosomes.** (a) Electron micrograph of Golgi hydrolase vesicles, which are bounded by membrane (M) and have an electron-dense core (C) composed of precursors of acid hydrolase enzymes. The membrane of this type of vesicle does not contain H⁺-ATPase. (b) Electron micrograph showing several endolysosomes, which are produced by fusion of Golgi hydrolase vesicles with endosomes. Endolysosomes have a membrane containing H⁺-ATPase, which can reduce pH to activate the hydrolases.

because of their common membrane H^+-ATPase, termed the **vacuolar ATPase**, which can decrease their luminal pH to 5. This low pH activates powerful acid hydrolase enzymes, which are derived from vesicles that bud from the Golgi.

The membrane proteins required for lysosomal function (particularly the membrane pump, which increases H^+ concentration to maintain the acid pH), are not present in the initial Golgi hydrolase vesicles (formerly called primary lysosomes), which appear as membrane-bound vesicles with a dense core measuring 200–400 nm in diameter (Fig. 2.17a).

A functional lysosome, fulfilling the definition of acid environment plus hydrolases, results from the fusion of hydrolase vesicles with endosomes that contain the correct membrane proteins to form an endolysosome (formerly termed a secondary lysosome). Endolysosomes are larger than Golgi hydrolase vesicles – 600–800 nm in diameter – and also have an electron-dense core (Fig. 2.17b). They can fuse with other endosomes derived from phagocytosis to form phagolysosomes. In this way, particulate matter brought into the cell is digested. Cells with a specific phagocytic function, such as certain white blood cells, have a well-developed acid vesicle system.

It is possible to demonstrate the presence of lysosomes by histochemical staining for acid hydrolases, the most reliable being the demonstration of acid phosphatases. Immunohistochemical reagents can also be used to detect specific hydrolases, for example cathepsin-B and β-glucuronidase.

Autophagy is a process used to eliminate cellular constituents

All cells have a requirement to turn over proteins and organelles. Effete organelles are eliminated from cells by first becoming wrapped in membrane derived from the ER. These bodies subsequently fuse with an endolysosome to form an autophagolysosome; this enables old or damaged organelles to be recycled in a process termed **autophagy**.

Proteins in the cell membrane also need to be eliminated, and this happens by the formation of multivesicular bodies. In this process, cell membrane containing the unwanted proteins is internalized into a body containing multiple bubble-like vesicles termed a multivesicular body. These bodies then fuse with vesicles containing lysosomal hydrolases, leading to protein degradation.

Following digestion of material by acid hydrolases, indigestible amorphous and membranous debris may be seen in large membrane-bound vesicles called residual bodies. The relationships between members of the acid vesicle system are shown in Figure 2.18.

 CLINICAL EXAMPLE
PEROXISOMAL DISORDERS

Several rare diseases are due to defects in the peroxisomal enzymes responsible for processing very long-chain fatty acids. The main clinical features of such diseases are metabolic disturbances associated with acidosis, or with the storage of abnormal lipids in susceptible cells, especially in cells of the nervous system.

The most common example is adrenoleukodystrophy, in which impaired β-oxidation of fatty acids results in abnormal lipid storage in the brain, spinal cord and adrenal glands, leading to intellectual deterioration (dementia) and adrenal failure.

Peroxisomes are membrane-bound vesicles important in metabolism of long fatty acids

Peroxisomes are small membrane-bound organelles containing enzymes involved in the oxidation of several substrates, particularly β-oxidation of very long-chain fatty acids (C18 and above).

Ultrastructurally peroxisomes are small spherical bodies 0.5–1 μm in diameter with an electron-dense core. In some animals, but not in man, there is a central paracrystalline core termed a 'nucleoid'.

Several enzymes in peroxisomes oxidize their substrate and reduce their O_2 to H_2O_2, whereas catalase, which is also present, decomposes H_2O_2 to O_2 and H_2O.

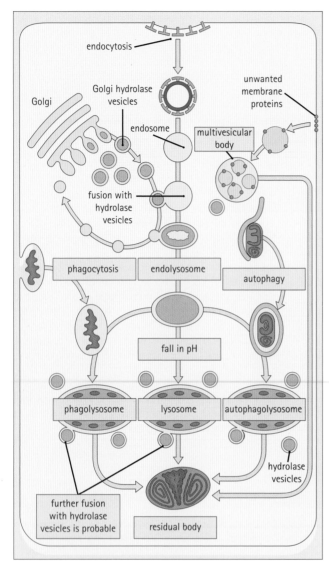

FIGURE 2.18 Acid vesicle system. The relationships between the 'digestive' organelles of the acid vesicle system. Endosome forms from cell membrane and fuses with hydrolase-containing vesicles derived from the Golgi to form endolysosomes. The special Golgi membrane that forms the hydrolase vesicles is recycled back to the Golgi. Autophagy eliminates unwanted organelles. Unwanted cell membrane proteins are internalized for destruction by forming multivesicular bodies.

CLINICAL EXAMPLE
LYSOSOMAL STORAGE DISORDERS

In the acid vesicle system, there are more than 30 defined and specific acid hydrolases, which not only degrade abnormal large molecules but also recycle or process normal cell constituents.

Genetic defects in the production of specific acid hydrolases lead to an inability to degrade specific classes of molecule, which then accumulate in the acid vesicle system. Most of these defects are inherited as single-gene autosomal recessive traits.

Lysosomal glycogen storage disease (acid maltase deficiency) leads to the accumulation of glycogen, which cannot be broken down (Fig. 2.19). Tay–Sachs disease results from a deficiency in an enzyme degrading one of the sphingolipids (hexosaminidase-A deficiency). Huge amounts of lipid accumulate in lysosomes and lead to severe neuronal degeneration.

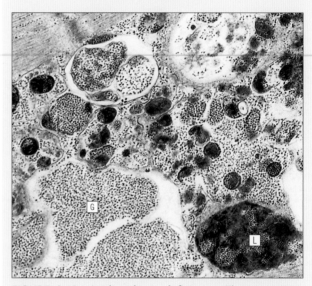

FIGURE 2.19 Acid maltase deficiency. Electron micrograph showing glycogen accumulation (G) in muscle cell cytoplasm and also within lysosomal bodies (L).

Cytoskeleton

The cytoskeletal proteins form filaments which brace the internal structure of the cell

Several functions of the cell are maintained by a set of filamentous cytosolic proteins, the cytoskeletal proteins, of which there are three main classes (depending on the size of their filaments):

- **Microfilaments** (5 nm in diameter), composed of the protein actin
- **Intermediate filaments** (10 nm in diameter), composed of six main proteins, which vary in different cell types
- **Microtubules** (25 nm in diameter), composed of two **tubulin** proteins.

These filamentous proteins become attached to cell membranes and to each other by anchoring and joining proteins to form a dynamic three-dimensional internal scaffolding in the cell. This scaffolding is in a continual state of assembly and disassembly, but periods of stability serve specific functional roles, such as maintaining cellular architecture, facilitating cell motility, anchoring cells together, facilitating transport of material around the cytosol and dividing the cytosol into functionally separate areas.

ADVANCED CONCEPT
ACTIN

In association with other proteins, actin filaments form a layer (the cell cortex, Fig. 2.20) beneath the cell membrane. The actin is arranged into a stiff cross-linked meshwork by linking proteins, the most abundant being filamin. This meshwork resists sudden deformational forces but allows changes in cell shape by reforming, which is facilitated by actin-severing proteins.

Actin filament networks can provide mechanical support to the cell membrane by attachment to it via membrane-anchoring proteins; the best characterized of these are spectrin and ankyrin in red blood cells (see Fig. 7.2c), but similar proteins are present in most other cells. In addition, actin can become linked to transmembrane proteins in specialized areas of the plasma membrane, termed adherent junctions or focal contacts (see Figs 3.9 and 3.10), which are externally attached to other cells or extracellular structures; thus the actin filament network of one cell can become linked to other cells or structures.

Actin filaments can form rigid bundles to stabilize protrusions of cell membrane termed microvilli (see Fig. 3.15). In these bundles actin is associated with small linking proteins, the most abundant being fimbrin and fascin.

In all cells, actin filaments interact with a protein called 'myosin' to generate motile forces. Myosin is an actin-activated ATPase composed of two heavy chains and four light chains arranged into a long tail and a globular head. These myosin heads can bind to actin and hydrolyse ATP to ADP. The interaction between actin and myosin to produce contractile forces is shown in Figure 5.3.

Polymerization of actin filaments is probably responsible for the forces that drive local outgrowths of cell cytoplasm, such as spikes and ruffles, which are particularly evident in motile cells and cells undergoing migration in embryogenesis.

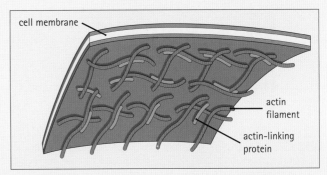

FIGURE 2.20 **Cell cortex.** The cell cortex is composed of a stiff cross-linked meshwork of actin and actin-linking proteins, the most abundant being filamin but also including spectrin acid. It forms a layer that lines the cytosolic face of the cell membrane.

Microfilaments are based on assemblies of the protein actin

Actin accounts for about 5% of the total protein in most cell types. It is a globular protein (G-actin), which polymerizes to form filaments (F-actin) with all the actin subunits facing in one direction (polar filaments).

There are several molecular variants (isoforms) of actin, which have specific distributions in different cell types, for example isoforms restricted to smooth muscle or skeletal muscle.

Microtubules brace internal organelles and guide movement in intracellular transport

Microtubules are present in all cells except red blood cells. They are formed from two protein subunits, α and β **tubulin**, which polymerize in a head-to-tail pattern to form protofilaments. These are arranged into groups of 13 to form hollow tubes 25 nm in diameter (Fig. 2.21).

Other cellular elements, such as centrioles and cilia, are also made up of tubulin in the form of doublet or triplet tubules (see below).

Microtubules are constantly polymerizing and depolymerizing in the cell and grow out from the microtubule-organizing centre. They are stabilized by associating with other proteins (microtubule-associated proteins or MAP,

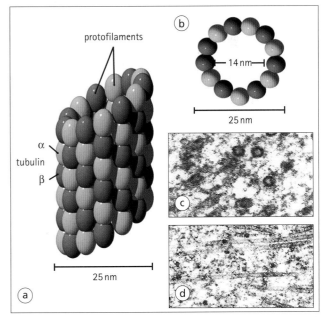

FIGURE 2.21 **Microtubules.** (a) Each microtubule is composed of 13 protofilaments of alternating α and β tubulin subunits. Microtubules are polar, with polymerization occurring at one end and depolymerization at the other. (b) In cross-section, each microtubule is 25 nm in diameter. (c) Electron micrograph showing the circular profiles of microtubules in cross-section. (d) Electron micrograph showing the faint parallel lines of microtubules in longitudinal section.

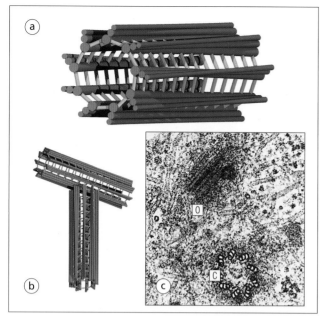

FIGURE 2.22 **Centriole.** (a) A centriole is composed of a cylindrical bundle measuring 200×400 nm composed of nine microtubule triplets arranged together by linking proteins. (b) In most cells, centrioles exist in pairs arranged at right-angles to each other. (c) In electron microscopic preparations, one centriole is usually visible in cross-section, revealing the circular (C) arrangement of tubules, whereas its partner is cut either longitudinally or slightly obliquely (O).

e.g. Tau protein), which convert the unstable microtubular network into a relatively permanent framework. Microtubules are also stabilized by proteins that cap the growing end and prevent depolymerization.

The centriole acts as a region which organizes the distribution of microtubules

Microtubules originate in the microtubule-organizing centre. This special region of the cell, known as the 'centrosome', is an organelle which contains a pair of centrioles (the centriole, Fig. 2.22).

Each centrosome, with its pair of centrioles surrounded by an amorphous electron-dense area of cytoplasm, acts as the nucleation centre for the polymerization of microtubules; these radiate from the centrosome in a star-like pattern called an 'aster'. The protein forming the amorphous area is highly conserved in evolution and is present in both animal and plant cells. Each centrosome can act as the centre for about 250 microtubules.

The centriole has several roles in the cell:
- It organizes the cytoplasmic microtubular network in both normal and dividing cells
- It organizes the development of specialized microtubules in motile cilia (see Fig. 3.17)
- It acts as the centre for cellular reorganization in the aggresomal response (see 'Advanced Concepts' box p. 29).

Intermediate filament	Localization
cytokeratins	epithelial cells
desmin	muscle (smooth and striated)
glial fibrillary acidic protein (GFAP)	astrocytic glial cells
neurofilament protein	neurons
nuclear lamin	nucleus of all cells
vimentin	many mesenchymal cells

FIGURE 2.23 **Intermediate filaments.** The location of different types of intermediate filament.

Intermediate filament proteins vary between different functional classes of cells

Intermediate filaments are a group of filamentous cytoskeletal proteins comprising six main types, which have a specific distribution in different cell types (Fig. 2.23). Ultrastructurally, they form relatively ill-defined bundles or masses in the cytosol of cells.

ADVANCED CONCEPT
MICROTUBULE FUNCTION

Microtubules form a network allowing transport around the cell, via the attachment proteins dynein, which moves down a microtubule toward the cell centre, and kinesin, which moves up a microtubule towards the cell periphery. These attachment proteins are associated with the membranes of vesicles and organelles and facilitate their movement around the cell. This process is particularly important in the transport of organelles down the long cell processes of nerve cells (see Chapter 6).

Microtubules also form a network (cytoskeleton) for membrane-bound cell compartments (e.g. they maintain the extended tubular arrangement of the ER).

Chromosomes are organized in cell division along the microtubular cell spindle (see Fig. 2.27).

Specialized motile components of the cell, cilia (see Fig. 3.17), are composed of microtubules bound together with other proteins.

KEY FACTS
CYTOSKELETON

- Microfilaments are made of actin and have roles in movement and membrane stabilization
- Microtubules are made of tubulin and have roles in intracellular transport as well as in scaffolding of internal membranes
- Intermediate filaments are made of proteins which vary between different cell types and function to link separate cells into structural units.

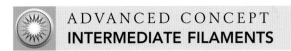

ADVANCED CONCEPT
INTERMEDIATE FILAMENTS

Intermediate filaments are anchored to transmembrane proteins at special sites on the cell membrane (desmosomes and hemidesmosomes, see Figs 3.11 and 3.12) and spread tensile forces evenly throughout a tissue, so that single cells are not disrupted.

Although intermediate filaments have several defined roles in cells as outlined below, detailed mechanisms of their function have not been elucidated, unlike those of the other cytoskeletal proteins.

In epithelial cells of the skin, keratin intermediate filaments become compacted with other link proteins to form a tough outer layer (see Fig. 3.28) and hence have an important structural role as an impermeable barrier, as well as being the main constituent protein of hair and nail.

In neurons, neurofilaments have long side arms, which probably help maintain the cylindrical architecture of nerve cell processes when subjected to lateral tensile forces in bending. They also anchor membrane ion channel proteins via a link protein 'ankyrin', to facilitate nerve conduction.

When cells are damaged, the intermediate filament network collapses around the centriole to form a perinuclear spherical mass associated with abnormal or damaged cellular proteins and elements of the ubiquitin–proteasome system used in protein degradation. This is termed the aggresomal response. It is possible that in this situation the intermediate filaments act to cocoon damaged cellular components in one spot for subsequent elimination by proteolysis and autophagy. Following cell recovery, the intermediate filament network re-expands. This phenomenon occurs in liver cells in response to persistent alcohol excess, when collapsed bundles of cytokeratin intermediate filaments (Mallory's hyaline) accumulate. This is also believed to be a response that happens in neurons in the brain in Parkinson's disease, where the accumulations of material are termed Lewy bodies.

In the nucleus, the nuclear lamins form a square lattice on the inner side of the nuclear membrane, which probably acts with other link proteins in the organization of the nucleus.

The cell-specific restriction of distribution of intermediate filament proteins may be used for the histological assessment of cell types, using immunohistochemical staining for the various filaments. This is particularly useful when small samples of malignant tumour are being assessed to determine their likely site of origin.

The detection of cytokeratin argues strongly for an epithelial origin, whereas the presence of desmin would suggest a muscle derivation, and glial fibrillary acidic protein (GFAP) is only seen in specialized central nervous system tumours.

Cell Inclusions and Storage Products

Accumulations of products within certain cells may occur in the form of cytoplasmic inclusions.

Lipofuscin pigment is mainly composed of phospholipid and is the result of 'wear and tear'

Lipofuscin appears as membrane-bound orange-brown granular material within the cytoplasm. Derived from residual bodies containing a mixture of phospholipids from cell degradation, lipofuscin is commonly referred to as 'wear and tear' pigment, as it becomes more prominent in old cells. It is particularly common in tissues from elderly persons, and is most evident in nerve, heart muscle and liver cells.

Lipid is stored in cells as non-membrane-bound vacuoles

Lipids may accumulate as non-membrane-bound vacuoles, which appear as large clear spaces in the cytoplasm because paraffin wax processing dissolves out the fat. If the tissues are frozen and cut in a freezing microtome, the fat can be stained with certain dyes. Large fat vacuoles are a special feature of fat storage cells called 'adipocytes' (see Fig. 4.20). Fat also accumulates in certain cells, such as hepatocytes in the liver in response to sublethal metabolic damage. The most common cause is chronic high alcohol ingestion.

Glycogen may impart a pale vacuolated appearance to cells

Glycogen, a polymer and storage product of glucose, forms as granules in the cell cytoplasm and is only visible by electron microscopy. Demands for energy are met by conversion of glycogen to glucose.

In certain cells, the presence of large amounts of glycogen causes pale staining or apparent vacuolation of cell cytoplasm. Glycogen can be stained by the PAS method.

Cell Division

Cell division for growth and renewal is achieved by the process of mitosis

An essential feature of development is the ability of cells to divide and reproduce. In addition, death of mature cells in the adult needs to be compensated for by the production of new cells.

Cells reproduce by duplicating their contents and dividing into two daughter cells. The phases involved in cell replication can be regarded as a cell cycle (Fig. 2.24). The phases of cell division are visible histologically and involve duplication of cellular cytoplasmic contents, duplication of DNA, separation of cellular DNA into two

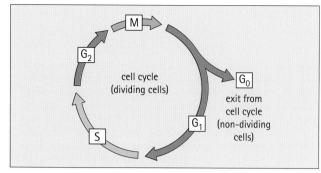

FIGURE 2.24 **Phases of cell cycle.** Cells can enter a phase of proliferation in which they divide. Cells that leave the cycle are said to be 'in the G_0 phase'.

separate areas of the cell (mitosis, Figs 2.25, 2.26) and finally cell division (cytokinesis).

Different cell populations can be defined according to their pattern of growth

In adults, not all cells are capable of division. Several different populations of cells can be defined based on their capacity to replicate:

- Static cell populations are cells which do not divide in the developed tissue
- Stable cell populations do not normally divide
- Renewing cell populations normally divide constantly.

Nerve cells and cardiac muscle cells, for example, divide and form tissues during embryogenesis, but once tissues are formed, the cells do not divide again in post-natal life and cells cannot be replaced if lost through disease. Stable cell populations, for example liver cells, do not normally divide in postnatal life but can prolifer-ate in order to replace cells lost through disease. Skin and gut lining cells are renewing cell populations that divide continually in postnatal life to replace shed cells. In a similar way, blood cell populations have a short lifespan and are constantly renewed.

Tissues that are regarded as being composed of static cell populations (e.g. heart and brain) have recently been shown to have a very low level of cell proliferation in postnatal life. However, this is currently not thought to contribute to functional renewal in postnatal life and for practical purposes, once cells have been lost from such tissues through disease, they are not replaced in adult life.

Stem cells are partly committed cells which function as a dividing population to produce a range of specialized cells

All cells in an adult must have originated from the single fertilized cell that originates from the fusion of the ovum and the sperm. Such a cell is regarded as being **totipo-tential**, as not only does it form the cells in the resulting adult, it also has the ability to form the extraembryonic tissues of the placenta.

In a developing embryo, there is a population of cells termed **embryonic stem cells** (ES cells) which are

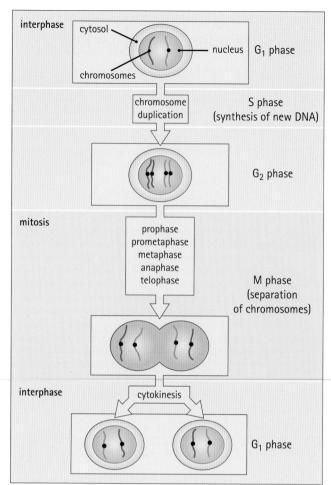

FIGURE 2.25 **The cell cycle.** The DNA of cells is only repli-cated during certain phases of a cell's growth pattern, which takes place in several stages. The cell cycle is divided into two main periods: mitosis and interphase, which includes G_1, S and G_2 phases. Cells which are not dividing are non-cycling or G_0 cells, whereas G_1 cells have just entered a phase of cellular growth. S-phase cells actively synthesize DNA, G_2 cells have a double complement of cellular DNA and are resting prior to cell division, and M-phase cells are in mitosis, which comprises five stages. In most tissues, only a small proportion of cells will be in the cell cycle, the majority being differentiated cells in a G_0 phase. Stem cells may be in a G_0 phase and only come to re-enter the cell cycle if there is a demand, for example follow-ing cell death. Progression through the cell cycle is carefully regulated by proteins such as cyclins that act at a series of checkpoints.

pluripotential and have the capacity to develop into any functional cell type. These cells have been isolated from either the inner cell mass of the developing blastocyst phase of an embryo or from fetal gonads, and cell lines have been established in tissue culture that retain the capacity for differentiation into any cell type.

It is the identification and characterization of ES cells that has suggested that they might be used therapeuti-cally, by transplantation, to treat a whole variety of dis-eases where there has been loss of permanent cells, for example nerve cells. However, because they originate and have to be harvested from an embryo, such work has led to ethical and moral debate, with some countries restricting or not allowing the development of therapeutic applications.

It is clear that in postnatal life there are populations of cells which are able to develop into a restricted set of different cell types and are regarded as **multipotential**. They then act as a pool of dividing cells to replenish more specialized cell populations. Such partly committed cells are called **multipotential stem cells**, and it is now known that they are the basis for continued renewal of many constantly dividing cell types.

Several types of renewing cell population are thought to originate from multipotential stem cells, for example the different cells of the blood originate from a common haemopoietic stem cell, and enterocyte stem cells probably give rise to the different cell types in the epithelial lining of the gut.

In some tissues, cells exist that serve to generate only one cell type, termed **committed progenitor cells**. An example of this type of cell is the 'epidermal stem cell', which is capable of forming new epithelial cells in skin. Such cells have also been classed as **unipotential stem cells**.

A stem cell must reproduce itself each time it divides to maintain a stem cell population. Following stem cell division, two types of cell may result: new stem cells to maintain the stem cell population, and committed cells, which differentiate along one cell line but may still divide in what are termed amplification divisions. Whereas stem cells typically have a low frequency of division, high rates of amplification divisions in committed cells are responsible for maintaining dynamic cell populations.

Multipotential stem cells typically represent a very small proportion of all cells in a tissue and on microscopy, they are generally very hard to see, as they lack differentiated features and appear as inconspicuous small cells. Their morphological anonymity belies their importance. Special markers have now been identified for some types of stem cell and this has allowed their isolation and study. It appears that the local environment of a stem cell and its attachments to the extracellular matrix influence its ability to divide and also influence the formation of specific committed cell types. The concept that the local microenvironment controls stem cell differentiation is acknowledged by describing each type of stem cell as being in a niche – a local microenvironment that defines growth and differentiation.

Finally, investigation of the fate of bone marrow stem cell transplants in humans and rodents has recently challenged the dogma that multipotential stem cells can only give rise to a limited set of cell types. It is evident that cells from bone marrow transplants have differentiated into liver cells, cardiac muscle cells and neuronal cells in the brain. Such findings are not fully explained but raise the possibility that, given the correct environment, certain multipotential stem cells can become pluripotential again. This concept is termed **adult stem cell plasticity**. The pathways that allow such adult plasticity, by characterizing the particular stimuli in specific niches that switch differentiation of resulting cells, are under intense investigation.

Cell division to produce gametes for reproduction is achieved through the process of meiosis

Normal cells have two sets of complementary (homologous) chromosomes derived from the maternal and paternal germ cells at fertilization and are therefore called **diploid**, or **2n** cells.

The germ cells (ova and spermatozoa), which are destined to fuse in fertilization to produce an embryo, have half the normal complement of chromosomes (i.e. are **haploid** – **n** – cells). They are the product of a modified form of cell division, **meiosis**.

In meiosis (Fig. 2.27), complementary chromosomes become paired on the mitotic spindle following the S phase of the cell cycle (see Fig. 2.25), with the maternal set attached to one pole and the paternal set attached to the opposite pole; the pole to which maternal- and paternal-derived chromosomes become attached is random for each chromosome. This is in contrast to mitosis, where complementary chromosomes do not align across the spindle.

Thus, in meiosis, maternal and paternal complementary chromosomes are separated, migrating to opposite ends of the spindle by a first meiotic division. Once they are segregated in this way, a second division (virtually identical to a mitotic division, see Fig. 2.26) separates replicated chromosomes. The result of meiosis is four daughter nuclei, each containing one set of chromosomes.

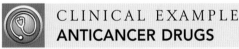

CLINICAL EXAMPLE
ANTICANCER DRUGS

Many drugs used to treat cancer act specifically on cells in the cell cycle (see Fig. 2.24), the aim being to remove abnormally growing cells.

Unfortunately, these drugs act on normal body cells as well as cancer cells and have adverse effects, particularly on renewing cell populations, which depend on a high proportion of cells being in cycle.

Thus, blood cell production, hair production and gut lining cell production are all impaired by the administration of such anticancer drugs.

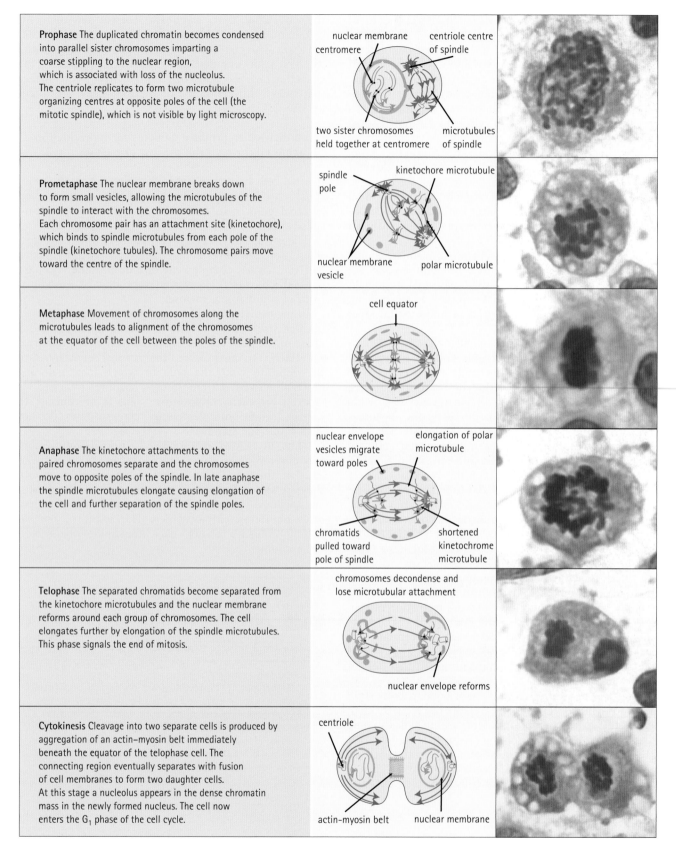

Prophase The duplicated chromatin becomes condensed into parallel sister chromosomes imparting a coarse stippling to the nuclear region, which is associated with loss of the nucleolus. The centriole replicates to form two microtubule organizing centres at opposite poles of the cell (the mitotic spindle), which is not visible by light microscopy.

nuclear membrane
centromere
centriole centre of spindle
two sister chromosomes held together at centromere
microtubules of spindle

Prometaphase The nuclear membrane breaks down to form small vesicles, allowing the microtubules of the spindle to interact with the chromosomes. Each chromosome pair has an attachment site (kinetochore), which binds to spindle microtubules from each pole of the spindle (kinetochore tubules). The chromosome pairs move toward the centre of the spindle.

spindle pole
kinetochore microtubule
nuclear membrane vesicle
polar microtubule

Metaphase Movement of chromosomes along the microtubules leads to alignment of the chromosomes at the equator of the cell between the poles of the spindle.

cell equator

Anaphase The kinetochore attachments to the paired chromosomes separate and the chromosomes move to opposite poles of the spindle. In late anaphase the spindle microtubules elongate causing elongation of the cell and further separation of the spindle poles.

nuclear envelope vesicles migrate toward poles
elongation of polar microtubule
chromatids pulled toward pole of spindle
shortened kinetochrome microtubule

Telophase The separated chromatids become separated from the kinetochore microtubules and the nuclear membrane reforms around each group of chromosomes. The cell elongates further by elongation of the spindle microtubules. This phase signals the end of mitosis.

chromosomes decondense and lose microtubular attachment
nuclear envelope reforms

Cytokinesis Cleavage into two separate cells is produced by aggregation of an actin–myosin belt immediately beneath the equator of the telophase cell. The connecting region eventually separates with fusion of cell membranes to form two daughter cells. At this stage a nucleolus appears in the dense chromatin mass in the newly formed nucleus. The cell now enters the G_1 phase of the cell cycle.

centriole
actin-myosin belt
nuclear membrane

FIGURE 2.26   **Mitosis.**

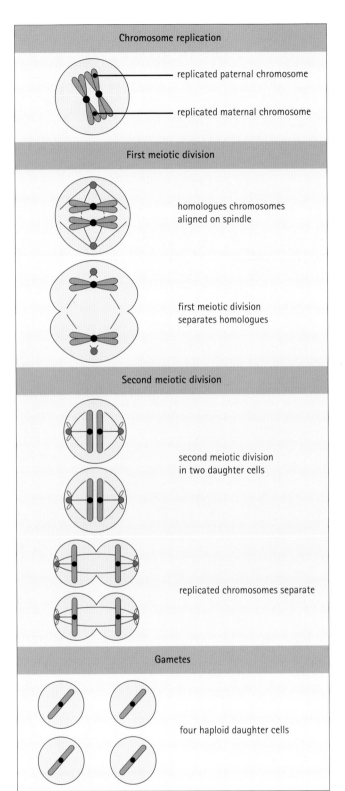

FIGURE 2.27 **Meiosis.** Meiosis results in the formation of four daughter cells, each with half the normal chromosomal complement (i.e. n, haploid).

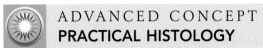

ADVANCED CONCEPT
PRACTICAL HISTOLOGY

General principles can be usefully applied when looking at cells either in cytological preparations or in tissue sections, to assess their activity, as outlined below:

Nucleus

A metabolically inactive cell has a compact round nucleus, which typically stains intensely as little chromatin is being transcribed. No nucleoli are visible, as ribosome production is minimal.

A protein-synthesizing cell has a large pale-staining nucleus with large or multiple nucleoli, reflecting active transcription of chromatin. Similar nuclear changes are evident in cells in an active phase of multiplication (see Fig. 2.25).

A dead cell has a shrunken nucleus, which appears as an amorphous compact mass of intensely staining material. This later fragments into separate particles and is completely lysed, leaving the cell devoid of any discernible nucleus.

Cytoplasm

Examination of cell cytoplasm should concentrate on the intensity and distribution of acidophilic (pink) and basophilic (blue) elements.

A granular, intensely pink-staining cytoplasm contains accumulations of organelles that take up acidic dye, which are usually mitochondria or secretory granules (e.g. neurosecretory granules, or specialized granules such as those seen in white blood cells).

A diffuse blue tint to the cytoplasm indicates the presence of cytoplasmic RNA in the form of ribosomes, and thus active protein production.

Large non-staining areas are generally large secretory vacuoles, such as those seen in the mucin-secreting cells. In some cell types, they may represent fat.

Cell Death

Programmed cell death is a normal means of controlling dividing cell populations

In many replicating tissues, and particularly during embryogenesis, control of the cell population is achieved by controlling the rate of cell death. Normal cells require a balance of signals that maintain their viability. In the absence of a correct pattern of signals, certain genes are switched on, which bring about carefully controlled dissolution of the cell. Because of the genetic control of this process it is referred to as 'programmed cell death', and contrasts with cell death that occurs in many diseases or is brought about by deleterious stimuli.

The most important form of programmed cell death is **apoptosis**. In this process, the cell shrinks, becomes fragmented and is ingested by adjacent cells (Fig. 2.28).

CLINICAL EXAMPLE
NUCLEAR CHANGES IN CANCER

A cell containing a very large nucleus relative to the amount of cytoplasm is generally in a phase of cell division. Cells with inappropriately large nuclei raise the suspicion of cancerous change. For example, cells on the surface of the uterine cervix should have small nuclei unless there is abnormal cell growth, such as that associated with the development of a malignancy.

In any specialized cell type, all the nuclei in adjacent cells should be roughly the same size and have the same staining characteristics. In cancer, however, nuclei vary in size and shape (nuclear pleomorphism) and commonly show dense-staining chromatin in a coarse, clumped pattern (nuclear hyperchromatism).

CLINICAL EXAMPLE
DIAGNOSTIC CYTOLOGY

Cytology is the study of cellular form and refers to an important specialty in laboratory medicine, which concentrates on establishing the diagnosis of disease by examination of small numbers of cells.

Cells for examination are obtained from patients either by scraping the surface of epithelia (e.g. the uterine cervix or gastric lining), by aspirating solid tissues with a needle or by collecting cells from body fluids such as sputum or urine.

The ultimate aim is to detect abnormalities in cell structure that point to the presence of disease. In clinical medicine, the most important aspect is the recognition of changes that herald the development of cancer (neoplastic changes).

ADVANCED CONCEPT
PROTEIN DEGRADATION IN CELLS

There is a constant need for protein turnover in cells. Proteins in the cell membrane, unwanted organelles, and proteins that enter cells from the extracellular space are degraded by the acid vesicle system, using lysosomal hydrolases.

In some cells, unwanted product in secretory vesicles is destroyed by the direct fusion of such secretory vesicles with lysosomes. This process is termed crinophagy. For example, when hormone-secreting cells in the pituitary gland no longer need to secrete their product, the secretory vesicles packed with hormone fuse with lysosomes and the hormone is degraded.

Cytosolic proteins are mainly degraded by a distinct mechanism called the ubiquitin–proteasome system. In this system, unwanted proteins are recognized by specific enzymes and subsequently tagged by the protein ubiquitin. The resulting ubiquitinated protein is then recognized by large multicatalytic proteases termed 'proteasomes' and degraded.

A highly efficient system for regulated elimination of proteins is essential for normal cell function. Certain proteins, such as those that control the cell cycle, those that activate transcription of genes or those that are intermediaries in intracellular signalling systems are eliminated rapidly by the ubiquitin–proteasome system. If they were not eliminated, their activities would persist and lead to adverse effects in the cell.

Normal cells are arranged in close contact with each other and are united by cell junctions. Early in the process of apoptosis there is synthesis of enzymes needed to cause cell dissolution, but this is not associated with structural changes. This is termed **priming**. In development many cells are primed for apoptosis and survive only if rescued by a specific trophic factor.

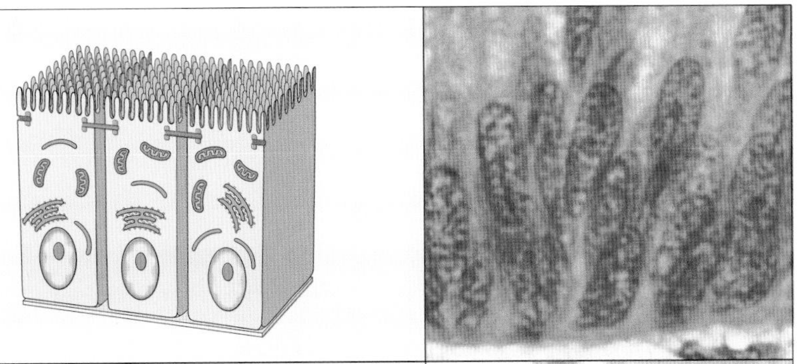

The apoptotic cells lose surface specializations and junctions, shrinking in size. The nuclear chromatin condenses beneath the nuclear membrane. In contrast to necrosis, cell organelles remain normal. Endonuclease enzymes cleave chromosomes into individual nucleosome fragments.

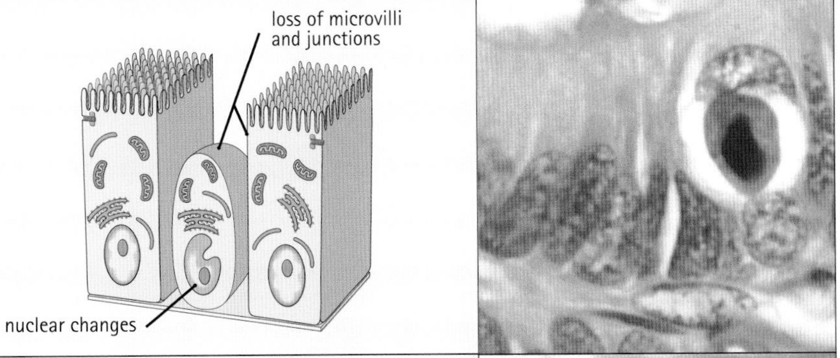

loss of microvilli and junctions

nuclear changes

There is splitting of the cell into several fragments known as **apoptotic bodies**. Nuclear fragmentation also occurs. Each fragment contains viable mitochondria and intact organelles. The process takes a few minutes only.

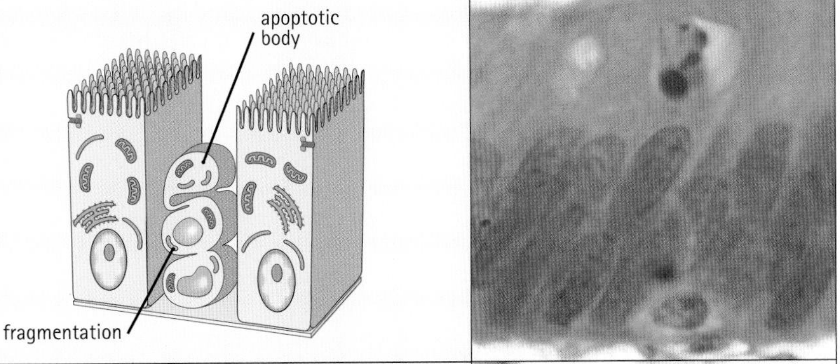

apoptotic body

fragmentation

Apoptotic fragments are recognized by adjacent cells, which ingest them by phagocytosis for destruction. Some fragments degenerate extracellularly, while others are ingested by local phagocytic cells, not shown on this diagram.

Although apoptosis is a physiological process, it can also be induced by pathological conditions.

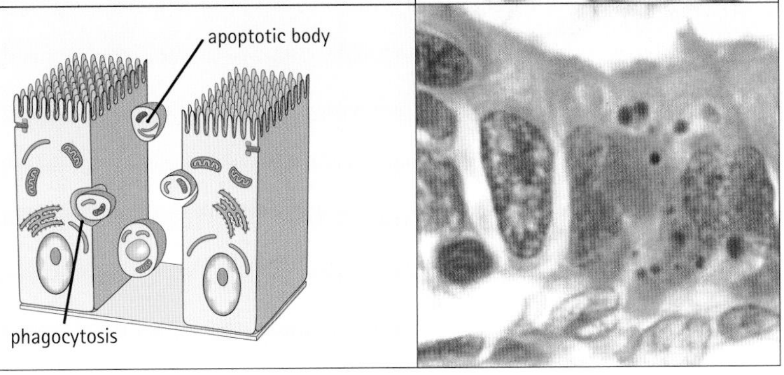

apoptotic body

phagocytosis

FIGURE 2.28 **Apoptosis.** Apoptosis of cells is a programmed and energy-dependent process designed specifically to eliminate them. This controlled pattern of cell death, termed 'programmed cell death', is very different from that which occurs as a direct result of a severe damaging stimulus to cells (termed 'necrosis').

For online review questions, please visit https://studentconsult.inkling.com.

END OF CHAPTER REVIEW

True/False Answers to the MCQs, as Well as Case Answers, can be Found in the Appendix in the Back of the Book.

1. **Which of the following features are seen in the cell membrane?**
   (a) It is structurally based on a lipid bilayer
   (b) Contains proteins which only act as enzymes
   (c) Surrounds the nucleus in a single layer
   (d) Surrounds individual ribosomes within the cell
   (e) It is maintained by vesicles derived from the Golgi

2. **Which of the following are features of mitochondria?**
   (a) Replicate independently from the cell
   (b) Are the main site for oxidative phosphorylation
   (c) Have a highly impermeable outer cell membrane
   (d) Vary in morphology between different cell types
   (e) Contain their own genetic material

3. **Which of the following features are present in lysosomes?**
   (a) Lysosomes have a membrane H^+-ATPase capable of maintaining an acid environment
   (b) The enzymes contained in lysosomes are also present in peroxisomes
   (c) Vesicles from the Golgi take acid hydrolases to lysosomes
   (d) Fusion of an endosome with a vesicle containing acid hydrolases forms an endolysosome
   (e) Lysosomal storage diseases are caused by lack of specific lysosomal enzymes leading to accumulation of a metabolic product

4. **Which of the following are seen in dividing cells?**
   (a) The nuclear membrane is fragmented during separation of chromosomes
   (b) The nucleolus is involved in ribosomal biogenesis and is a prominent structure in dividing cells
   (c) Prophase and metaphase both occur in the S phase of the cell cycle
   (d) The final daughter cells which derive from meiosis are haploid
   (e) Control of the overall population may be regulated by apoptosis

CASE 2.1   A CHILD WITH MUSCLE WEAKNESS

A 12-year-old child is admitted to hospital because his parents are concerned that he has been experiencing difficulty with simple things like running, walking and lifting. He has felt weak and easily fatigued. Examination reveals proximal muscle weakness but no evidence of muscle tenderness. There is no clinical evidence that the peripheral nerves are involved. Routine blood investigations are normal. In particular, serum creatine kinase levels are normal.

A biopsy of muscle shows excessive glycogen in muscle fibres, with large numbers of lysosomes also containing glycogen. Assay of muscle showed no detectable acid maltase, a lysosomal enzyme. Subsequent echocardiogram shows abnormally thick cardiac muscles.

Q. Describe the functional and structural basis of this case. In particular, classify this type of disease within the spectrum of causes of disease. Why do you think the heart is found to be abnormal?

CASE 2.2   A TUMOUR OF UNKNOWN ORIGIN

A 37-year-old man has been referred to hospital for investigation. He had noted a swelling in his neck and his own doctor felt that this was due to enlarged lymph nodes. On examination, he had several palpable enlarged lymph nodes in the right lower cervical region. Detailed imaging confirmed enlarged lymph nodes but no obvious associated lesions in other organs. A surgeon has removed an enlarged node and sent it for histological examination to determine the cause of disease. A poorly-differentiated tumour is discovered but its origin is not clear from initial histology.

Q. How might immunohistochemical assessment using antibodies to different cell constituents help in diagnosis? Concentrate on how expression of intermediate filaments could help with the diagnosis. What other cellular markers might be considered?

Chapter 3

Epithelial Cells

Introduction

Epithelial cells are a specialized component of many organs. They are characterized by common structural features, especially their arrangement into cohesive sheets, but have diverse functions made possible by many specialized adaptations. Many of the physical properties of epithelial cells rely on their attachment to each other, which is mediated by several types of cell junctions. The specialized functions of epithelial cells are mediated both through structural modifications of their surface and by internal modifications, which adapt cells to manufacture and secrete a product.

Epithelial cells are specialized for absorption, secretion or to act as a barrier

Epithelial cells form very cohesive sheets of cells, called 'epithelia', which function mainly as:
- A covering or lining for body surfaces, e.g. skin, gut and ducts
- The functional units of secretory glands, such as salivary tissue and liver.

Epithelial cells are firmly joined together by adhesion specializations. These special structures serve to anchor the cytoskeleton of each epithelial cell to its neighbours and to anchor the epithelium to underlying or surrounding extracellular matrix materials.

Epithelial cells are further specialized by modifications of their surfaces to fulfil their specific role, which may be absorption or secretion or to act as a barrier (see p. 39).

The classification of epithelial cells is based on their shape and how they are stacked together

The traditional nomenclature and classification of different types of epithelium are based on the two-dimensional shape of cells as observed by early light microscopy, and ignore any specialized functional attributes. Thus, the nomenclature now appears rather simplistic, given the present detailed knowledge of the biology of these cells.

Traditionally, cells are classified into three main cell groups according to their shape. These groups are: **squamous** (flat plate-like, Fig. 3.1); **cuboidal** (height and width similar, Fig. 3.2); and **columnar** (height 2–5 times greater than width, Fig. 3.3).

Epithelial cells form either a single layer in which all of the cells contact underlying extracellular matrix (simple epithelium), or several layers, where only the bottom layer of cells is in contact with the extracellular matrix (stratified epithelium, Fig. 3.4).

Pseudostratified epithelium (Fig. 3.5) contains epithelial cells that appear to be arranged in layers but which are all in contact with the extracellular matrix. A transitional epithelium is a further special type of stratified epithelium, which is mainly restricted to the lining of the urinary tract (see Ch. 15), and varies between cuboidal and squamous depending on the degree of stretching.

Epithelia are also grouped according to whether they occur as a surface or glandular component.

The traditional morphological classification has limitations. In the past, great emphasis was placed on the distribution of the different morphological types of epithelium and whether they were stratified or simple, surface or glandular; such classification is now outmoded. Although two epithelia may be described as cuboidal, their function and biology may be so different that it is misleading to equate them.

However, provided this limitation of nomenclature is realized, the use of a morphological classification of epithelia is still descriptively valuable.

The traditional terms used to describe epithelia are found throughout this book, but are always qualified to give insight into their function.

Epithelial Cell Junctions

Specialized structures are present in epithelia, which link the individual cells together into a functional unit.

The structural integrity of epithelium is maintained by adhesion of the constituent cells, both to each other and to structural extracellular matrix. These adhesions are mediated by two main systems:
- Cell membrane proteins acting as specialized cell adhesion molecules
- Specialized areas of cell membrane incorporated into cell junctions.

There are three types of cell junctions: **occluding junctions** link cells to form an impermeable barrier; **anchoring junctions** link cells to provide mechanical strength; and **communicating junctions** allow movement of molecules between cells.

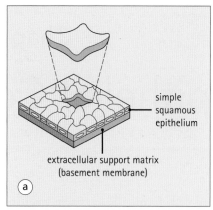

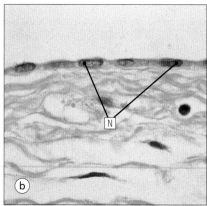

FIGURE 3.1 **Simple squamous epithelium.** (a) A simple squamous epithelium is composed of a single layer of cells, which are flat and plate-like. (b) In histological sections, the nuclei (N) appear flattened and the cytoplasm is indistinct. Although 'squamous' refers to any flat epithelium, its use is restricted as many flat epithelia are given more specific names, the flat epithelium lining blood vessels being called 'endothelium', and that lining the abdominal and pleural cavities, 'mesothelium'.

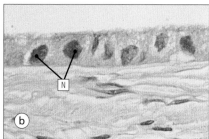

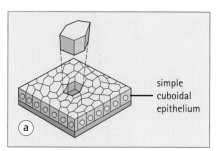

FIGURE 3.2 **Simple cuboidal epithelium.** (a) A simple cuboidal epithelium is composed of a single layer of cells whose height, width and depth are the same. Note that they are not strictly cuboidal. (b) In histological section, such cells usually have a centrally placed nucleus (N).

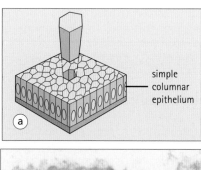

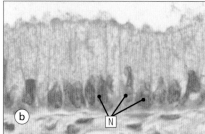

FIGURE 3.3 **Simple columnar epithelium.** (a) A simple columnar epithelium is composed of cells whose height is 2–3 times greater than their width. (b) The nuclei (N) of columnar cells are basal and arranged in an ordered layer.

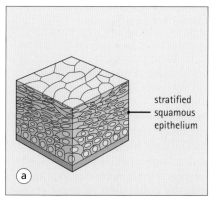

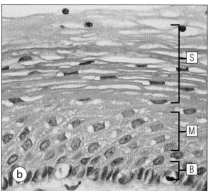

FIGURE 3.4 **Stratified squamous epithelium.** (a) A stratified squamous epithelium is composed of several layers, such that cells high up in the epithelium are not in contact with the underlying extracellular matrix. (b) Stratified squamous epithelium derives its name from the flattened (squamous) appearance of cells in the superficial part of the epithelium (S). Cells in the basal (B) and middle (M) layers of this type of epithelium are in fact pyramidal or polygonal and are not flattened.

Occluding junctions bind cells together and maintain the integrity of epithelial cells as a barrier

Occluding junctions have two main functions:
- Prevention of diffusion of molecules between adjacent cells, thereby contributing to the barrier function of the epithelial cells in which they are present

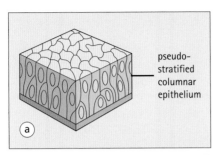

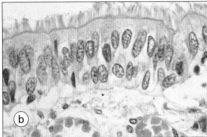

pseudo-stratified columnar epithelium

FIGURE 3.5 **Pseudostratified columnar epithelium.** (a) In a pseudostratified columnar epithelium, several layers of nuclei suggest several layers of cells, but in fact, all cells are in contact with the underlying extracellular matrix. (b) Routine histological preparations show several layers of nuclei.

- Prevention of lateral migration of specialized cell membrane proteins, thereby delineating and maintaining specialized cell membrane domains.

The occluding function is performed by intramembranous proteins (Fig. 3.6), which mediate the adhesion of adjacent cells.

Ultrastructurally, an occluding junction is seen as a focal area of close apposition of adjacent cell membrane. This has led to its alternative name of **tight junction**.

Occluding junctions are particularly well-developed in the epithelial cells lining the small bowel, where they:
- Prevent digested macromolecules from passing between the cells
- Confine specialized areas of the cell membrane involved in absorption or secretion to the luminal side of the cell.

Occluding junctions are also important in cells that actively transport a substance, for example the active transport of an ion, against a concentration gradient. In this situation, occluding junctions prevent back-diffusion of the transported substance (Fig. 3.7).

Anchoring junctions link the cytoskeleton of cells both to each other and to underlying tissues

Anchoring junctions (Fig. 3.8) provide mechanical stability to groups of epithelial cells so that they can function as a cohesive unit.

The actin network interacts with two separate types of junction:
- Adherent junctions link the actin filament network between adjacent cells (Fig. 3.9)

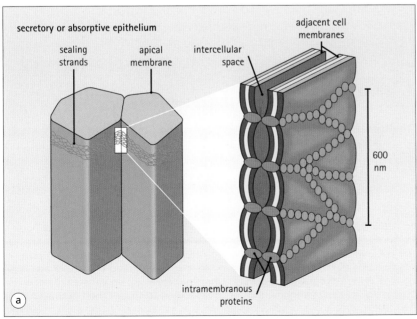

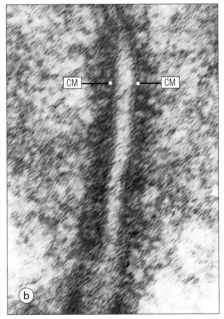

FIGURE 3.6 **Occluding junction (tight junction).** (a) Occluding junctions are particularly evident between epithelial cells that have secretory or absorptive roles. A collar of occluding junction is present between each cell, sealing individual cells into a tight barrier. The intramembranous proteins that form these junctions are arranged as serpiginous intertwining lines (sealing strands), which stitch the membrane of adjacent cells together. The proteins involved include occluding and claudin. (b) An occluding junction is seen ultrastructurally as an area of close apposition of adjacent areas of cell membrane (CM) corresponding to the site of membrane attachment proteins.

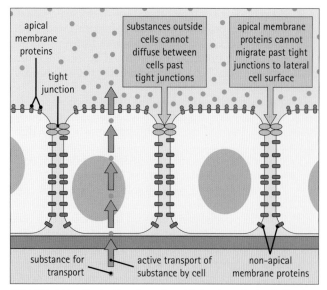

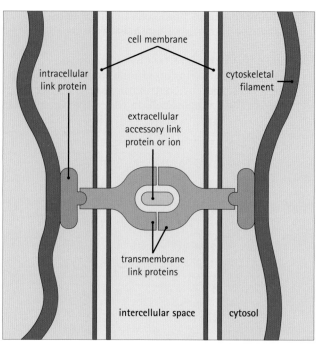

FIGURE 3.7 Occluding junction (tight junction). Cells that transport molecules against a concentration gradient have occluding junctions to prevent back-diffusion of the transported substance. The protein claudin is mainly responsible for this diffusion barrier. In addition, it is desirable to concentrate specialized cell membrane components into certain areas of the cell, for example a transport protein in the apical cell membrane. Cells use occluding junctions to prevent lateral migration of specialized membrane proteins, thus establishing specialized membrane domains.

FIGURE 3.8 Anchoring junction (general structure). Cytoskeletal filaments of adjacent cells are joined through intracellular link proteins, which attach the filaments to transmembrane link proteins. These can then interact with similar proteins on adjacent cells. The extracellular interaction may be mediated by additional extracellular proteins or ions, such as Ca^{2+}. Different (or multiple) link proteins and transmembrane proteins operate for the different classes of junction. An important class of proteins in this group are the cadherins, which link between adjacent cells using Ca^{2+}.

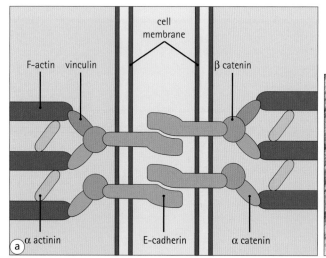

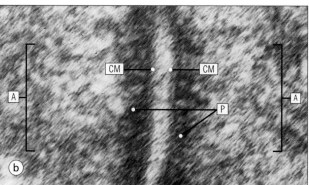

FIGURE 3.9 Adherent junction. In this type of junction: (a) F-actin fibres in adjacent cells are linked by actin-binding proteins, fibre including α and β catenins, vinculin and α actinin to a transmembrane protein, which is one of a group of the cadherin family of cell surface glycoproteins (E-cadherin), which links cells in the presence of Ca^{2+}. Ultrastructurally: (b) an adherent junction is a fuzzy plaque (P) of electron-dense material adjacent to the cell membrane (CM), corresponding to the location of α actinin and vinculin, into which actin filaments (A) are inserted. The intercellular junctional component (i.e. extracellular component of adjacent E-cadherin molecules and Ca^{2+}) is not visible, but is evident as a lucent area between the adjacent membranes.

- Focal contacts link the actin filament network of a cell to the extracellular matrix (Fig. 3.10).

The intermediate filament network interacts with two separate types of junction:

- Desmosomes connect the intermediate filament networks of adjacent cells (Fig. 3.11)
- Hemidesmosomes connect the intermediate filament network of cells to extracellular matrix (Fig. 3.12).

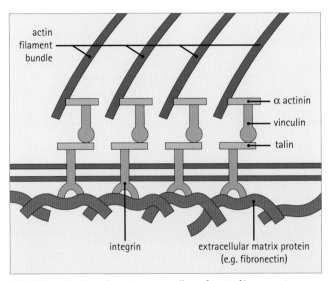

FIGURE 3.10 **Focal contact.** Bundles of actin filaments interact with actin-binding proteins (α actinin, vinculin and talin) to link with a transmembrane link protein, which is one of a class of cell adhesion molecules termed an 'integrin' (see also Fig. 4.10).

Adherent junctions are most common toward the apex of adjacent columnar and cuboidal epithelial cells, where they link submembranous actin bundles into a so-called **adhesion belt**. They are prominent in the cells lining the small intestine, where they form a zone visible by light microscopy as an eosinophilic band (the **terminal bar**).

In embryogenesis, adherent-type junctions transmit motile forces generated by the actin filaments across whole sheets of cells. They are thus essential in mediating the folding of epithelial sheets to form early organs in the embryo.

Desmosomes provide mechanical stability in epithelial cells subject to tensile and shearing stresses, and are particularly well-developed in stratified squamous epithelium covering the skin.

Desmosomes are so characteristic of epithelial cells that their detection in malignant tumours of uncertain nature is indicative of an epithelial as opposed to a lymphoid or support cell origin.

A **junctional complex** is the close association of several types of junction between adjacent epithelial cells and is a manifestation of the requirement for several types of epithelial cell attachment in order to maintain structural and functional integrity (Fig. 3.13).

Bullous pemphigoid is a blistering disease in which autoantibodies form and are directed against proteins in hemidesmosomes. These proteins have been termed 'bullous pemphigoid antigens 1 and 2' (BPAG1 and BPAG2). These proteins normally link cytokeratin intermediate filaments with integrin proteins that bind the cell to the basal lamina. In bullous pemphigoid, binding of antibody to these normal proteins leads to

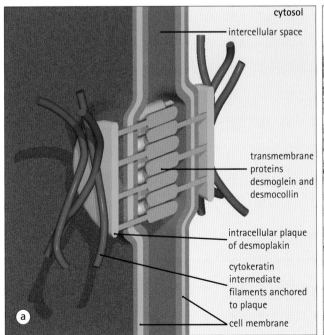

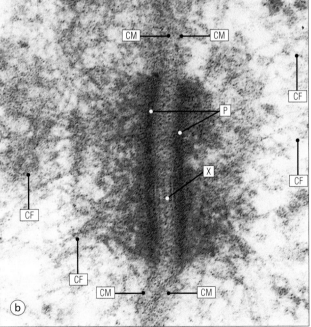

FIGURE 3.11 **Desmosome.** (a) Each desmosome consists of an intracellular plaque composed of several link proteins, the main type being desmoplakin associated with plakoglobin and plakophilin, into which cytokeratin intermediate filaments (tonofilaments) are inserted. The cell adhesion is mediated by transmembrane proteins: desmoglein and desmocollin, which are members of the cadherin family of cell adhesion proteins. (b) The disc-shaped adhesion plaques (P) in adjacent cells are seen as electron-dense areas into which cytokeratin filaments (CF) are inserted. The cell membranes (CM) between adhesion plaques are about 30 nm apart and there may be an electron-dense band between cells in some desmosomes (X).

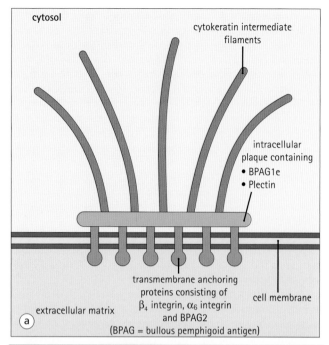

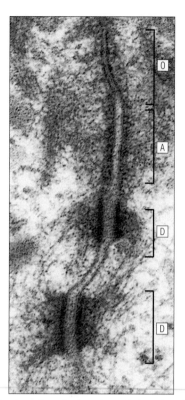

FIGURE 3.13 **Junctional complex.** A junctional complex is commonly seen towards the apex of cuboidal and columnar cells. Immediately below the cell apex, an occluding junction (O) is followed by an adherent junction (A), and below this, by desmosomes (D). This example is obtained from cells lining the small bowel, where such complexes are well-developed. In other epithelia, particularly those in which occluding junctions are not required, such fully-developed complexes are uncommon.

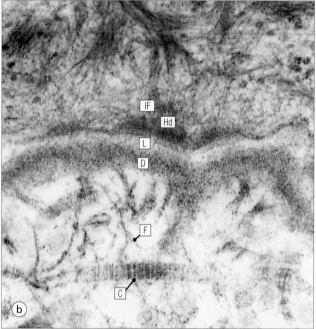

FIGURE 3.12 **Hemidesmosome.** (a) A hemidesmosome is similar to a desmosome, except that it interacts with the extracellular matrix rather than with an adjacent desmosome on another cell. In contrast to a desmosome, the cytokeratin filaments (tonofilaments) commonly terminate end-on rather than looping through. The proteins in the hemidesmosome differ from those in desmosomes. The intracellular plaque contains the proteins: plectin and BPAG1e. The transmembrane anchoring proteins comprise β_4 integrin, α_6 integrin and BPAG2 (BPAG, bullous pemphigoid antigen). (b) Ultrastructurally a hemidesmosome (Hd) consists of a dense plaque composed of intracellular link proteins into which the cell's cytokeratin intermediate filaments (IF) are inserted. This plaque links to the basement membrane, which consists of two layers: lamina lucida (L) and lamina densa (D), with an external ill-defined fibroreticular lamina. Fine anchoring fibrils (F), composed of type VII collagen, anchor the lamina densa to external collagen fibres (C).

CLINICAL EXAMPLE
DISEASE OF CELL JUNCTIONS – PEMPHIGUS

In pemphigus, the body produces abnormal antibodies to the proteins forming desmosome junctions in the skin; this prevents normal adhesion between the desmosomes. Affected people develop widespread skin and mucous membrane blistering as the desmosomal junctions between adjacent squamous cells of the skin fall apart. Immunohistochemical staining can be used to demonstrate the abnormal antibodies adhering to the intercellular space between the diseased epidermal cells.

inflammation and separation of the epithelium from the basal lamina, causing blistering.

Communication junctions allow direct cell–cell communication

Communication junctions (gap junctions) allow selective diffusion of molecules between adjacent cells and facilitate direct cell–cell communication (Fig. 3.14).

Gap junctions are usually present at relatively low density in most adult epithelia, but are found in large numbers during embryogenesis, when they probably have a role in the spatial organization of developing cells. Gap junctions are also important in cardiac and smooth

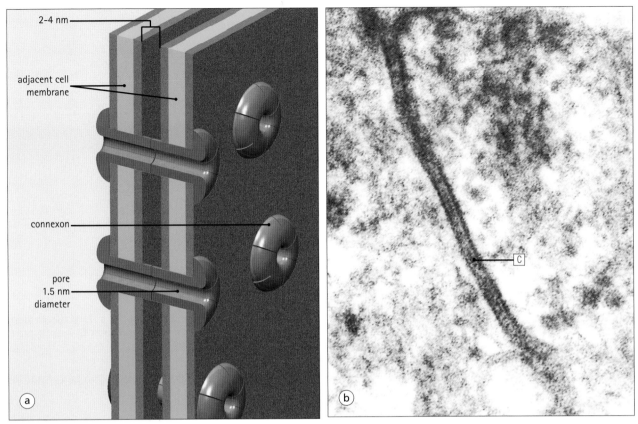

FIGURE 3.14 **Gap (communication) junction.** (a) A small part of a gap junction. Each junction is a circular patch studded with several hundred pores, each formed by six protein subunits traversing the cell membranes and termed a 'connexon'. Pores on adjacent cells are aligned, allowing small molecules to move between cells. (b) Ultrastructurally, a cross-section of a gap junction is seen as a flat area of closely apposing cell membranes, between which the connexons (C) can just be seen as dot-like granules.

muscle cells, where they pass signals involved in contraction from one cell to another.

The basement membrane anchors epithelial cells to underlying tissues

The attachment of epithelial cells to underlying support tissues at hemidesmosome and focal contacts is mediated by a specialized layer of extracellular matrix materials, the basement membrane (see Fig. 4.11). Basement membrane contains a special form of matrix protein called type IV collagen, which is synthesized by the epithelial cells.

Using light microscopy, basement membrane is just visible as a linear structure at the base of epithelia. It can be stained with the PAS technique.

Epithelial Cell Surface Specializations

The surface of epithelial cells can be adapted to allow a specialized function

The surface of epithelial cells is highly developed to fulfil specialized functions:
- The main adaptation requirement is for increased surface area, which in different cell types is sub-

served by microvilli, basolateral folds and membrane plaques
- The need to move substances over their surface is met by motile cell projections termed 'cilia'.

Microvilli are surface specializations to increase the surface area of cells

Microvilli are finger-like projections of the apical cell surface (Fig. 3.15). Small microvilli are found on the surface of most epithelial cells but are most developed in absorptive cells, such as kidney tubule cells and small bowel epithelium.

The shape of microvilli is maintained by a bundle of actin filaments, which form a core running through each villus; it is anchored to the actin cortex of the cell. In epithelial cells of the small bowel, the actin core is also linked to the actin network of adherent junctions between adjacent cells.

The cell membrane that covers microvilli bears specific cell surface glycoproteins and enzymes involved in the absorptive process. This cell surface specialization is just about visible ultrastructurally as a fuzzy coating, but is much more evident when enzyme histochemistry or immunohistochemistry is used to detect specific proteins, such as lactase and alkaline phosphatase (see Fig. 3.19).

Stereocilia are extremely long forms of microvilli and, despite their name, have nothing to do with true

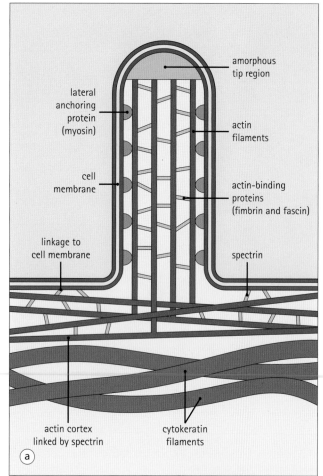

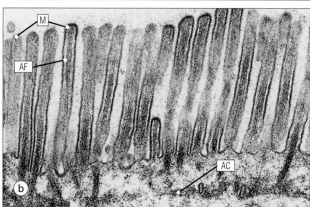

FIGURE 3.15 **Microvilli.** (a) Each microvillus is a finger-like extension of cell membrane, which is stabilized by a bundle of actin filaments held rigidly 10 nm apart by actin-binding proteins. The actin bundle is bound to the lateral surface of the microvillus by a helical arrangement of myosin molecules, which bind on one side to the actin and on the other to the inner surface of the cell membrane. The bundle is also adherent to the apex of the microvillus in an amorphous area of anchoring proteins, which may represent capping proteins for the actin filaments to prevent their depolymerization. At the base of the microvillus, the entering actin bundle is stabilized by the actin/spectrin cell cortex, under which are cytokeratin intermediate filaments. (b) Electron micrograph showing the surface of a cell lining the small bowel. Microvilli (M) form finger-like projections, each having an actin filament (AF) core that enters the cell and merges with the actin cortex (AC), which is also known as the terminal web.

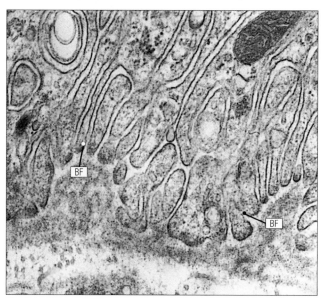

FIGURE 3.16 **Basal folds.** Electron micrograph showing deep infolding of basal cell membrane (BF) of a distal tubule kidney cell. This facilitates cell membrane transport of ions by greatly increasing cell surface area.

cilia. They are found on epithelial cells lining the epididymis and are the sensors of cochlear hair cells (see Ch. 19).

Basolateral folds increase cell surface area

Basolateral folds are deep invaginations of the basal or lateral surface of cells (Fig. 3.16). They are particularly evident in cells involved in fluid or ion transport, and are commonly associated with high concentrations of mitochondria, which provide the energy for ion and fluid transport. The presence of basal folds and mitochondria imparts a striped appearance to the basal cytoplasm of such cells, giving rise to the descriptive term 'striated epithelial cells'.

Basal folds are seen in renal tubular cells (see Fig. 15.18) and in the ducts of many secretory glands.

Cell surface area can be similarly increased by folding of the lateral cell membrane, which can be seen in some epithelial cells, particularly absorptive cells lining the gut.

Membrane plaques are a specialized structure seen in the urothelium

Membrane plaques are rigid areas of the apical cell membrane found only in the epithelium lining the urinary tract. They can fold down into the cell when the bladder is empty and unfold to increase the luminal area of the cell when the bladder is full (see Fig. 15.33).

Cilia are motile surface projections of cells involved in transport

Cilia are hair-like projections, 0.2 μm in diameter, which arise from the surface of certain specialized cells and

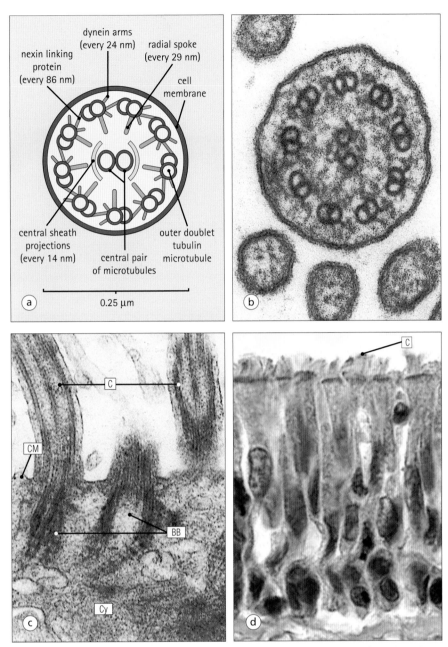

FIGURE 3.17 **Cilia.** (a) Cross-section of a cilium. The nine outer doublet tubules are made of tubulin, whereas arms composed of the protein dynein occur every 24 nm down the length of the cilium and interact with adjacent doublets as a 'molecular motor' to produce bending. Links composed of another protein, nexin, are more widely spaced (every 86 nm) and hold the microtubules in position. Radial spokes extend from each of the nine outer doublets toward a central pair of tubules at 29 nm intervals, and the central sheath projections are present every 14 nm. (b) Ultrastructural appearance of a cilium in cross-section. Because the different constituent proteins are periodically spaced at different intervals along the length of the axoneme, not all are visible in any one plane of section. (c) In longitudinal section, the base of each cilium (C) is seen to arise as a specialized derivative of the centriole (the basal body, BB). Here, the outer doublets of the cilium arise directly from the outer triplet of the centriole (CM, cell membrane; Cy, cytoplasm.) (d) Micrograph of a ciliated epithelium. Cilia (C) form a hair-like layer at the apical cell surface. As they are very fragile, they may not be well preserved in poorly fixed or processed tissue.

have a role in moving fluid over the surface of the cell or to confer cell motility.

Each cilium is a highly specialized extension of the cytoskeleton and is composed of an organized core of parallel microtubules (the axoneme). These microtubules are bound together with other proteins to produce energy-dependent movement of the filaments, which results in side-to-side beating (Fig. 3.17).

Cilia are particularly evident in:
• Epithelium lining the respiratory tract, where they move mucus over the cell surfaces (see Fig. 10.2)
• Epithelium lining the fallopian tube, where they convey released ova to the uterine cavity (see Fig. 17.12).

A similar axonemal structure to that of cilia is found in the flagellum of spermatozoa (see Fig. 16.8).

CLINICAL EXAMPLE
CILIAL DEFECTS AND DISEASE

Genetic defects in genes coding for ciliary proteins give rise to uncoordinated or absent ciliary beating in ciliated epithelia. This causes the immotile cilia syndrome.

Ultrastructurally, elements of the cilia may be absent or abnormal (Fig. 3.18).

There are several possible consequences of such abnormality:

- In embryogenesis, the defective cilia are unable to move cell layers correctly and the major organs do not assume their normal anatomic positions, e.g. right-sided heart
- Development of air sinuses in the skull, which is dependent on normal cilial action, is impaired
- Failure of mucus removal from the lung results in recurrent and severe chest infections. Eventually, prolonged stagnation of secretions and recurrent bacterial infections lead to permanent dilation of the large air passages, which fill with stagnant infected secretions and lead to premature death
- Infertility is common because ovum transport along the fallopian tube depends on normal ciliary function and ciliary proteins make up the motile tail of spermatozoa.

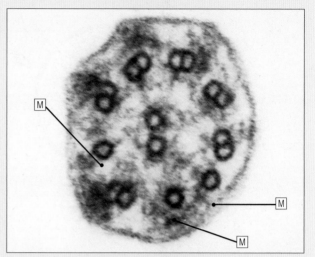

FIGURE 3.18 **Immotile cilia syndrome.** Electron micrograph of cilia from a person with recurrent chest infections since childhood. The outer dynein arms are absent and there are abnormal single microtubules (M), which prevent normal motility. Compare with Figure 3.17b.

Cell surface proteins can act as enzymes or adhesion molecules or be used for cell recognition

The surface of epithelia is invested with a layer of protein, glycoprotein and sugar residues which, in many cells, can be resolved ultrastructurally as an amorphous fuzzy coating to the cell membrane. Because of the sugar content, it is stainable by techniques, such as the PAS method (see p. 6). This coating is the **glycocalyx**.

Enzyme histochemical and immunohistochemical methods can be used to detect specific enzymes in this surface coating (Fig. 3.19), and it is apparent that epithelial cells at different sites have different functional attributes in terms of enzyme activity, despite similarities in their morphology.

Surface proteins are also used in a variety of cell recognition and adherence mechanisms, often of great importance to the function of the immune system.

Secretory Adaptations

Some organelles develop to adapt a cell for secretion of macromolecules

Certain epithelial cells have structural specializations related to their role in the production and secretion of

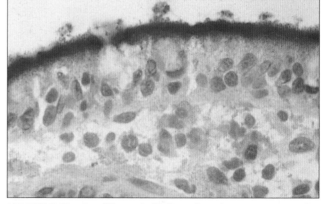

FIGURE 3.19 **Small bowel alkaline phosphatase activity.** The localization of cell membrane-associated alkaline phosphatase on the surface of epithelial cells lining the small bowel is shown. Note that the enzyme activity (demonstrated as a red stain deposit) is confined to the apical surface of the cells.

macromolecules, such as enzymes, mucins and steroids. In addition, epithelial cells can be adapted for the secretion and transport of ions. Such cells are characterized by an expansion of the specific organelle systems involved in the elaboration and secretion of the respective macromolecules (see pp. 47-48).

PRACTICAL HISTOLOGY

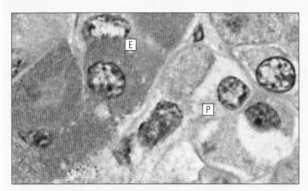

FIGURE 3.20 **Protein-secreting epithelial cells.** The cells shown in this micrograph are from the pituitary gland and are producing different peptide hormones, which impart different staining characteristics to the cells (E, eosinophilic; P, pale staining).

Protein-secreting epithelial cells have large nuclei and abundant rough endoplasmic reticulum (ER)

Although all cells contain the apparatus to produce structural proteins, certain cells are specialized to secrete a protein product and have the following characteristics:

- A well-developed rough ER, which often results in blue colouration of the cytoplasm in H&E-stained sections (see plasma cell, Ch. 8)

- Distinct polarity with basal rough ER, a supranuclear Golgi just visible as an ill-defined lucent area of the cytoplasm, and an apical zone containing granules filled with packaged protein ready for secretion by exocytosis.

The staining characteristics of the apical portion of the cells depend on the nature of this protein (Fig. 3.20).

Mucin-secreting epithelial cells have a greatly expanded Golgi system

Mucins (mixtures of glycoproteins and proteoglycans) have important functions in body cavities, for example as a lubricant in the mouth and as a barrier in the stomach.

Cells that produce and secrete mucin (Fig. 3.21) are characterized by the following features:

- A well-developed basal rough ER makes the protein core of mucins and imparts a faint blue colour to the basal cytoplasm
- A well-developed supranuclear Golgi is the main site of protein glycosylation, but is not clearly visible by light microscopy
- Large secretory vesicles of mucin at the cell apex impart an unstained vacuolated appearance to the apical cell cytoplasm.

Mucin-secreting cells may be part of a surface epithelium, when they are termed goblet cells, for example in epithelia lining the gut (see Fig. 11.44) and respiratory tract. In addition, mucin-secreting cells can be aggregated into specialized glands, for example in the genital tract, respiratory tract and intestinal tract.

PRACTICAL HISTOLOGY

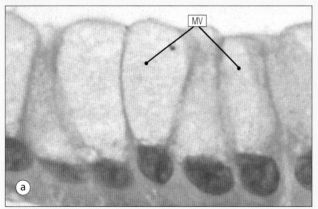
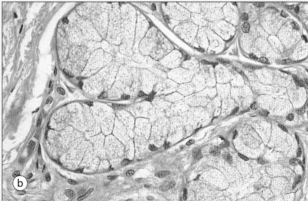

FIGURE 3.21 **Mucin-secreting epithelial cells.** (a) Micrograph of mucin-secreting surface epithelium showing the blue basal cytoplasm due to well-developed basal endoplasmic reticulum, and the unstained vacuolated appearance of the apical cytoplasm due to large secretory vesicles of mucin (MV). (b) Micrograph of mucin-secreting epithelial cells aggregated into a gland.

Steroid-secreting epithelial cells have an extensive smooth endoplasmic reticulum system

Cells producing steroid hormones (Fig. 3.22) are mainly found in the adrenal gland, ovary and testis, and have the following characteristics:

- A well-developed smooth ER, which gives the cytoplasm a granular pink appearance
- Free lipid (lipids are the precursors of the steroid hormones) in vacuoles in the cell cytoplasm, which imparts a fine vacuolated appearance to the cells
- Prominent mitochondria with tubular rather than flattened cristae. Mitochondria are involved in the biosynthesis of steroids from lipid, but the functional significance of the tubular shape of their cristae is not clear.

PRACTICAL HISTOLOGY

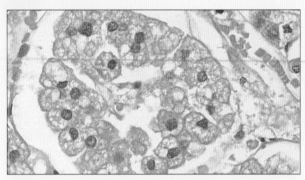

FIGURE 3.22 **Steroid-secreting epithelial cells.** According to their cytoplasmic composition, steroid-secreting cells vary in appearance in H&E-stained sections from granular pink-staining cells, which contain many mitochondria and little lipid, to pale pink-staining and vacuolated cells, which contain abundant lipid and dilated smooth endoplasmic reticulum. The cells shown here are from the adrenal gland and have a pale and finely vacuolated appearance.

Ion-pumping epithelial cells have many mitochondria and a large surface area

Cells in the kidney tubules and in the ducts of some secretory glands transport ions and water, whereas acid-producing cells of the stomach transport H⁺ ions (see Fig. 11.29). Ion transport is mediated by membrane ion pumps; these use ATP as a source of energy for the exchange of ions between cytosol and extracellular space.

The structural specializations of ion-pumping epithelial cells (Fig. 3.23) are as follows:

- The cell membrane is folded to increase the active surface area of membrane containing the membrane protein that acts as the ion pump
- Large numbers of mitochondria are closely apposed to the membrane folds to supply ATP
- Tight junctions between the cells prevent back-diffusion of pumped ions.

In cells of the intestine, gallbladder and kidney, the ion pumps move sodium and water from the apical surface to be absorbed, whereas in secretory glands, the cells move ions and fluid out of the apex of the cell, resulting in secretion of watery fluid (e.g. sweat).

PRACTICAL HISTOLOGY

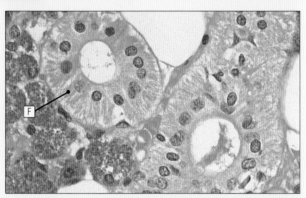

FIGURE 3.23 **Ion-pumping epithelial cells.** Micrograph of striated duct epithelial cells from salivary gland. Folding of the cell membrane (F) containing the active membrane protein produces a fine, striped appearance, whereas the large numbers of mitochondria impart a granular pink-staining appearance to the basal part of the cell. Tight junctions are only visible ultrastructurally.

Epithelial secretion is divided into four types

There are four mechanisms of secretion of cell product by epithelial cells: **merocrine, apocrine, holocrine and endocrine** (Fig. 3.24).

Secretions from the apex of the cell on to a surface or into a lumen are termed 'exocrine', whereas secretions from the side or base of the cell, which enter the bloodstream directly, are termed 'endocrine'.

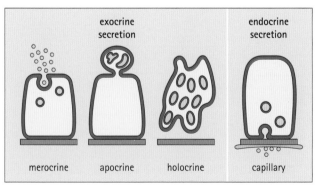

FIGURE 3.24 **Types of cell secretion.** Secretion of cell products may occur by exocytosis from the cell apex into a lumen (merocrine secretion); pinching off apical cell cytoplasm containing cell product (apocrine secretion); shedding of the whole cell containing the cell product (holocrine secretion); or endocytosis from the cell base into the blood stream (endocrine secretion, see also Fig. 14.1).

Epithelial cells are grouped into glands to allow focused production of a secreted product

A gland is an organized collection of secretory epithelial cells. In many epithelia, secretion is performed only by occasional specialized cells (e.g. mucin-secreting goblet cells) scattered among other, non-secretory cells (Figs 3.25, 3.26).

When more secretions are required, the surface area of secretory epithelium can be increased by invagination of the surface, to form straight tubular glands or by the formation of more complex coiled or branched glands, which may be divided into specialized zones for the secretion of different products.

The most structurally refined glands are those that have a branched architecture with secretory cells arranged in islands termed 'acini'. Transport of secretion from this type of exocrine gland is via a series of ducts lined by columnar epithelium, with apical junctional complexes to prevent escape of the secretions (Fig. 3.27).

Whereas most glands form part of other tissues (e.g. mucous glands in the respiratory tract), many are anatomically distinct (e.g. salivary glands, pancreas, liver).

Gland secretions are under hormonal and innervatory control, and all glands have a rich vascular supply to provide the necessary metabolites.

Barrier Function of Epithelium

Many epithelia function as a barrier, and this role is associated with certain specializations.

- Occluding junctions prevent diffusion of molecules between cells and therefore prevent diffusion of substances from one side of an epithelium to the other
- The apical cell membrane of epithelial cells lining the urinary tract (i.e. urothelial transitional epithelium) contains a high proportion of sphingolipids. These not only form membrane plaques (see p. 310), but are also believed to resist fluid and electrolyte movements out of the cells in response to the osmotic effect of concentrated urine
- Desmosomal and hemidesmosomal junctions provide a tight mechanical linkage between cells and extracellular matrix to resist shearing forces and allow an epithelium to function as a mechanical barrier
- Stratified squamous epithelial cells may undergo keratinization, a process in which the cytoskeleton of superficial cells of the epithelium becomes tightly condensed with other specialized proteins into a resilient mass. This results in cell death and the formation of a tough impervious and protective layer (keratin) from the remaining cell membranes and cytoplasmic contents (Fig. 3.28).

Keratinization ultimately transforms the cells into non-living proteinaceous material, which remains attached to underlying cells by existing anchoring junctions. The surface keratin layer is mechanically strong, but flexible; it is relatively inert and acts as a physical barrier, particularly preventing ingress of microorganisms. The intercellular phospholipid renders the epithelium impermeable to water.

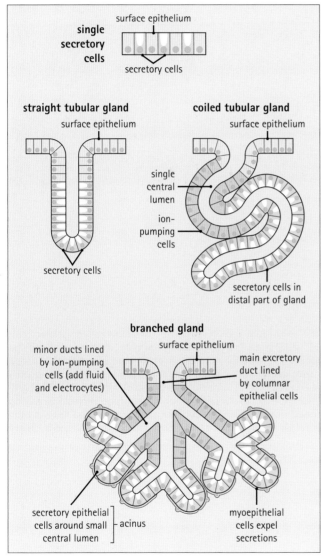

FIGURE 3.25　**Secretory cells and glands.**

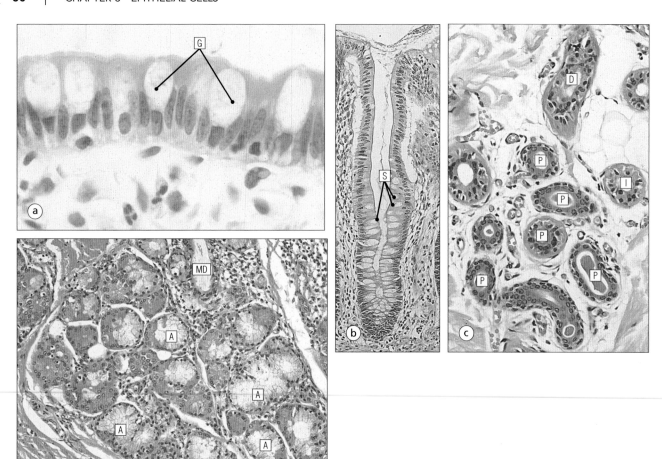

FIGURE 3.26 **Secretory cells and glands.** (a) Single cells in a surface epithelium secreting mucin. These are called 'goblet cells' (G). (b) H&E-stained section showing a straight tubular colonic gland, which is typical of glands in the gut. Secretory cells (S) line straight tubules and discharge their mucin secretions on to the surface. (c) H&E-stained section of a sweat gland from the skin showing the arrangement of a coiled tubular gland. Secretory cells are present in the distal part and there is zoning of secretory function, with an area of protein-secreting cells (P) being followed by an area of ion-pumping cells (I), which add fluid to the secretion in the lumen. The distal part of the gland, (D), has no secretory function but is specialized for transporting secretions, having tight junctions to prevent back diffusion of ions; such tubules are termed ducts. (d) H&E section of a branched gland showing the arrangement of secretory epithelial cells into acini (A), and main excretory duct (MD). The myoepithelial cells (see Fig. 5.13) are not readily visible at this low magnification.

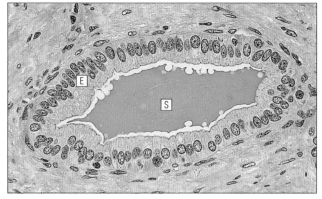

FIGURE 3.27 **Gland duct.** Ducts carry exocrine secretion from a gland and discharge it on to an epithelial surface or into a body cavity. Ducts are lined by a tall columnar epithelium (E) and contain no specialized secretory cells. Note pink-stained secretion (S) in the lumen.

FIGURE 3.28 **Keratinization.** (a) Basal cells of keratinizing squamous epithelium are anchored by hemidesmosomes and desmosomes to basement membrane and adjacent cells, and contain abundant cytokeratin intermediate filaments (tonofibrils). As the cells differentiate and move up the stratified epithelium, they remain tightly bound by desmosomal junctions, but the cytokeratin proteins change to higher molecular weight forms and the cells develop lamellar bodies. Lamellar bodies are membrane-bound granules containing phospholipids, which are secreted by exocytosis into the extracellular space and form a lamellar sheet between cells in the upper epithelium. Cells in the upper part of the epithelium express genes coding for a variety of specialized proteins which interact with the cytokeratin filaments and the cell membrane to produce a resilient and mechanically robust compact mass (keratin). Small granules (keratohyaline granules) contain some of these specialized proteins. A prominent protein (involucrin) associates with and thickens the cell membrane. (b) H&E section of keratinized squamous epithelium. Note the purplish keratohyaline granules (KHG) and the absence of nuclei in the surface keratin layer (K). (c) Keratinizing squamous epithelium stained to show involucrin (brown), which is only present in the upper keratinizing part of the epithelium.

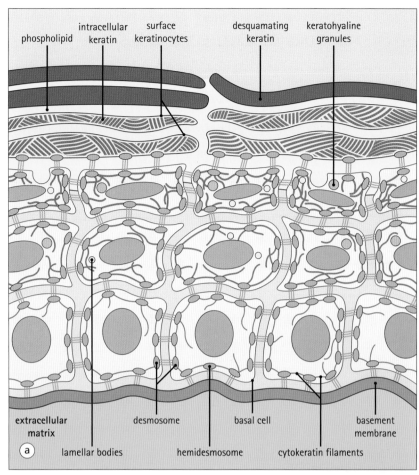

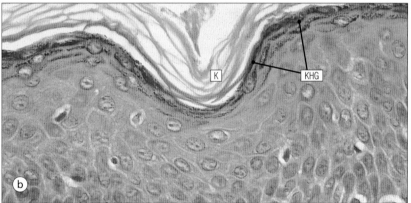

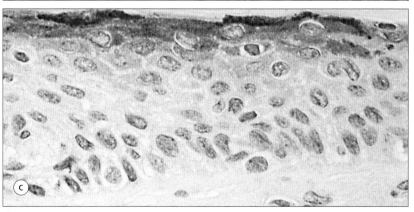

CLINICAL EXAMPLE
TUMOURS OF EPITHELIAL CELLS

Cells may lose their normal growth control mechanisms and give rise to a tumour (neoplasm). Many such abnormal growths remain localized (benign neoplasms), but some invade adjacent tissues and metastasize to other parts of the body (malignant neoplasms).

A malignant neoplasm arising from squamous epithelial cells is termed a 'squamous carcinoma', whereas carcinoma derived from glandular epithelium is called an 'adenocarcinoma' (Fig. 3.29).

In most cases, cells of a carcinoma resemble those of their tissue of origin. The diagnosis of malignancy is based on the presence of abnormal cytology, and by locating cells that have invaded other tissues.

In some cases, a carcinoma bears little resemblance to its cell of origin (undifferentiated carcinoma); such tumours commonly present with metastases and their site of origin may not be clear. In this situation, it is essential to use immunohistochemistry and electron microscopy to confirm the diagnosis.

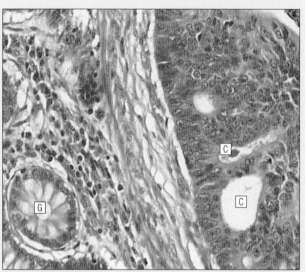

FIGURE 3.29 **Adenocarcinoma.** H&E section of colonic epithelium, showing normal glandular epithelium (G) and carcinoma (C) forming gland-like structures (i.e. adenocarcinoma).

CLINICAL EXAMPLE
IMMUNOCHEMISTRY OF EPITHELIA

Immunohistochemical techniques can identify epithelial cells and are useful in biopsy diagnosis of cancer.

In diagnostic histopathology, biopsy samples are looked at by a pathologist to diagnose disease. A common clinical problem is the evaluation of a biopsy of an abnormal growth, the commonest type of which is malignant growth of epithelial cells as a carcinoma. The pathologist has to try and answer the following questions:

1. Is the tissue normal or abnormal?
2. If the tissue is abnormal, does it represent an abnormal growth of cells, a tumour?
3. If the abnormality is a tumour, what is the cell of origin? Is it epithelial?
4. If the abnormality is an epithelial tumour, is it one that would be predicted only to grow locally (benign – termed 'adenoma' or 'papilloma'), or is it one that would be predicted to spread by invasion or metastasis (malignant – termed 'carcinoma').

To answer these questions about a tumour of epithelial cells, the pathologist first uses conventional staining, usually haematoxylin and eosin (H&E), and evaluates the tissue architecture. This will often give the diagnosis of the type of epithelial tumour and usually predicts behaviour.

- Benign growths closely resemble normal tissues, have few mitoses and cells have a uniform morphology
- Malignant growths do not resemble normal tissues closely, have increased numbers of mitoses, and cells vary in morphology – usually showing variation in size, with variation in size and density of staining of nuclei.

In some instances, a carcinoma shows few distinguishing features using standard histological techniques. The pathologist then faces a problem in diagnosis. Different types of carcinoma require different types of treatment, as clinical trials have shown that certain types of epithelial tumour respond better to certain types of therapy. This is most important in situations where a tumour first presents by spread, for example as a mass in a bone or a lymph node, and where imaging shows no clear origin. Histology shows a carcinoma but there is no known primary site. In this case, the clinical team will be asking the pathologist to try and state the likely primary site of origin of the tumour, to help direct the further investigations and treatment.

Fortunately, the availability of antibodies that detect specific cellular components has transformed diagnostic histopathology in the last several decades. It is now possible to stain tissue sections with specific antibodies using immunohistochemistry (see p. 7), and depending on the pattern of expression of different antigens, predict the cell type of the tumour and predict a likely primary site for a carcinoma.

For very poorly-differentiated malignant tumours, it may first be necessary to discriminate between cells of different histogenesis, using a broad panel of antibodies.

- Leucocyte common antigen detects if the tumour is lymphoid in origin
- Muscle-specific actin detects a tumour of muscle
- S100 protein detects tumours of melanocytes.

Epithelial cells have the following characteristics, detectable by immunohistochemical techniques:

- Expression of the cytokeratin class of intermediate filament proteins. This is not a feature of other classes of cells, for example support cells or lymphoid cells
- Expression of a class of cell surface glycoprotein (epithelial membrane antigen, EMA).

Once a broad panel of antibodies has established that a malignant tumour is of epithelial origin, and is a carcinoma, further panels of antibodies may be employed to predict the likely primary site of origin of the tumour. Examples include:

- Possession of a specialized stainable epithelial product by some epithelia, for example prostate-specific antigen and prostate-specific acid phosphatase in the ducts and acini of the prostate gland, thyroglobulin in cells of the thyroid gland, and gamma-gamma-enolase in cells of neuroendocrine lineage
- Cytokeratin 7 and cytokeratin 20 are differentially expressed in epithelia of different types and are commonly used in predicting the site of origin of carcinomas of glandular tissue, termed 'adenocarcinomas'
- Carcinoembryonic antigen (CEA) is strongly expressed in many tumours derived from glandular epithelium of the gastro-intestinal tract
- Thyroid transcription factor 1 (TTF-1) is a protein located primarily in the nucleus of epithelial cells in lung tissue. TTF-1 has been shown to be present in a variety of lung and thyroid tumours and is not present in most other carcinomas
- Tumours derived from mesothelial cells show a high frequency of staining for cytokeratins 5/6, thrombomodulin and calretinin
- Tumours of hepatic epithelial cells show a high frequency of staining for Hep Par 1 (hepatocyte paraffin 1 monoclonal antibody), alpha fetoprotein and CD10 antigen
- Carcinoma of the breast may show immunoreactivity for oestrogen receptor, and this may direct therapy with anti-oestrogenic agents.

After evaluation of a panel of antibodies covering a variety of possible tumour sites, a pathologist is usually able to give a diagnosis and opinion on which is clinically useful in directing further investigation and patient management.

For online review questions, please visit https://studentconsult.inkling.com.

END OF CHAPTER REVIEW

True/False Answers to the MCQs, as Well as Case Answers, Can be Found in the Appendix in the Back of the Book.

1. Which of the following are distinct features of epithelial cells?
   (a) Squamous epithelial cells are flat and plate-like
   (b) A pseudostratified epithelium has all its cells in contact with the underlying extracellular matrix
   (c) A simple columnar cell is typically two to three times higher than its width
   (d) Cell division occurs at all layers in a stratified squamous epithelium
   (e) Transitional epithelium is a characteristic cell lining the urinary tract

2. Which of the following features are present in epithelial cell junctions of varying types?
   (a) Occluding junctions prevent lateral diffusion of membrane proteins
   (b) Adherent junctions interact with the actin filaments in cells
   (c) Desmosomal junctions interact with the actin filaments in cells
   (d) Hemidesmosomes anchor cells to basement membrane
   (e) Gap junctions have a role in intercellular communication

3. Which of the following features are seen in epithelial cells?
   (a) Microvilli are braced by the actin cytoskeleton
   (b) Membrane plaques are a feature of transitional epithelium
   (c) Cilia are based on the intermediate filaments
   (d) The glycocalyx is seen within the rough ER and stores lipids
   (e) The characteristic type of intermediate filament is cytokeratin

Continued

4. Which of the following is true for the secretory role of epithelial cells?
(a) Endocrine secretion occurs when a cell enters the bloodstream
(b) Mucin-secreting cells have a well-developed Golgi, this being the main site of protein glycosylation
(c) Ion-pumping cells have many lysosomes to export transported solutes
(d) Merocrine secretion occurs when a secreted product is exocytosed from the cell on to a surface or into a lumen
(e) Apocrine secretion occurs when the whole cell is shed as the secreted product

CASE 3.1   NODULES ON THE LIVER

A 62-year-old man is admitted to hospital with abdominal pain. On examination, he has an enlarged liver and investigations show multiple nodules in the liver. Although a diagnosis of cancer spreading to the liver is strongly suspected, detailed imaging reveals no obvious site for a primary tumour. Under image guidance, a needle biopsy of one of the liver lesions is performed. This reveals unusual cells in the liver that are characterized by large, densely-stained nuclei, variation in nuclear size and many mitoses.

Q. What do the histological features suggest as a likely diagnosis? What other histological assessments could be done to help refine the diagnosis? Concentrate on why these features do not fit with normal histology. What stains can be used to help determine cellular differentiation?

CASE 3.2   A GIRL WITH A BLISTERING RASH

A 6-year-old girl is referred to a dermatology clinic because she has developed a recurrent blistering rash. It seems that she has always developed blisters on the hands and feet in response to trauma. A skin biopsy shows separation of the epidermis from the dermis at the level of the basement membrane. Further investigation shows mutation in the gene coding for one of the keratin intermediate filaments.

Q. Explain the possible structural basis for blistering in this condition. Concentrate on how cytokeratin filaments normally stabilize the epithelium and anchor skin via basement membrane. What other molecular/structural defects in the basement membrane/epidermis might be responsible for blistering disease?

Chapter 4

Support Cells and the Extracellular Matrix

Introduction

The cells that form tissues can be divided into two types: **parenchymal cells**, which subserve the main function of a tissue, and **support cells**, which provide the structural scaffolding of a tissue. Support cells comprise a set of highly developed cell types with complex metabolic functions and produce an extracellular matrix, which largely defines the physical characteristics of a tissue.

Support cells and their associated extracellular matrix are commonly termed **connective tissue**. However, we believe that this term does not emphasize the highly specialized nature of this class of tissues.

This chapter covers the general characteristics and types of support cell, and describes the main components of the extracellular matrix materials that form the essential support scaffolding to tissues.

Support cells have common characteristics that distinguish them from other classes of cell

Support cells are vital in providing mechanical stability to tissues. These are included in the class of connective tissue cells and have the following common characteristics:
- Embryological derivation from mesenchyme (Fig. 4.1)
- Production of a variety of extracellular matrix materials
- When mature, formation of sparsely cellular tissues in which the matrix is the main component
- Cell adhesion mechanisms that interact with extracellular matrix materials rather than other cells.

There are five main classes of support cell

The support cells (see p. 63) are as follows:
- **Fibroblasts** secrete the extracellular matrix components in most tissues, usually collagen and elastin
- **Chondrocytes** secrete the extracellular matrix components of cartilage
- **Osteoblasts** secrete the extracellular matrix components of bone
- **Myofibroblasts** secrete extracellular matrix components and also have a contractile function
- **Adipocytes** are specially adapted lipid-storing support cells which not only act as an energy store, but also have a cushioning and padding function.

Extracellular Matrix

The extracellular matrix is mainly composed of fibrillar proteins surrounded by glycosaminoglycans

The extracellular matrix produced in most support cells is composed of two major materials: glycosaminoglycans (GAG) and fibrillar proteins. In addition, there are small amounts of structural glycoprotein present in the extracellular matrix, with important roles in cell adhesion.

The general structure of support tissue is a scattered network of support cells producing an organized, abundant extracellular network of fibrillar proteins arranged in a hydrated gel of GAG. Other cells (e.g. epithelial cells, contractile cells) are anchored to this tissue by cell matrix-anchoring junctions (see p. 61).

Glycosaminoglycans are large polysaccharides which help give turgor and determine the diffusion of substances through extracellular matrix. These polysaccharides link to backbone proteins to form proteoglycans. Many of the proteins that form the backbone of proteoglycans have been isolated and characterized.

GAG are large, unbranched polysaccharide chains composed of repeating disaccharide units (70–200 residues).

ADVANCED CONCEPT
GAG HAVE THE FOLLOWING PROPERTIES

A high negative charge, because in all GAG one of the repeating units is an amino sugar (N-acetylglucosamine or N-acetylgalactosamine), which is commonly sulfated (SO_3-), and in most GAG, the second sugar is uronic acid with a carboxyl group ($COO-$).

Strongly hydrophilic behaviour because they cannot fold into compact structures and therefore have a large, permanently open coil conformation.

Retention of positive ions (e.g. Na^+) together with water, thereby maintaining tissue architecture by virtue of an inherent turgor, which tends to prevent deformation by compressive forces.

With the exception of hyaluronic acid, covalent attachment to proteins to form proteoglycans, which are huge molecules capable of maintaining a large hydration space in the extracellular matrix. The spatial organization and charge of proteoglycans facilitate selective diffusion of different molecules, probably by allowing variation in pore size of the matrix gel. This is particularly important in the basement membranes of the kidney glomerulus (see Fig. 15.7).

They can be divided into four groups according to their structure: hyaluronic acid, chondroitin sulfate and dermatan sulfate, heparan sulfate, and heparin and keratan sulfate (Fig. 4.2). They form the hydrated gel matrix of support tissues, the properties of which are determined by their charge and spatial arrangement. There is great variability in GAG distribution in different tissues, reflecting local requirements for specific pore sizes and charges in the extracellular matrix.

Fibrillar proteins determine the tensile properties of support tissues

There are four major proteins that form fibrils in the extracellular matrix:
- Collagen
- Fibrillin
- Elastin
- Fibronectin.

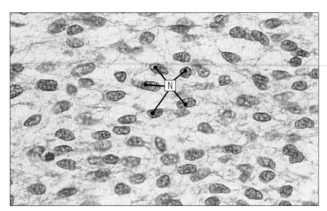

FIGURE 4.1 **Embryonic mesenchyme.** Mesenchyme is an embryonic tissue and may develop from any of the three germ layers. It is characterized by spindle-shaped cells with large nuclei (N), which develop into a variety of cell types in embryonic life, thus forming the family of support cells.

The role of these fibrillar proteins is to provide different tensile properties to support tissues and to provide anchorage for other cellular elements in tissues.

The collagens are a large family of proteins and comprise the most important fibrillar extracellular matrix components

The collagens are a family of closely-related proteins, which can aggregate to produce either filaments, fibrils or meshwork, which then interact with other proteins to provide support in the extracellular matrix. There are at least 20 types of collagen polypeptide chains (α chains) produced from different genes, which combine to produce different morphological forms (Fig. 4.3). The collagens can be divided into several families according to the types of structure they form:
- **Fibrillar collagens**: types I, II, III, V, XI
- **Facit collagens** (fibril-associated collagen with interrupted triple helix): types IX, XII, XIV
- **Short-chain collagens**: types VIII, X
- **Basement membrane collagens**: type IV
- **Other collagens**: types VI, VII, XIII.

Collagen types I, II and III are arranged as rope-like fibrils and are the main forms of fibrillar collagen.

Collagen fibres (type I collagen) resist tensile stresses in tissues, thus their orientation and cross-linking vary according to the local environment. In histological preparations collagen fibres appear as pink-staining material and have a dominant role in providing tensile strength to tissues (Fig. 4.4). Reticular fibres (also called 'reticulin') are thin fibrils (about 20 nm in diameter) of type III collagen (Fig. 4.5). They form a loose mesh in many support tissues and are particularly evident in a zone beneath basement membranes, where they are thought to have a support function as part of the fibroreticular lamina (see Fig. 4.12c).

Reticular fibres can be considered as a fine scaffolding supporting specialized extracellular matrix components. In lymph nodes, spleen and bone marrow, reticular

Glycosaminoglycan	Sulfation	Protein-linked	Distribution
Hyaluronic acid	no	no	cartilage, synovial fluid, skin, support tissue
Chondroitin sulfate	yes	yes	cartilage, bone, skin, support tissue
Dermatan sulfate	yes	yes	skin, blood vessels, heart
Heparan sulfate	yes	yes	basement membrane, lung arteries
Heparin	yes	yes	lung, liver, skin, mast cell granules
Keratan sulfate	yes	yes	cartilage, cornea, vertebral disc

FIGURE 4.2 **Glycosaminoglycans.** There are four main groups of glycosaminoglycans which have different tissue distributions. Sulfation causes the molecules to be highly negatively charged and contributes to their ability to retain Na^+ ions and water. With the exception of hyaluronic acid, the glycosaminoglycans become linked to proteins to form proteoglycans. The presence of specific types of glycosaminoglycan in different tissues confers special attributes to the extracellular matrix, particularly with regard to diffusion or binding of other extracellular substances.

Type	I	II	III	IV	V	VI	VII	VIII	IX	X	XI
Morphology	large banded collagen fibre	small banded collagen fibre	small banded collagen fibre	sheet-like layers	thin fibrils	thin fibrils	short striated fibrils	chains and lattices	fibril	short chain	fibril
Distribution	skin dermis, tendon, bone, ligaments, fascia, fibrous cartilage, cornea, loose fibrous tissue	hyaline and elastic cartilage, vertebral discs, vitreous of eye	blood vessels, parenchymal organs, bone marrow, lymphoid tissues, smooth muscle, nerves, lung, fetal skin	basement membranes, external laminae, lens capsule	basement membrane of placenta, smooth and skeletal muscle	ubiquitous	anchoring fibrils in basement membrane of skin and amnion	Descemet's membrane (cornea)	cartilage	mineralizing cartilage	cartilage

FIGURE 4.3 **Important molecular forms of collagen.**

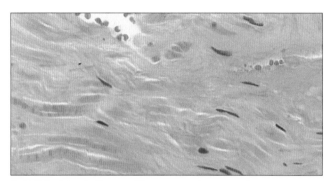

FIGURE 4.4 **Collagen fibres.** In H&E-stained preparations, collagen fibres appear as pink-stained material, which is often difficult to delineate from other structures that stain equally pink (e.g. support cells, walls of blood vessels). Special stains can be used to stain collagen (see also Fig. 4.14). Immunohistochemical staining can also be performed for different molecular types of collagen, but is seldom used in the routine examination of tissues.

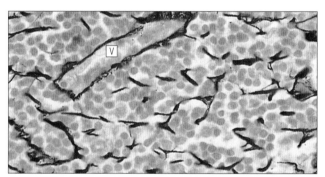

FIGURE 4.5 **Reticular fibres.** Reticular fibres cannot be seen in H&E sections, but can be stained by silver impregnation methods. In this micrograph, reticular fibres in a lymph node are seen as fine black lines, with lymphoid cells stained red in the background (V, vessel).

fibres form the main extracellular matrix fibres supporting the haemopoietic and lymphoid tissues. In parenchymal organs, such as the liver and kidney, reticular fibres form a network supporting specialized epithelial cells.

Type IV collagen assembles into a meshwork rather than fibrils and is restricted to basement membrane formation (see p. 60).

Type VII collagen forms the anchoring fibrils of some basement membranes.

Type VIII collagen forms a hexagonal lattice in Descemet's membrane in the cornea of the eye.

Although collagen is mainly produced by fibroblasts (see p. 63), it can be produced by other mesenchyme-derived cells of the support cell family, as well as by a variety of epithelial and endothelial cells that produce the type IV collagen of basement membranes. Collagen fibres are constructed of precursor proteins (α chains) wound together to form rigid linear triple helix structures, which are then secreted by fibroblasts. After proteolytic cleavage, the triple helical portions are assembled into long filaments and incorporated into cross-linked fibres and bundles (Fig. 4.6).

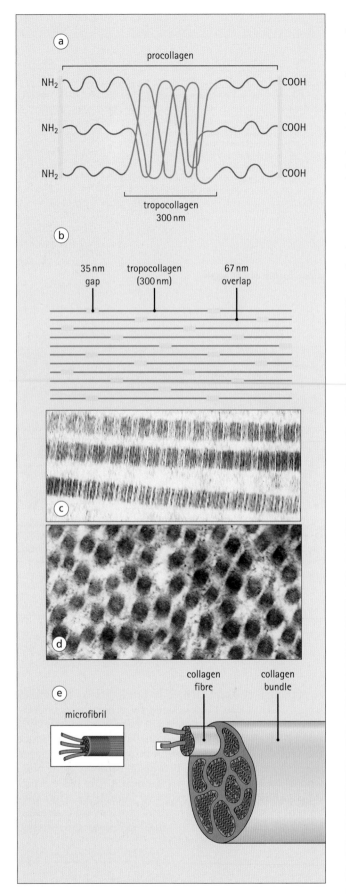

FIGURE 4.6 **Fibrillar collagen.** (a) Fibrillar collagen is formed from three polypeptide chains, which are initially secreted with both amino and carboxyl terminal extensions to prevent collagen forming inside cells. Initial assembly of these chains is into a triple helix (procollagen). (b) Cleavage of the amino and carboxyl extensions to leave the functional mid domains (tropocollagen) allows the molecules to align themselves into linear arrays to form long filaments. The individual collagen molecules are 300 nm long and are arranged with a 67 nm overlap between adjacent molecules. This gives rise to a periodicity of 67 nm. (c) Electron micrograph of collagen showing the periodicity of 67 nm. (d) Electron micrograph of collagen in transverse section. (e) The initial filaments (collagen microfibrils) become arranged into fibres, and the fibres into larger bundles by tight cross-linking between adjacent molecules via lysine residues; this contributes to the mechanical strength of collagen fibres in tissues, seen as fine black lines, with lymphoid cells stained red in the background (V, vessel).

CLINICAL EXAMPLE
DISEASES DUE TO DISORDERS OF COLLAGEN

There are several inherited diseases caused by mutations in the genes coding for collagen. The main effect is reduced tensile strength in support tissues, leading to abnormal tissue laxity or susceptibility to injury.

Ehlers–Danlos syndromes are characterized by abnormal skin laxity and hypermobility of joints, which can predispose to recurrent joint dislocations. There are several genetic subtypes of disease and six main forms have been described, characterized by distinct clinical associations. In some individuals, disease is caused by mutation in a collagen gene or in an enzyme related to collagen metabolism. Figure 4.7 shows a patient with Ehlers–Danlos syndrome who kindly demonstrated the remarkable joint laxity characteristic of the condition by bending the hand backwards.

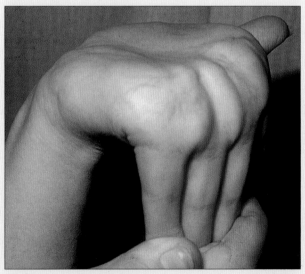

FIGURE 4.7 **Hyperextensibility of finger joint in Ehlers–Danlos syndrome.**

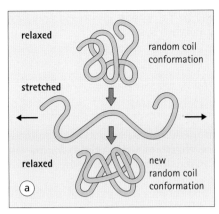

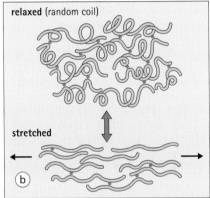

FIGURE 4.8 **Elastin.** (a) In the relaxed state, elastin has a random coil structure that can stretch but which reforms as a different random coil on relaxation. (b) Elastin molecules are covalently linked into arrays, which can reversibly stretch and recoil, and may be arranged as fibres or sheets.

Elastin is a protein which assembles into stretchable and resilient fibres and sheets

Elastin is a hydrophobic protein which assembles into filaments and sheets by cross-linking (Fig. 4.8) and is the main component of elastic fibres. Like collagen, elastin is produced by fibroblasts.

Elastic fibres are formed by the interaction of elastin and fibrillin. The fibrillin microfibrils appear to organize secreted elastin so that it is deposited between the microfibrils to form distinct elastic fibres (Fig. 4.9). As their name implies, they confer elasticity to tissues and allow them to recoil after stretching. Elastic fibres are important constituents of many support tissues.

Microfibrils contain fibrillin and are important components of elastic fibres

Fibrillin is a fibril-forming glycoprotein and the main component of extracellular microfibrils. Microfibrils, 8–12 nm in diameter, are one constituent of elastic fibres (see Fig. 4.9). They are also found in the extracellular matrix of renal glomeruli (mesangium) and the suspensory fibres of the lens.

Microfibrils are prominent in elastic-containing extracellular matrix, particularly in lung, skin and blood vessel walls. The microfibrils are believed to mediate adhesion between different components of the extracellular matrix.

CLINICAL EXAMPLE
MUTATIONS IN GENES FOR FIBRILLIN CAUSE MARFAN'S SYNDROME

People who have Marfan's syndrome are unusually tall, have a very wide arm span, are prone to develop subluxation of the lens and are also prone to develop rupture of the aorta. It is believed that the composer Sergei Rachmaninov had Marfan's syndrome.

The abnormality in this condition has been associated with the absence of fibrillin, which interacts with elastin in tissues. It is easy to understand why the lens dislocates, as its suspensory fibres normally contain fibrillin. It is also easy to understand how a lack of elastic recoil in the aorta would weaken the wall and predispose to rupture. It is assumed that the growth of long bones is somehow constrained by the presence of fibrillin, and hence bones grow longer in its absence.

Fibronectin mediates adhesion between a wide range of cells and extracellular matrix components

Fibronectin is a multifunctional glycoprotein and exists in three main forms. These are:
- A circulating plasma protein
- A protein that transiently attaches to the surface of many cells
- Insoluble fibrils forming part of the extracellular matrix, when fibronectin dimers cross-link to each other by disulfide bonds.

The functional importance of fibronectin stems from its ability to adhere to several different tissue components because it possesses sites that bind collagen and heparin, as well as cell adhesion molecules.

Extracellular structural glycoproteins link cells and extracellular matrix

Several non-filamentous proteins mediate interaction between cells and extracellular matrix and interact with specific receptors on the cell surface. The distribution of such proteins varies between different tissues. The best characterized of these proteins are laminin, tenascin and entactin.

Laminin, a sulfated glycoprotein, is a major component of basement membranes. It is produced by most epithelial and endothelial cells, and is a cross-shaped molecule with binding sites for specific cell receptors (integrins) (Fig. 4.10), heparan sulfate, type IV collagen and entactin (see below). The multiple binding ligands for laminin make it a major extracellular link molecule between cells and extracellular matrix. There are several forms specific to different tissues.

ADVANCED CONCEPT

Fibronectin is recognized by fibronectin receptor proteins in cell membranes, allowing cell adhesion to extracellular matrix. Such a fibronectin receptor is one of the class of cell surface receptors called 'integrins' (Fig. 4.10). When tissues grow, fibronectin binds to cell surfaces via integrins and is thought to have an important role in organizing the subsequent deposition and orientation of early collagen fibrils through its collagen attachment sites.

Because fibronectin receptors are linked to intracellular actin, the orientation of the internal cytoskeleton of a cell influences the orientation of the extracellular matrix.

Entactin is a sulfated glycoprotein that is a component of all basement membranes and binds with laminin. It is thought to function as a link protein binding laminin to type IV collagen.

Tenascin, an extracellular glycoprotein involved in cell adhesion, is particularly expressed in embryonic tissue and thought to be important to cell migration in the developing nervous system.

Basement Membrane and External Lamina

Basement membranes and external lamina are specialized sheets of extracellular matrix that lie between parenchymal cells and support tissues

Basement membranes and external lamina are specialized sheet-like arrangements of extracellular matrix proteins and GAG, and act as an interface between parenchymal cells and support tissues.

They are associated with epithelial cells, muscle cells and Schwann cells, and also form a limiting membrane around the central nervous system. Basement membrane and external lamina have similar structures.

Basement membranes have five major components: type IV collagen (Fig. 4.11), laminin, heparan sulfate, entactin and fibronectin. With the exception of fibronectin, these are synthesized by the parenchymal cells. In

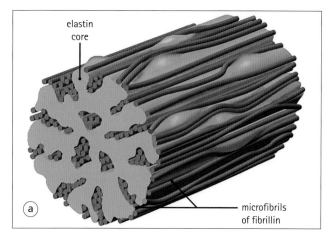

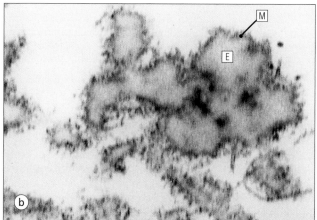

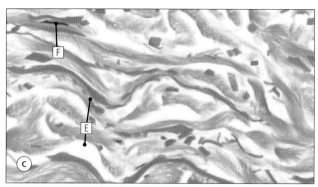

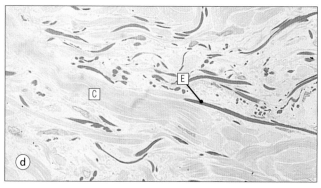

FIGURE 4.9 **Elastic fibre.** (a) Elastic fibres are composed of glycoprotein microfibrils (fibrillin) surrounding and organizing a core region of cross-linked elastin. (b) Ultrastructurally, the elastin core appears as an electron-dense area (E) with microfibrils (M) arranged peripherally. The microfibrils are prominent in early formed elastic tissue, and decrease in number with ageing. (c) In H&E-stained tissues, elastic fibres (E) stand out as glassy, bright pink-stained structures, taking up acidic dyes such as eosin with much greater avidity than collagen fibres (F, fibroblast). (d) Elastic fibres can be stained by special techniques. In this thin acrylic resin section, elastic fibres (E) in the dermis of the skin are stained blue by toluidine blue and contrast with the pale-staining collagen (C).

addition, there are numerous minor and poorly characterized protein and GAG components.

The general structure of basement membrane has been well characterized (Fig. 4.12). Superimposed on this, minor protein and carbohydrate components are specific to certain tissues. Thus, for example, the renal basement membrane differs from that of the skin.

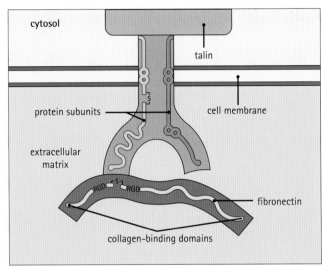

FIGURE 4.10 **Integrins.** Integrins are a class of cell adhesion molecule each comprised of two protein subunits. An 'a' subunit is composed of two protein chains and has a globular head. The 'b' subunit extends through the membrane and binds via link proteins to the actin cytoskeleton. The fibronectin receptor shown in the diagram is the best characterized of the integrin family, possessing a cytosolic domain binding to actin (via talin), a transmembrane domain, and extracellular domains binding to fibronectin. Thus, this molecule links the intracellular actin network with extracellular matrix at focal contacts (see also Fig. 3.10). The laminin receptor also belongs to the integrin family. Integrins may bind to other cell surface proteins, thus acting as intercellular adhesion molecules. In addition, some integrins bind to extracellular matrix components and allow cell–matrix adhesion, the main extracellular matrix ligands being fibronectin, laminin, collagens, tenascin and thrombospondin.

The main functions of basement membrane are cell adhesion, diffusion barrier and regulation of cell growth

Basement membrane has three main functions:

First, it forms an adhesion interface between parenchymal cells and underlying extracellular matrix, the cells having adhesion mechanisms to anchor them to basement membrane, whereas basement membrane is tightly anchored to the extracellular matrix of support tissues, particularly collagen. Where such an interface occurs in non-epithelial tissues, for example around muscle cells, it is referred to as an **external lamina**.

Second, the basement membrane acts as a molecular sieve (permeability barrier) with pore size depending on the charge and spatial arrangement of its component GAG. Thus, the basement membrane of blood vessels prevents large proteins leaking into the tissues, that of the kidney prevents protein loss from filtered blood during urine production, and that of the lung permits gaseous diffusion.

Third, basement membrane probably controls cell organization and differentiation by the mutual interaction of cell surface receptors and molecules in the extracellular matrix. These interactions are the subject of intense research, particularly in the investigation of mechanisms that might prevent the spread and proliferation of cancer cells throughout the body.

Cell Adhesion to Extracellular Matrix

Adhesion of cells to the extracellular matrix is mediated by four main types of junction

The organization of cells into functional tissues and organs depends on the support functions of the extracellular matrix and the cells that produce it. Although various types of intercellular junctions tie cells together (see p. 37), the junctions between cells and

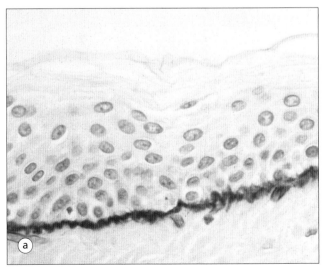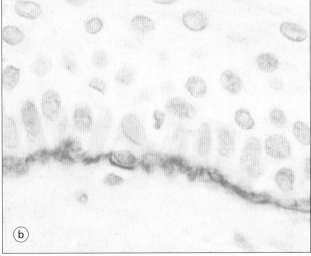

FIGURE 4.11 **Basement membrane.** The basement membrane can be demonstrated by immunostaining for constituent proteins such as (a) laminin and (b) type IV collagen.

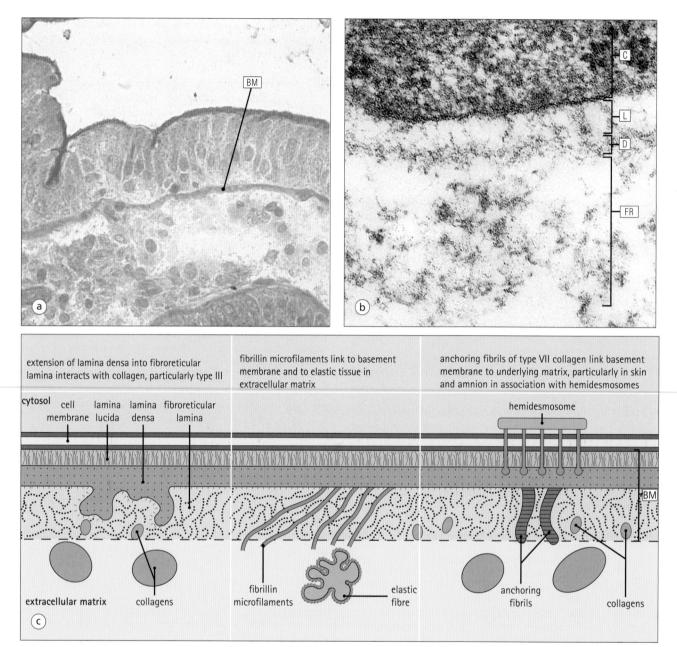

FIGURE 4.12 Basement membrane. (a) H&E preparations fail to show a distinct basement membrane because it is only 0.05 mm thick and stains poorly; however, a high content of glycoprotein renders it stainable with PAS, when it appears as a faint magenta-stained line (BM). Specific components of basement membrane can be detected with immunohistochemical staining, for example laminin and type IV collagen. (b) On electron microscopy, basement membrane resolves into several layers (laminae). The lamina densa (D) is a dark-staining band 30–100 nm thick. Between this and the attached cell (C) is a lucent zone, the lamina lucida (L), which is usually 60 nm wide. On the other side of the lamina densa is a rarefied layer of variable thickness, the fibroreticular lamina (FR), which merges with fibrous proteins of the extracellular matrix. The structure seen by light microscopy with PAS and silver stains and referred to as basement membrane is a combination of all these laminae, but particularly the fibroreticular lamina. The term 'basal lamina' should strictly refer to the lamina densa as an ultrastructural feature. However, with the detection of specific basal lamina components by light microscopy using immunohistochemistry, the terms 'basement membrane' and 'basal lamina' are commonly used interchangeably. (c) The fibroreticular lamina anchors the basement membrane to adjacent extracellular matrix by three main mechanisms, which vary according to site and are illustrated in this figure.

the extracellular matrix are equally important in maintaining structural integrity.

Junctions between cells and extracellular matrix include the following:

- Hemidesmosomes (see Fig. 3.12) – anchor the intermediate filament cytoskeleton of cells to basement membrane
- Focal contacts (see Fig. 3.10) – anchor the actin cytoskeleton to basement membrane. The interaction is mediated through the fibronectin receptor (see Fig. 4.10)
- Laminin receptors (see Fig. 4.10) – anchor cells to basement membrane where laminin is a major component
- Non-integrin glycoproteins (possessed by many cells) – bind to collagen and other cell matrix components.

Support Cell Family

Support cells derive from embryonic mesenchyme

During embryogenesis, a proportion of developing mesenchymal spindle-shaped cells differentiate into the following types of support cell: fibroblasts, myofibroblasts, lipoblasts, osteoblasts and chondroblasts.

The addition of 'blast' to the root name of a support cell indicates that the cell is actively growing or secreting extracellular matrix material. Support cells in a quiescent phase in tissues are indicated by the use of the suffix 'cyte' (e.g. fibrocyte, osteocyte, chondrocyte).

Fibroblasts and fibrocytes populate fibrocollagenous tissue, which is the most important of the support tissues

Fibroblasts (Fig. 4.13) produce fibrocollagenous (fibrous) tissue, which is composed mainly of collagen fibres associated with GAG, elastic fibres and reticular fibres (Fig. 4.14). Fibrocollagenous tissue is described as loose when collagen fibres are thin, haphazardly arranged and widely spaced, or dense when collagen fibres are broad and virtually confluent. The degree of organization and collagen orientation varies from site to site according to local tissue stresses. Highly organized dense fibrocollagenous tissue forms tendons and ligaments.

Fibrocollagenous tissue is the major support tissue in most organs, and has the following specific functions:

- Support of nerves, blood vessels and lymphatics; vessels and nerves are a conspicuous feature, particularly in loose fibrocollagenous support tissue
- Separation of functional layers in organs and tissues (e.g. separation of mucosa from underlying tissues). Its loose arrangement and variable elastic content allow mobility and stretching
- Support for transient and resident immune cell populations (i.e. macrophages, lymphocytes, plasma cells, mast cells)
- Formation of fibrous capsule, which surrounds most parenchymal organs, such as the liver, spleen and kidneys
- Formation of fibroadipose tissue, which is a component of most tissues, by enclosing and blending with adipocytes.

Fibroblasts are extremely robust and resist the damaging stimuli that kill most other cell types, such as nerves, epithelial cells or muscle. They are important in tissue repair (see p. 64).

Myofibroblasts have features that overlap between fibroblasts and smooth muscle cells

Myofibroblasts resemble fibroblasts on light microscopy, but ultrastructurally contain aggregates of actin fibres associated with myosin to subserve a contractile function (see p. 71). They are not prominent in support tissues, being found only in small numbers, and are identifiable by immunohistochemical or ultrastructural methods.

Chondroblasts and chondrocytes form cartilage

Chondroblasts elaborate a special support tissue called 'cartilage', which is composed mainly of GAG associated with collagen fibres. Developing from embryonic mesenchyme, chondroblasts first appear as clusters of vacuolated cells with a rounded morphology. These contrast with the spindle-shaped cells of surrounding undifferentiated mesenchyme, which develop into fibroblasts and form a confining sheet of cells termed the **perichondrium**.

Chondroblasts contain abundant glycogen and lipid and their active synthesis of extracellular matrix proteins is indicated by their basophilic cytoplasm, which is due

---

CLINICAL EXAMPLE
TUMOURS OF SUPPORT CELL FAMILY

Tumours may arise from support cells and these may be either benign or malignant.

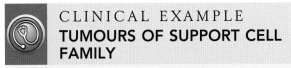

Cell type	Benign	Malignant
Fibroblast	Fibroma	Fibrosarcoma
Chondrocyte	Chondroma	Chondrosarcoma
Adipocyte	Lipoma	Liposarcoma
Osteocyte	Osteoma	Osteogenic sarcoma

ADVANCED CONCEPT
MYOFIBROBLASTS

Myofibroblasts develop during repair after tissue damage, and may originate either from tissue fibroblasts through the effects of PDGF, TGF-β, and FGF-2 released by macrophages at the wound site, or they can also originate from bone marrow precursors (fibrocytes) or from epithelial cells, through the process of epithelial-to-mesenchymal transition.

Myofibroblasts express smooth muscle α-actin and vimentin, they produce collagen and their contractile properties contribute to wound retraction and shrinkage of early fibrocollagenous scar tissue.

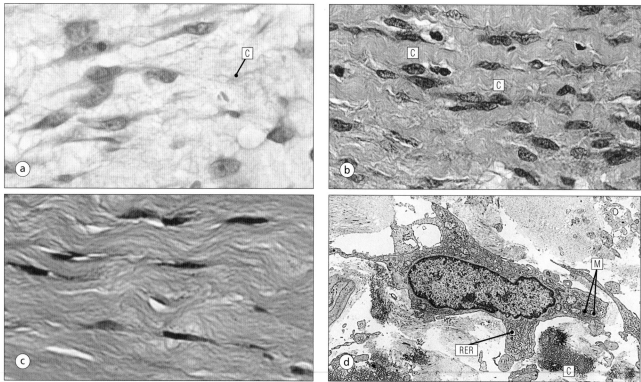

FIGURE 4.13 **Fibroblasts and fibrocytes.** (a) In the embryo, collagen-secreting cells develop from mesenchyme and appear as plump, spindle-shaped cells separated by early secreted collagen (C), which stains pink in H&E preparations. (b) In the adult, active collagen-secreting cells are called 'fibroblasts' and are characterized by a large oval nucleus and large nucleolus, a tapering spindle-shaped morphology with small additional cell processes, and basophilic cytoplasm reflecting active collagen synthesis. The collagen (C) is seen as pink-stained fibrillar material between fibroblasts. (c) Once collagen secretion has stopped, the fibroblasts lose their voluminous basophilic cytoplasm and the nucleus shrinks, reflecting non-transcription of DNA. The cells are now called 'fibrocytes' to indicate this inactivity. The collagen appears more compact and has, and is aligned in, parallel bundles. (d) Ultrastructurally, fibroblasts have a well-developed rough endoplasmic reticulum (RER), Golgi and secretory vesicles, reflecting active collagen secretion. Mitochondria (M) are numerous. Collagen fibres (C) are visible adjacent to the cells. Fibroblasts also secrete elastic and reticular fibres, and when they form reticular fibres in lymphoid tissue and bone marrow, they have a highly branched stellate shape and are often called 'reticulum cells'.

CLINICAL EXAMPLE
TISSUE DAMAGE IS REPAIRED BY PROLIFERATION OF SUPPORT CELLS AND SECRETION OF MATRIX TO FORM SCAR TISSUE

Following tissue damage (e.g. by infection), the loss of specialized cells can be rectified by regrowth only if the architecture of the support tissues (particularly basement membrane) is preserved; for example, epithelial cells lining the lung can regrow following some types of pneumonia (e.g. lobar pneumonia caused by *Streptococcus pneumoniae*).

If damage has been severe and the specialized support tissue architecture is destroyed, such regrowth is usually not possible and the area of dead tissue is repaired by means of the growth of non-specialized support tissue, which forms a fibrous scar.

Chemical mediators produced by damaged tissue attract phagocytic cells, such as neutrophils and monocytes (see Chapter 7) from the blood into the tissue. These cells ingest the dead cells, whereas inactive support cells, particularly fibroblasts, are stimulated to proliferate by the secretion of growth factors (e.g. platelet-derived growth factors and fibroblast growth factor).

The stimulated support cells are multipotential and can differentiate into endothelial cells, myofibroblasts and fibroblasts, the damaged area being replaced by a mixture of these cell types, which form new blood vessels and lay down collagen. The resulting fibrocollagenous tissue is termed a **fibrous scar**.

During this process of healing by fibrous repair, which is one of the basic responses to cell death in most body tissues, active fibroblasts assume a multipotential role and behave in a similar manner to the primitive mesenchyme from which they were derived, by differentiating into a variety of cell types.

This ability to transform into a variety of cell types in adult life to facilitate healing and repair is an important attribute of the support cell family.

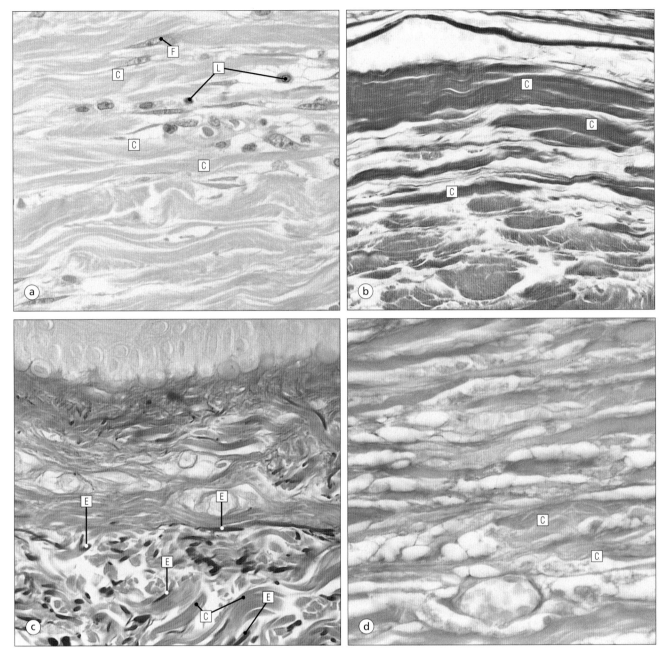

FIGURE 4.14 **Fibrocollagenous (fibrous) tissue.** (a) Fibrocollagenous tissue contains many extracellular matrix components, with collagen fibres being predominant. Only collagen (C) is evident in H&E sections, staining light pink. Fibroblasts (F) are widely scattered and inconspicuous. Immune cells (i.e. lymphocytes (L), plasma cells, macrophages, mast cells) are occasionally found. (b) The collagen fibres (C) in loose fibrocollagenous tissue can be stained by dyes with affinity for collagen (e.g. van Gieson's, shown here). The bundles are haphazardly arranged and of varying thickness. (c) In most loose fibrocollagenous tissues, elastic fibres are present, but are usually inconspicuous in H&E preparations. They are revealed by special stains (elastic stain) as wavy black-staining fibres (E), which contrast with the orange-stained collagen (C). Elastic fibres form a minor and variable component of most fibrocollagenous tissues. (d) Stains for the GAG component of fibrocollagenous tissue reveal that the unstained areas of the H&E preparations are rich in this extracellular material (seen here stained blue with Alcian blue stain) (C, collagen). In contrast with loose fibrocollagenous tissue, dense irregular fibrocollagenous tissue has little space for GAG and appears uniformly pink with few architectural features. Collagen-secreting fibroblasts are widely spaced and inconspicuous.

to a high content of rough endoplasmic reticulum (Fig. 4.15a).

Growth of cartilage results from proliferation of chondroblasts within established matrix (interstitial growth) and also by the development of new chondroblasts from the perichondrium (appositional growth). After depositing cartilage matrix, chondroblasts become less

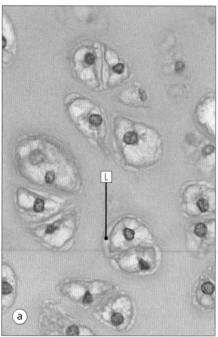

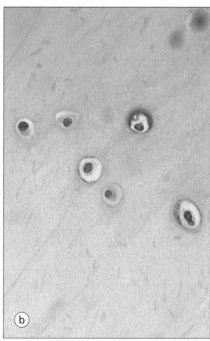

FIGURE 4.15 **Chondroblasts and chondrocytes.** (a) Chondroblasts are metabolically active and have large vesicular nuclei with prominent nucleoli. Their cytoplasm is pale and vacuolated because of a high lipid and glycogen content, and tends to draw away from the extracellular matrix when fixed and embedded in paraffin, forming a space called a 'lacuna' (L). (b) Chondrocytes are smaller than chondroblasts, with densely staining nuclei and less cytoplasm, reflecting their low level of metabolic activity.

metabolically active and have small nuclei with pale, indistinct cytoplasm (i.e. they become chondrocytes; Fig. 4.15b).

ADVANCED CONCEPT

Cartilage has two main extracellular components:

- Fibrous proteins (predominantly type II collagen), which confer mechanical stability
- Abundant GAG, which resist deformation by compressive forces.

The collagen fibres are thin and arranged in an interwoven lattice, which merges into the extracellular matrix of adjacent support tissues. The major GAG are hyaluronic acid, chondroitin sulfate and keratan sulfate, which are bound to a core protein called 'aggrecan' to form a large proteoglycan. These are attached to the collagen lattice by so-called link protein.

Because of its high content of sulfated GAG, cartilage stains with basic dyes such as haematoxylin, which gives it a slightly blue colour in H&E preparations; this is particularly evident around the chondrocytes.

The arrangement of extracellular matrix in cartilage confers important properties:

- The tightly bound proteoglycans form a hydrated matrix with an inherent turgor that resists deformation by compressive forces
- Small molecules can diffuse freely through the extracellular matrix.

Different types of cartilage contain different fibrous proteins

The three types of cartilage: hyaline, fibrocartilage and elastic, are distinguished by their fibrous protein content. **Hyaline cartilage** contains type II collagen only (Fig. 4.16). In fetal development, it forms the temporary skeleton until it is replaced by bone; it forms the growing point in long bones in childhood, the articular surface in joints (see Chapter 13), and in the respiratory passages, it acts as a support tissue (see Fig. 10.10).

Fibrocartilage contains both type II and type I collagen (Fig. 4.17) and is a component of intervertebral discs, tendon attachments to bones and the junctions between the flat bones of the pelvis. **Elastic cartilage** contains elastic fibres in addition to type II collagen (Fig. 4.18). It is located in the auricle of the ear, the walls of the external auditory canal and eustachian tubes (see Chapter 19) and in the epiglottis of the larynx (see Fig. 10.8).

Osteoblasts and osteocytes form bone, which contains an extracellular matrix material termed osteoid

Osteoblasts elaborate the support matrix of bone – osteoid – which subsequently calcifies to form bone.

Osteoid is composed mainly of type I collagen, which is associated with the extracellular GAG chondroitin

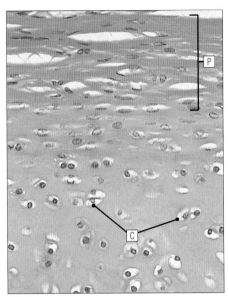

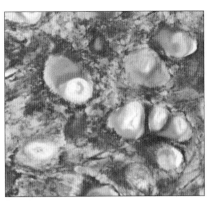

FIGURE 4.18 **Elastic cartilage (elastic stain).** The structural arrangement of elastic cartilage is similar to that of hyaline cartilage, with a perichondrial layer and chondrocytes set in an extracellular matrix, but differs because it contains elastic fibres. These appear as black-staining linear bundles running between cells and confer great resilience and elastic recoil in the cartilage.

FIGURE 4.16 **Hyaline cartilage.** This hyaline cartilage is from a child and therefore in a state of growth. The perichondrium (P) is a layer of spindle-shaped fibroblasts with associated type I collagen, which merges with the outer layer of the pink-staining extracellular matrix of the hyaline cartilage. New chondroblasts develop from the perichondrium and allow appositional growth. The chondroblasts show artifactual vacuolation, forming the characteristic lacunae around the cell bodies. Many in this sample are in small clusters (C), which will eventually move apart as the cells secrete extracellular matrix material during interstitial growth. Hyaline cartilage is associated with perichondrium in most sites except where it lines synovial joints.

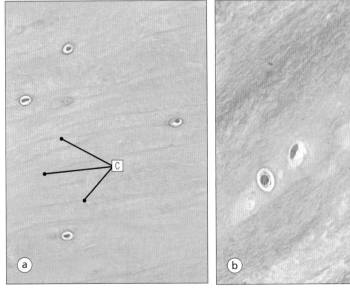

FIGURE 4.17 **Fibrocartilage.** (a) In this H&E section of fibrocartilage, small inactive chondrocytes are dispersed in a pink-stained extracellular matrix, in which coarse collagen fibres (C) are visible. These are type I collagen fibres, and merge with the type I collagen fibres in surrounding fibrocollagenous support tissue. (b) The presence of type I collagen is highlighted in this van Gieson-stained section of fibrocartilage, in which it stains red.

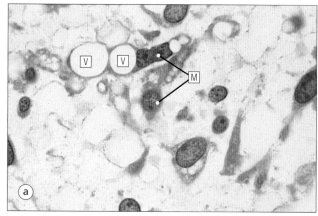

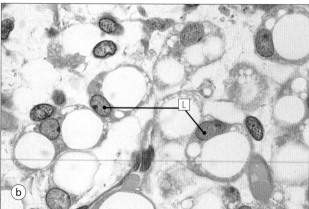

FIGURE 4.19 **Lipoblasts.** (a) In the fetus, the first indication of differentiation into a fat-storing cell is when the spindle-shaped mesenchymal cells (M) accumulate fat in their cytoplasm in multiple small vacuoles (V). (b) The vacuoles fuse to form a larger perinuclear vacuole and the cell is recognized as a maturing lipoblast (L), losing its spindle shape. With increased fat storage, the cytoplasm becomes attenuated around a single huge lipid vacuole and the nucleus is displaced to one side. Each developing lipoblast produces extracellular matrix material and a basement membrane forms around each cell.

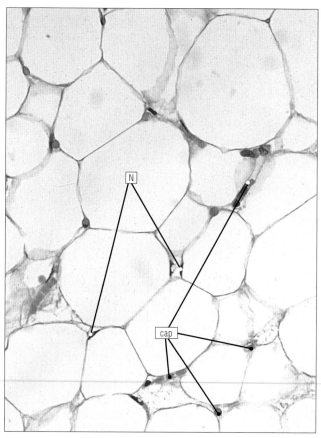

FIGURE 4.20 **Unilocular adipose tissue.** Unilocular (white) adipose tissue cells (adipocytes) are 50–150 μm in size and polyhedral in shape. In H&E-stained preparations, as here, they appear as stringy wisps of cytoplasm surrounding an empty vacuole because embedding in wax involves immersion in lipid solvents, which remove all of the fat. Close examination reveals inconspicuous flattened nuclei (N) to one side of the cells. Numerous fine arborizing capillary vessels (cap) transfer metabolites to and from the cells.

sulfate and keratan sulfate. Two glycoproteins, sialoprotein and osteocalcin, are mainly found in the bone matrix and bind calcium, hence they may have a role in bone mineralization. The cytology and structure of bone and its matrix are discussed in Chapter 13.

Adipose tissue stores fat and has a role in heat regulation in the young

Adipocytes are characterized by their intracellular storage of fat. There are two types of fat-storing tissue: unilocular and multilocular.

Unilocular adipose tissue ('white fat') develops from embryonic mesenchyme with the formation of spindle-shaped cells (lipoblasts) containing small fat vacuoles (Fig. 4.19). These mature into adipocytes, storing fat which is used as a source of energy by other body tissues (Fig. 4.20).

Ultrastructurally, adipocytes have prominent smooth endoplasmic reticulum and numerous pinocytotic vesi-

cles, these being involved in lipid biosynthesis and transport.

Each cell is surrounded by an external lamina and there is an extracellular matrix composed of reticular fibres (type III collagen).

Multilocular adipose tissue ('brown fat') is most prominent in the newborn, its development in the fetus being separate from that of unilocular adipose tissue. Its function is to metabolize fat to produce heat in the neonatal period (Fig. 4.21).

Ultrastructurally, multilocular adipose cells contain huge numbers of mitochondria in addition to lipid vacuoles; this correlates with their function of heat generation through mitochondrial metabolism of fatty acids.

The high mitochondrial density is responsible for both the eosinophilia seen histologically and the brown colour seen macroscopically, which gives this tissue its alternative name of 'brown fat'. Multilocular adipose tissue does not usually persist in adult life: it becomes lost during

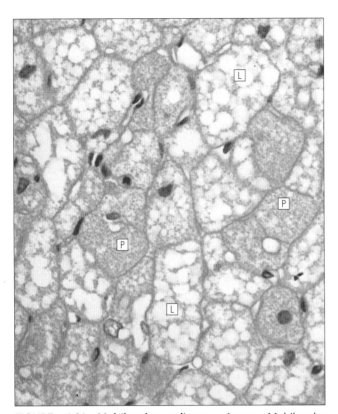

FIGURE 4.21 **Multilocular adipose tissue.** Multilocular adipose tissue is so-called because cells contain multiple small lipid droplets. It develops as a cluster of plump eosinophilic cells differentiating from fetal mesenchyme, and has a restricted distribution, being concentrated in support tissues in the neck, shoulders, back, perirenal and para-aortic regions. As shown in this micrograph, two populations of cells can be seen: lipid-rich cells (L) with a central nucleus and multiple small unstained vacuoles, and polyhedral-shaped cells (P) with a granular, pink-stained cytoplasm, a central nucleus and only occasional lipid vacuoles. A capillary vascular supply, together with thin fibro-collagenous septa, divides the tissue into small lobules.

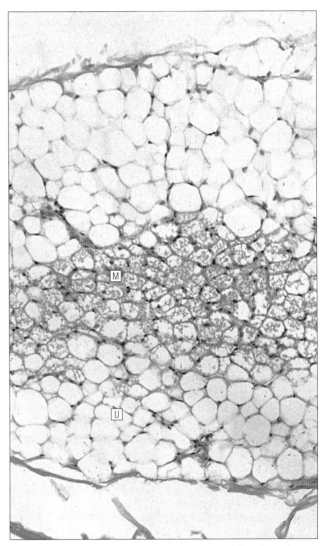

FIGURE 4.22 **Mixture of unilocular and multilocular adipose tissue.** Certain adipose tissue, particularly in the subcutaneous tissue over the back and shoulders, contains a mixture of both unilocular (U) and multilocular (M) adipose tissue.

childhood, although small amounts may remain in certain sites (Fig. 4.22).

Adipose tissue has a secretory and endocrine function

In addition to their energy-storage role, it is evident that adipocytes have an important secretory role. In this way, adipocytes modulate energy metabolism and influence general metabolism in coordination with hormones, such as insulin to regulate body mass.

Adipose tissue is also responsible for the secretion of several proteins into the blood, collectively known as **adipocytokines** that regulate general metabolism. These include leptin, adipsin, resistin, adiponectin, tumour necrosis factor alpha (TNF)-α, and plasminogen-activator inhibitor type 1.

 ADVANCED CONCEPT

Unilocular adipose tissue is the main form of fat-storing cell in the adult, and is adapted as a support tissue and as an energy store by means of:

- Receptors for growth hormone, insulin, glucocorticoids, thyroid hormones and norepinephrine (noradrenaline) that modulate the uptake and release of fat
- A rich capillary blood supply and innervation by the autonomic nervous system. Local release of noradrenaline stimulates the release of stored fat into the blood
- Organization into pads by sheets of fibrocollagenous tissue at certain sites to act as deformable shock-absorbing support tissues, particularly in the soles of the feet, the buttocks, around the kidneys and in the orbit around the eye.

For online review questions, please visit https://studentconsult.inkling.com.

END OF CHAPTER REVIEW

True/False Answers to the MCQs, as Well as Case Answers, Can be Found in the Appendix in the Back of the Book.

1. **Which of the following features is true of collagen?**
   (a) Type I is the main collagen in skin
   (b) Type IV is the main type in bone
   (c) Type III is the main type in reticulin
   (d) Is secreted by fibroblasts as procollagen molecules
   (e) Is one of the matrix components of osteoid

2. **Which of the following is true for glycosaminoglycans?**
   (a) Are composed of repeating sugar residues
   (b) Are weakly hydrophilic
   (c) May be attached to proteins to form proteoglycans
   (d) Include hyaluronic acid, dermatan sulfate, heparin and fibronectin
   (e) Have a very dense folded structure which gives turgor to the tissue extracellular matrix

3. **Basement membranes have which of the following features?**
   (a) Contains type I collagen
   (b) Contains laminin
   (c) Contains glycosaminoglycans
   (d) Links to epithelial cells via integrin receptors
   (e) Acts as a permeability barrier

4. **Which of the following features are seen in the specific type of support tissue specified?**
   (a) Fibrocollagenous tissue is the major support tissue in most organs
   (b) Chondroblasts elaborate the specialized extracellular matrix of cartilage
   (c) Hyaline cartilage contains type II collagen and forms the main component of the auricle of the ear
   (d) Unilocular adipose tissue produces heat in the neonatal period
   (e) Following severe tissue damage, fibrocollagenous tissue is formed in healing to produce a fibrous scar

CASE 4.1 INFANT WITH BROKEN FEMUR

Parents bring their 1-year-old daughter to the hospital as an emergency. They give a history that after a bath she had been pulling up to stand, when there was a 'popping' noise and she collapsed, screaming out in pain. She lay on the floor crying with pain. Her leg looked deformed and appeared broken.

An X-ray confirms a fractured femur. In the hospital there was a suspicion of non-accidental injury. However, further detailed investigation showed that the child had a genetic abnormality in type I collagen formation, of the type known to be associated with 'brittle bones'.

Q. Explain how this molecular defect relates to abnormal bone fragility. Knowing that there are many types of collagen, each with a different gene and tissue distribution, predict which organs and tissues may be affected by genetically abnormal collagen.

Chapter 5

Contractile Cells

Introduction

Several cell types are specialized to generate motile forces through contraction. This chapter presents an overview of the main types of contractile cell. The general structure of each type of cell is described, together with details of their fine structure and how this relates to the molecular basis of contraction.

There are four main groups of contractile cell

Contractile cells are specially adapted to generate motile forces by the interaction of the proteins actin and myosin (contractile proteins).

There are four groups of contractile cell: muscle cells, myofibroblasts, pericytes and myoepithelial calls. Muscle cells are the main type and comprise striated (voluntary) muscle, cardiac muscle and smooth (involuntary) muscle. Myofibroblasts have a contractile role in addition to being able to secrete collagen. Pericytes are smooth, muscle-like cells that surround blood vessels. Myoepithelial cells are an important component of certain secretory glands.

Different arrangements of actin and myosin in each type of contractile cell, together with important structural adaptations, modulate and control contraction.

Skeletal Muscle

Skeletal muscle cells form the structural basis of muscles (see Chapter 13), which are responsible for voluntary movement under the influence of the nervous system, and for maintenance of posture. The attachment of muscle to the skeletal system is discussed in Chapter 13.

Each skeletal muscle fibre is a multinucleate syncytium formed by the fusion of individual cells in development

In embryogenesis, each skeletal muscle cell forms from the fusion of many hundreds of precursor cells (myoblasts), so in the adult each is a syncytium containing hundreds of nuclei, which are located just beneath the cell membrane. Each skeletal muscle cell is a long thin cylindrical structure, typically 50–60 μm in diameter in an adult and up to 10 cm long, depending on its location (Fig. 5.1).

In adult muscle, there is a resident population of muscle precursor cells (satellite cells) which can divide to form new muscle cells after tissue damage.

In addition to contractile proteins, skeletal muscle cell cytoplasm contains numerous mitochondria, as well as abundant glycogen to provide energy. Each muscle cell is surrounded by an external lamina (see p. 60).

Because of long usage, special terms are often used to describe skeletal muscle cell components. These are: sarcolemma (cell membrane), sarcoplasm (cell cytoplasm) and sarcoplasmic reticulum (endoplasmic reticulum).

Skeletal muscle contracts as a result of organized assemblies of actin and myosin

The contractile elements of skeletal muscle cells (myofibrils) are thin cylindrical structures 1–2 μm in diameter. They are composed of overlapping, repeating assemblies of thick (mainly myosin) and thin (mainly actin) filaments.

Any one muscle fibre has hundreds of myofibrils running parallel along its length, the alternating zones of thick and thin filaments giving rise to the descriptive term 'striated muscle' (Fig. 5.2a).

Ultrastructurally, the thick and thin filaments are held in place by plates of accessory proteins, visible as lines, which divide the myofibrils into functional units called 'sarcomeres' (Fig. 5.2b). Sarcoplasm, mitochondria and other cellular elements are packed between the myofibrils.

There is a regular arrangement of contractile proteins within each sarcomere, with each thick filament being surrounded by six thin filaments (Fig. 5.2c,d). Contraction of muscle occurs as thick and thin filaments slide past each other (Fig. 5.3), and is therefore accompanied by a decrease in the width of the light bands. The width of the dark bands remains unchanged.

Accessory proteins maintain the alignment of actin and myosin filaments

Skeletal muscle function depends on a precise alignment of actin and myosin filaments within each myofibril. This is achieved by accessory proteins, which link the different components and hold them in register with each other. These proteins can only be visualized using immunohistochemical techniques.

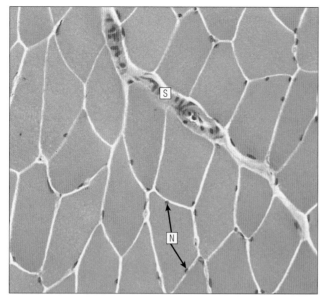

FIGURE 5.1 **Skeletal muscle.** In cross-section, skeletal muscle cells have a roughly hexagonal profile with individual cells moulded together. Nuclei (N) are arranged beneath the cell membrane. Fibrocollagenous septa (S) contain blood vessels.

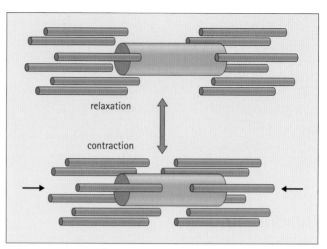

FIGURE 5.3 **Muscle contraction.** During muscle contraction the thin filaments of the myofibrils slide over the thick filaments. This is reversed on muscle relaxation.

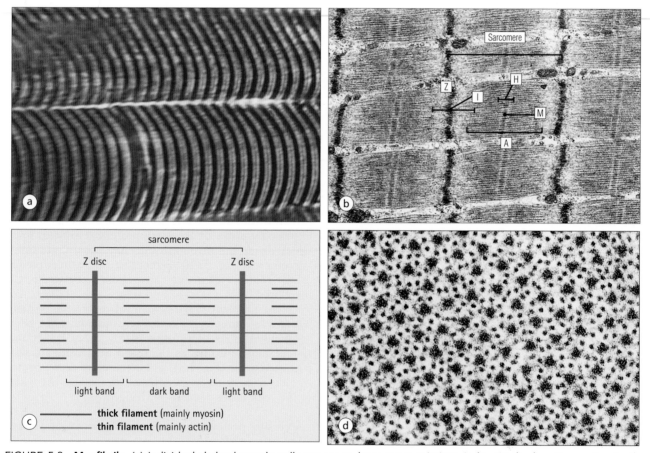

FIGURE 5.2 **Myofibrils.** (a) Individual skeletal muscle cells appear to have cross-striations in longitudinal section owing to the presence of stacks of myofibrils composed of alternating, overlapping zones of thick (dark-stained) and thin (light-stained) filaments. (b) Ultrastructurally, several zones of staining can be discerned along myofibrils. The A (dark) band refers to the thick filament band and includes a zone where the thin filaments overlap the thick filaments. The H zone is a pale-staining area in the centre of the A band and indicates where no thin filaments overlap the thick filaments. The I (light) band is the zone of thin filaments that does not overlap the thick filaments, while the Z line is a dark band in the centre of the I band and the M line runs down the centre of the H band. The unit delineated between two Z discs is termed a 'sarcomere'. (c) The arrangement of filaments in a sarcomere. The thin filaments are composed mainly of actin, the thick filaments mainly of myosin. (d) When viewed in cross-section at the level of overlap between the A and I bands as in (b), each myofibril is seen to have a regular spaced arrangement of thick and thin filaments, such that each thick filament is surrounded by six thin filaments arranged in an approximately hexagonal lattice.

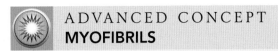

ADVANCED CONCEPT
MYOFIBRILS

Thin Filaments are Mainly Formed from Actin

Thin filaments are 8 nm in diameter and composed mainly of the protein actin. Each thin filament (F-actin) is formed by the polymerization of many single molecules of globular actin (G-actin). These actin filaments are polar, all G-actin molecules pointing in the same direction.

To form a complete thin filament, two actin filaments become attached by their tail ends to α actinin in the Z line so that they face in opposite directions (i.e. away from the Z line).

Thick Filaments are Mainly Formed from Myosin

Thick filaments are composed mainly of the protein myosin. Like the actin filament, the myosin filament is polar. To form a complete heavy filament, two myosin filaments become attached by their tail ends so that they face in opposite directions (i.e. away from the M line) (Fig. 5.4). Different molecular types (isoforms) of myosin are present in different types of skeletal muscle fibre.

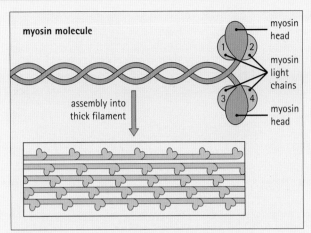

FIGURE 5.4 **Myosin molecule.** Each myosin molecule is composed of two tadpole-shaped heavy chains, the tails of which coil around each other, with four small light chains attached to the head portions. The coiled, rod-like tail portions of many myosin molecules aggregate and pack together in a regular staggered array to form the filament, while the head portions project out in a regular helical pattern.

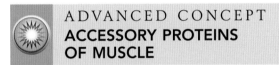

ADVANCED CONCEPT
ACCESSORY PROTEINS OF MUSCLE

Actinin holds actin filaments in a lattice arrangement in the Z disc. Other Z disc proteins include filamin, amorphin and Z protein.

Nebulin is associated with actin-containing thin filaments.

Myomesin holds myosin filaments in a lattice arrangement in the region of the M line, associated with creatine kinase and M protein.

Titin (connectin) is an extremely long elastic protein, which runs parallel to the filament array and links the ends of the thick filaments to the Z disc, maintaining their ends in register with the lattice of thin filaments.

Desmin filaments (one of the class of intermediate filament proteins) link adjacent myofibrils to each other and maintain their register. In addition, they link myofibrils to the cell membrane.

C protein is a myosin-binding protein localized in seven stripes running parallel to the M band in the first half of the A band.

Contraction of skeletal muscle is mediated by a cycle of binding and release between actin and myosin

In muscle contraction, the actin filaments slide along the myosin filaments. This is driven by the heads of the myosin molecules, which bind to actin and, in a sequence of binding and release movements, 'walk' along the actin filament. This repetitive binding and release is powered by the hydrolysis of ATP (Fig. 5.5), and myosin can be regarded as an ATPase that is activated by the binding of actin.

Control of muscle contraction is achieved by proteins that bind to actin and prevent muscle contraction by blocking the myosin–actin interaction (Fig. 5.6). This is reversed by high concentrations of Ca^{2+} ions in the cell cytoplasm (Fig. 5.7).

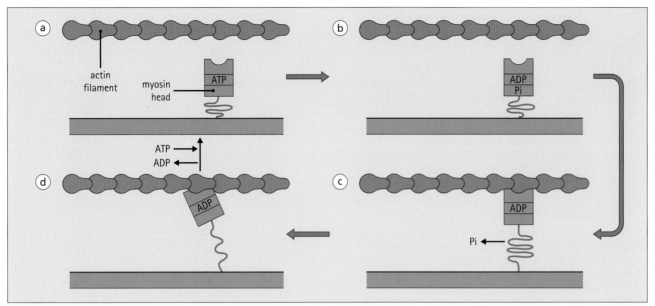

FIGURE 5.5 **Use of ATP by myosin binding to actin.** A myosin molecule uses the energy of ATP to move along an actin filament. (a) ATP bound to myosin is hydrolysed to ADP and phosphate (Pi). (b) This causes myosin to bind loosely to actin. (c) Pi is released and myosin binds tightly to actin. (d) This binding initiates molecular folding of the myosin molecule to cause the movement of the molecule relative to the actin filament. ADP is released, fresh ATP binds and the myosin returns to its non-attached state. The cycle repeats and the myosin head 'walks' along the actin filament.

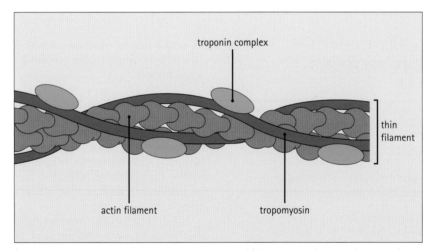

FIGURE 5.6 **Control of muscle contraction.** Tropomyosin is a long rod-like protein that winds around an actin filament to stabilize and stiffen it. The troponin complex, which regulates the binding of actin to myosin, is attached to tropomyosin and composed of three separate polypeptides termed 'troponins T, I and C'. Troponin T binds the complex to tropomyosin and positions the complex on the actin filament at the site where actin would bind to myosin. Troponin I physically prevents myosin binding to actin. Troponin C binds Ca^{2+} ions, which cause a confrontational change in the troponin complex, allowing myosin access to the actin filament.

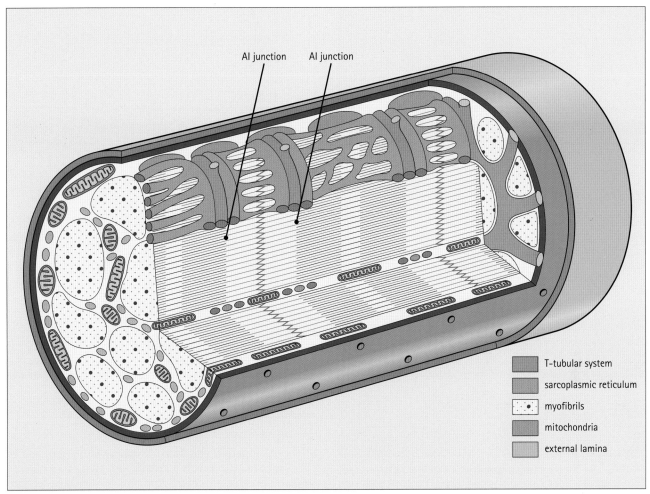

AI junction   AI junction

T-tubular system

sarcoplasmic reticulum

myofibrils

mitochondria

external lamina

FIGURE 5.7 **Muscle cell excitation and intracellular Ca^{2+} ions.** Following a nerve signal, excitation of the muscle cell membrane is conveyed to the interior of the cell via a series of membranous channels (the transverse tubular system of T tubules) that extend from the muscle surface to surround each myofibril. Running alongside each T tubule are two portions of sarcoplasmic reticulum, called terminal cisternae, which contain a high concentration of Ca^{2+} ions and have electrically sensitive Ca^{2+} ion channels in their wall. Membrane excitation of the T tubular system causes these Ca^{2+} ion channels to open, thus allowing Ca^{2+} ions to flood into the sarcoplasm. In the resting state, muscle cells have few intracellular free Ca^{2+} ions, and a sudden increase in free cytosolic Ca^{2+} ions initiates muscle contraction. Membrane pumps (Ca^{2+}-ATPase) in the sarcoplasmic reticulum pump the Ca^{2+} ions back into the sarcoplasmic reticulum rapidly (within about 30 ms) and stop contraction. The close association of T tubules and sarcoplasmic reticulum forms three tubules in cross-section (a membrane triad). In human muscle, there is a membrane triad surrounding every myofibril in the AI junction region; thus there are two triads to each sarcomere.

ADVANCED CONCEPT
THE FORCE OF MUSCLE CONTRACTION IS TRANSMITTED TO THE EXTRACELLULAR MATRIX BY A SERIES OF LINK PROTEINS

The cytoskeleton of each skeletal muscle fibre is linked to the external lamina by a series of link molecules. Actin filaments inside the cell are linked to the protein dystrophin. Dystrophin then links with a complex composed of several glycoproteins that bridge through the muscle cell membrane to the cell surface. On the outer surface of the muscle cell, the glycoprotein complex links to the protein merosin, which is a laminin component of the basement membrane. In this way, forces generated inside the muscle are transferred to the extracellular matrix in the external lamina.

If there is a genetic absence of one of the linking proteins, then muscle fibres are prone to undergo tearing on contraction and the affected person develops one of the many forms of muscular dystrophy.

It is being increasingly recognized that the different forms of muscular dystrophy can be related to defects in structural proteins in the muscle fibres. Duchenne muscular dystrophy is described on page 242.

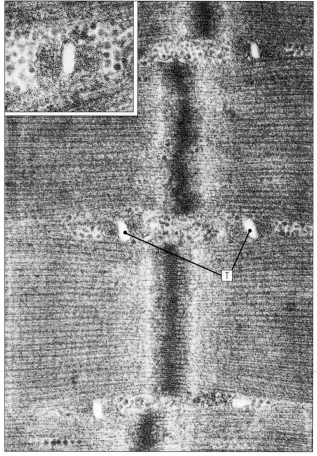

FIGURE 5.8 **Electron micrograph of a skeletal muscle triad.** The T tubule is seen as a small open tube (T) and on each side are extensions of the sarcoplasmic reticulum. In humans, the sarcoplasmic reticulum contains electron-dense material, making these relatively indistinct structures in comparison to illustrations taken from animal material. A single triad is shown at higher magnification in the inset.

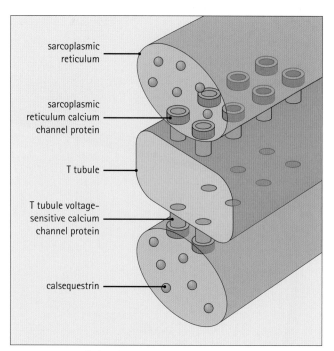

FIGURE 5.9 **Skeletal muscle triad.** The sarcoplasmic reticulum (SR) Ca^{2+} channel protein lines up with the Ca^{2+} channel protein in the T-tubular system. Depolarization of the T-tubular system causes opening of the SR calcium channels. Calcium, which is held in the SR lumen by calsequestrin, can then be released into the muscle cytoplasm.

of the AI junction (Fig. 5.8). Running alongside, and in close apposition to each T tubule, are two extensions of the sarcoplasmic reticulum containing a very high calcium concentration. In cross-section these three tubes form a triad (Fig. 5.9).

In response to membrane depolarization in the T-tubular system calcium channels in the membrane of the sarcoplasmic reticulum release calcium into the cytosol of the muscle fibre, causing contraction.

Cardiac Muscle

Cardiac muscle is a form of striated muscle but differs significantly from skeletal muscle

Like skeletal muscle, cardiac muscle is a type of striated muscle and is characterized by a similar arrangement of actin and myosin filaments to mediate contraction. The important differences between cardiac muscle and skeletal muscle are as follows:

- Cardiac muscle cells are mononuclear and much shorter than those of skeletal muscle;
- Long cardiac muscle fibres are produced by linking numerous cardiac muscle cells end to end via anchoring-type cell junctions;
- A population of cardiac resident c-kit-positive stem or progenitor cells, analogous to satellite cells of skeletal muscle (see p. 71), is present in cardiac muscle, but regeneration following damage does not significantly repair or restore lost cardiac tissue in most disease states.

Special internal membrane systems called triads control muscle contraction by regulating calcium release

There is a specialized internal membrane system in skeletal muscle called the 'T-tubular system'. This extends from the surface membrane as thin tubules which extend deep through the muscle fibre running along the region

KEY FACTS
SKELETAL MUSCLE

- Each muscle fibre is surrounded by an external lamina
- Striated muscle is based on close alignment of actin and myosin filaments
- Actin is arranged as thin filaments anchored to the Z line
- Myosin is arranged as thick filaments anchored to the M line
- Membrane triads couple membrane excitation to calcium release into the cytoplasm
- Cytosolic calcium regulates contraction.

Individual cardiac muscle cells are linked into long chains by specialized cell junctional systems

Instead of fusing to form syncytia as for skeletal muscle (see p. 71), cardiac muscle cells align into long chains and develop cell junctions, which anchor each cell to its neighbour (Fig. 5.10).

In the adult, a cardiac muscle cell is about 15 μm in diameter and about 100 μm long, with a centrally positioned nucleus. Intercellular junctions, which can be seen in light microscopic preparations as faint lines running transversely across fibres, are termed intercalated discs. These contain three types of cell junction:

- Desmosomal junctions tightly link adjacent cells via anchors involving the intermediate filaments (see Fig. 3.11)
- Adherent-type junctions anchor the actin fibres of the sarcomeres to each end of the cell (see Fig. 3.9)
- Communicating gap junctions (see Fig. 3.14) facilitate the passage of membrane excitation (communication) and thereby synchronization of muscle contraction.

The molecular basis of contraction of cardiac muscle is very similar to that of skeletal muscle

Contraction of cardiac muscle cells is regulated by cytosolic Ca^{2+} ion concentration in a manner virtually identical to that for skeletal muscle (see Figs 5.5 and 5.6), but:

- The cardiac muscle transverse (T) tubular system consists of much wider invaginations of the cell surface
- Sarcoplasmic reticulum associated with the T tubules is neither as regular nor as well organized as in skeletal muscle
- The association of cardiac sarcoplasmic reticulum with T tubules takes the form of dyads rather than triads, and is located in the region of the Z lines rather than the AI junction.

Smooth Muscle

Smooth muscle is the main contractile cell in the walls of viscera and in blood vessels

Smooth muscle cells have a much less organized system of contractile proteins than striated skeletal and cardiac muscle cells. Forming the contractile portions of the wall of most hollow viscera (e.g. gut, urinary bladder and uterus), as well as the contractile elements in blood vessel walls and secretory gland ducts, smooth muscle cells are found in situations requiring sustained slow or rhythmic contractions not under voluntary control.

Individual smooth muscle cells are anchored together into functional units by basement membrane material.

Smooth muscle cells are typically spindle-shaped and, depending on site, vary in size from 20 μm (small blood vessels) to 400–500 μm (uterus). Each cell has a single, centrally located nucleus, which is elongated or elliptical in shape (Fig. 5.11).

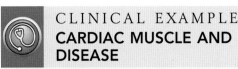

CLINICAL EXAMPLE
CARDIAC MUSCLE AND DISEASE

The cardiac muscle is the most hard-worked muscle in the body; it contracts and relaxes 60–100 times per minute from intrauterine life until death, often 80–90 years later, without rest. Stress and physical activity can increase the number of beats per minute to well above 120, often for long periods. The cardiac muscle in the wall of the left ventricle has a particularly heavy workload, having to force oxygenated arterial blood all around the body. It is not surprising that any factor affecting the function of the cardiac muscle has the major impact on the left ventricle and its function. The most important factor affecting the function of the cardiac muscle is inadequate oxygenation, usually the result of an inadequate coronary artery supply. Once a cardiac muscle cell dies, other cells have to increase their size and work output to compensate (these cells undergo hypertrophy).

- Other causes of cardiac muscle hypertrophy are given in the Clinical Example box on page 81.
- The structural and functional consequences of failure of oxygenation of cardiac muscle cells are given in the Clinical Example box on page 161.
- Genetic disorders, which affect the structure and function of cardiac muscle (primarily myosin heavy chains) are termed cardiomyopathies.

The heart does contain stem cells but this population is not able to proliferate and replenish large areas of tissue loss due to infarction. Experimental techniques are currently being investigated to stimulate in situ stem cell growth or to grow stem cells ex vivo and inject them back into damaged hearts. These trials show promise but are very early in their development.

In cross-section, smooth muscle cells have polygonal profiles, but in longitudinal section they appear as linear bundles.

Each smooth muscle cell is surrounded by an external lamina to which cell membranes adhere; small groups of cells are organized into bundles by fine collagenous tissue containing blood vessels and nerves.

Contraction of smooth muscle cells is mediated by a dispersed arrangement of actin and myosin which is very different from that of striated muscle

Ultrastructurally, smooth muscle does not show the highly organized system of contractile proteins (i.e. myofilaments) seen in striated muscle, but has an arrangement whereby bundles of contractile proteins criss-cross the cell and are inserted into anchoring points (focal densities). Focal densities are similar to adherent junctions and are studded around the cell membrane (Fig. 5.12).

Tension generated by contraction is transmitted through the focal densities to the surrounding network of external laminae, thus allowing a mass of smooth muscle cells to function as one unit. The abundant intermediate filaments of smooth muscle, desmin, are also inserted into the focal densities.

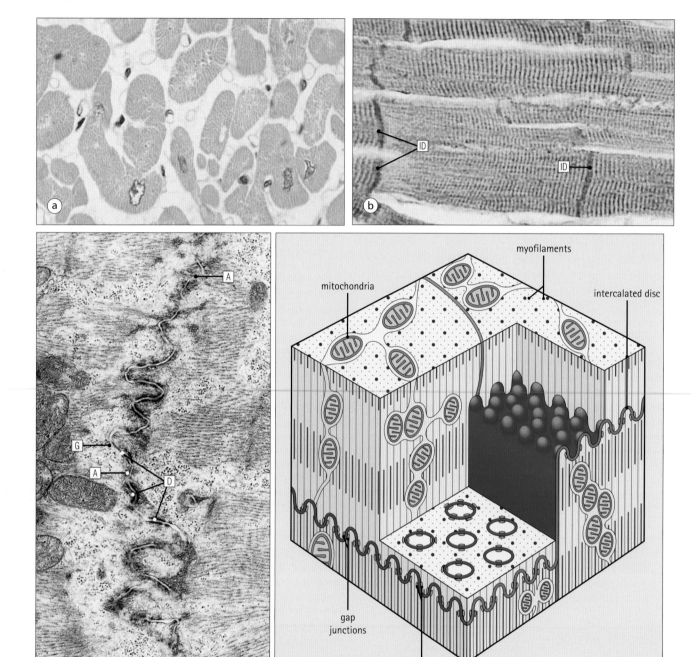

FIGURE 5.10 **Cardiac muscle.** (a) Cardiac muscle cells appear as elliptical or lobulated structures in transverse section. Their nuclei are centrally placed and have irregular shapes, and fibrocollagenous septa containing small blood vessels run between fibres. Between individual cardiac muscle cells, there is a rich capillary blood supply. (b) In longitudinal section, cardiac muscle appears as a series of anastomosing cords of cells, which branch and join with adjacent fibres at cell junctions (intercalated discs, ID), seen as dark lines by the immunocytochemical method for α-B crystallin. (c) Ultrastructurally, cardiac muscle cells contain myofibrils with thick and thin filament systems virtually identical to those in skeletal muscle, but composed of different structural isoforms. Mitochondria are prominent and make up a much larger proportion of cell volume than in skeletal muscle. Several regions of the intercalated disc structure can be resolved, showing desmosome-like junctions (D), adherent-type junctions (A) and, in the lateral portions of the intercalated disc, prominent communicating gap junctions (G). (d) The structural arrangement of adjacent cardiac muscle cells. Cells are bound together by desmosomal junctions at interdigitating areas at the ends of adjacent cells to form the intercalated disc. Gap junctions facilitate transmission of the contractile stimulus between cells.

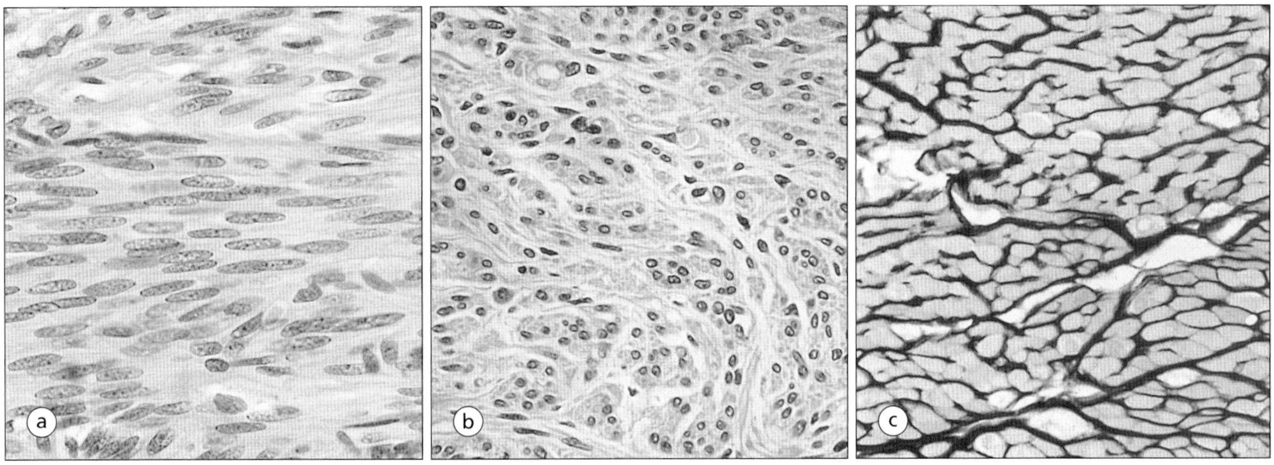

FIGURE 5.11 **Smooth muscle (light microscopy).** (a) In longitudinal section, smooth muscle cells occur in linear bundles. The cells have abundant pink-staining cytoplasm and central elongated nuclei. (b) In transverse section, the smooth muscle cells have polygonal profiles. (c) This special stain demonstrates (in black) the external laminae that surround each smooth muscle cell and to which the cell membranes adhere. The laminae are composed of type IV collagen and glycoproteins, and bind individual cells into a functional mass.

Energy is supplied by numerous mitochondria, which tend to be located, along with endoplasmic reticulum and other organelles, around the nucleus, in an area devoid of contractile filaments.

Although each smooth muscle cell is surrounded by an external lamina, this is deficient where the cells communicate with each other via gap junctions. These junctions, which are also termed 'nexus junctions' in smooth muscle, are widespread and allow spread of membrane excitation between cells.

A characteristic feature of smooth muscle cells is the presence of numerous invaginations of cell membrane forming structures that resemble caveolae. It is thought that these invaginations function in a similar way to the specialized transverse (T) tubular system of striated muscle by controlling the entry of Ca^{2+} ions into the cell following membrane excitation. Terminal sacs of Ca^{2+} ion-containing endoplasmic reticulum terminate beneath the cell membrane close to these vesicles.

The molecular basis of contraction in smooth muscle differs from that in skeletal muscle

The contraction mechanism of smooth muscle differs from that for striated muscle. Because the contractile proteins are arranged in a criss-cross lattice inserted circumferentially into the cell membrane, contraction results in shortening of the cell, which assumes a globular shape in contrast to its elongated shape in the relaxed state (Fig. 5.12f).

ADVANCED CONCEPT
SMOOTH MUSCLE CONTRACTION

Thin filaments of actin (an isoform specific to smooth muscle) are associated with tropomyosin (see Fig. 5.6) but, in contrast to striated muscle, there is no troponin.

The thick filaments are composed of myosin, but of a different type to that in skeletal muscle and will only bind to actin if its light chain is phosphorylated; this phenomenon does not occur in skeletal muscle.

Although Ca^{2+} ions in smooth muscle cells cause contraction as in striated muscle, the control of Ca^{2+} ion movements is different. In relaxed smooth muscle, free Ca^{2+} ions are normally sequestered in sarcoplasmic reticulum throughout the cell. On membrane excitation, free Ca^{2+} ions are released into the cytoplasm and bind to a protein called 'calmodulin' (a calcium-binding protein). The calcium–calmodulin complex then activates an enzyme called 'myosin light-chain kinase', which phosphorylates the myosin light chain and permits it to bind to actin. Actin and myosin subsequently interact by filament sliding to produce contraction in a similar way to that for skeletal muscle.

In the cell membrane of smooth muscle cells are calcium channels, which can open and let calcium into the cell. Some of these channels are activated by hormones (ligand-gated channels), whereas others are activated by membrane depolarization (voltage-gated channels). These channels provide another mechanism for initiation or modulation of contraction.

Contraction of smooth muscle can be modulated by surface receptors activating internal secondary messenger systems. Expression of different receptors allows smooth muscle in different sites to respond to several different hormones.

Compared with skeletal muscle, smooth muscle is able to maintain a high force of contraction for very little ATP usage.

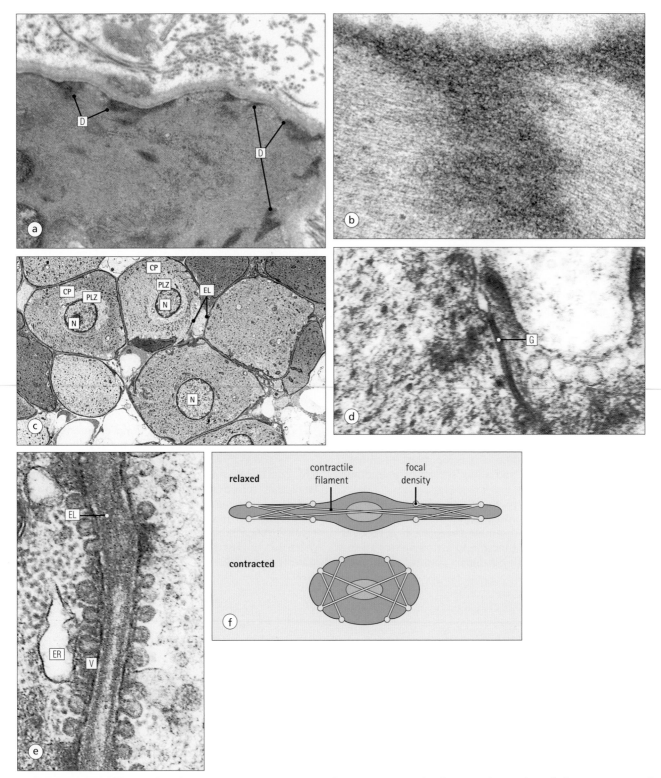

FIGURE 5.12 **Smooth muscle (ultrastructure).** (a) Low-power electron micrograph of a smooth muscle cell showing scattered focal densities (D) around the cell membrane. (b) High-power electron micrograph of one of the focal densities in (a), showing the insertion of large numbers of very fine contractile filaments into it. (c) Very low-power electron micrograph of smooth muscle fibres in transverse section showing central nucleus (N), distinct surrounding external laminae (EL), the bulk of the cytoplasm occupied by tightly packed contractile protein filaments (CP), and a perinuclear lucent zone (PLZ) in which most of the mitochondria and non-contractile organelles reside. (d) Gap junctions (G) connect adjacent cells at defects in the external lamina. (e) A terminal sac of the endoplasmic reticulum (ER) lies close to caveolae-like endocytotic vesicles (V) on the surface. External lamina material (EL) lies between two adjacent smooth muscle cells. (f) Contractile protein filaments are inserted into focal densities around the cell membrane. With contraction of the tethered filaments, each cell assumes a short, rounded shape.

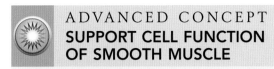

Smooth Muscle Cells have to Secrete Elements of Their Extracellular Matrix

Depending on the site, smooth muscle cells produce collagen, elastin and other components of the extracellular matrix. Thus, they have a support cell function as well as a contractile cell function. In most situations, this support cell function is limited to manufacturing extracellular matrix to anchor the smooth muscle.

Smooth muscle can be arranged into two functional types termed unitary and multiunit

Most smooth muscle is present in the walls of hollow viscera (e.g. gut, ureter, fallopian tube), where it is arranged in sheets with cells aligned circumferentially or longitudinally, with contraction resulting in reduction of the luminal diameter.

In these so-called unitary smooth muscles, cells tend to generate their own low level of rhythmic contraction, which may also be stimulated by stretch, and is transmitted from cell to cell via the gap junctions. Such smooth muscle is richly innervated by the autonomic nervous system (see Chapter 6), which increases or decreases levels of spontaneous contraction rather than actually initiating it. Physiologically, this is termed tonic smooth muscle and is characterized by slow contraction, no action potentials, and a low content of fast myosin.

A second arrangement of smooth muscle is typified by that in the iris of the eye. Here, rather than simply modulating spontaneous activity, autonomic innervation controls contraction precisely, resulting in opening and closing of the pupil. Similar neurally controlled or multiunit smooth muscle is found in the vas deferens and some large arteries. Physiologically, this is termed 'phasic smooth muscle' and is characterized by rapid contraction associated with distinct action potential, and a high cell content of fast myosin.

Myofibroblasts

Myofibroblasts are important in tissue responses to injury

Myofibroblasts are spindle-shaped cells that secrete collagen (i.e. fibroblast-like), but also have well-defined contractile properties similar to those of smooth muscle.

In conventional histological sections, myofibroblasts cannot be readily distinguished from fibroblasts, but immunohistochemical detection of their content of smooth muscle actin and desmin (not seen in fibroblasts) and ultrastructural demonstration of contractile proteins shows that they are distinct. Myofibroblasts lack an external lamina, in contrast to true smooth muscle cells.

Cells, including muscle cells of all types, can adapt to handle a heavier workload. They can do this by either increasing the size of the cell, and hence its work output, or by increasing the number of cells doing the job. Increasing a cell's capacity for work by increasing its size is called hypertrophy, and by increasing the number of cells is called hyperplasia. For hyperplasia to occur, the mature functioning cells must be capable of cell division, and neither skeletal muscle nor cardiac muscle cells are capable of cell division so can only increase their output by hypertrophy. Smooth muscle cells are capable of cell division and can therefore increase their work output by both hypertrophy and hyperplasia.

Similarly, muscle which has to deal with greatly reduced workload can adapt by each cell becoming smaller (atrophy).

Here are some examples:

Skeletal muscle undergoes hypertrophy in increased physical exercise, e.g. in athletes, but undergoes atrophy when the muscles are underused, for example in someone who is immobilized by paralysis or limb injury.

Cardiac muscle can undergo hypertrophy in many circumstances, both as a result of increased physiological demand (again in athletes) and as a result of some disease processes. For example, if the aortic outflow lumen in the heart is reduced by valve disease (see Chapter 9), the cardiac muscle fibres of the left ventricle will undergo hypertrophy to increase the force with which blood can be pushed through the partially obstructed outflow. Hypertrophy of cardiac muscle cells makes the heart big.

Atrophy of cardiac muscle cells is commonly seen in elderly people who have been physically inactive for a long time. It makes the heart small.

Smooth muscle can undergo both hypertrophy and hyperplasia and usually responds to increased demands by doing both, although hypertrophy is usually the major component. A good example is the smooth muscle of the uterus (myometrium), which increases enormously in both bulk and power during the 9 months of pregnancy in preparation for the immense contractile effort required at childbirth. Atrophy of uterine smooth muscle occurs after the menopause, indicating that the status of uterine smooth muscle is under hormonal control.

- Spindle-shaped cells surrounded by external lamina
- Main contractile cell of hollow viscera, blood vessels and airways
- Contractile proteins inserted into focal densities around cell periphery
- Contraction modulated by neuronal and endocrine factors
- Two main smooth muscle types (tonic and phasic) characterized by arrangement and speed of contraction.

In normal tissues, myofibroblasts are inconspicuous and commonly form an inactive population of cells, for example in the alveolar septa of the lung and around the crypts of glands in the gut. They also form a sparse population in loose collagenous support tissue.

CLINICAL EXAMPLE
MYOFIBROBLASTS IN DISEASE

As well as being prominent in wound healing and in the normal processes of repair, myofibroblasts are also found in several diseases characterized by fibrosis of tissues, for example fibrosis of the lung following damage by immune-mediated diseases, atheroma in the lining of arteries (see Fig. 9.6) and cirrhosis of the liver (see Fig. 12.8). In these diseases, the stimuli that cause myofibroblast proliferation are uncertain, but include local production of growth factors.

During wound healing, however, myofibroblasts become active and proliferate, and their role appears to be to repair defects resulting from tissue damage. They secrete collagen to provide a firm scaffold to consolidate a damaged area (fibrous scar). As healing proceeds, myofibroblasts contract and pull the extracellular matrix together to reduce the physical size of the damaged area.

Pericytes

Pericytes are found around vessels and can act as mesenchymal stem cells

Pericytes are spindle-shaped cells which are found circumferentially arranged around capillaries and venules (see Fig. 9.11). They are surrounded by external lamina and, in normal tissues, show little cytoplasmic differentiation ultrastructurally, but contain actin and myosin immunohistochemically, suggesting a contractile function.

Following tissue injury, pericytes proliferate and assume the role of primitive mesenchymal cells, being able to differentiate into myofibroblasts, as well as mesenchymal tissue, which develops into collagenous support tissue and new blood vessels.

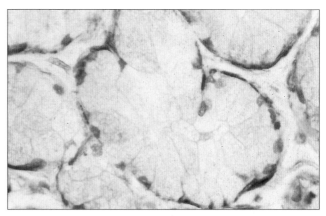

FIGURE 5.13 **Myoepithelial cells.** Myoepithelial cells in this section from a salivary gland can be shown by an immunoperoxidase technique that demonstrates desmin, which is the muscle-specific intermediate filament and stains brown.

Myoepithelial Cells

Secretions from glands are expelled by the contractile function of myoepithelial cells

Myoepithelial cells are found in exocrine glands, including highly developed glands, such as the breast, where they form a major population surrounding glandular acini and ducts, and squeeze secretions from the glandular lumina.

Myoepithelial cells are generally inconspicuous in routine H&E sections, appearing as a layer of flat cells running around acini and ducts. They have dark-staining, rounded nuclei and clear or vacuolated cytoplasm.

Around acini, myoepithelial cells have a stellate, multiprocessed morphology in three dimensions and form a contractile meshwork, which encloses secretory units of glands. Around ducts they are fusiform in shape and surround the periphery of ducts in a way analogous to barrel hoops.

Ultrastructurally, myoepithelial cells contain contractile proteins arranged in a similar manner to that in smooth muscle and have numerous desmosomal connections with adjacent cells.

Immunohistochemically, they can be detected by their content of the muscle-specific intermediate filament desmin (Fig. 5.13).

Myoepithelial cells are controlled by the autonomic nervous system and on stimulation contract and expel glandular secretions.

For online review questions, please visit
https://studentconsult.inkling.com.

END OF CHAPTER REVIEW

True/false Answers to the MCQs, as well as Case Answers, can be Found in the Appendix in the back of the Book.

1. **Which of the following features are seen in the skeletal muscle cells?**
   (a) Have thin filaments made of actin which are anchored to the Z band
   (b) Have thick filaments made of desmin which are anchored to the M band
   (c) Regulate contraction by control of calcium release from sarcoplasmic reticulum
   (d) Are surrounded by an external lamina
   (e) Contain multiple nuclei in each cell

2. **Which of the following are true of cardiac muscle cells?**
   (a) Are mononuclear and linked by intercellular junctions to form a fibre
   (b) Are striated in a similar way to skeletal muscle
   (c) Can regenerate following cell damage
   (d) Regulate contraction by release of calcium from sarcoplasmic reticulum
   (e) Have communicating junctions linking fibres to facilitate contraction

3. **Which of the following features are specific for smooth muscle cells?**
   (a) Have single nuclei
   (b) Use actin and myosin to develop contractile forces
   (c) Are surrounded by an external lamina
   (d) Have membrane receptors for hormones
   (e) May generate their own level of rhythmic contraction

4. **Myofibroblasts, pericytes and myoepithelial cells are all types of specialized contractile cells with which of the following features?**
   (a) Myoepithelial cells are found in exocrine glandular tissue such as the breast
   (b) Myoepithelial cells are stellate cells, with multiple processes, which surround secretory units of glands
   (c) Myoepithelial cells are controlled by autonomic innervation
   (d) Pericytes may assume the role of primitive mesenchymal cells
   (e) Myofibroblasts proliferate and are involved in repair following tissue damage

CASE 5.1 SUDDEN CARDIAC DEATH

A 24-year-old male is brought into hospital by ambulance having collapsed while running in a local half-marathon. Paramedics had attended and he was found to have no cardiac output and was in asystole. He was pronounced dead and an autopsy requested to establish the cause of death.

The pathologist found that the heart was greatly enlarged and showed hypertrophy of the left ventricle. The left ventricular wall was much thicker than normal. Histology showed that myocardial cells were greatly enlarged and had an abnormal pattern of myofibres. A diagnosis of hypertrophic cardiomyopathy was made. Further genetic testing showed a mutation in one of the genes coding for cardiac-specific myosin.

Q. Explain the relationship between the mutation in the gene and cardiac disease.

Chapter 6

Nervous Tissue

Introduction

The nervous system allows rapid and specific communication between widely spaced areas of the body by the action of specialized nerve cells (neurons), which gather and process information and generate appropriate response signals.

The nervous system is divided into two main parts:
- The **central nervous system** (CNS) comprising the brain and spinal cord
- The **peripheral nervous system** (PNS) comprising the nerves which run between the CNS and other tissues, together with nerve 'relay stations' termed 'ganglia'.

Nerve Cells (Neurons)

Nerve cells are responsible for direct communications between different groups of cells

Neurons form a network of highly specific connections between different groups of cells in order to:
- Gather information from sensory receptors
- Process information and provide a memory
- Generate appropriate signals to effector cells.

A neuron is divided into several regions, each with a different function

Neurons (Fig. 6.1) are characterized by:
- A cell body containing the nucleus and most of the organelles responsible for maintaining the cell
- A long cell process (**axon**) stretching from the cell, often over a long distance, which is responsible for transmitting signals from the neuron to other cells
- Numerous short cell processes (**dendrites**) which increase the surface area available for connecting with axons of other neurons
- Specialized cell junctions (**synapses**) between its axon and other cells to allow direct cell communication.

The functional attributes of the nervous system are determined mainly by the network of connections between neurons rather than by specific structural features of individual neurons.

Neurons have a characteristic cytology reflecting a high metabolic activity

Neurons are highly metabolically active as they not only maintain a massive surface area of cell membrane, but also constantly require energy to develop electrochemical gradients. This activity is reflected in their histological appearance (Fig. 6.2), in which the nucleus is typically large and rounded, with a large central nucleolus, reflecting a high degree of transcriptional activity. There is abundant rough endoplasmic reticulum, which synthesizes the necessary proteins, and is visible in the cytoplasm in H&E sections as blue-stained granules, the so-called **Nissl substance**, which is present in the cell body (perikaryon) and dendrites but not the axon. There is also a well-developed Golgi to produce secretory products, and large numbers of mitochondria to supply the high energy requirements. Lysosomes are numerous because of a high turnover of cell membrane and other cell components, and residual bodies containing lipofuscin are often prominent, particularly in the elderly.

Neurons have different shapes reflecting differences in function

Several types of neuron can be identified according to the pattern of axons and dendrites (Fig. 6.3). These appearances are only apparent when special staining methods are used to highlight cellular anatomy.

Motor neurons have a large cell body to provide metabolic support for the large axon. They also have many dendritic processes and are therefore classed as multipolar neurons.

Sensory neurons are commonly unipolar cells, which are characterized by the possession of one major process. This divides into two branches, one running to the central nervous system and one to a sensory area of the body.

Interneurons are generally small, simple cells with short processes that provide local connections within the central nervous system. Many such cells are bipolar in type, having two main processes of equivalent size, one dendritic and one axonal.

In addition to these general types of neuron, there are many types of neuron that are unique to a particular part

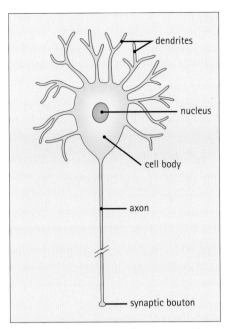

FIGURE 6.1 **General structure of a neuron.** Neurons consist of a cell body, axon and dendrites, the axon carrying impulses to its terminal, the synaptic bouton, which makes contact with another cell. The dendrites connect with synaptic boutons from other neurons.

ADVANCED CONCEPT

THE CYTOSKELETON OF THE NEURON IS VITAL FOR AXONAL TRANSPORT

The cytoskeleton of neurons is highly organized to maintain the unique shape of these cells, and particularly axons, which may be up to 1 m long.

Neurofilament protein, the intermediate filament of nerve cells, is thought to act as an internal scaffold to maintain the shape of the axon and cell body. In the axon, certain membrane proteins are anchored in place in an organized pattern by attachment to cellular neurofilaments.

There is also a highly organized network of microtubules, which transport substances and organelles up and down the axon.

The metabolic maintenance of the long cell process of the axon requires a transport system for organelles, enzymes and metabolites from the cell body, which is largely directed by the microtubular cytoskeleton. Enzymes and elements of the cytoskeleton are transported down the axon at a speed of 1–5 mm/day by an unknown mechanism (slow axonal transport). Membrane-bound organelles, such as neurosecretory vesicles, are transported at speeds of 400 mm/day (anterograde fast axonal transport). This method is mediated by microtubular transport mechanisms using the molecule kinesin as a molecular motor.

The return of effete organelles as well as recycled membrane from the synaptic ending back to the neuronal cell body for processing occurs at a rate of 300 mm/day (retrograde fast transport). This is mediated by microtubular transport mechanisms using the molecule dynein as a molecular motor.

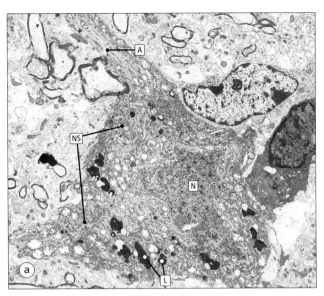

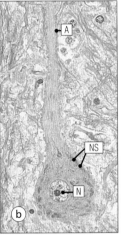

FIGURE 6.2 **Neuron.** (a) Electron micrograph of a neuron showing the axon (A) containing mitochondria and cytoskeletal filaments, and the cell body containing a nucleus (N), dark-staining lysosomal bodies (L) and abundant rough endoplasmic reticulum (Nissl substance) (NS). (b) Micrograph showing a neuron with a large nucleus (N) containing a prominent nucleolus. Within the cell body, blue-staining Nissl substance (NS), composed of rough endoplasmic reticulum, can be seen. The axon (A) stretches away from the cell body.

of the brain, for example the Purkinje cells, which are large multiprocessed cells in the cerebellum (see Fig. 6.27b).

Neurons transmit signals by changes in the electrical polarity of the cell membrane

Neuron signalling is controlled by an electrical (ionic) gradient across the cell membrane. Firing is associated with depolarization of the cell membrane which, in a resting axon, has a negative membrane potential (−70 mV). This depolarization is propagated along the axon of the cell at up to 100 m/s.

The cell membrane of neurons is divided into several regions, each containing highly specialized membrane proteins. **Membrane ion pumps** maintain the baseline electrical gradient between the outside and inside of the

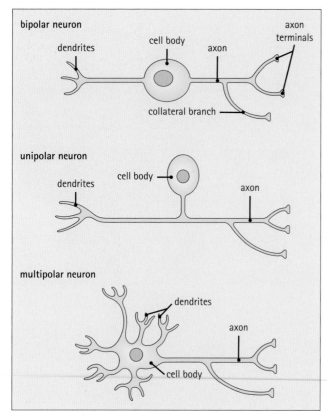

FIGURE 6.3 **Types of neuron.** There are many different types of neuron, which are shaped according to their function. Bipolar cells are commonly interneurons, whereas unipolar cells tend to be sensory neurons and multipolar cells are often motor neurons.

cell and are widely distributed in the cell membrane. **Ion channel proteins** modify the electrochemical gradient across the neuron cell membrane by forming pores or gates, which can switch their permeability to ions in response to specific signals (gated channels).

- **Ligand-gated channels** close or open in response to binding to chemical transmitter substances and are located mainly in synapses
- **Voltage-gated channels** are involved mainly in the explosive and rapid depolarization that occurs as nerve cells fire, and are widely distributed in the cell membrane.

If an area of the axon membrane is locally depolarized and the current is small, then no gated channels will open. The current flows down the axon by passive local spread for a small distance before dissipating because of leakage from the membrane. In this situation, the axon behaves like an electrical cable, simply conducting a current along its surface with the speed of conduction related to the resistance and capacitance of the axon.

If an area of axon membrane is depolarized and the current is large, Na^+ and K^+ gated channels open and lead to an explosive change in the membrane potential, termed an **action potential**.

The opening of voltage-gated channels to produce an action potential can be considered as a local amplification system for membrane depolarization; the current does not now dissipate over a small length of the axon,

but propagates to the end of the axon by causing a chain reaction triggering of gated ion channels along the way.

Action potentials propagate along an axon at the speed of passive local spread, which is determined by the resistance and capacitance of the axon: the larger the diameter of the axon, the greater the speed of propagation.

KEY FACTS
THE NEURON

- Divided into cell body, axon, dendrites, terminal bouton
- Highly metabolically active cell with abundant lysosomes and rough endoplasmic reticulum (termed Nissl substance)
- Cytoskeleton is vital for function, especially neurofilaments (architecture) and microtubules (axonal transport)
- The axon is specialized for conduction of electrical depolarization (action potential) mediated by ion channels in the cell membrane.

Nerve cells signal to each other through structures called synapses

A 'synapse' is a special type of cell junction that allows direct communication between cells; a transmitter substance is secreted in a highly localized fashion by one cell and received uniquely by the other.

CLINICAL EXAMPLE
MOTOR NEURON DISEASE

Motor neuron disease is a progressive disease, mainly seen in old age, in which symptoms include weakness of voluntary muscles caused by the death of motor neurons. The disease progresses to severe paralysis, leading to death in 2–3 years. The reason for the peculiar susceptibility of motor neurons to spontaneous death is not known. All motor neurons are vulnerable, and the particular symptoms in each case depend on which groups of motor neurons are most severely involved. Death of motor neurons in the brain stem produces the symptom complex called **progressive bulbar palsy**; that of the lower motor neurons of the spinal cord produces **progressive muscular atrophy**. The most common pattern is called amyotrophic lateral sclerosis and is due to death of motor neurons in the cerebral cortex, brain stem and spinal cord.

Each synapse has vesicles containing neurotransmitter substances

The terminal end of an axon is swollen to form a synaptic bouton, which is closely applied to the surface of a target cell, leaving a small gap 20 nm wide (the synaptic cleft). The cell membrane on each side of the synaptic cleft contains special membrane proteins and receptors involved in neurotransmission.

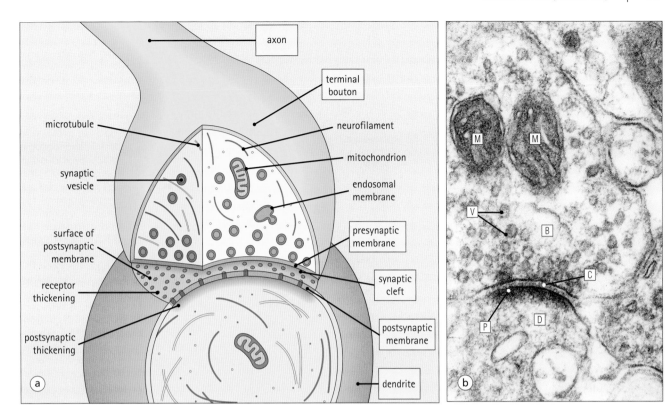

FIGURE 6.4   Synapse. (a) An axon terminating as a synaptic bouton on the surface of a neuron. The postsynaptic membrane bears arrays of receptors for the neurotransmitter contained in the synaptic vesicles. Vesicles are released into the synaptic cleft by exocytosis. (b) Electron micrograph showing the synaptic bouton (B) making contact with dendrite (D). The bouton contains small vesicles (V), mitochondria (M) and cytoskeletal filaments. The synaptic cleft (C) contains faint granular material above the thickened postsynaptic membrane (P).

Ultrastructurally, the cell membrane on each side of the synaptic cleft is slightly thickened and the synaptic bouton contains mitochondria, microtubules and neurofilaments, as well as membrane-bound vesicles 40–65 nm in diameter (neurosecretory vesicles, Fig. 6.4). The appearance of these vesicles is variable; most are small and round with a clear centre, others are elliptical. Certain neurosecretory granules (dense-core granules) have an electron-dense core with a pale 'halo' beneath the membrane.

In tissue sections, it is possible to detect transmitter substances in neurons and their terminals by immunochemistry, using antibodies specific for the transmitter.

Neurosecretory granules also contain unique non-transmitter proteins, which are vital to their function. Again, these may be detected by immunochemistry, for example synaptophysin, which is a glycoprotein in the membrane of neurosecretory granules, and chromogranins, proteins involved in the packaging of transmitter into dense-core vesicles.

Neurosecretory vesicles release transmitter by fusion with the presynaptic membrane

When a wave of depolarization reaches the synaptic bouton, it triggers the release of a transmitter substance from the neurosecretory granules by exocytosis (Fig. 6.5). The transmitter substance then diffuses across the synaptic cleft and is able to interact with receptors in the postsynaptic membrane of the target neuron.

The membrane of the synaptic vesicle is recovered as a coated pit and recycles back to an endosome compartment in the nerve terminal. There is thus a constant recycling of membrane in the nerve terminal. Neurosecretory vesicles also arrive in the axon terminal by transport from the cell body, but others are formed locally by budding off from the endosome compartment in the synapse. Neurotransmitter substances can be imported into vesicles formed from the endosome compartment of the nerve terminal by reuptake systems.

Three possible effects of transmitter release are depolarization, hyperpolarization or altered cell sensitivity

When a released transmitter binds to receptors on the postsynaptic cells, there are three possible effects: depolarization, hyperpolarization or altered cell sensitivity.

The target cell **depolarizes** if the transmitter substance binds to a ligand-gated receptor (i.e. Na^+ ion channel protein) and causes it to open, allowing ions to diffuse into the neuron. If many receptors are activated at the same time, the alteration in membrane potential causes activation of voltage-gated ion channels, leading to an action potential.

Only a small group of transmitter substances act in this way, which generally results in rapid neural transmission. These include acetylcholine, which is the major transmitter in this group, and glutamate.

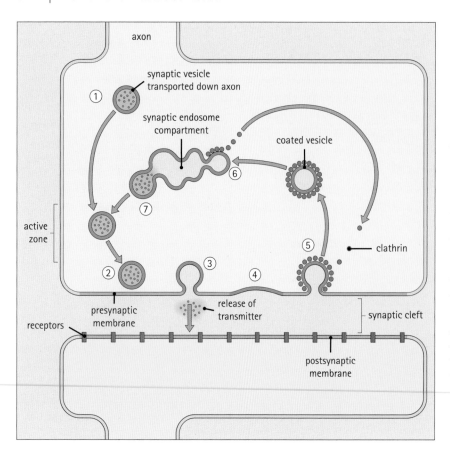

FIGURE 6.5 **Turnover of synaptic vesicles.** Synaptic vesicles (NSV) are formed in the neuronal cell body and are transported down the axon (1). Once in the terminal bouton, proteins in the NSV membrane direct vesicles to an area just above the presynaptic membrane termed the 'active zone'. Vesicles from the active zone bind to special docking proteins in the presynaptic membrane and become primed for exocytosis (2). Exocytosis is associated with the release of the transmitter substance into the synaptic cleft (3) and integration of the membrane of the vesicle with the presynaptic membrane (4). The protein clathrin associates with vesicle membrane and forms coated vesicles which recycle the vesicle membrane back into the nerve terminal (5). Recycled vesicle membrane fuses with an endosome membrane compartment in the nerve terminal (6) and clathrin is released. New synaptic vesicles can bud off from the endosome compartment (7). Transmitter substances which are free in the nerve terminal can be imported into these recycled vesicles via special membrane pumps.

ADVANCED CONCEPT
NEUROSECRETION IS MEDIATED BY PROTEINS IN THE SYNAPTIC VESICLE AND PRESYNAPTIC MEMBRANE

Many of the proteins involved in neurosecretion have now been characterized (Fig. 6.6).

The membrane of the synaptic vesicle contains an anchoring protein (synaptobrevin) which ties the vesicle to a docking protein in the presynaptic membrane (syntaxin) by a group of linking proteins (composed of proteins called 'SNARE, αSNAP, βSNAP, SNAP25 and NSF').

The membrane of the synaptic vesicle and the adjacent presynaptic membrane contain proteins which can bring about membrane fusion and allow exocytosis. In the resting state, a calcium-sensitive trigger protein (synaptotagmin) prevents the linking complex from allowing membrane fusion.

If an action potential reaches the terminal bouton, voltage-sensitive calcium channels open and increase the concentration of calcium in the nerve terminal. This releases the trigger protein and allows membrane fusion to take place, leading to exocytosis.

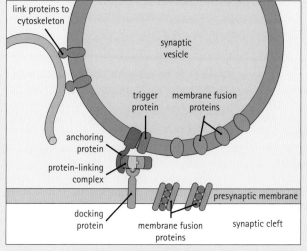

FIGURE 6.6 **Synaptic docking and exocytosis.** Many of the proteins involved in the exocytosis of synaptic vesicles are characterized. Fusion of vesicle to presynaptic membrane only takes place when an increase in calcium causes an alteration in the configuration of proteins involved in docking.

The target cell **hyperpolarizes** if the transmitter substance binds to a ligand-gated receptor that admits small negative ions into the cell. Hyperpolarization inhibits depolarization.

The main transmitter substances causing hyperpolarization are γ-aminobutyric acid and glycine.

The overall **sensitivity of a cell** to stimulation is altered if the transmitter substance binds to one of the class of non-channel-linked receptors. These receptors generate secondary messengers (e.g. cAMP) within the target neuron, to modify the overall sensitivity of the cell to depolarization mediated by the ligand-gated receptors. Such behaviour is called 'neuromodulation'.

Many of the transmitters causing altered cell sensitivity are monoamines (e.g. dopamine, serotonin), but some are small neuropeptides.

In any given nerve terminal, more than one transmitter substance may operate.

Synapses form different patterns of connection between neurons

Within the CNS, synapses form in a diversity of combinations between axons and dendrites, axons and cell bodies, axons and other axons (Fig. 6.7).

Because axons may be excitatory, inhibitory or modulatory, certain synapses are formed from the coincidence

of many axons from different neurons on to one part of a target neuron. The target neuron can then integrate the overall input into an appropriate output. Such functional clusters of synapses are commonly isolated from the adjacent nervous system by support cells of the brain, such as astrocytes.

The neuromuscular junction or motor endplate (see Chapter 13) is a specialized form of synapse between a motor nerve axon and skeletal muscle.

Myelin

Myelin wraps around axons and increases speed of conduction

The speed of conduction along nerves is limited by the electrical capacitance and resistance of the axon.

Because wide axons have a lower capacitance than narrow ones, increasing their diameter is a useful means of increasing the speed of nerve conduction. This is inefficient, however, as giant axons require high metabolic upkeep.

The speed of conduction along axons can also be increased if leakage of current from the membrane is minimized by insulation.

The two functions of insulation and reduction of electrical capacitance are performed by a substance called **myelin**, which is produced by specialized support cells. These cells, which wrap layers of membrane containing the lipid-rich insulating layer around axons, are called **oligodendrocytes** in the CNS and **Schwann cells** in the PNS.

A Schwann cell myelinates only one axon, but an oligodendrocyte may myelinate several adjacent axons. Although largely identical in structure, there are minor differences in the composition of myelin formed by these two cell types.

Myelin can be stained by histological methods with affinity for the lipid or protein components of the myelin sheath, and such methods highlight the structural difference in the CNS between neuron-rich areas low in myelin (grey matter) and tracts of axons with abundant myelin (white matter).

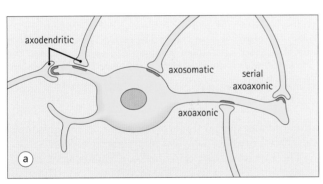

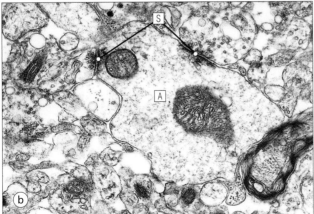

FIGURE 6.7 **Patterns of synapse.** (a) The combination of synapses. Synapses can form between axons and dendrites, axons and cell bodies, axons and other axons. (b) Electron micrograph showing two axoaxonic synapses (S) on to the same axon (A). Firing of (A) will depend on the integration of these separate inputs.

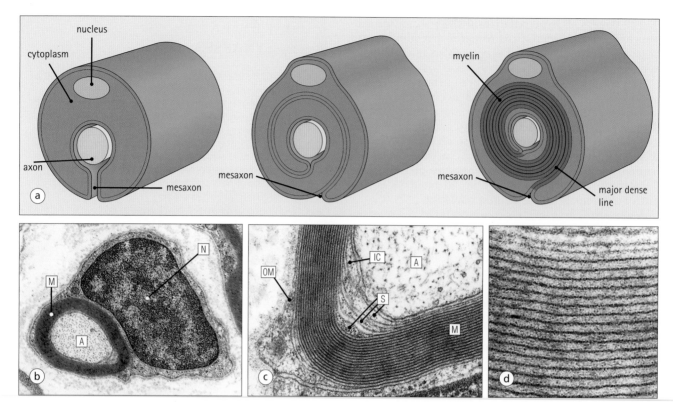

FIGURE 6.8 Myelin. (a) Myelin formation. First, an axon invaginates a myelin-forming cell and the outer leaflets of the myelin-forming cell's membrane fuse to form the mesaxon. The myelin-forming cell then wraps layers of the mesaxon around the axon; the inner cytoplasm is lost when the inner leaflet of the cell membrane fuses to form the major dense line. Myelin forms into numerous lamellae of fused membrane, the lamellae being separated by alternating major dense lines and mesaxon (intraperiod line). (b) Low-power electron micrograph showing an axon (A) surrounded by myelin (M) and the nucleus (N) of a Schwann cell. (c) Medium-power electron micrograph showing the fine structure of myelin. The axon (A) is surrounded by myelin lamellae (M). Note the outer mesaxon (OM). The areas of cytoplasm in the myelin represent Schmidt–Lanterman incisures (S) (see Fig. 6.9) and the inner collar of cytoplasm (IC). (d) High-power electron micrograph showing the fine detail of myelin lamellae; the dark lines are the major dense lines, whereas the intraperiod lines are barely visible in between.

Myelin is a spiral layer of closely apposed cell membranes

The myelin sheath is formed by the oligodendrocytes or Schwann cells wrapping spiral layers of cell membrane around the axon. Each layer of cell membrane is linked to its neighbour by specialized cell adhesion proteins.

Myelination begins with the invagination of a single axon into the support cell, which brings its outer cell membranes into close apposition and seals them together to form a sheet of internal membrane (the mesaxon; Fig. 6.8). The line of fusion is mediated by proteins in the outer surfaces of the cell membrane, and ultrastructurally forms a line (the intraperiod line). Myelination then proceeds as the support cell wraps numerous layers of the mesaxon around the axon. A tight spiral composed of double-thickness cell membrane fused together forms because the cytoplasm of the support cell is excluded from most of the space between the membrane layers.

The inner surfaces of the cell membranes also fuse together and form a dense line, the **major dense line**.

The thickness of the myelin sheath depends on the number of layers (lamellae) wrapped around the axon.

In addition to the specialized cell adhesion proteins, the cell membrane of the support cells that forms myelin also contains special lipids – for example the glycolipid galactocerebroside, which is abundant in myelin.

The myelin insulation is not continuous along axons, being limited by the size of the myelinating cell. The small bare areas of axon between myelin sheaths are termed the **nodes of Ranvier** and are physiologically important.

Myelin is maintained by extensions of cytoplasm from the parent myelin-forming cell

The cell membranes forming myelin are a dynamic structure. The cytoplasm of the myelin-forming support cell remains in the myelin sheath at three sites to maintain the cell membrane. These sites are located:

- Adjacent to the axon (**inner collar**)
- Between the internodal myelin lamellae of peripheral nervous system myelin formed by Schwann cells (**Schmidt–Lanterman incisures**)
- At each end of the myelin segment adjacent to the nodes of Ranvier (**paranodal area**, see below)
- Adjacent to the cell body on the outer aspect of the myelin (**outer collar**).

The cytoplasm in all these areas is in continuity with that of the cell body of the support cells so that the membrane forming the myelin can be maintained (Fig. 6.9).

ADVANCED CONCEPT
CELL MEMBRANES IN MYELIN ARE LINKED TOGETHER BY SPECIALIZED PROTEINS

The layers of cell membrane which are wrapped to form myelin are tightly bound together by special proteins. The proteins involved are different for CNS myelin and PNS myelin.

In the myelin of the CNS, proteolipid protein (PLP) links the exoplasmic surfaces of myelin membranes together. The cytoplasmic surfaces are linked through interactions with another protein called 'myelin basic protein' (MBP).

In the PNS, P0 protein associates with myelin basic protein to form the major dense line. P0 protein accounts for about 50% of protein in PNS myelin.

Myelin-associated glycoprotein (MAG) is expressed on the surface of oligodendrocytes and is a member of the family of immunoglobulin-like proteins, acting as a cell surface ligand-binding protein.

Peripheral myelin protein-22, like P0 is also involved in the formation and maintenance of myelin in the PNS.

CLINICAL EXAMPLE
ABNORMALITIES IN MYELIN PROTEINS CAUSE DISEASE OF THE NERVOUS SYSTEM

Several inherited diseases of the nervous system are now recognized to be caused by abnormalities in the genes coding for myelin-related proteins.

Dominantly inherited hereditary motor and sensory neuropathy type 1 (HMSN-1) is caused by mutations in peripheral myelin protein-22 (PMP-22) in 90% of affected families. Patients develop weakness and impaired sensation caused by degeneration of the myelin in peripheral nerves.

Deletion of the gene for peripheral myelin protein-22 (PMP-22) gives rise to hereditary neuropathy, with liability to pressure palsies. Patients are unusually susceptible to nerve damage following relatively trivial pressure to nerves.

Mutations in the proteolipid protein (PLP) gene can cause two disorders. In Pelizaeus–Merzbacher disease, affected children develop degeneration of their CNS myelin and develop progressively severe mental disability. Other mutations can cause degeneration of myelin in the spinal cord, leading to spastic paraparesis. The gene for PLP is on the X chromosome and so these diseases are manifest in males.

The nodes of Ranvier contain bare areas of axon devoid of myelin

Myelination of an axon is not continuous along its length, but occurs in small units 1–2 mm long, each unit being formed by an individual support cell. The small space between each unit of myelin is the node of Ranvier and

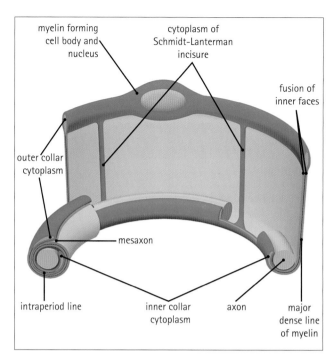

FIGURE 6.9 **Cytoplasmic compartments in myelin.** If the myelin around an axon is theoretically unwrapped, the relationships between the cytoplasmic compartments become evident. The inner collar and outer collar run along and parallel to the axon, whereas the cytoplasm of the Schmidt-Lanterman incisures is wrapped around the axon in between myelin lamellae. These zones of cytoplasm are continuous with the cell body of the myelin-forming cell and serve to maintain the membrane forming the myelin.

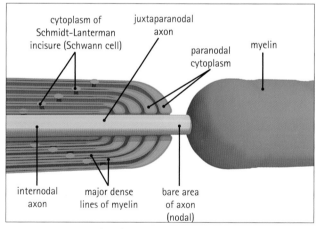

FIGURE 6.10 **Node of Ranvier.** A node of Ranvier in longitudinal section. At the end of a myelin segment, the myelin lamellae give way to a series of paranodal loops containing cytoplasm. The adjacent bare area of axon is generally slightly wider than the internodal axon and is the region containing the voltage-gated Na^+ channels, which are necessary for the formation of action potential. Compare the Schmidt-Lanterman incisures in this plane, with those in Figure 6.9.

has an important physiological role in increasing the efficiency of nerve conduction (Fig. 6.10).

At the node of Ranvier, the myelinating cells form paranodal loops of cytoplasm in continuity with the cell body.

In the CNS, the axons in the nodes of Ranvier are bare, whereas those in the PNS are partly covered by tongues of cytoplasm from adjacent Schwann cells.

The axon at the node of Ranvier is slightly thicker than in the internodal regions and contains most of the Na^+ gated channels of the axonal cell membrane, which is reflected ultrastructurally as a fuzzy thickening of the membrane. These gated channels are anchored via the link protein, ankyrin, to the cytoskeleton. There are no gated channels in the internodal region beneath the myelin sheath.

Depolarization at a node of Ranvier is followed by rapid passive spread of the depolarization current along the axon beneath the myelin to the next node, because leakage of current is minimized by the insulation. As the membrane capacitance is low, which is also the result of the myelin, only a small change is required to cause a significant voltage difference.

When such passively spread conduction encounters the zone of highly concentrated gated channels in the next node of Ranvier along the axon, there is further local depolarization. Thus, the depolarization progresses in a series of jumps, with passive spread of charge in between.

Depolarization in a myelinated nerve is much more efficient metabolically than in a non-myelinated nerve, because the restricted entry of Na^+ ions to small areas, instead of to the whole axonal surface, reduces the demand for energy to pump the ions back out again.

KEY FACTS
MYELIN

- Is formed by Schwann cells in the PNS and oligodendrocytes in the CNS
- Ultrastructurally is seen as a spiral of membrane wrapped around an axon
- Contains special cell adhesion proteins and lipids which differ between the CNS and PNS
- Functions to increase the speed of conduction along axons
- Occurs in small units with a space between termed the node of Ranvier.

Central Nervous System

The central nervous system (CNS) comprises the brain and spinal cord. These contain nerve cells and their processes, together with a series of specialized support cells.

The specialized support cells of the CNS are collectively called glia

The CNS contains numerous non-neural support cells. These are astrocytes, oligodendrocytes, ependyma and microglial cells (Fig. 6.11), which are collectively called the **glia**.

Astrocytes are stellate cells with roles in embryogenesis, fluid transport and structural support

Astrocytes are large, multiprocessed cells with several functions:
- In embryological development, they form a structural framework to guide the migration of developing nerve cells
- In the developed brain, they form a structural scaffolding for the more specialized neural elements
- Certain astrocytes transport fluid and ions from the extracellular space around neurons to blood vessels.

Astrocytes are characterized by oval or slightly irregular nuclei with an open chromatin pattern, and a spectacular stellate morphology with numerous fine processes radiating in all directions. These processes contain a specific form of cytoskeletal intermediate filament called **glial fibrillary acidic protein** (GFAP).

The stellate morphology is not evident in conventional H&E sections because the processes merge with the processes of other cells, but is seen with special staining methods (Fig. 6.12).

Two types of astrocyte have been identified. **Fibrous astrocytes** are most evident in the white matter and have long cell processes, which are rich in bundles of GFAP. **Protoplasmic astrocytes** are most evident in the grey matter of the brain and have long thin processes containing few bundles of GFAP.

ADVANCED CONCEPT
MOLECULAR ORGANIZATION AROUND THE NODE OF RANVIER

Myelin-producing cells (Schwann cells or oligodendrocytes) organize the cell membrane of the axon into four specific functional areas.

The node of Ranvier: the axonal membrane in this region is enriched in Na^+ channels held in a molecular complex with ankyrin G and cell adhesion molecules NrCAM and neurofascin.

The paranodal region: this part of the axon lies beneath the paranodal loops of cytoplasm derived from the myelinating cell. This area is characterized by membrane-associated cell junctional proteins, such as caspr/paranodin and contactin that bind the paranodal loops of the myelinating cell to the axon. These junctions are known as the 'paranodal septate junctions'. As well as anchoring myelin loops to the axon; these specialized junctions form a diffusion barrier into the periaxonal space; and help to maintain the specialized axonal domains by preventing cell membrane diffusion.

The juxtaparanodal region: this part of the axon lies just beyond the paranodal region, with overlying compact myelin. This region has a high concentration of the delayed-rectifier K^+ channels Kv1.1, Kv1.2, which are believed to mediate repolarization together with caspr2, a second member of the caspr family.

The internodal region: this region of the axon is not specifically enriched in specialized proteins. Some proteins concentrated in the paranode and juxtaparanode, such as caspr, contactin, Kv1.1, and Kv1.2, extend into the internodal axon membrane as a narrow spiral aligned with the inner mesaxon of the myelinating cell.

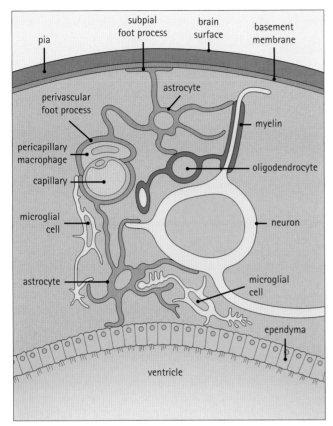

FIGURE 6.11 **Support cells of the CNS.** The support cells of the CNS are called 'glia' and have several roles. Astrocytes not only form a scaffolding for the other cells, but also extend foot processes around capillaries to maintain a blood–brain barrier. At the surface of the brain, astrocytes line a basement membrane and form the glia limitans, which surrounds the whole CNS. Oligodendrocytes myelinate the axons of the nerve cells, and a vast network of antigen-sensing microglial cells is present throughout the CNS. Phagocytic macrophages, which also have an immune defence role, reside in the perivascular space, outside the CNS substance. The ependymal cells form an epithelial sheet which, unlike other epithelia, does not lie on a basement membrane. This sheet lines the fluid-filled ventricular cavities of the brain and the central canal of the spinal cord.

One important structural adaptation of astrocytes is seen in their interaction with the blood vessels of the brain, which they surround by forming flat plates termed end feet (see Fig. 6.11). The interaction induces changes in the structure of the cerebral vascular endothelium, rendering it highly impermeable, so that it acts as a barrier to diffusion between the blood and the brain.

Oligodendrocytes are the myelin-forming cells of the CNS

Oligodendrocytes produce myelin within the CNS, each cell sending out several cell processes and myelinating several nearby axons (Fig. 6.13).

In routine histological preparations of oligodendrocytes, their branching morphology is not seen, but they do show a rounded nucleus with moderately dense-staining chromatin and, in most preparations, a cytoplasm containing a clear 'halo' around the nucleus. Such a halo is an artefact of preparation because oligodendrocytes are fragile and contain few cytoskeletal elements.

Immunohistochemical staining for myelin-related proteins, for example myelin basic protein, can be used specifically to identify oligodendrocytes (Fig. 6.13c).

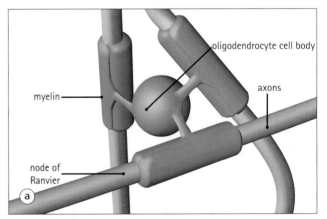

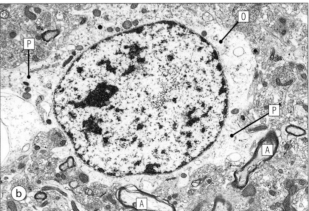

FIGURE 6.13 **Oligodendrocytes.** (a) Oligodendrocytes myelinate several adjacent axons within the CNS. (b) Ultrastructurally, the oligodendrocyte (O) has abundant mitochondria and Golgi but few cytoskeletal elements. Note processes (P) myelinating nearby axons (A).

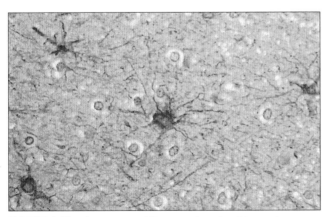

FIGURE 6.12 **Astrocytes.** Micrograph stained by an immunoperoxidase method to show glial fibrillary acidic protein (GFAP), the intermediate filament of astrocytes. The astrocyte is stained brown and shows the characteristic stellate morphology.

Continued

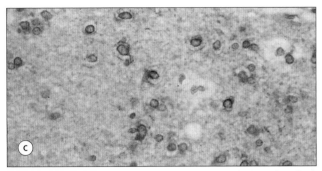

FIGURE 6.13, cont'd (c) Oligodendrocytes can be identified by immunochemical staining for specific proteins, in this instance highlighting oligodendrocytes (brown), but not other cells such as microglia or astrocytes.

CLINICAL EXAMPLE
DISEASES AFFECTING MYELIN

Multiple Sclerosis

The myelin of the CNS is the target for attack by the immune system in multiple sclerosis (Fig. 6.14), which is of unknown cause.

Myelin is vital for the CNS to function effectively, and its destruction in multiple sclerosis results in severe functional deficits, such as paralysis, loss of sensation and/or loss of coordination. The nature of the deficit depends on the area of the CNS affected.

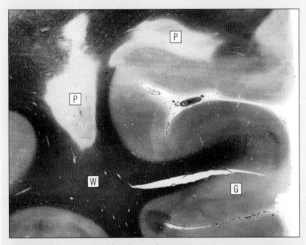

FIGURE 6.14 **Multiple sclerosis.** Low-power micrograph of cerebral cortex from a patient with MS. Tissue is stained with Luxol fast blue to demonstrate myelin in the white matter (W) while the grey matter (G) contains cell bodies and capillaries. Two pale areas, called MS plaques (P), demonstrate focal areas of myelin loss.

CLINICAL EXAMPLE
GLIOSIS

When neurons die, the dead cells are removed by macrophages, by phagocytosis. The damaged area is then repaired by proliferation of astrocytic cells, which fill the defect and form an astrocytic scar in a process termed gliosis.

CLINICAL EXAMPLE
LEUKODYSTROPHY

Several inherited diseases of metabolism result in defective production of myelin within the nervous system. Such disorders are called 'leukodystrophies'. Affected children have severe neurological deficits and progressive degeneration of myelin. Some of these diseases are due to lysosomal defects preventing normal metabolism of myelin lipids.

Ependymal cells are epithelial-like and have cilia

Ependymal cells are epithelial in type and line the cavities in the brain (ventricles) and the central canal of the spinal cord, forming a sheet of cuboidal cells in contact with the cerebrospinal fluid.

Each ependymal cell has a small oval basal nucleus with dense chromatin, and many are ciliated (Fig. 6.15).

Ultrastructurally, the cells are bound to each other by prominent desmosomal junctions and have apical microvilli in addition to cilia.

Unlike other epithelial cells, the ependymal cells do not lie on a basement membrane but have tapering processes, which merge with the processes of underlying astrocytic cells.

Microglia are specialized immune cells in the CNS

The CNS has its own unique set of immune cells, the main type being the microglial cells, which are specialized macrophages.

In conventional H&E preparations microglial cells are not easily seen, appearing only as rod-shaped nuclei, with no discernible cytoplasmic borders. Immunohistochemical staining (Fig. 6.16), however, shows that they have extensive fine ramifying processes and form a widespread network of cells throughout the brain.

The phenotype of microglia suggests that they are similar to dendritic antigen-presenting cells, having a low level of phagocytic activity and expressing class II major histocompatibility molecules.

In disease states, microglial cells become activated and increase in size and number. Under these circumstances, they are usually supplemented by monocytes, which enter the brain from the blood and form macrophagic cells.

In addition to the microglial cells, which are intrinsic to the brain, there are large numbers of macrophages in the perivascular spaces outside the brain substance, and these cells can also act as immune effector cells.

The brain appears to have only a very small traffic of lymphoid cells in the normal state.

The meninges are membrane systems covering and supporting the CNS

The CNS is invested by three protective coats, the meninges, which are composed of fibrocollagenous support

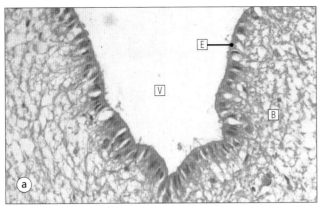

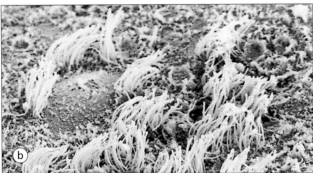

FIGURE 6.15 **Ependyma.** (a) Micrograph showing ependymal cells (E) lining the lateral ventricle (V) of the brain. They are cuboidal epithelial cells and rest on underlying glial processes in the brain (B). (b) Scanning electron micrograph showing that many of the ependymal cells bear tufts of surface cilia.

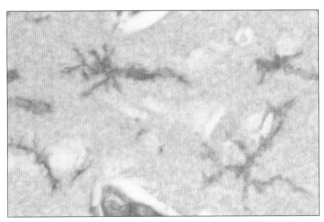

FIGURE 6.16 **Microglia.** Micrograph of brain stained by a lectin technique using Ricinus communis agglutinin, which binds to a sugar on the surface of microglial cells and endothelial cells in the brain. Microglial cells (brown) have a rod-shaped or elliptical dark-staining nucleus and a fine ramified dendritic morphology consisting of numerous extremely fine cell processes. They can also be immunocytochemically stained by many of the antisera that react with surface markers expressed by macrophages.

tissue and epithelial cells (Fig. 6.17). There are three meningeal layers: the dura, the arachnoid and the pia.

The **dura** is a tough fibrocollagenous layer, which forms the outer coat of the CNS. It blends with the periosteum of the skull and is attached to the periosteum of the vertebral canal by the dentate ligaments. It is covered on its internal surface by an incomplete layer of flat epithelial cells.

The dura is reflected down from the skull to form sheets of tissue, the tentorium cerebelli and the falx cerebri, which separate the structures of the brain. The venous sinuses of the brain run at the base of these sheets of dura.

The **arachnoid** is a layer of fibrocollagenous tissue covered by inconspicuous flat epithelial cells and is located beneath, but not anchored to, the dura. Web-like strands of fibrocollagenous tissue extend down from the arachnoid into the subarachnoid space, which contains the cerebrospinal fluid. The main arteries and veins to and from the brain run in the subarachnoid space.

The **pia** is a delicate layer of epithelial cells associated with loose fibrocollagenous delicate tissue. It lies external to a basement membrane which completely invests the CNS. This basement membrane is formed by a special set of astrocytes, termed the **limiting glia (glia limitans)**.

The choroid plexus is responsible for production of cerebrospinal fluid

The choroid plexuses are located in the ventricular system of the brain and produce cerebrospinal fluid. Each choroid plexus consists of a vascular stroma covered by columnar epithelial cells, which form large frond-like masses (Fig. 6.18). The epithelial cells are anchored by junctional complexes, rest on a basement membrane, have apical microvilli and are adapted for secretion.

The cerebrospinal fluid produced in the ventricles flows out through exit foramina at the base of the brain and circulates in the subarachnoid space. It is reabsorbed by the venous sinuses in the dura.

CLINICAL EXAMPLE
MENINGEAL SPACES IN DISEASE

There are several spaces defined by the meninges that are of clinical importance. These are the subdural space, the subarachnoid space and the extradural space.

Extradural Haematoma

Fracture of the skull can cause an accumulation of blood outside the dura in the extradural space.

Subdural Haematoma

Following trauma, bleeding may occur from venous channels into the space between the dura and the arachnoid (subdural space).

Subarachnoid Haemorrhage

Rupture of arteries running on the surface of the brain causes bleeding into the subarachnoid space between the arachnoid and the pia.

Meningitis

The cerebrospinal fluid in the subarachnoid space is the site of bacterial and occasionally viral infection in meningitis.

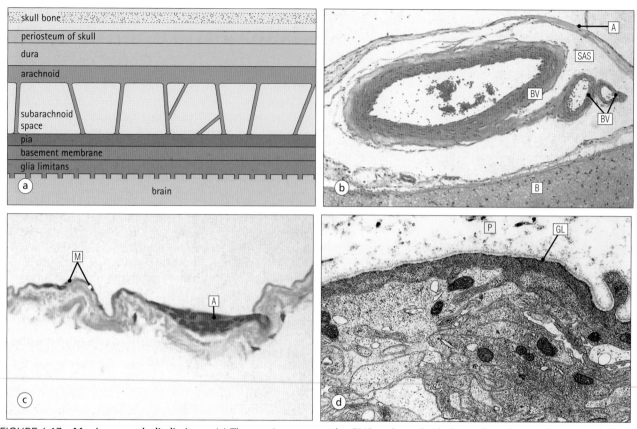

FIGURE 6.17 **Meninges and glia limitans.** (a) The meninges cover the CNS and are divided into three layers: the dura, arachnoid and pia. Below the pia, there is a basement membrane giving rise to a set of astrocytic cells, which form a barrier around the CNS, termed the 'glia limitans'. The subarachnoid space contains the cerebrospinal fluid. (b) Micrograph showing the arachnoid (A), subarachnoid space (SAS) and underlying brain (B). Blood vessels (BV) run in the subarachnoid space. (c) Meningothelial cells are normally flat, inconspicuous cells that line the dura, arachnoid and pia, but with age, some of these cells become histologically prominent; in this micrograph from the arachnoid of a 60-year-old man, the meningothelial cells (M) form a small aggregate (A). (d) Electron micrograph showing the glia limitans (GL), which forms an outer barrier investing the whole of the CNS. It is composed of a basement membrane, which is seen just beneath the pia collagen (P), and is produced by a sheet of closely adherent foot processes from astrocytic cells in the underlying brain.

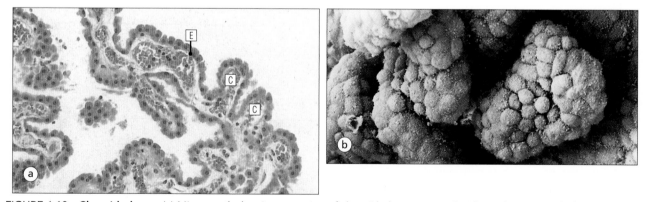

FIGURE 6.18 **Choroid plexus.** (a) Micrograph showing a portion of choroid plexus covered with a columnar epithelium (E), which is arranged as papillae over vascular stromal cores (C). (b) Scanning electron micrograph showing the convoluted surface of the choroid plexus, which is thrown into deep folds, and the fine microvilli on the apical surface of the covering epithelium.

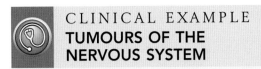

TUMOURS OF THE NERVOUS SYSTEM

Gliomas

Primary brain tumours are most commonly derived from the glial cells and are collectively termed gliomas.

The most common glioma is derived from astrocytes (astrocytoma), and varies from a slow-growing lesion, which diffusely infiltrates the brain over many years, to a rapidly growing lesion that soon compresses vital structures.

Ependymomas commonly arise in the region of the ventricles and are recognized histologically by their epithelial characteristics. Oligodendrogliomas are most common in the temporal lobe, where they may be a cause of temporal lobe epilepsy.

Certain tumours of the CNS resemble the primitive embryonic cells of the developing brain and are grouped together as primitive neuroectodermal tumours (PNET). These are commonest in childhood and may show differentiation towards neuronal, astrocytic or ependymal cells.

Meningiomas

The epithelial cells of the meninges (meningothelial cells) may form tumours termed 'meningiomas'. These tumours appear macroscopically as rounded nodules, typically 3–4 cm in size, but can be much larger. Histologically, meningiomas are made up of sheets of meningothelial cells which characteristically form spherical whorls.

Confirming the Diagnosis

The diagnosis of CNS tumours must be confirmed by histology of tumour biopsies, and immunohistochemistry is used increasingly in the laboratory to identify cell types within a tumour. Finding glial fibrillary acidic protein (GFAP) is a strong indication that a tumour is of glial origin.

Blood vessels entering the CNS are surrounded by a perivascular space

The brain is supplied with blood from major arteries that form an anastomotic link around the base of the brain. From this region, the arteries run in the subarachnoid space before turning and dipping down into the brain.

Around the large vessels within the brain is a perivascular space, called, eponymously, the **Virchow–Robin space**. In humans, this space is sealed from the subarachnoid space by reflections of the pia on to the blood vessels as they enter the brain (Fig. 6.19), and is therefore continuous with the potential subpial space.

The perivascular space is bounded externally by the basement membrane of the glia limitans (see Fig. 6.17d) and extends as far as the capillaries, where the vascular and glial basement membranes fuse.

A blood–brain barrier prevents diffusion of materials into the CNS from the blood

The microvascular system in the nervous system is highly specialized. The endothelial cells of brain capillaries are joined by occluding junctions and are not fenestrated, hence they form a barrier to the diffusion of substances from the blood to the brain. The brain endothelial cells have systems for active transport of substances, such as glucose into the brain.

External to the capillary endothelium is a basement membrane and external to this is a layer composed of the foot processes of astrocytes (see Fig. 6.11).

These three layers (endothelium, basal lamina, astrocyte foot processes) form a functional **blood–brain barrier**, which is important in the physiology of CNS function. There is considerable evidence that in embryogenesis, it is the interaction of astrocyte foot processes that is responsible for induction of the special properties of the cerebral capillary endothelial cells.

Peripheral Nervous System

The peripheral nervous system is made up of nerve cells and support cells

The peripheral nervous system is described in terms of nerves and ganglia.

A **nerve** is a collection of axons, linked together by support tissue into an anatomically defined trunk. The axons may be either motor or sensory, myelinated or non-myelinated.

A **ganglion** is a peripheral collection of nerve cell bodies together with efferent and afferent axons, and support cells. Ganglia may be sensory (e.g. spinal sensory ganglia) or contain the cell bodies of autonomic nerves (i.e. sympathetic or parasympathetic ganglia).

Peripheral nerves are bundles of axons associated with support tissues

A peripheral nerve is composed of:
- Axons
- Schwann cells, which make myelin
- Spindle-shaped fibroblast support cells, which produce fibrocollagenous tissue
- Blood vessels.

The endoneurium, perineurium and epineurium are composed of support tissues

There are three types of support tissue in a nerve trunk: the endoneurium, perineurium and epineurium (Fig. 6.20).

Endoneurium is composed of longitudinally orientated collagen fibres, extracellular matrix material rich in glycosaminoglycans, and sparse fibroblasts. It surrounds the individual axons and their associated Schwann cells, as well as capillary blood vessels.

Perineurium surrounds groups of axons and endoneurium to form small bundles (fascicles). It is composed of seven to eight concentric layers of epithelium-like flattened cells separated by layers of collagen. The cells are joined by junctional complexes, and each layer of cells is surrounded by an external lamina.

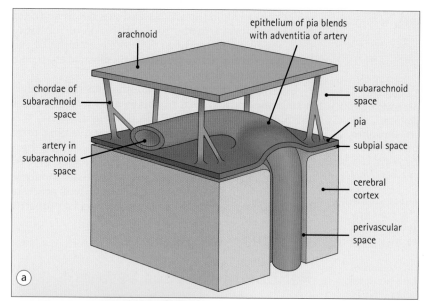

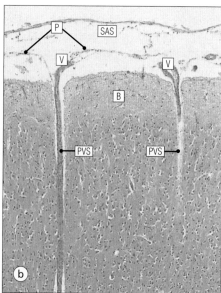

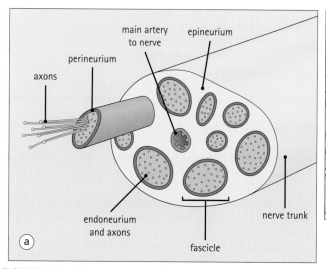

FIGURE 6.19 **Vascular arrangement in the brain.** (a) Arteries running in the subarachnoid space penetrate the pia, which is reflected up on to the wall of the vessel, thus isolating the perivascular space from the subarachnoid space. The layer of pia reflected on to the vessel is composed of a single layer of flat meningothelial cells anchored by junctional complexes. The perivascular space is continuous with the potential subpial space. (b) Micrograph showing vessels (V) penetrating the surface of the brain (B) from the subarachnoid space (SAS). The pia (P) is reflected on to the vessel wall and separates the subarachnoid space from the perivascular space (PVS). (c) Scanning electron micrograph showing the subarachnoid space (SAS) with an artery (A) becoming invested by pia (P). Note the underlying subpial space (SPS) and brain (B).

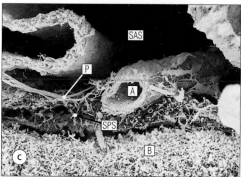

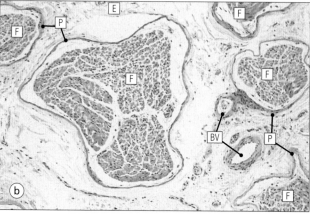

FIGURE 6.20 **Support tissue of peripheral nerve.** (a) The arrangement of support tissue in a peripheral nerve. Individual axons and their associated Schwann cells are surrounded by endoneurium and bound into fascicles by the epithelial-like perineurium. The epineurium binds individual fascicles into a nerve trunk, and may contain the main muscular artery supplying the nerve trunk. (b) Micrograph showing nerve fascicles (F) surrounded by perineurium (P) and grouped into a nerve trunk by epineurium (E). Note blood vessels (BV).

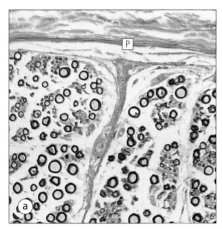

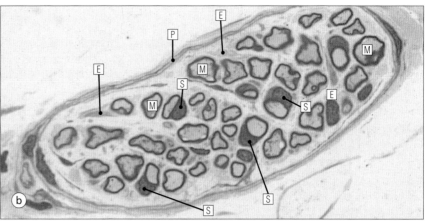

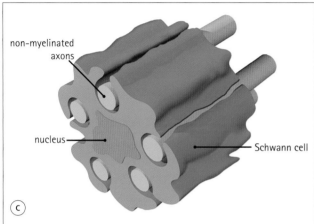

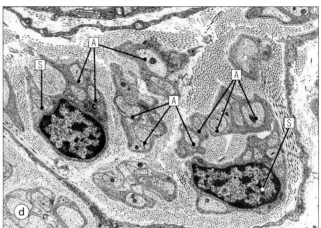

FIGURE 6.21 **Peripheral nerve.** (a) Micrograph of the edge of a single fascicle from a peripheral nerve stained with osmium, which stains myelin black. The perineurium (P) surrounds the fascicle. The myelinated axons appear as circular profiles with the central non-staining area occupied by axon. Non-myelinated fibres are not visible. (b) Micrograph of a small nerve fascicle embedded in resin and stained with toluidine blue. The increased resolution allows myelinated axons (M) to be seen with associated Schwann cell nuclei (S) and endoneurial support tissue (E). The perineurium (P) is visible as two to three thin cell and collagen layers. (c) Non-myelinated fibres are buried into and thereby supported by the cytoplasm of Schwann cells. (d) Electron micrograph showing non-myelinated axons (A) of a peripheral nerve embedded in the cytoplasm of Schwann cells (S).

Epineurium is an outer sheath of loose fibrocollagenous tissue which binds individual nerve fascicles into a nerve trunk. The epineurium may also include adipose tissue, as well as a main muscular artery supplying the nerve trunk.

Schwann cells support both myelinated and non-myelinated axons in the PNS

Within a peripheral nerve, there are both myelinated and non-myelinated axons, which are both supported by Schwann cells. Each Schwann cell has a well-defined external lamina, which separates the cell from the endoneurium.

The myelin of peripheral nerve differs from that in the CNS, as it has a different set of myelin-related proteins. Each Schwann cell produces myelin for one axon, and this contrasts with oligodendrocytes in the CNS (p. 93).

In addition to producing myelin, Schwann cells also support non-myelinated axons, which bury themselves into the Schwann cell cytoplasm (Fig. 6.21).

Nerves vary in their relative composition of myelinated and non-myelinated fibres from one anatomic site to another. Myelinated fibres in a typical peripheral nerve in the lower limb of an adult vary in diameter from 2 to 17 μm (including myelin), there being a bimodal distribution with peaks around 5 μm and 13 μm.

Ganglia are neuronal relay centres in the PNS

A ganglion is composed of:
- Neuron cell bodies
- Support cells (satellite cells and Schwann cells)
- Axons
- Loose fibrocollagenous support tissue (Fig. 6.22).

The neuron cell bodies are large; they have abundant cytoplasm containing Nissl substance and large nuclei with prominent nucleoli.

Satellite cells are small support cells resembling Schwann cells that surround the neuron cell bodies.

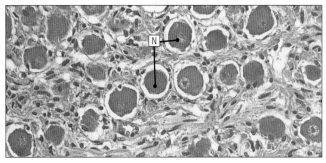

FIGURE 6.22 **Ganglion.** Micrograph showing a peripheral sensory ganglion containing neurons (N) with large nuclei and prominent nucleoli, surrounded by small darkly-stained satellite support cells. Axons running to and from the ganglion are supported by Schwann cells and a loose fibrocollagenous stroma.

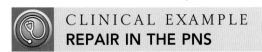

CLINICAL EXAMPLE
REPAIR IN THE PNS

The axons of neurons can regenerate following damage if the cell body remains alive.

Following section of a nerve supplying a muscle, the axons and myelin beyond the area of damage degenerate and are removed by Schwann cell lysosomes and by macrophages which migrate into the nerve. This is called Wallerian degeneration. The neuron cell body accumulates large amounts of neurofilaments, and the Nissl substance and nucleus migrate peripherally, so that it appears pale and swollen with an eccentric nucleus (chromatolysis).

The Schwann cells proliferate and form longitudinal columns of cells in the distal damaged nerve. At the proximal end the damaged axons regrow by sprouting, the sprouts growing down the cords of Schwann cells at 2–5 mm/day. One fibre may eventually connect with the muscle, become remyelinated and re-establish innervation (Fig. 6.23). The cell body then resumes a normal appearance.

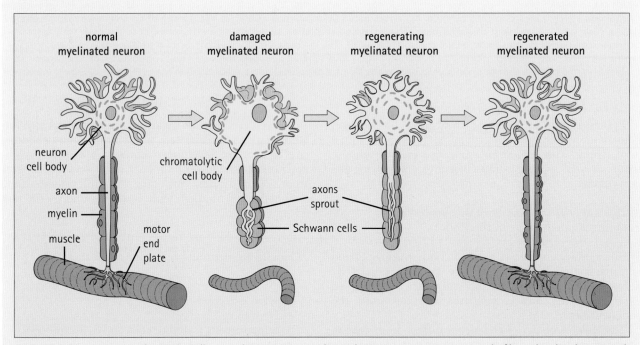

FIGURE 6.23 **Repair in the PNS.** Following damage to a myelinated neuron innervating a muscle fibre, the distal axon and myelin are phagocytosed by proliferating Schwann cells. The muscle fibre, devoid of innervation, undergoes wasting, while the cell body of the neuron undergoes chromatolysis, with swelling, lateral migration of the nucleus and loss of Nissl substance. Axons then sprout from the damaged end of the nerve and grow down the column of Schwann cells, eventually restoring innervation of the muscle. The Schwann cells remyelinate the axon, but the myelin segments are much shorter than before the damage.

PRACTICAL HISTOLOGY

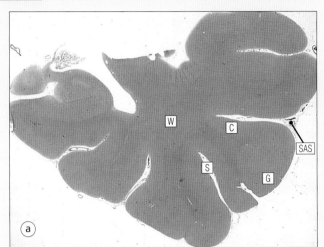

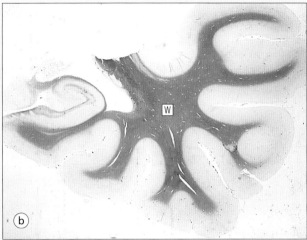

FIGURE 6.24 **Cerebral hemispheres.** (a) Micrograph of a section through the temporal lobe of the brain at low magnification. The cerebral hemisphere is thrown into a series of convolutions, the gyri (G), which are separated by intervening sulci (S). The arachnoid covers the brain and is just visible at this magnification over the subarachnoid space (SAS). The white matter (W) contains the axons of nerve cells which run to and from the cortex (C). The cortex is composed of nerve cells and does not contain myelin. In H&E preparations, the white matter stains more intensely with eosin (pink) than the cortex. (b) Micrograph of the same section shown in (a) after staining with a dye with an affinity for myelin. Such a dye delineates the white matter (W) but does not stain the cortex (grey matter).

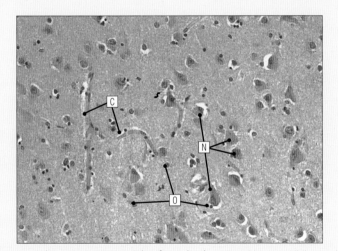

FIGURE 6.25 **Cerebral cortex.** High-power micrograph of cerebral cortex. Neurons (N) vary in size and shape according to their function, which is specific for different levels in the cortex, and in most of the cerebral cortex there are six distinct layers of different neuronal types. Capillary vessels (C) are plentiful. The small, densely-stained nuclei belong to a mixture of glial cells, of which oligodendrocytes (O) are most prominent. Cortical oligodendrocytes do not make myelin, but act as support cells for axons and neurons. The oligodendrocytes adjacent to neurons are called 'satellite cells'. The pink-stained background is a mat of neuronal and glial cell processes (neuropil).

PRACTICAL HISTOLOGY

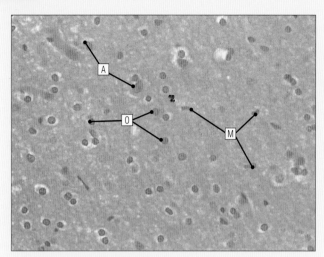

FIGURE 6.26 **White matter.** High-power micrograph of white matter, in which it is generally not possible to perceive individual nerve fibres or cell processes because they merge into the pink-staining background of the neuropil. The nuclei of glial cells are prominent but again details of the cytoplasm merge into the neuropil. Different glial types can be distinguished by the character of their nuclei. Oligodendrocytes (O) are most numerous and have rounded nuclei, which are often surrounded by an ill-defined clear perinuclear halo. Astrocytes (A) are fewer in number and are characterized by larger polygonal nuclei, which commonly contain central nucleoli. The nuclei of microglial cells (M) are frequently rod- or comma-shaped and stain more densely than those of the other glia.

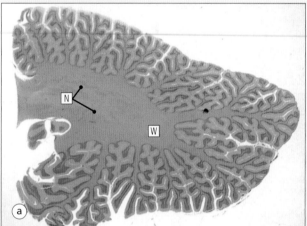

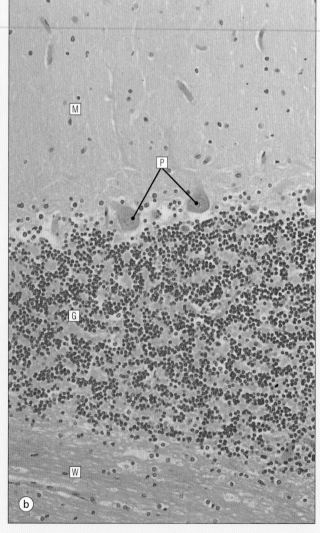

FIGURE 6.27 **Cerebellum.** (a) Micrograph of cerebellum, which is a distinct part of the brain and is characterized by complex folding of cerebellar cortex, generating a pattern of pleats (cerebellar folia). The folia contain the nuclei of nerve cells, which produce a blue-staining ribbon at this low magnification. The centre of the cerebellum is composed of white matter (W), in which a serpiginous aggregate of nerve cells, termed a 'nucleus' (N), is seen. (b) Higher-power micrograph of cerebellum showing that the outer part of the cerebellar cortex is composed of nerve cell processes with scanty glial cells (the molecular layer, M), whereas the bulk of the blue-staining ribbon is formed by a band of small nerve cells with dark-staining rounded nuclei (the granular layer, G). Below the granular layer is the white matter (W), which contains myelinated fibres. At the junction of the molecular layer with the granular layer, is a row of large nerve cells (Purkinje cells, P) characterized by a vast branching pattern of dendrites in the molecular layer, but this is only visible by special staining methods.

PRACTICAL HISTOLOGY

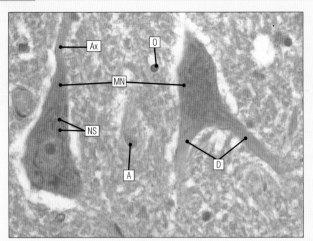

FIGURE 6.28 **Motor neurons of spinal cord.** Micrograph of spinal motor neurons (MN), which send axons (Ax) out to supply voluntary muscles and lie in the anterior part of the spinal cord. These neurons are large because they maintain an axon that may be up to 1 m long. The nucleus is large with a prominent nucleolus and the cytoplasm is packed with blue-staining Nissl substance (NS). Motor neurons make multiple connections with the axons of other neurons via large dendrites (D). The axon of a motor neuron passes out through the spinal nerve roots and eventually forms part of a peripheral nerve. The background in this micrograph is composed of a neuropil of nerve cell and glial processes and cannot be resolved with this type of preparation. The nuclei of oligodendrocytes (O) and astrocytes (A) are visible.

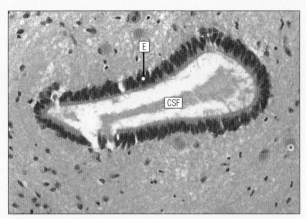

FIGURE 6.30 **Central canal of spinal cord.** Micrograph showing the central canal of the spinal cord. It is lined by ependymal cells (E) and contains cerebrospinal fluid (CSF).

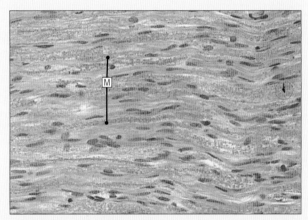

FIGURE 6.31 **Peripheral nerve.** In this micrograph of a longitudinally sectioned peripheral nerve, myelin (M) is just visible as long tapering profiles with a granular or foamy texture. The nuclei of the Schwann cells, which make the myelin, are the most conspicuous feature, and are typically long and tapering.

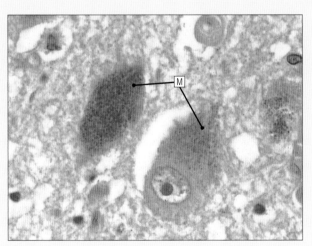

FIGURE 6.29 **Neuromelanin-containing neurons.** Micrograph of neurons containing brown neuromelanin pigment (M). Such cells are part of the substantia nigra, so named because of its black colour imparted by the melanin, and contain transmitter substance dopamine, which is responsible for coordination and fluidity of movement. Destruction of these neurons results in Parkinson's disease, which is characterized by rigid, slow movement and a tremor.

For online review questions, please visit https://studentconsult.inkling.com.

END OF CHAPTER REVIEW

True/False Answers to the MCQs, as well as Case Answers, can be Found in the Appendix in the Back of the Book.

1. **Which of the following features are seen in neurons?**
   (a) Dendrites carry signals away from the cell body
   (b) There are few lysosomes
   (c) The smooth endoplasmic reticulum is termed 'Nissl substance'
   (d) Slow anterograde transport down the axon is mediated by microtubules
   (e) The terminal bouton is located at the end of the axon

2. **Which of the following are present in a synapse?**
   (a) Synaptic vesicles are derived solely from transport down the axon
   (b) Release of neurotransmitter is mediated by voltage-sensitive calcium channels in the nerve terminal
   (c) Release of transmitter substance is via diffusion through the presynaptic membrane
   (d) The postsynaptic membrane is fused to the presynaptic membrane by cell adhesion proteins
   (e) Membrane from synaptic vesicles becomes transiently incorporated into the presynaptic membrane

3. **Which of the following features are attributable to myelin?**
   (a) Completely ensheaths myelinated axons throughout their length
   (b) Is formed by Schwann cells in the CNS
   (c) May regenerate after damage in the PNS
   (d) Reduces the conduction speed in very large diameter axons
   (e) In the PNS has a different biochemical composition to that in the CNS

4. **In the PNS which of the following are true?**
   (a) The perineurium surrounds a group of nerve fascicles
   (b) The epineurium is composed of flattened, epithelial-like cells
   (c) Axons are all myelinated
   (d) Nodes of Ranvier are areas of bare axon between segments of myelination
   (e) Ganglia contain neuronal cell bodies, axons, Schwann cells and satellite cells

CASE 6.1 POSSIBLE EPILEPTIC SEIZURE

A 52-year-old man is admitted to hospital because he has collapsed with a possible epileptic seizure. Clinical examination suggests that he has mild weakness of the right side of the body. A CT scan shows an abnormal area in the left cerebral hemisphere, which is felt to be a possible brain tumour.

Q. What cells can give rise to tumours affecting the brain?

CASE 6.2 DIABETES-RELATED NEUROPATHY

A 45-year-old patient with diabetes mellitus complains of numbness in the hands and feet. He has developed ulcers on the toes that are painless. Clinical examination shows reduced sensation to pain, touch and vibration in the hands and feet. A nerve conduction study shows a reduced speed of conduction. A diagnosis of peripheral neuropathy is made.

Q. Describe the structural elements of peripheral nerve that may have become abnormal. Given that there is a reduced nerve conduction velocity, what component is most likely to be affected?

Chapter 7

Blood Cells

Introduction

The blood is a mixture of cellular elements, fluid, proteins and metabolites

Blood has four major elements:
- **Red blood cells** (erythrocytes) transport oxygen from the lungs to the peripheral tissues
- **White blood cells** (leukocytes) have a defensive role, destroying infecting organisms, such as bacteria and viruses, as well as assisting in the removal of dead or damaged tissues
- **Platelets** (thrombocytes) are the first line of defence against damage to blood vessels, adhering to defects and participating in the blood clotting system
- **Plasma** is the proteinaceous solution in which the above-mentioned cells circulate, and carries nutrients, metabolites, antibodies, hormones, proteins of the blood clotting system and other molecules throughout the body.

In postnatal life, under normal circumstances, the formation of the cellular elements of the blood (**haemopoiesis**) occurs in the **bone marrow** in various bones (see p. 117). Most of the proteins in the plasma are made by the liver.

Bone Marrow Derived Stem Cells

The bone marrow contains at least two kinds of stem cells

One population, called 'haematopoietic stem cells' can form all of the types of blood cells in the body. These are the cells useful clinically for bone marrow transplants.

A second population is called 'bone marrow stromal stem cells' or 'mesenchymal stem cells'. These non-haematopoietic stem cells make up a small proportion of the stromal cell population in the bone marrow, and can generate bone, cartilage, fat, cells that support the formation of blood and fibrous connective tissue. These cells are under study as sources of different cell types for regenerative medicine.

Methods of Studying the Blood Cells

Blood is readily accessible by sampling with a needle and syringe. The name for the two main types of cells in blood derives from what is seen if blood is prevented from clotting and left to stand in a tube. Blood settles into several layers: a thick layer of clear plasma is seen at the top of the tube, beneath which is a very thin layer of white material on top of a thick layer of red material. The cells in the white material are called 'white cells' and the cells in the red material 'red cells'.

The usual way to look at blood is to make a very thin smear on a glass slide. The names applied to the white cells are largely derived from the stains used to examine blood smears. The main staining method used (Romanovsky stain) involves applying several dyes which have an affinity for different cellular constituents (Fig. 7.1).

Under the microscope it is possible to count the proportion of different cell types in blood and, as it has been found that this reflects disease processes, a blood count is a valuable diagnostic tool. In modern laboratory practice, routine counting of cells in blood is done electronically on preparations of cells in suspension. Smears of blood are still examined for morphological abnormalities of cells.

Red Blood Cells

Red blood cells are highly deformable and are specialized for carrying oxygen

The red blood cells are responsible for oxygen transport. Red cells in peripheral blood smears (Fig. 7.2a,b) appear as rounded, bright pink-stained cells. They are 6.5–8.5 μm in diameter and have a biconcave shape, appearing paler in the centre and darker at the periphery. The biconcave shape maximizes their surface area/volume ratio and thereby maximizes oxygen exchange. The bright pink colour (acidophilia) is due to the content of oxygen-carrying haemoglobin, which binds the acidic eosin dye used in staining. Red cells do not have a nucleus, as this is lost during formation. In paraffin-processed tissue sections, red cells appear smaller and the biconcave shape is generally not discernible.

Ultrastructurally, red cells have a cell membrane which surrounds an electron-dense cytoplasm that contains haemoglobin. There are no discernible organelles as these have been lost during differentiation. Despite a lack of organelles, red cells are metabolically active and derive energy by anaerobic metabolism of glucose, and through ATP generation by the hexose monophosphate shunt.

Functionally, red cells are highly deformable and are able to squeeze through small blood vessels down to

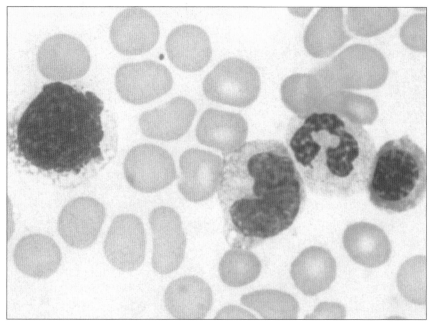

FIGURE 7.1 **Blood film.** A blood film is made by smearing a sample of peripheral blood, which has been previously mixed with an anticoagulant, on a slide and staining it with a mixture of dyes. Four white blood cells (nucleated) of various types are seen against a background of numerous smaller anucleate red blood cells.

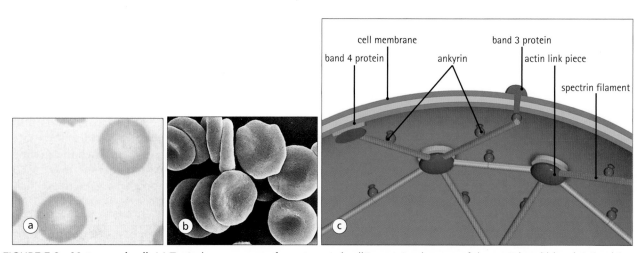

FIGURE 7.2 **Mature red cell.** (a) Typical appearance of a mature red cell in a stained smear of the peripheral blood. It is a biconcave disc 1.8 μm thick and ranges from 6.5 to 8.5 μm in diameter, the size decreasing slightly with age. Its main cytoplasmic constituent is the protein complex haemoglobin, which results in its characteristic acidophilic staining property. Because of its biconcave shape, which facilitates oxygen exchange, the centre of the cell appears pale. (b) Scanning electron micrograph showing the typical biconcave structure of a mature red cell. (c) The red cell cytoskeleton, which maintains its distinct shape. A filamentous skeleton of the protein spectrin is anchored to the cell membrane by three main proteins (band 3 protein, ankyrin and band 4 protein), with short actin pieces, about 15 actin monomers long, linking spectrin to the band 4 protein. Other proteins are also involved, but have been omitted for clarity.

3–4 μm in diameter. The cell membrane is braced by an actin/spectrin-containing cytoskeletal meshwork, which is largely responsible for maintaining the distinctive biconcave shape (Fig. 7.2c).

Red cells have a limited lifespan and are eventually destroyed in the spleen

Red cells have a lifespan of 100–120 days in the circulation. The mature red cell is unable to synthesize new enzymes to replace those lost during normal metabolic processes. Diminishing efficiency of ion pumping mechanisms is probably the main factor in red cell ageing, the cell becoming progressively less deformable until it is unable to negotiate the splenic microcirculation and is removed by phagocytosis. The spleen, liver and bone marrow all dispose of aged and defective red cells, but their relative contributions under normal conditions is uncertain; the spleen appears to be the most active.

CLINICAL EXAMPLE
HEREDITARY SPHEROCYTOSIS

Hereditary spherocytosis is caused by an abnormal arrangement of the internal cytoskeleton of red cells. Normally the internal surface of the cell membrane is braced by cytoskeletal proteins via interactions between ankyrin and spectrin (Fig. 7.2c). In hereditary spherocytosis, a defect in spectrin or the ankyrin binding of spectrin is the main underlying abnormality. As a result, the red cell membrane is not braced and is easily deformed.

In hereditary spherocytosis, red cells do not form their normal biconcave disc shape, but appear round and convex (Fig. 7.3). They are abnormally brittle and less deformable than normal red cells, and so do not pass easily through the splenic microcirculation (see Fig. 8.16). They are trapped there and rapidly destroyed in large numbers; this excessive breakdown of red blood cells is called **haemolysis**.

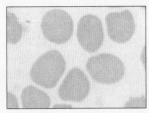

FIGURE 7.3 **Hereditary spherocytosis.** Micrograph showing the abnormal round convex blood cell of hereditary spherocytosis. Compare with Figure 7.2a.

CLINICAL EXAMPLE
ANAEMIA

The most common blood disorder is anaemia, in which an inadequate haemoglobin supply causes weakness, pallor and, sometimes, breathlessness. It may be the result of either impaired red cell formation or excessive red cell destruction.

The most common cause is **deficiency of iron**, which is essential for the formation of haemoglobin. Red cells are released into the circulation containing much less haemoglobin than normal, and are therefore pale staining (hypochromic) and small (microcytic) (Fig. 7.4).

Excessive red cell destruction usually occurs because the red cells are structurally abnormal and therefore more liable to damage while circulating. Such cells are removed prematurely and in excess by the spleen, causing **haemolytic anaemia**. This can be due to a genetic abnormality of red cell structure, and occurs in hereditary spherocytosis (see Fig. 7.3). Point mutations in the haemoglobin gene may cause abnormal red cells. Sickle cell anaemia is caused by such a mutation, leading to precipitation of haemoglobin in red cells subject to hypoxia, which causes a sickle shape instead of the biconcave disc. Sickled cells become disrupted and can also block blood vessels.

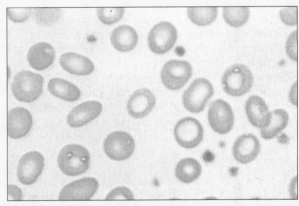

FIGURE 7.4 **Hypochromic, microcytic anaemia.** Micrograph of blood smear showing the hypochromic, microcytic red cells of iron deficiency anaemia. Compare with Figure 7.2a.

KEY FACTS
RED CELLS

- Biconcave shape for high surface area/volume ratio
- Main function is oxygen and carbon dioxide transport
- Contain haemoglobin
- Have no cell organelles
- Cell membrane is braced by an actin/spectrin-containing cytoskeleton which maintains shape.

White Blood Cells

There are five main types of white blood cells

White cells use the blood for transport from the bone marrow to their major sites of activity. The majority of the functions of white blood cells take place when they leave the circulation to enter tissues. The total number of white cells in peripheral blood is normally $4.0–11.0 \times 10^9/L$.

There are five types of white cells, and their names and relative proportions in the circulation are as follows:
- Neutrophils 40–75%
- Eosinophils 5%
- Basophils 0.5%
- Lymphocytes 20–50%
- Monocytes 1–5%.

If there is a requirement for increased activity of any one cell type in the peripheral tissues, the number and proportion of that cell type rises accordingly.

Neutrophils, eosinophils and basophils are known as **granulocytes** because their cytoplasm contains prominent granules, and may also be referred to as myeloid cells because of their origin from bone marrow. Neutrophils are also commonly called polymorphonuclear leukocytes or polymorphs because of their multilobed nucleus.

Lymphocytes and monocytes are classed as white blood cells because they are a constituent of the blood and ultimately originate from bone marrow. They are found mainly in tissues such as lymph nodes and spleen. In the tissues, monocytes transform into macrophages.

Neutrophils are the most common type of white blood cell

Neutrophils (Fig. 7.5) are the most abundant of the circulating white cells. They circulate in a resting state but, with appropriate activation, leave the blood and enter

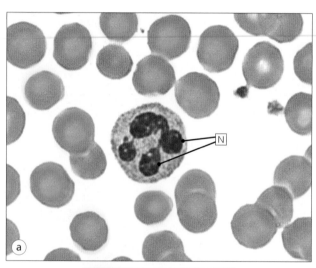

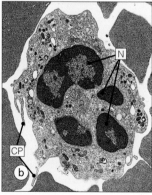

FIGURE 7.5 **Neutrophil.** (a) A mature neutrophil is 12–14 μm in diameter and has a characteristic multilobed nucleus (N) and pale-staining cytoplasm, in which only a few of the many granules it contains can be seen in a routine stain. (b) Electron micrograph of a neutrophil from the blood, showing its characteristic multilobed nucleus (N), cytoplasmic processes (CP) and a mixture of granule types within its cytoplasm. At this magnification, individual granule types cannot be identified.

tissues, where they become highly motile, phagocytic cells. Their primary function is to ingest and destroy invading microorganisms in tissues. They play a central role in the early stages of the acute inflammatory response to tissue injury and are the major constituent of pus.

There are normally $1.5–10 \times 10^9$/L neutrophils in peripheral blood; a rise to above 10×10^9/L is called **neutrophilia** and is usually an indication of bacterial infection or tissue necrosis (e.g. myocardial infarction). A reduction in numbers of circulating neutrophils below 1.5×10^9/L is called **neutropenia** or agranulocytosis; this reduction in numbers can be due to decreased production in the bone marrow or to increased destruction in the tissues. The danger of persistent neutropenia is that the patient becomes very vulnerable to severe bacterial infections.

The neutrophil nucleus has several lobes

The characteristic neutrophil nucleus is composed of 2–5 distinct lobes, joined to one another by fine strands of nuclear material, the lobulation developing with cellular maturity. The chromatin is highly condensed, reflecting a low degree of protein synthesis.

In females, about 3% of nuclei exhibit a small, condensed nuclear appendage (drumstick chromosome), which represents the quiescent X chromosome (Barr body).

ADVANCED CONCEPT

WHITE CELL TRAFFIC FROM BLOOD VESSELS IS MEDIATED BY CELL ADHESION MOLECULES

Normally, white cells circulate in the blood in an inactive state. To leave a capillary vessel and enter tissues, white cells have first to stick to the endothelium lining capillaries and then pass into the tissues by traversing the vessel wall. The adhesion to endothelium is mediated by complementary cell adhesion molecules expressed on the white cell surface and the surface of the endothelium. In the healthy state, such molecules are not strongly expressed and so there is little traffic. In disease states, cytokines cause activation of both white cells and endothelium, there is high expression of adhesion molecules, and cells stick firmly to the endothelium. Further cell signals then cause white cells to become motile and gain the ability to actively migrate into the tissues.

Neutrophils contain three types of granules

Neutrophil cytoplasm contains three types (i.e. primary, secondary and tertiary) of membrane-bound vesicles (granules) (Fig. 7.6).

Primary granules are similar to lysosomes in other cells. They are the first granules to appear during neutrophil formation, but as the cell matures, their number falls with respect to secondary granules (see below), making them difficult to see with light microscopy. With electron microscopy, they are large and electron-dense. As with lysosomes, primary granules contain acid

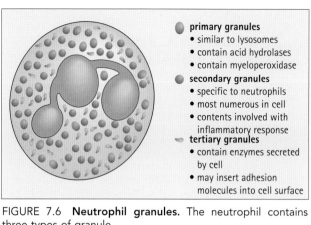

FIGURE 7.6 **Neutrophil granules.** The neutrophil contains three types of granule.

hydrolases, but in addition they also contain antibacterial and digestive substances, most notably myeloperoxidase, which can be detected by the peroxidase stain. Myelo-peroxidase is therefore a useful light microscopic marker not only for these granules, but also in establishing cell lineage in the diagnosis of leukaemias (see p. 113).

Secondary granules are specific to neutrophils and twice as numerous as primary granules. With a diameter of 0.2–0.8 μm (i.e. smaller than primary granules), they are barely visible by light microscopy.

Ultrastructural studies have shown secondary granules to be variable in size, shape and density and to contain substances involved in the mobilization of inflammatory mediators and complement activation. These substances are secreted into the extracellular environment.

Tertiary granules have only recently been described and contain enzymes (e.g. gelatinase) secreted into the extracellular environment. They also insert some glyco-proteins into cell membranes, and this may promote cellular adhesion and hence may be involved in the phagocytic process.

ADVANCED CONCEPT
NEUTROPHILS ARE ADAPTED FOR ANAEROBIC METABOLISM

The neutrophil cytoplasm contains few organelles apart from granules. There are only a few scattered profiles of rough endoplasmic reticulum and free ribosomes, with the remnants of the Golgi complex involved in granule packaging earlier in development. Although mitochondria are also few, they provide about 50% of energy needs.

Once activated, neutrophils need to be able to operate in devascularized tissue, where oxygen and glucose may be in short supply. They therefore contain abundant glycogen for anaerobic metabolism, which occurs mainly via the glycolytic pathway. Energy production may also take place via the hexose monophosphate shunt, but this is used to generate microbicidal oxidants rather than for general cellular upkeep.

Once neutrophils have become activated in tissues, they do not live for long. The neutrophil cytoplasm also contains various antioxidants to destroy potentially toxic peroxides that may be generated during lysosomal activity.

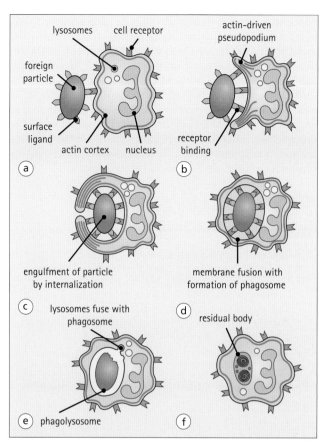

FIGURE 7.7 **Neutrophil phagocytosis.** (a) Neutrophils have membrane receptors, mainly for the Fc portion of antibodies, complement factors bound to foreign particles, and bacterial polysaccharides. Neutrophils do not phagocytose material to which they do not bind. (b) As the first step in phagocytosis the neutrophil binds to the abnormal particle by its specific recep-tors. The cell pushes out pseudopodia to surround the particle, driven by assembly and disassembly of actin filaments. (c) The pseudopodia fuse to enclose completely the abnormal particle and form an endocytotic vesicle. Special proteins probably allow final sealing of the membrane. (d) The internalized par-ticle in the endocytotic vesicle is called a 'phagosome'. (e) The phagosome fuses with neutrophil granules, particularly primary granules, which discharge their contents, exposing the particle to a potent mixture of lysosomal enzymes. If the particle is a bacterium, killing is enhanced by hydrogen peroxide and super-oxide generated by the enzymatic reduction of oxygen by respiratory burst oxidase (RBO), a membrane enzyme. (f) Foreign particle destruction is associated with the formation of a residual body containing degraded material.

Neutrophils migrate into areas of tissue damage, where they have a defensive role

Phagocytosis (Fig. 7.7) is the process whereby cells ingest extracellular particles for destruction. Neutrophils have a role in the phagocytosis of bacteria and dead cells.

To reach an area of infection or tissue damage, neu-trophils leave the circulation by adhering to endothelial cells using adhesion molecules expressed in response to local secretion of cytokines, and move through the endo-thelium and basement membrane.

Once in the extravascular tissue, neutrophils respond to chemicals (chemotaxins), moving towards the highest concentration. Chemotaxins include degradation products of complement, products leaking from dead cells, and bacterially derived polysaccharides in the extracellular space. Neutrophil motility is derived from the assembly and disassembly of cellular actin filaments.

Neutrophils typically die soon after phagocytosis, as this highly energy-dependent process uses up their glycogen reserve. When they die, their lysosomal enzymes are released into the extracellular space, causing liquefaction of adjacent tissue. The collection of dead neutrophils, tissue fluid and debris is termed 'pus'.

KEY FACTS
NEUTROPHILS

- One of the myeloid series of white blood cells
- One of the granulocyte type of white blood cells
- Main role in phagocytosis and bacterial killing
- Contains three types of granule in cytoplasm
- Cells marked by myeloperoxidase
- Increase in number in blood in bacterial infection and inflammation ('neutrophilia').

Eosinophils have a bilobed nucleus and acidophilic granules

Eosinophils have a bilobed nucleus and contain strongly eosinophilic granules (Fig. 7.8). They are phagocytic, with a particular affinity for antigen–antibody complexes, but have less microbicidal activity than neutrophils.

After production in the bone marrow, eosinophils are stored for approximately 8 days before release into the circulation, where they remain for 6–12 h before preferentially migrating to the skin, lungs and gastrointestinal tract where they reside for 1–2 weeks. They may enter lung and gut secretions via lymphatics or by direct migration.

Circulating eosinophil numbers show a marked diurnal variation, being maximal in the morning and minimal in the afternoon. They increase greatly in many types of parasitic infestation, and protection against parasitic disease appears to be one of their main functions.

Tissue (and sometimes blood) eosinophil numbers are also increased in certain allergic states, for example in the nasal and bronchial mucosae in hay fever and asthma, and in adverse reactions to drugs. Eosinophils do not usually re-enter the circulation after tissue migration.

Basophils and mast cells have common lineage and similar functions

Basophils are the least common white cell in the blood. They are characterized by large, intensely basophilic, cytoplasmic granules, and share a common lineage with tissue mast cells, with which they have many structural and functional similarities (Fig. 7.9).

The granules of basophils and mast cells contain the sulfated proteoglycans heparin and chondroitin sulfate, together with histamine and leukotriene 3.

Both basophils and mast cells have highly specific membrane receptors for the Fc segment of IgE produced

ADVANCED CONCEPT
EOSINOPHIL PHAGOCYTOSIS AND DEGRANULATION

Like neutrophils, eosinophils move chemotactically in response to bacterial products and complement components. They are preferentially attracted by substances released from mast cells, notably histamine and eosinophil chemotactic factor of anaphylaxis (ECF-A), as well as by activated lymphocytes (see Chapter 8).

All eosinophils have surface receptors for IgE (not found on neutrophils), which may be involved in the destruction of parasites. Only a few eosinophils have IgG Fc receptors, but these increase markedly in eosinophilia.

Phagocytosis involves the usual endocytotic process, but if the object is too large to be engulfed (e.g. a parasite), the eosinophil appears to release its granule contents into the external environment.

Eosinophils may function to localize the destructive effect of reactions causing secretion of mast cell granules (hypersensitivity allergic reactions) by:

- Neutralizing histamine
- Producing a factor (eosinophil-derived inhibitor) which is probably composed of prostaglandins E1 and E2, and is thought to inhibit mast cell degranulation.

Activated eosinophils inhibit vasoactive substances (e.g. leukotriene 3, formerly called 'SRS-A'), which are produced by basophils and mast cells.

in response to allergens (see Chapter 8). Exposure to allergens results in rapid exocytosis of their granules, thereby releasing histamine and other vasoactive mediators, and resulting in **an immediate hypersensitivity (anaphylactoid)** reaction. Such a reaction causes allergic rhinitis (hay fever), some forms of asthma, urticaria and anaphylaxis.

Mast cells reside in support tissues, especially those beneath epithelia, around blood vessels and lining serous cavities. They are long-lived (weeks to months) and can proliferate in the tissues. In mucosae, but not in other sites, proliferation appears to depend on interaction with T lymphocytes.

Monocytes are part of a cell network, the monocyte–macrophage system

Monocytes are the blood- and bone marrow-located precursors of the macrophages found in tissues and lymphoid organs, and are members of a single functional unit, the monocyte–macrophage system (mononuclear phagocyte system). This system consists of the bone marrow precursors (monoblasts and promonocytes), circulating monocytes and tissue macrophages, both free and fixed (histiocytes). Also included in this system are:

- Kupffer cells of the liver
- Sinus lining cells of the spleen and lymph nodes (see Chapter 8)
- Pulmonary alveolar macrophages
- Free macrophages in synovial, pleural and peritoneal fluid
- Dendritic antigen-presenting cells (see Chapter 8).

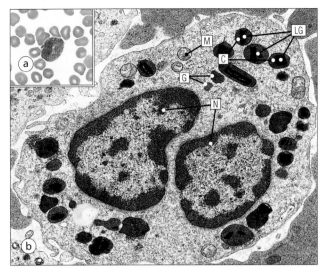

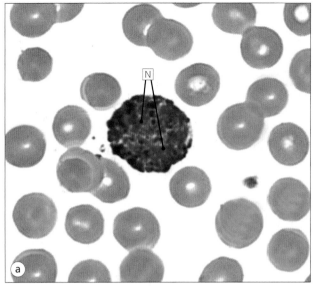

FIGURE 7.8 **Eosinophil.** (a) The eosinophil is 12–17 μm in diameter in blood films and is easily recognizable by its large granules, which stain bright red. Most have a bilobed nucleus, but nuclear detail is often obscured by the numerous overlying densely packed granules. (b) Electron micrograph of an eosinophil from blood showing its characteristic bilobed nucleus (N), scattered mitochondria (M) and cytoplasmic glycogen. The characteristic granules (LG) are large and ovoid in shape (0.15–1.5 μm long and 0.3–1.0 μm wide), and contain a central electron-dense crystalloid (C), surrounded by a less dense matrix. In humans, the crystalloid has a cubic lattice structure and consists of an extremely alkaline (basic) protein called 'major basic protein', as well as other basic proteins, hydrolytic lysosomal enzymes and peroxidase, which has a different substrate specificity from the neutrophil myeloperoxidase. Smaller granules (G) 0.1–1.5 μm in diameter are also present in mature eosinophils and contain acid phosphatase and aryl sulfatase, which is eight times more concentrated than in other white cells and appears to be secreted in the absence of phagocytosis and degranulation.

Monocytes are large motile, phagocytic cells. In blood films, they often have vacuolated cytoplasm (Fig. 7.10).

Ultrastructurally, monocyte cytoplasm contains numerous small lysosomal granules and cytoplasmic vacuoles. The granules are electron dense, homogeneous and membrane bound, and are of two types. One type represents primary lysosomes; they contain acid phosphatase, aryl sulfatase and peroxidase, and are analogous to the primary granules of neutrophils. The content of the other group of granules is less certain. Numerous small pseudopodia extend from the monocyte, reflecting its phagocytic ability and amoeboid movement.

Monocytes respond chemotactically to the presence of necrotic material, invading microorganisms and inflammation, and leave the blood to enter the tissues, where they are called macrophages.

Monocyte numbers are depressed by corticosteroid administration

Monocytes express high levels of MHC class II molecules on their surface. They are an important site for the formation of the cytokine interleukin (IL)-1, which has an important role in mediating systemic responses in acute inflammation.

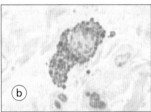

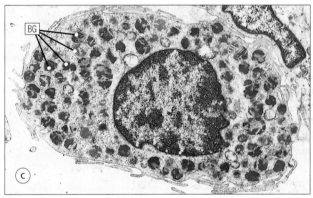

FIGURE 7.9 **Basophil and mast cell.** (a) The basophil is 14–16 μm in diameter. Its nucleus (N) is bilobed, the two lobes exhibiting marked chromatin condensation. The cytoplasmic granules are large, dark-blue staining and often obscure the nucleus. (b) Mast cells in tissues are ovoid or elongated spindle cells with a non-segmented nucleus. Their granule content imparts a diffuse purplish colour to the cytoplasm in H&E paraffin sections, unless special stains are used to demonstrate individual granules (as here). In thin resin H&E sections, the granules can be resolved by light microscopy. (c) Ultrastructurally, mast cell granules (BG) are round or oval, membrane bound, and contain dense particles and less dense matrix. There is also a small population of smaller uniform granules found near the nucleus. Mast cell cytoplasm also contains free ribosomes, mitochondria and glycogen, and the cell membrane exhibits blunt, irregularly-spaced surface projections.

Lymphocytes are responsible for generating specific immune responses

In adults and older children lymphocytes are the second most numerous white cell in the blood, their numbers increasing in response to viral infections; they are the

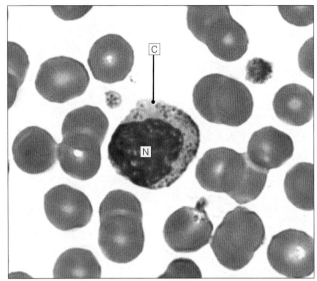

FIGURE 7.10 **Monocyte.** This monocyte is a large cell, up to 15–20 μm in diameter, with a pale-staining vacuolated cytoplasm (C), which often contains granules. The nucleus is often reniform with a distinct indentation or it can be irregular in shape as in this case, with this monocyte and an irregular nucleus (N), often with a deep indentation on one side.

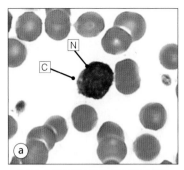

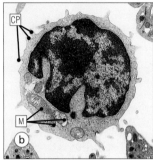

FIGURE 7.11 **Lymphocyte.** (a) In small lymphocytes, which have a diameter of 6–9 μm, the nucleus (N) occupies about 90% of the cell. The cytoplasm (C) appears only as a narrow rim and is slightly basophilic, owing to the presence of free ribosomes (RNA); rough endoplasmic reticulum is minimal. (b) Ultrastructurally, lymphocyte cell membrane shows small cytoplasmic projections (CP), which appear as short microvilli with the scanning electron microscope, and are most numerous on B lymphocytes. Cytoplasm is sparse and contains only a few mitochondria (M) and occasional aggregates of glycogen.

most numerous white cell in young children. Most circulating lymphocytes are small (Fig. 7.11), but about 3% are large, with a diameter of 9–15 μm. Their nuclei are ovoid or kidney-shaped, with the dense chromatin typical of cells with little biosynthetic activity. There are two main types of lymphocyte, termed B and T cells, which perform different but linked roles in the generation of specific immune responses (see Chapter 8).

The small mature lymphocytes circulating in the blood emigrate into tissues and into special organs of the immune system. They are responsible for immune surveillance, constantly sampling their environment for foreign material. Lymphocytes then transform into active cells, mediating the immune responses, particularly in specialized lymphoid tissues (see Chapter 8). Large lymphocytes may be seen in the blood, representing such activated lymphocytes en route to the tissues.

Plasma cells are formed from B lymphocytes and secrete immunoglobulin

Plasma cells are a differentiated form of B lymphocyte (Chapter 8) and actively synthesize immunoglobulin.

Plasma cells form a small population in normal marrow and are usually seen in support tissues and specialized lymphoid organs. In health, they are not found in the blood.

Plasma cells are large and have an eccentrically located, round or oval nucleus with the chromatin coarsely clumped in a characteristic cartwheel or clock-face pattern, reflecting active transcription.

Their cytoplasm is moderately basophilic owing to its large content of ribosomal RNA in abundant rough endoplasmic reticulum, required to manufacture the immunoglobulin protein. A well-developed Golgi complex displaces the nucleus and is visible as a paranuclear halo or pale zone (Fig. 7.12).

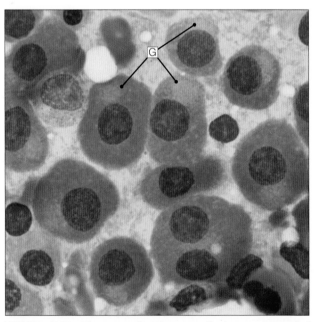

FIGURE 7.12 **Plasma cell.** Plasma cells have a rounded nucleus, with a speckled chromatin pattern and a central nucleolus, which is often likened to a clock-face. The cytoplasm is deeply purple staining, reflecting the RNA content. Note the clear, pale-stained area next to the nucleus, which is the area occupied by the Golgi complex (G).

CLINICAL EXAMPLE
WHITE BLOOD CELL ABNORMALITIES

Analysis of the peripheral blood is an important part of diagnosing disease in sick patients. Part of a full blood count lists the numbers of white cells in the peripheral blood. The number of circulating white blood cells is altered in many disease processes and changes in different cell types are associated with different diseases.

Increased numbers of white cells appear in the peripheral blood in a variety of disorders and provide a useful clue to underlying disease. For example, although in these cases the white cells are qualitatively normal, there is:

- A considerable and sustained increase of circulating neutrophils in bacterial infections (neutrophilia)
- An increase of circulating eosinophils in parasitic infestations and some allergies (eosinophilia)
- An increase in circulating lymphocytes in certain viral infections (lymphocytosis).

Reduction in the number of white blood cells can also be detected in certain conditions. Reduction in the number of circulating neutrophils (neutropenia or agranulocytosis) can be caused by:

- Disorders that damage the bone marrow, for example following infiltration and replacement by tumour or following treatment for malignancy using chemotherapy
- Increased destruction of neutrophils seen in several conditions, for example in severe sepsis, in association with some autoimmune diseases, and in diseases where the spleen is enlarged causing hypersplenism.

Reduction in the number of lymphocytes (lymphopenia) can be seen in association with some autoimmune diseases, such as systemic lupus erythematosus, in some infections, such as typhoid and brucellosis, and in association with rare inherited diseases.

The most important and life-threatening disorders of white cells are the leukaemias, in which there is a malignant proliferation of the white cell precursors in the bone marrow. This produces vast numbers of white cells and their precursors, many of which spill over into the blood.

Leukaemias are classified according to the cell line involved (i.e. granulocytic, monocytic, lymphocytic) and also according to their degree of malignancy.

In chronic leukaemias (Fig. 7.13a), the proliferating cells are partly or completely differentiated, for example myelocytes, metamyelocytes, band forms and neutrophils in granulocytic leukaemias. The diseases are slowly progressive and the residual bone marrow still produces some normal elements.

In acute leukaemias (Fig. 7.13b), the proliferating cells are often the virtually undifferentiated precursor cells, for example myeloblasts in acute granulocytic leukaemia and lymphoblasts in acute lymphoblastic leukaemia. Acute leukaemias are rapidly progressive. In this type of disease, there is failure of bone marrow resulting in reduction in formation of normal red cells, platelets and white cells. Clinical presentation is often dramatic as a result of symptoms of anaemia due to lack of red cells or bleeding due to loss of platelets.

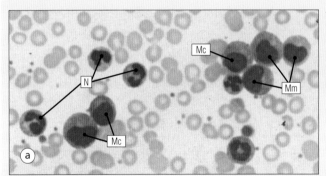 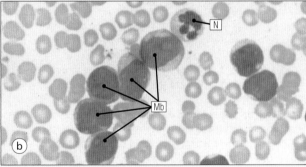

FIGURE 7.13 **Leukaemia.** (a) In this blood film from a patient with chronic granulocytic leukaemia, there are increased numbers of mature white cells, mainly neutrophils (N), as well as precursor cells, mainly myelocytes (Mc) and metamyelocytes (Mm), which have escaped from the marrow into the blood. (b) In this typical blood film from a patient with an acute granulocytic leukaemia, the malignant cells are immature granulocyte precursors, mainly myeloblasts (Mb). Very few mature neutrophils (N) are being formed.

Platelets

Platelets are small cell fragments derived from megakaryocytes and are important in haemostasis

Platelets (also called 'thrombocytes') are small, disc-shaped anuclear structures (Fig. 7.14) that are formed by the cytoplasmic fragmentation of huge precursor cells (megakaryocytes) in the bone marrow (see p. 120).

Platelets contain mitochondria, microtubules, glycogen granules, occasional Golgi elements and ribosomes, as well as enzyme systems for aerobic and anaerobic respiration. Their most conspicuous organelles, however, are their granules, of which there are three types:

- α granules are variable in size and shape and are believed to be heterogeneous in content and function. Various α granules can contain: PF4 (platelet factor 4), vWF(von Willebrand Factor),

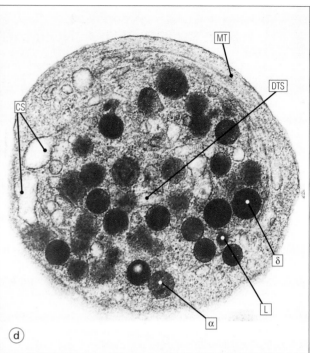

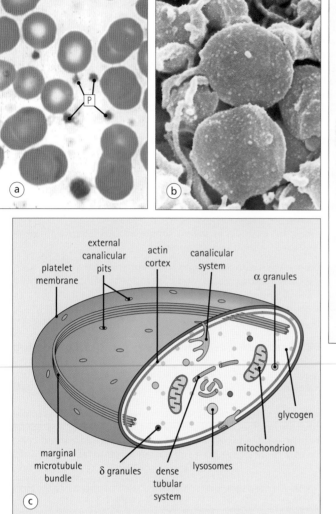

FIGURE 7.14 **Platelets.** (a) Platelets (P) are 1.5–3.5 μm in diameter in peripheral blood. (b) Scanning electron micrograph showing the smooth disc shape of an inactive platelet. The surface canalicular pores (see below) cannot be seen at this magnification. (c) Platelet structure. Platelet cell membrane, which has a prominent glycocalyx that includes cell adhesion molecules for platelet adhesion, contains many external pits which connect a system of interconnected canalicular membrane channels with the external environment. The cytoplasmic aspect of these membranes is associated with an actin cortex (see p. 27). This canalicular system secretes the contents of the α granule, whereas the contractile proteins in the actin cortex (previously called thrombosthenin), are involved in clot retraction and extrusion of granule contents. A well-developed cytoskeleton incorporates a marginal band of microtubules arranged beneath the cell periphery; these polymerize into component filaments at the onset of platelet aggregation. Deep to the marginal band of microtubules and also scattered throughout the cytoplasm is the dense tubular system (DTS), consisting of narrow membranous tubules containing a homogeneous electron-opaque substance. Although histochemical studies have shown a platelet-specific isoenzyme of peroxidase within the DTS, the function of this system is poorly understood; there is some evidence that it may be the site of prostaglandin synthesis. (d) Electron micrograph of a platelet. The circumferential band of microtubules (MT) and elements of the dense tubular system (DTS) and canalicular system (CS) can be seen, as well as a selection of granules, including α and δ granules and some lysosomes (L).

and platelet derived growth factor, fibrinogen, fibronectin, vitronectin and thrombospondin
- Dense granules (δ granules) are electron-dense and contain small molecules such as ADP, serotonin and calcium. These components are critical for platelet activation and vasoconstriction
- Lysosomes are membrane-bound vesicles containing lysosomal enzymes (e.g. cathepsins and hexosaminidase).

Platelets aggregate together and degranulate in haemostasis

Platelets are essential to normal haemostasis, undergoing aggregation in the process (Fig. 7.15).

Haemostasis is achieved by the following steps:

After loss of the lining endothelium of blood vessels, platelets adhere to exposed collagen by interacting with

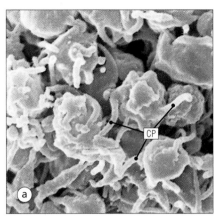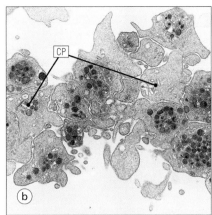

FIGURE 7.15 **Aggregating platelets.** (a) Scanning electron micrograph of platelets in the early stages of aggregation. They show extensive alteration in shape, becoming spherical. They also develop numerous long thin cytoplasmic processes (CP). Compare with Figure 7.14b. (b) Transmission electron micrograph of aggregating platelets. Note the interlinking of some cytoplasmic processes and the decrease in granule numbers in some platelets. Compare with Figure 7.14d.

glycoprotein receptors for von Willebrand Factor attached to it.

Platelet actin, myosin and microtubules cause reversible platelet moulding and adhesion along a broad surface. They then irreversibly release the contents of their granules through the canalicular system, in a secretion reaction, and synthesize thromboxane.

Thromboxane, ADP and Ca^{2+} ions mediate adhesion of other platelets. Platelet phospholipids (with Ca^{2+} ions) activate the blood clotting cascade, leading to the formation of fibrin.

CLINICAL EXAMPLE
PLATELET DISORDERS

A severe reduction in the number of platelets well below 150×10^9/L in circulating blood is called 'thrombocytopenia'. It causes spontaneous bleeding because of the failure of platelets to plug microscopic breaches in vessel walls, resulting from minor trauma.

In the skin, this manifests as a reddish-purple blotchy rash, either small blotches (purpura) or larger, bruise-like patches (ecchymoses).

Severe thrombocytopenia may be a stand-alone condition, for example idiopathic thrombocytopenic purpura. It may also be part of a wider failure of haemopoietic bone marrow, when it is associated with a reduction in the number of circulating neutrophils (neutropenia) and red cells. This may arise, for example, when normal haemopoietic marrow is suppressed by tumour invasion in acute leukaemia (see Fig. 7.13b) or caused by drugs, such as the cytotoxic drugs used in cancer therapy.

The presence of excessive numbers of circulating platelets is called 'thrombocytosis', and frequently occurs as a transient phenomenon when a general burst of bone marrow hyperactivity follows acute blood loss. A more persistent thrombocytosis occurs as a part of so-called 'myeloproliferative disorder', an uncontrolled clonal proliferation of the blood-forming cell colonies in the bone marrow. Thrombocytosis is an important predisposing factor in the development of pathological thrombosis.

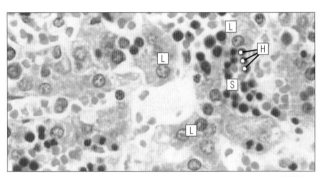

FIGURE 7.16 **Haemopoiesis in fetal liver.** Micrograph showing haemopoietic cells (H) in the sinusoidal spaces (S) between plates of liver cells (L) in a fetus.

Haemopoiesis

Blood cells are made in the bone marrow in adult life

The site of blood cell formation (haemopoiesis) changes several times during fetal development, the earliest sites being the yolk sac and then the liver (Fig. 7.16) and spleen. At 5 months, the fetal bone marrow begins to produce white cells and platelets, whereas red cell production by bone marrow starts later, at around 7 months.

At birth, the bone marrow is the main site of red cell production and almost all bones in the body are involved.

Over the next few years, with the rapid increase in bone size, the haemopoietic capacity of the bone marrow expands far beyond even emergency requirements, and so the haemopoietic bone marrow occupies less of the marrow space available. By skeletal maturity, only the marrow of the vertebrae, ribs, skull, pelvis and proximal femurs is haemopoietic, the rest having been replaced by adipose tissue, although retaining its capacity to resume haemopoiesis should the need arise.

In adult life, cell formation from the bone marrow is enough to meet normal requirements. If there is disease

ADVANCED CONCEPT
HAEMOPOIETIC PROGENITOR CELLS

The different types of progenitor cell and their relationship to each other are shown in Figure 7.17. The nomenclature that applies to stem cells refers to their ability to form differentiating colonies of committed cells in culture, termed colony-forming units (CFU), the stem cells being termed colony-forming cells (CFC).

Two main types of multipotential progenitor cell derive from the pluripotential haemopoietic stem cell:

- Lymphoid progenitor cells, which give rise to the different types of lymphocyte (B and T cell types)
- Granulocyte/erythroid/monocyte/megakaryocyte (CFU-GEMM or CFU-MIX) progenitor cells, which give rise to the main types of blood cell.

The types of committed progenitor cell derived from the multipotential CFU-GEMM (CFU-MIX) cells are:

- Erythroid (CFU-E), which give rise to red cell precursor cells
- Granulocyte/monocyte progenitor cells (CFU-GM), which give rise to granulocytes and monocytes by forming further subsets of specific progenitor cells (CFC-G and CFC-M)
- Eosinophil (CFU-Eo), which give rise to eosinophils
- Basophil (CFU-Bas), which give rise to basophils
- Megakaryocytic (CFC-Meg), which give rise to megakaryocytes (and so platelets).

of the bone marrow, such that it can no longer make adequate numbers of blood cells, then haemopoietic activity may develop once again in the liver and spleen; this is termed extramedullary haemopoiesis.

Pluripotential stem cells give rise to all of the different types of blood cells

All cellular elements of the blood originate from a common pluripotential progenitor stem cell (haemopoietic stem cell, HSC, Fig. 7.17). These pluripotential stem cells are found in very small numbers in sites of blood cell formation, and even smaller numbers can be found in the peripheral blood. Histologically, they resemble lymphocytes, but can be identified by immunohistochemical techniques as they have distinctive cell-surface antigens. The pluripotential cells divide and give rise to cells with a more restricted line of growth.

It is possible to divide blood-forming cells into four groups depending on their capacity for self-renewal, cell division and ability to form different cell types (Fig. 7.18). **Pluripotential stem cells** are capable of forming any type of blood cell; **multipotential progenitor** cells are capable of forming a specific but wide range of blood cells; **committed progenitor cells** are capable of forming only one or two types of blood cell and **maturing cells** are undergoing structural differentiation to form one cell type and so are incapable of division.

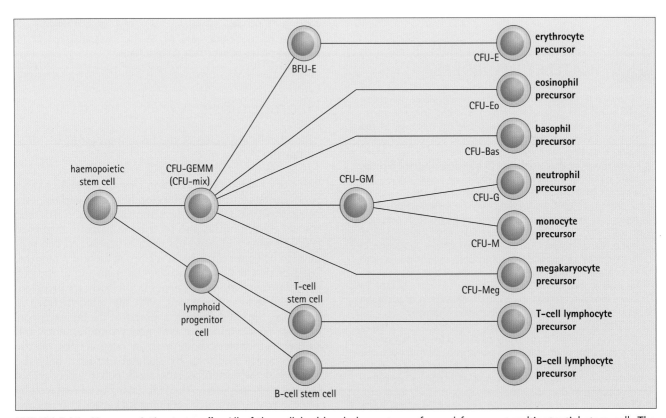

FIGURE 7.17 **Haemopoietic stem cells.** All of the cellular blood elements are formed from one multipotential stem cell. The progenitor cells are termed colony-forming units (CFU) after the ability of cells to form colonies in cell culture. Red cell precursors are capable of rapid bursts of cell growth in culture and a 'burst-forming-unit' (BFU-E) precursor can be identified.

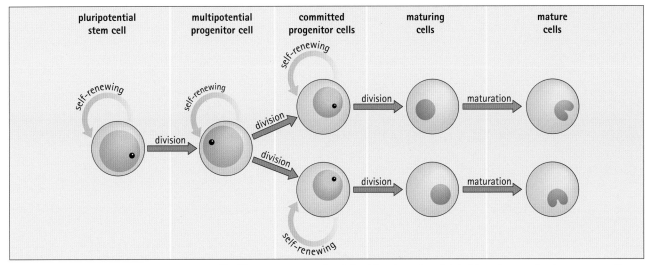

FIGURE 7.18 Haemopoietic precursor cells. The precursor cells of the blood can be divided into four main classes according to their ability to differentiate into different cell types and their capacity for self-renewal.

Growth control of blood stem cells is through secreted growth factors and local cell contacts

The best-understood mechanism of control of growth of the different types of haemopoietic stem cells is the action of growth factors. These substances are secreted systemically or locally and modulate three aspects of cell growth:

- Proliferation
- Differentiation
- Maturation.

The names and activities of the main factors are listed in Figure 7.19. It is apparent that each factor has more than one activity, some acting in synergy to promote a specific aspect of cell development. Many of these substances can now be synthesized and are being used in the treatment of diseases of the blood.

Less well understood in the control of blood cell formation is the role of local cell–cell contacts. Stromal cells in the bone marrow appear to be important in the control of differentiation and maturation; however, the signals involved are at present unknown.

Bone Marrow

The bone marrow is the main site of haemopoiesis

Bone marrow occupies the spaces between the trabeculae of medullary bone (see Chapter 13) and consists of highly branched vascular sinuses and a reticulin scaffolding, with the interstices packed with haemopoietic cells (Fig. 7.20).

In addition to its haemopoietic function, the bone marrow, along with the spleen and liver, contains fixed macrophagic cells, which remove aged and defective red cells from the circulation, by phagocytosis. It also plays a central role in the immune system, being the site of maturation of B lymphocytes, which produce antibodies (see Chapter 8).

Bone marrow has a highly developed set of vascular sinusoids

Bone marrow is supplied by medullary branches derived from the nutrient artery of the bone, which pierces the cortical bone through a nutrient canal, giving off a series of small branches to the cortical and medullary bone. This is augmented by smaller vessels from the muscle and periosteum surrounding the bone, which similarly penetrate the cortical bone. A capillary network opens into a well-developed series of thin-walled sinusoids, which empty into a large central sinus. Blood leaves the bone via the nutrient canal.

The bone marrow sinusoids are lined by flat cells (endothelial cells), which normally line blood vessels, and these lie on a discontinuous basement membrane. In places, the cytoplasm of endothelial cells is so thin that the endothelial barrier is little more than the inner and outer layers of endothelial cell membrane. Mature blood cells probably adhere to the marrow sinusoidal endothelium before being released into the circulation.

The bone marrow support cells have important roles in haemopoiesis

Outside the endothelium and basement membrane of the marrow sinusoids is a discontinuous layer of fibroblast-like support cells (reticular cells) that synthesize collagenous reticulin fibres (see Fig. 4.5), extracellular matrix materials and certain growth factors. Reticular cells have extensive branched cytoplasmic processes, which enclose well over 50% of the outer surface area of the sinusoid wall. The reticular cells also ramify throughout the haemopoietic spaces, forming a regular sponge-like matrix, a meshwork to support the haemopoietic cells.

By accumulating lipid, the reticular support cells may transform into the adipocytes found in bone marrow.

The extracellular matrix in the haemopoietic compartment contains coarse collagen fibres, as well as

Cytokine	Cells of origin	Activity
Granulocyte–macrophage colony-stimulating factor (GM-CSF)	Endothelium, macrophages, T cells	Proliferation and activation of granulocyte and monocyte precursors Proliferation of multilineage progenitor cells
Granulocyte colony-stimulating factor (G-CSF)	Monocytes, endothelium, fibroblasts	Proliferation and maturation of precursors of granulocytes
Macrophage colony-stimulating factor (M-CSF)	Endothelium, monocytes, fibroblasts, endometrium	Proliferation and activation of monocyte precursors
Stem cell factor	Marrow stromal cells, endothelial cells, fibroblasts	Proliferation of early and committed progenitor cells in synergy with other cytokines
Erythropoietin	Kidney, liver	Proliferation of erythroid and megakaryocyte precursors
IL-1	Monocytes, endothelium, fibroblasts	Induces stem cells to enter cycle Induces G-CSF, GM-CSF, M-CSF, IL-3 production Release of neutrophils from marrow
IL-2	T cells	Proliferation and activation of T cells, NK cells, monocytes
IL-3	T cells	Proliferation of early and committed haemopoietic stem cells, especially megakaryocytes
IL-5	T cells	Proliferation and activation of eosinophil and basophil precursors
IL-6	Monocytes, fibroblasts, T cells	Induces stem cell proliferation, especially megakaryocyte progenitors
IL-8	Endothelium, monocytes, fibroblasts	Neutrophil activation
IL-9	Monocytes	Proliferation of erythroid and mast cell precursors Maturation of megakaryocytes
IL-11	Fibroblasts	Proliferation of monocyte progenitors and early committed progenitor cells

FIGURE 7.19 **Growth factors involved in haemopoiesis.** IL, interleukin.

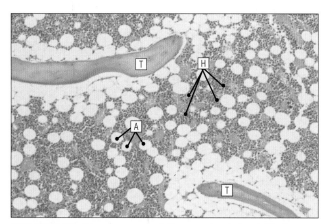

FIGURE 7.20 **Bone marrow.** Micrograph of decalcified vertebra showing haemopoietic bone marrow (H) in the spaces between the bony trabeculae (T) of the ilium. Some of the space is also occupied by adipocytes (A).

laminin and fibronectin, which facilitate adhesion of the haemopoietic cells to the marrow stroma. The associated proteoglycans, chondroitin sulfate, hyaluronic acid and heparan sulfate, may also bind growth factors, which control haemopoiesis.

There is an intimate contact between developing blood cells and stromal cells in the marrow. It is believed that such cell–cell contacts are important in the control of haemopoiesis.

Erythropoiesis is associated with the formation of distinct precursor cells termed erythroblasts

Red cells are the terminal differentiated progeny of one cell line of pluripotent bone marrow stem cells which is committed to erythropoiesis only.

CFU-GEMM (CFU-Mix) cells give rise to progenitor cells that form 'bursts' of erythroid cells in culture (BFU-E), and these give rise to cells (CFU-E) responsive to the

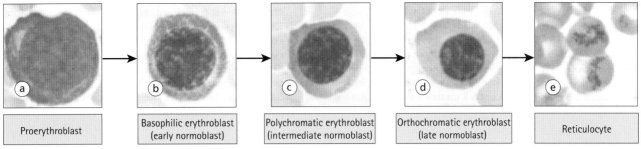

| Proerythroblast | Basophilic erythroblast (early normoblast) | Polychromatic erythroblast (intermediate normoblast) | Orthochromatic erythroblast (late normoblast) | Reticulocyte |

FIGURE 7.21 **Morphological stages in erythropoiesis.** Red blood cells constantly develop from a dividing population of erythropoietic cells in the bone marrow. Differentiation into mature red cells is associated with distinctive morphological and functional changes. A proerythroblast divides to form 8–16 cells. As seen in the micrographs, as cells mature they decrease in size from 25 µm for a proerythroblast to 10 µm for a reticulocyte. Nuclei in the dividing blast cells are large, with prominent nucleoli. With differentiation, the nucleus becomes condensed and smaller and is eventually extruded. Stippled material in reticulocytes is not nuclear material. As a red cell matures, it accumulates haemoglobin in the cytoplasm, giving increasing eosinophilia. This contrasts with dividing cells that have basophilic cytoplasm, reflecting large amounts of RNA from the protein synthetic machinery of the cell. A pale-staining perinuclear halo is the result of a Golgi apparatus. Reticulocytes mature into red cells in 24–48 h and leave the bone marrow via the sinusoids.

growth factor erythropoietin. The erythroid stem cells are few in number and cannot be identified in routine bone marrow smears. Immunochemical techniques have allowed the characterization of erythroid progenitor cells, which have large nucleoli, many polyribosomes and large mitochondria. Differentiation of these stem cells into mature red cells is associated with:

- Decreasing cell size
- Haemoglobin production
- Gradual decrease and eventual loss of all cell organelles
- Changing cytoplasmic staining, from intense basophilia due to large numbers of polyribosomes to eosinophilia due to haemoglobin
- Condensation and eventual extrusion of the nucleus.

Along the path of red cell differentiation, certain morphological cell types can be distinguished in routine marrow smears: proerythroblast, basophilic erythroblast, polychromatic erythroblast, orthochromatic erythroblast and reticulocyte (Fig. 7.21).

Red cell formation occurs in small cellular islands in the marrow

Red cells are formed in small erythroblastic islands consisting of one or two specialized macrophages surrounded by red cell progenitor cells. The macrophages have long cytoplasmic processes and deep invaginations to accommodate the dividing erythroid cells, which migrate outwards along the cytoplasmic process as they differentiate.

When mature, the red cell contacts nearby sinusoidal endothelium and passes out to enter the circulation.

Red cell production is controlled by erythropoietin

The term **erythron** describes the whole mass of mature red cells and their progenitors. It functions as a dispersed organ, the number of red cells in the circulating blood being regulated to meet oxygen-carrying needs, and the rate of red cell production varying with changing rates of their removal from the circulation.

This behaviour is mediated by a number of factors, but particularly by the growth factor **erythropoietin**, which adjusts red cell production to match oxygen demand. Erythropoietin is secreted mainly by the kidneys in adults and by the liver in the fetus.

Erythropoietin (EPO) production is stimulated by low tissue oxygen tension (e.g. hypoxia), whatever the cause; the most common stimulus is anaemia, but other causes of tissue hypoxia, such as heart or lung disease, can also increase the production of erythropoietin. Erythropoietin increases the number and proliferative activity of erythroid colony-forming units (CFU-E, see p. 116). Erythropoietin deficiency is a common feature of chronic kidney disease, leading to chronic anaemia, which can be corrected by treatment with synthetic human erythropoietin.

Certain factors are required by the bone marrow for the formation of red cells, notably iron (as a component of haemoglobin), folic acid and vitamin B_{12}. Lack of any of these factors leads to defective red cell formation and the development of anaemia (p. 107).

Granulopoiesis occurs with the formation of distinctive cell types in marrow

The formation of granulated white cells is termed 'granulopoiesis'. This takes place under the influence of cytokines. The first recognizable precursor of neutrophil formation is the myeloblast. The stages of subsequent maturation through promyelocyte, myelocyte, metamyelocyte and band cell are shown in Figure 7.22.

Maturation from myeloblast to neutrophil takes about 7–8 days and involves five cell divisions between myeloblast and metamyelocyte stages, after which no further multiplication divisions take place and chemotactic ability, complement and Fc receptors are acquired.

Structurally mature neutrophils remain in the marrow for about 5 days and are then released into the blood. After circulating for about 6 h they migrate into the peripheral tissues, where they survive for 2–5 days unless destroyed earlier as a result of their phagocytic activity.

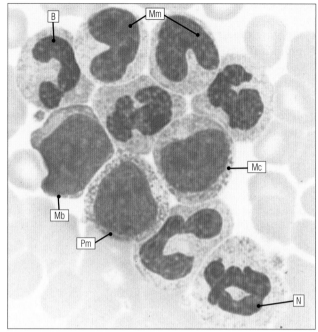

FIGURE 7.22 Morphological stages in neutrophil granulopoiesis. Micrograph showing granulocyte precursors at various stages of maturation. The myeloblast (Mb) is a large cell largely occupied by a nucleus in which nucleoli are prominent; its scanty cytoplasm contains a few granules. The promyelocyte (Pm) contains more abundant cytoplasm and more primary granules; nucleoli are still present. The myelocyte (Mc) shows early flattening or invagination of one face of the nucleus, from which the nucleoli have disappeared. Its cytoplasm contains a mixture of a few primary granules and smaller secondary granules. The metamyelocyte (Mm) shows more advanced invagination of the nucleus to a reniform shape, and a later stage, the band or stab form (B), has a horseshoe-shaped nucleus. Increasing lobation of the nucleus produces the mature neutrophil (N), which features a multilobed nucleus and abundant cytoplasm containing small secondary granules.

Increase in numbers of circulating neutrophils may occur by two mechanisms

A huge pool of stored neutrophils is maintained, loosely adherent to the sinusoidal endothelium in the bone marrow. This pool can be mobilized rapidly when there is a disease process. Stimuli cause a sudden outpouring of granulocytes from the bone marrow, leading to an increase in the number of blood neutrophils (neutrophilia, see p. 108). This mechanism copes with a sudden demand for neutrophils.

If it is necessary to maintain a high blood neutrophil count, for example during bacterial infection, there is increased proliferation of the granulocyte precursors in the marrow. This is regulated by systemic secretion of cytokines, especially IL-1, GM-CSF and G-CSF.

Eosinophil and basophil formation resembles neutrophil granulopoiesis morphologically

Eosinophils are derived from CFU-Eo progenitor cells under the influence of cytokines. Eosinophil myeloblasts resemble neutrophil myeloblasts, and there are comparable subsequent developmental stages. Eosinophils are readily distinguishable from neutrophils at the early myelocyte stage by the appearance of their larger granules, most of which are eosinophilic, but a few are initially basophilic.

Basophils are formed from CFU-B progenitor cells. Basophil myeloblasts resemble neutrophil myeloblasts; development then proceeds through analogous stages to those of neutrophils and eosinophils. Basophil granules are distinguishable at the early myelocyte stage.

Monocytes leave the marrow soon after formation, with no marrow pool

Monocytes are derived from CFC-M cells under the influence of cytokines. Two morphological monocyte precursors are recognized: the monoblast and the promonocyte. At least three cell divisions occur before the mature monocyte stage is reached. Mature monocytes leave the bone marrow soon after their formation and there is no reserve pool. They spend about 3 days in the blood before migrating into the tissues in an apparently random fashion; they are then unable to re-enter the circulation.

Lymphoid precursors migrate to peripheral lymphoid tissues

The bone marrow is the site of formation of primitive lymphocyte precursors, which subsequently give rise to both T and B lymphocytes at different sites.
- B cells undergo initial maturation in the bone marrow and move on to colonize peripheral lymphoid tissues
- T cells migrate to the thymus, where they undergo initial maturation before moving on to colonize peripheral lymphoid tissues.

Lymphoid cells are capable of division in adult life, when expansion of selected clones is desirable to mount a specific immune response. **Lymphoblasts** are recognizable dividing lymphocytes, having a large open nucleus, a prominent nucleolus and a small amount of cytoplasm. This cell division takes place in the specialized peripheral lymphoid tissues, discussed in Chapter 8.

Megakaryocytes are large multinucleate cells which give rise to the platelets

Megakaryocytes (Fig. 7.23) are the largest cells seen in bone marrow aspirates, and produce platelets by cytoplasmic fragmentation.

The precursor of the megakaryocyte in bone marrow is the megakaryoblast, which duplicates its nuclear and cytoplasmic constituents up to seven times without cell division, each causing increased ploidy, nuclear lobulation and cell size.

Cytoplasmic maturation involves the elaboration of granules, vesicles and demarcation membranes (see below), and progressive loss of free ribosomes and rough endoplasmic reticulum.

Megakaryocyte cytoplasm is divided into three zones. First, the perinuclear zone contains the Golgi and

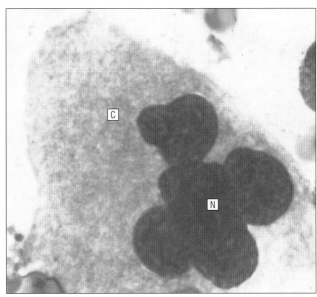

FIGURE 7.23 **Megakaryocyte.** Megakaryocytes are huge polyploid cells 30–100 μm in diameter with a large irregular, multilobular nucleus (N), which contains dispersed chromatin and is devoid of nucleoli. Their extensive cytoplasm (C) is filled with fine basophilic granules, reflecting their profusion of cytoplasmic organelles. With light microscopy the cell margin is often difficult to define clearly, owing to the presence of numerous disaggregating platelets, cytoplasmic processes, ruffles and blebs.

associated vesicles, rough and smooth endoplasmic reticulum, developing granules, centrioles and spindle tubules. It remains attached to the nucleus after platelet shedding. Second, the intermediate zone contains an extensive system of interconnected vesicles and tubules (the demarcation membrane system, DMS), which is in continuity with the cell membrane and has the function of delineating developing platelet fields (i.e. potential platelets) which, like platelets, are uneven in size. Finally, the marginal zone is filled with cytoskeletal filaments and traversed by membranes connecting with the DMS.

 For online review questions, please visit https://studentconsult.inkling.com.

END OF CHAPTER REVIEW

True/False Answers to the MCQs, as Well as Case Answers, Can be Found in the Appendix in the Back of the Book.

1. **Which of the following features are seen in red blood cells?**
   (a) A biconcave shape which maximizes the surface/volume ratio for gas transfer in capillary vessels
   (b) No mitochondria
   (c) A membrane-associated cytoskeleton which maintains their shape
   (d) A lifespan in peripheral blood of about 20 days
   (e) They are removed, when aged, by cells in the spleen

2. **Neutrophils have which of the following features?**
   (a) A regular, spherical nucleus
   (b) Perform their main functions in the peripheral blood
   (c) Contain the enzyme myeloperoxidase, which is important for bacterial killing
   (d) Express cell adhesion molecules on their surface to allow them to adhere to endothelium prior to emigration into tissues
   (e) Receptors on their surface which recognize foreign material for internalization by phagocytosis

3. **Which of the following are specialized roles of white blood cells?**
   (a) Basophils emigrate into tissues and form plasma cells
   (b) Monocytes emigrate into tissues and form macrophages
   (c) Lymphocytes of certain types can secrete immunoglobulin
   (d) Eosinophils are increased in number in the tissues and blood in allergic reactions
   (e) Neutrophils have a long half-life of about 30 days once they are activated and have entered tissues

Continued

4. Which of the following is true regarding the blood cells generated by haemopoiesis?

(a) All blood cells derive from a common haemopoietic stem cell

(b) Both granulocytes and monocytes derive from a common committed progenitor cell

(c) Each of the cytokines that control and modulate haemopoiesis acts very specifically on one cell line

(d) Platelets are formed from myeloid cells

(e) Committed progenitor cells are not self-renewing

CASE 7.1   A MAN WHO WAS TIRED AND WEAK

A 62-year-old man is admitted to hospital for investigation. He had gone to his family physician feeling generally unwell and tired. A full blood count had shown a greatly reduced red cell count together with a reduction in the number of circulating white cells and platelets. Red cells were of normal size (normocytic) and contained normal amounts of haemoglobin (normochromic).

The neutrophil count was 0.5×10^9/L

The platelet count was 20×10^9/L

A diagnosis of pancytopenia was made and further investigations were performed. A biopsy of the bone marrow was taken and showed a low cellularity affecting all precursors. A diagnosis of aplastic anaemia was made.

Q. Describe the structural and histological background to this case. Concentrate on describing the normal formation of the cells in the blood and describe the functional complications that may be expected from disease.

Chapter 8

Immune System

Introduction

The immune system is part of an array of defence systems used to combat disease

The body must constantly protect itself from invasion by a variety of living organisms and other foreign bodies, which may gain entry via the skin, gut, respiratory tract and other routes. This protection is provided by the following two basic mechanisms:

- Innate immunity
- Adaptive immune response.

Innate immunity involves the non-specific mechanisms of surface protection (barrier functions), such as provided by keratin in the skin, mucus in the respiratory and alimentary tracts and by an acid environment in the vagina.

The innate immune response is a non-specific process that proceeds in the same way, whatever the initiating factor. Foreign agents are destroyed or neutralized by complement, interferon, cytokines, natural killer cells, neutrophils and macrophages.

In contrast, the adaptive immune response is highly specific and targeted to compounds on invading organisms or foreign particles.

Lymphocytes are one of the most important cells in the adaptive immune response

The immune response is served by specialized tissues and cells which form the immune system. This system depends on the recognition of exogenous materials as foreign to the body: any foreign substance so recognized is known as an **antigen**. Such recognition then activates the immune system to neutralize or destroy the antigen, with **lymphocytes** playing the central role. The immune response is highly antigen specific, but may employ the phagocytic cells of the non-specific tissue defence system (see p. 107) in initial antigen presentation or to effect final antigen destruction.

The two main types of immune response are termed cell-mediated and humoral

The immune response is served by several types of cells acting synergistically. Exogenous agents (commonly microorganisms) are first recognized by **antigen-presenting cells** (APC), which constantly patrol their local environment and are similar to macrophages. The exogenous agents are broken down within the APC into key components. These act as antigens, which are then presented to specialized effector cells (lymphocytes). Lymphocytes recognize the foreign antigens by specifically binding to them. Such lymphocytes then proliferate and are able to mount an immune response, which may be one of two main types:

- **Cell-mediated immunity** – characterized by the joint action of lymphocytes and macrophages to destroy or neutralize the foreign agent
- **Humoral immunity** – characterized by the secretion of proteins (antibodies) by one type of lymphocyte. Antibodies neutralize foreign agents by specifically binding to the antigen (see Key Facts box, below).

These two systems usually work together in the elimination of a foreign agent.

Whereas the immune response occurs in all body tissues, the growth, maintenance and programming of immune cells takes place preferentially in the lymph nodes, spleen, thymus gland and bone marrow, which are the special organs of the immune system.

Different cells of the immune system can be identified by characteristic markers

Many markers are cell-surface receptors or their ligands and have roles in signalling or cell adhesion. The many cytoplasmic and cell membrane proteins that characterize cells of the immune system have been given names according to an international system, which relates them to proteins (antigens) expressed at different phases of cell maturation. These are called 'CD (cluster designation) molecules' (Fig. 8.1). Antibodies to the different CD molecules can be used to identify specific subtypes of lymphoid cell using immunohistochemical staining.

CD molecules can be considered in three main groups:

- Markers which are expressed by a cell line throughout its life
- Markers which are expressed transiently during one phase of differentiation
- Markers which are expressed when cells are activated.

KEY FACTS
ANTIBODIES

- Are synthesized by B lymphocytes (as plasma cells) and bind to specific antigens
- Are also known as immunoglobulins, and fall into five different structural classes: IgG, IgA, IgD, IgM and IgE
- Have two main components, immunoglobulin light chain (κ or λ) and immunoglobulin heavy chains (γ, α, δ, μ or ε)
- Have heavy and light chains with highly variable regions (antigen-binding sites) and constant regions, which form the main part of the molecules
- May circulate in the blood and body fluids or remain bound to the B lymphocyte surface, where they activate the B cell on meeting the appropriate antigen

Lymphocytes

The three main types of lymphocyte are termed 'B cells', 'T cells' and 'natural killer (NK) cells'.

B cells turn into plasma cells and secrete antibodies

B lymphocytes (B cells) are mainly concentrated within the specialized lymphoid organs. They also circulate in the peripheral blood – accounting for between 5% and 15% of blood lymphocytes – and migrate through body tissues. Thus, the constant movement of this type of lymphoid cell means they are readily available for immune defence. When stimulated by an appropriate antigen, B cells undergo proliferation and convert into plasma cells, which then secrete specific proteins called immunoglobulins. B cells, plasma cells and antibodies in the blood and body fluids are the basis of the **humoral response**.

ADVANCED CONCEPT

CD	Function/identity	Expression
CD1	class I-like glycoprotein	cortical thymocytes, Langerhans' cells, some B cells
CD2	LFA-3 receptor	T cells, some NK cells
CD3	T-cell receptor complex	T cells
CD4	MHC class II receptor	some T cells (T helper), monocytes
CD5	scavenger receptor	T cells and some B cells
CD8	MHC-class I receptor	some T cells (T cytotoxic)
CD10	CALLA	pre-B cells
CD16	FcγRIIIA	NK cells and monocytes
CD19		B cells
CD20	L26	B cells
CD21	CR2, C3d receptor	mature B cells
CD22	BL-CAM	B cells
CD35	CR1	B cells, monocytes
CD40	cell signalling	B cells
CD45	leukocyte common antigen	lymphocytes, granulocytes, macrophages
CD45RA	restricted leukocyte common antigen	T$_S$ cells, monocytes, B cells
CD45RO	restricted leukocyte common antigen	T$_H$ cells, monocytes, B cells
CD56	NCAM	NK cells
CD79a	Igα	B cells
CD79b	Igβ	B cells

FIGURE 8.1 **CD markers.** The most common CD markers in routine diagnostic laboratory use.

All developing B cells have common genes coding for the production of immunoglobulins. At this stage they are called 'germline' B cells. During B-cell maturation, and after antigen stimulation, these genes undergo rearrangement to produce different unique immunoglobulin proteins, which can specifically interact with antigen. In this way, the diversity of the humoral immune response is generated. Cells that produce an immunoglobulin recognizing a normal body (self) antigen are eliminated during development. Some activated cells become dormant and remain as so-called 'memory cells'. These can rapidly proliferate on repeated encounter with the same antigen.

B cells originate in haemopoietic tissues and later colonize lymphoid tissues

B cells mature from small inactive cells to large immunoglobulin-secreting cells. Their cytological appearance varies according to their activity.

Originating in the haemopoietic tissues of the liver and bone marrow, B cells develop from lymphoid stem cells. They leave their site of development and populate specialized lymphoid tissues (lymph nodes, spleen and gut mucosa in particular). In birds, B cells develop in a structure called the 'bursa of Fabricius', hence the origin of the term B (bursal) cell.

Inactive B cells are small cells, 6–8 μm in diameter, with barely discernible cytoplasm. The nucleus is rounded with compact chromatin, reflecting a lack of DNA transcription.

When B cells become activated and proliferate, they develop large nuclei with prominent nucleoli and moderate amounts of cytoplasm. These cells are termed **lymphoblasts**, **centroblasts** and **immunoblasts**.

The fully differentiated immunoglobulin-secreting B cell is termed a 'plasma cell', and has cytological features that reflect its function as a protein-secreting cell (see Fig. 7.12). The cytoplasm is basophilic because of a high content of rough endoplasmic reticulum, and there is a clear area near the nucleus corresponding to the Golgi complex. The nucleus has an open chromatin pattern, said to resemble a clock-face, and a large central nucleolus.

T cells are responsible for cell-mediated immunity

T lymphocytes (T cells) are found concentrated within the specialized lymphoid organs but they also circulate in the peripheral blood and migrate through body tissues.

When stimulated by an appropriate antigen, T cells undergo proliferation. They become able to direct and recruit other cells of the immune system, as well as attacking diseased cells directly. T cells have cell-surface receptors, which recognize specific antigen in a similar way to that of antibodies. Activated T cells also secrete cytokines (lymphokines) (Fig. 8.2).

T cells, T-cell receptors and cytokines are the basis of the **cell-mediated immune response** as well as being essential for organizing many aspects of the humoral response.

The T-cell receptor proteins are assembled with proteins of CD3 to form a complex which sits on the T-cell surface (T-cell receptor complex). During maturation, genetic mechanisms (somatic mutation and T-cell receptor gene rearrangement) generate the diversity of T cells needed to respond to different antigens. Cells that recognize a normal body (self) antigen are eliminated during development.

T cells can be divided into two types depending upon the type of antigen receptor

All developing T cells have common genes coding for the production of T-cell receptor proteins. At this stage, they are called 'germline T cells'. The T-cell receptors have variable regions which, like antibodies, can bind to different antigens. The receptors are assembled as pairs (dimers) of antigen-binding peptides. There are two types of resulting T-cell receptor (TCR), termed 'TCR-1' and 'TCR-2':
- TCR-2$^+$ cells express α and β chains together (αβ T-cell receptor) and account for about 90% of lymphocytes in the blood
- TCR-1$^+$ cells express γ and δ chains together (γδ T-cell receptor) and account for about 10% of lymphocytes in the blood.

TCR-1$^+$ cells are present in large numbers in mucosal tissues.

T cells undergo maturation in the thymus gland

T cells originate from stem cells in the haemopoietic tissues of the liver and bone marrow and are so named because they undergo maturation in the thymus gland.

Cytokine	Cells of origin	Activity
granulocyte–macrophage colony-stimulating factor (GM-CSF)	endothelium, macrophages, T cell precursors	proliferation and activation of granulocyte and monocyte proliferation of multilineage progenitor cells
granulocyte colony-stimulating factor (G-CSF)	monocytes, endothelium, fibroblasts	proliferation and maturation of precursors of granulocytes
macrophage colony-stimulating factor (M-CSF)	endothelium, monocytes, fibroblasts, endometrium	proliferation and activation of monocyte precursors
stem cell factor	marrow stromal cells, endothelial cells, fibroblasts	proliferation of early and committed progenitor cells in synergy with other cytokines
erythropoietin	kidney, liver	proliferation of erythroid and megakaryocyte precursors
IL-1	monocytes, endothelium, fibroblasts	induces stem cells to enter cycle induces G-CSF, GM-CSF, M-CSF, IL-3 production release of neutrophils from marrow
IL-2	T cells	proliferation and activation of T cells, NK cells, monocytes
IL-3	T cells	proliferation of early and committed haemopoietic stem cells, especially megakaryocytes
IL-5	T cells	proliferation and activation of eosinophil and basophil precursors
IL-6	monocytes, fibroblasts, T cells	induces stem cell proliferation, especially megakaryocyte progenitors
IL-8	endothelium, monocytes, fibroblasts	neutrophil activation
IL-9	monocytes	proliferation of erythroid and mast cell precursors maturation of megakaryocytes
IL-11	fibroblasts	proliferation of monocyte progenitors and early committed progenitor cells

FIGURE 8.2 **Cytokines.** A major function of T cells is to synthesize proteins called 'cytokines' (lymphokines), which mediate interactions between cells. Cytokines, however, are not unique to lymphoid cells and are secreted by other cell types to influence the growth and differentiation of cells (IL, interleukin).

From the thymus gland, T cells leave to populate specialized lymphoid tissues (lymph nodes, spleen and gut mucosa, in particular).

T cells have a varied morphology

The histological appearance of T cells depends on their activity.

Inactive T cells can be of two morphological types. The most common form in peripheral blood, accounting for between 60% and 90%, is called a **small lymphocyte**. This is 6–7 μm in diameter, with barely discernible cytoplasm and a rounded nucleus with compact chromatin (see Fig. 7.11a). The second type of inactive T cell is called a **large granular lymphocyte** (Fig. 8.3). These cells are 7–10 μm in diameter; they have a moderate amount of cytoplasm, which contains small numbers of granules that stain with azure dyes (**azurophilic granules**).

T cells that have been stimulated to divide as part of an immune response are larger than the inactive cells and have a moderate amount of basophilic cytoplasm. The nucleus is large, with a convoluted appearance (in contrast to that of B cells) and an open vesicular

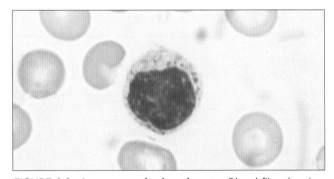

FIGURE 8.3 **Large granular lymphocyte.** Blood film showing a large granular lymphocyte. Note that the nucleus is larger than in a small lymphocyte and that there is a moderate amount of cytoplasm with small numbers of pink-staining (azurophilic) granules.

chromatin pattern and a visible nucleolus, reflecting gene transcription.

Lymphokine-secreting activated T cells have basophilic cytoplasm owing to their high content of rough endoplasmic reticulum (ER), and a large nucleus with a convoluted contour.

The three functional subsets of T lymphocyte are termed helper, cytotoxic and suppressor types

There are several subsets of T cells, which can be defined by their expression of specific markers and their functional activity. TCR-2$^+$ cells can be divided into three groups:

- Helper T cells or Th cells
- Cytotoxic T cells or Tc cells
- T suppressor cells or Ts cells.

Th cells, which express the CD4 molecule, help other lymphocytes perform their effector functions. Their assistance is necessary to induce B cells to produce antibody and to activate macrophage defence systems. This type of cell recognizes antigen when it is presented on cells that also express class II major histocompatibility complex (MHC) molecules.

Tc cells, which express CD8 molecule, are able to kill target cells. This type of cell recognizes antigens when presented on cells in association with class I MHC molecules.

Ts cells, which express either CD8 or CD4 molecules, are capable of inhibiting the response to Th cells and thus modulate the immune response.

TCR-1$^+$ cells generally do not express CD4 or CD8, although some may express CD8. These types of lymphocyte are particularly abundant in mucosal-associated lymphoid tissues (MALT, p. 140) and generally have cytotoxic functions. The relationships between these forms of T cell are shown in Figure 8.4.

Natural killer cells are activated to become cytotoxic lymphocytes

NK cells are the third main type of lymphocyte and in the peripheral blood have the morphology of large granular lymphocytes (see Fig. 8.3). As well as forming a population in the blood, they are also present in the spleen. This type of cell is capable of activation by interleukin (IL)-2, as it carries an IL-2 receptor and has the ability to kill other cells (**cell-mediated cytotoxicity**). The main role of this type of cell is in the elimination of virus-infected cells and some tumour cells. When activated, NK cells may also release cytokines, such as IL-1 and GM-CSF, to modulate other immune responses.

CLINICAL EXAMPLE
HIV INFECTION AND THE IMMUNE SYSTEM

The virus that causes the acquired immune deficiency syndrome (AIDS), HIV-1, gains entry to cells by using the CD4 surface protein as a receptor. One of the most important markers of progression in HIV infection is reduction in the number of CD4+ cells in the blood.

NK cells can be recognized by immunochemical techniques, as they do not express CD3 (part of the T-cell receptor complex). However, they do express CD16 (a surface receptor involved in activation) and CD56 (a cell adhesion molecule). Many NK cells express CD2.

ADVANCED CONCEPT
HELPER T CELLS

Subtypes of Th cell have been identified according to the cytokines they secrete.

- ThP cells are unstimulated and secrete IL-2
- Th0 cells are cells that have just been stimulated by antigen and secrete IL-2, IL-4, IL-10 and IFN-γ
- Th1 cells secrete IL-2, IL-3, granulocyte–macrophage colony-stimulating factor (GM-CSF) and IFN-γ
- Th2 cells secrete IL-3, IL-4, IL-10 and GM-CSF
- ThM cells are inactive memory cells that secrete IL-2
- The Th cell population can also be divided into two subtypes based on the expression of different CD molecules
- A subtype that promotes the activity of both T cells and B cells expresses CD29 and CD45RO
- A subtype that induces CD8 cells to become suppressor/cytotoxic cells expresses CD45RA.

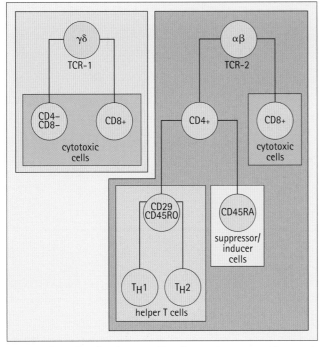

FIGURE 8.4 **T-cell subtypes.** T cells may be grouped according to their T-cell receptor into TCR-1 and TCR-2 types. Cytotoxic cells, helper cells and suppressor cells are associated with the expression of other surface markers.

ADVANCED CONCEPT
CYTOTOXIC LYMPHOCYTES

Cytotoxic lymphocytes may be artificially stimulated to enhance their activity. When lymphocytes from blood or spleen are incubated in vitro with IL-2, a population of cells develops with enhanced cellular cytotoxicity. These are termed lymphokine-activated killer cells or LAK cells. They are believed to develop from large granular lymphocytes, which are a mixture of TCR-1⁺, TCR-2⁺ and CD8+ cells and NK cells. This technique of enhancing immune function is being tested in patients with cancer. Patients' own blood lymphocytes are cultured with IL-2 and then returned to the bloodstream in the hope that the host will develop immunity to the disease and the LAK cells will kill cancer cells.

KEY FACTS
LYMPHOCYTES

- There are three main types: T cells, B cells and NK cells
- There are two morphological types of inactive lymphocyte: small lymphocytes and large granular lymphocytes
- The different types of lymphoid cell are identified using immunochemical techniques to detect specific markers
- B cells mature into plasma cells and secrete immunoglobulin
- T cells have several roles as cytotoxic cells, helper cells and suppressor cells
- NK cells have a primary cytotoxic role.

Macrophages and Dendritic Cells

Macrophages and dendritic cells are part of the mononuclear phagocyte system

Macrophages and dendritic cells are derived from monocytes (see p. 110) which become resident in tissues where they may assume a variety of morphological appearances, as they differentiate to serve specialized roles:
- They may form a population of cells adapted mainly for phagocytosis (fixed tissue macrophages or histiocytes)
- They may be stimulated by T cells to secrete cytokines that control local cellular immune responses
- They may form specialized immune surveillance cells (i.e. dendritic antigen-presenting cells, APC).

The cells adapted mainly for phagocytosis remove or store material by assuming a rounded morphology with short broad pseudopodia. They contain large numbers of lysosomes (Fig. 2.17).

Secretory-type macrophages are large cells with voluminous pink-staining cytoplasm due to expansion of the Golgi complex and smooth ER. They are seldom seen in normal tissues, but are important in T cell-mediated immune responses, when they are termed **epithelioid**

cells because of their superficial resemblance to epithelial cells.

APC are characterized by elongated ramified cell processes and a low content of lysosomal enzymes.

Fixed tissue macrophages, secretory macrophages, epithelioid cells and APC are often grouped together with blood monocytes to form the **mononuclear phagocytic** system.

Macrophagic cells are widely distributed in most tissues

The morphology of macrophages is variable according to their site and function.

Macrophages are an important component of the specialized organs of the immune system. They are also particularly abundant in loose fibrocollagenous support tissue, which is found in most parts of the body (see Fig. 8.5).

Specialized macrophages are seen in the lung (alveolar macrophages, see p. 178), liver (Kupffer cells, see Fig. 12.3), brain (microglial cells, see Fig. 6.16) and skin (Langerhans' cells, see Fig. 18.9).

Most antigen-presenting cells are a special form of macrophage

APC phagocytose antigenic material, process it and present the fragments to lymphocytes.

Most APC are monocyte derived and express markers of white cell lineage (leukocyte common antigen). Some non-monocyte derived cells also function as antigen-presenting cells, for example the follicular dendritic cells of lymph nodes.

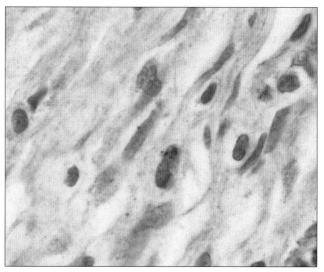

FIGURE 8.5 **Macrophages.** Macrophages are particularly abundant in the loose fibrocollagenous support tissue found in most organs. In this site they are adapted for major phagocytic activity, which is reflected in their high lysosome content. In H&E sections, normal macrophages are inconspicuous, but they may be detected by histochemical staining for acid phosphatase or immunochemical staining for lysosomal enzymes, as here.

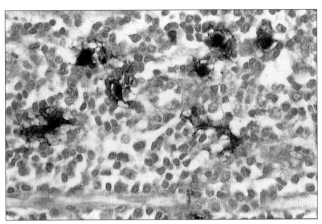

FIGURE 8.6 Dendritic antigen-presenting cells. Micrograph showing the ramifying cell processes of dendritic antigen-presenting cells from one area (paracortex) of a lymph node. This section is stained by an immunoperoxidase method, which detects a protein specific to this cell type.

APC have fine ramifying cytoplasmic processes, which increase the surface area of cell membrane interacting with other cells and antigen. These give rise to their descriptive name, dendritic antigen-presenting cells (Fig. 8.6).

Although actively pinocytotic, APC have low levels of lysosomal enzymes, unlike other monocyte-derived cells specialized for phagocytosis. They have high levels of class II MHC molecules (HLA-Dr): this feature is essential for presenting new antigen to T cells. The follicular dendritic cells differ in this respect as they present antigen to B cells and lack class II MHC expression.

Cells that can be classified as dendritic APC are:
- Langerhans' cells of the skin
- Dendritic reticulum cells of lymph nodes
- Follicular dendritic cells
- Interstitial dendritic cells, which form a population of dendritic cells in the support tissues of most organs
- Veiled cells of the blood, which are thought to be circulating forms of dendritic APC in transit between tissues
- Microglia of the central nervous system (see Fig. 6.16).

KEY FACTS
THE IMMUNE RESPONSE

- Occurs in specialized tissues and organs of the immune system, particularly lymph nodes and spleen
- Is initiated when antigen interacts with lymphocytes; this usually involves APC
- Activates lymphocytes to proliferate; some will mature to become memory T and B cells which respond rapidly to the antigen by proliferation and activation on re-exposure.

Despite certain common attributes, each of these cell types is microenvironmentally specialized and each has slightly different cell-surface receptors and proteins which adapt them to antigen presentation in different sites.

In addition to this group of cells, which have a primary role in antigen presentation, several other cells, particularly the non-specific phagocytic macrophages, can present antigen.

Bone Marrow

The bone marrow is the site of origin of B- and T-cell precursors and of macrophages, and is discussed in detail in Chapter 7.

Thymus

The thymus is the site of T-cell development

Immunologically naive lymphocytes from bone marrow differentiate into mature T cells in the thymus. During this process, the immune system distinguishes self from foreign antigens and develops self-tolerance.

The thymus is also an endocrine organ, secreting hormones and other soluble factors, which not only control T-cell production, differentiation and maturation in the thymus, but also regulate T-cell function and interactions in peripheral tissues.

The thymus is the first lymphoid organ to develop, and is derived from the endoderm and a small ectodermal element of the ventral wing of the third pharyngeal pouch on each side.

The thymus is a soft lobulated organ located in the superior and anterior mediastinum

At birth, the thymus is pinkish-grey in colour and weighs 10–15g, increasing to 30–40g by puberty. Thereafter, it undergoes progressive involution and extensive fatty infiltration, and assumes a yellowish colour.

In children, the thymic parenchyma is divided into an outer, highly cellular cortex and a pale-stained central medulla. The cortex is divided into irregular lobules 0.5–2.0 mm in diameter by fine septa extending in as far as the corticomedullary junction from a loose fibrocollagenous capsule. The less cellular medullary tissue forms a continuous central core. The main cell types in the thymus are epitheliocytes, lymphocytes and macrophages (Fig. 8.7).

The thymic epitheliocytes are true epithelial cells

The epitheliocytes form the stromal meshwork of the thymus and have a variety of ultrastructural and immunohistochemical features. At least four distinct cell types are recognizable: the subcapsular cortical, inner cortical, medullary and Hassall's corpuscle cells.

Beneath the **capsule**, the epitheliocytes form a continuous layer, which is carried deeply into the thymus to

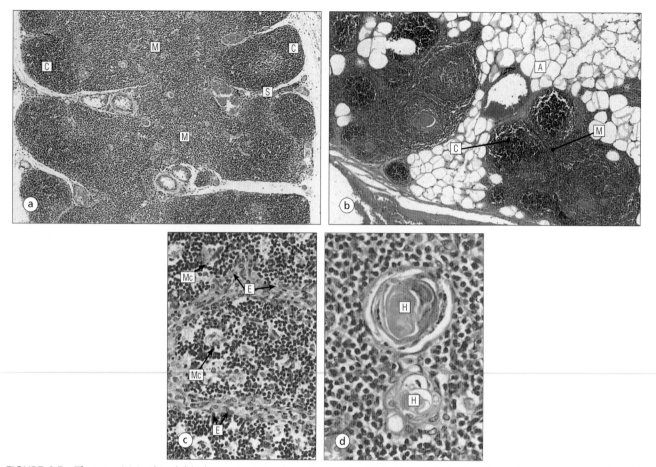

FIGURE 8.7 **Thymus.** (a) In the child, the cortex (C) of the thymus is divided into lobules by fibrocollagenous septa (S) and is surrounded by adipose tissue of the mediastinum. The medulla (M) is less cellular. (b) In the adult, there is involution of the thymus, with replacement by adipose tissue (A). The division into a cellular cortex (C) and a less cellular medulla (M) is still apparent. (c) The dominant feature of the thymic cortex is its vast number of densely packed lymphocytes, which range in size from small to large, depending on their activity. Most, if not all, of the lymphocytes are in direct contact with epitheliocytes (E), which permeate the whole gland and act as a supporting framework. They are difficult to identify in the sea of lymphoid cells, but are visible where they surround blood vessels entering the gland. Numerous macrophages (Mc) are scattered throughout the cortex and contain the phagocytosed debris of eliminated lymphocytes. (d) The dominant feature of the thymic medulla is its epithelial component, the cells having large pale nuclei and abundant eosinophilic cytoplasm. Lymphocytes are less densely packed than in the cortex; most are T cells probably en route to the general circulation. Hassall's corpuscles (H) are derived from epitheliocytes, which first appear during fetal development and form continuously thereafter. The process begins with the enlargement of a single medullary epitheliocyte, which undergoes progressive degenerative changes characterized by nuclear disintegration and increasing cytoplasmic eosinophilia. Vacuoles appear in the cytoplasm, taking up the nuclear debris. This process is repeated in nearby epithelial cells, which form concentric lamellae around a central hyalinizing mass. Hassall's corpuscles may grow as large as 100 μm in diameter and undergo a variety of degenerative changes, becoming infiltrated by lymphocytes, macrophages and eosinophils; they may also show cystic change or calcification.

invest the septa and vessels entering and leaving the organ.

Within the **cortex**, the epitheliocytes form a sponge-like structure containing an extensive network of spaces which becomes colonized by lymphocytes (see Fig. 8.7c).

In the medulla, sheets of epitheliocytes converge to form a coarser, more solid structure with smaller interstices accommodating much smaller numbers of lymphocytes.

Deep in the medulla, the epitheliocytes form bulky cords and whorls, some of which contain lamellated structures (**Hassall's corpuscles**, see Fig. 8.7d).

Thymic epitheliocytes have pale-staining oval nuclei and eosinophilic cytoplasm and can be readily identified in the medulla. In the cortex, however, their fine cytoplasmic extensions make them difficult to identify within the mass of lymphocytes.

With the electron microscope, typical desmosomes (see Fig. 3.11) are seen to bind the epithelial cells, which contain bundles of intermediate (cytokeratin) filaments.

Epitheliocytes in the cortex are in close contact with thymic lymphocytes and are called nurse cells

In much of the thymic cortex, the epitheliocytes are in intimate contact with the lymphocytes, and completely enclose them by deep infolding of surface membrane. Described as **thymic nurse cells**, these cells are thought to eliminate immature T cells that recognize self-antigens.

Epitheliocytes also promote T-cell differentiation, proliferation and subset maturation. In addition, they secrete hormones and other substances that regulate T-cell maturation and proliferation within the thymus and other lymphoid organs.

The thymic lymphocytes are T cells undergoing development

Most thymic lymphocytes are T cells in various stages of differentiation. B cells are also present, but in smaller numbers. Although the term 'thymocyte' is often used as a generic term for thymic lymphocytes, it strictly applies to immature lymphocytes of T-cell lineage.

Clones of T cells are produced by cell division in the outer part of the thymic cortex and undergo maturation as they are pushed deep into the cortex toward the medulla.

In the medulla, the maturing T cells enter blood vessels and lymphatics to join the pool of circulating T cells. They subsequently populate peripheral lymphoid tissues, where they reach full immunological maturity.

Only a small minority of lymphocytes generated in the thymus are believed to reach maturity. These are clones of T cells with the ability to recognize foreign antigens. The rest of the lymphocytes are thought to recognize self-antigens and are eliminated; this results in immunological self-tolerance.

The thymus has a rich vascular supply which allows migration of lymphoid cells

The thymus receives its arterial supply via many small branches of the internal thoracic and inferior thyroid arteries, which enter the thymus mainly via the interlobular septa.

In the region of the corticomedullary junction, the vessels give rise to small radially arranged arterioles and capillary loops to supply the cortex and medulla.

The cortical capillaries have continuous endothelium (see Chapter 9), whereas those of the medulla and septa may be fenestrated.

At the corticomedullary junction, which is the site of lymphocyte migration into the thymus, the postcapillary venules have a taller endothelium with features of high endothelial venules.

Venous tributaries follow the course of the arterial vessels in the septa, some forming a plexus within the thymic capsule before draining via the thymic veins into the left brachiocephalic, internal thoracic and inferior thyroid veins.

The thymus receives no afferent lymphatics, but the medulla and corticomedullary area give rise to efferent lymphatics, which follow the course of the arteries and veins.

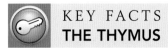

KEY FACTS
THE THYMUS

- Functions for the development and maturation of T cells
- Is composed of lymphoid cells, thymic epithelial cells, macrophagic cells and stromal cells
- Is divided into cortex and medulla
- Undergoes involution after puberty.

The thymus undergoes involution after puberty

The thymus reaches its maximum weight at puberty, declining thereafter, so that in old age, it may be so small as to be unrecognizable. Involution involves replacement of the gland by adipose tissue (fatty infiltration) and a decline in its lymphocyte content.

Fatty infiltration begins at birth, but accelerates after puberty. Adipocytes increase in number in the perivascular compartment. Initially, this is most apparent in the septa, thus the cortex is involved first and then the process is extended into the medulla (see Fig. 8.7b).

Lymphocyte depletion begins after 1 year of age and thereafter continues at a constant rate, independent of puberty. It results in progressive collapse of the sponge-like epitheliocyte framework, which nevertheless remains intact, so that cords of epitheliocytes can be seen histologically, even in the most atrophic thymic remnants. Such cells probably continue to secrete thymic hormones into old age.

Despite the progressive decrease in their number with involution, thymic lymphocytes continue to differentiate and proliferate, thus maintaining a supply of T cells throughout life.

Lymph Nodes

The lymph nodes are an important site for generation of immune responses

Lymph nodes are small organs found in groups or chains at sites where lymphatic vessels draining an anatomic region converge to form larger lymphatic vessels, for example in the neck, axillae, groins and para-aortic area. They have two main functions.

Phagocytic cells within the nodes act as non-specific filters for particulate matter, such as microorganisms and carbon, preventing them from reaching the general circulation.

They provide an elegant mechanism whereby lymphocytes can interact with new antigens and APC at an interface between lymph and the blood. Starting with only a small number of lymphocytes recognizing an antigen, lymph nodes facilitate proliferation of activated cells and consequently amplification of the immune response by forming clones of lymphocytes.

When relatively inactive, each lymph node is only a few millimeters in length, but they may become greatly enlarged when functional demands are increased.

The cells of the lymph node can be divided into three functional types: lymphoid cells, immunological accessory cells, and non-immunologically active stromal cells.

Lymphoid cells in lymph nodes include lymphocytes of all types and their derivatives. Most of the lymphocytes enter the node via the blood, but a few enter via lymph draining from the tissues.

Immunological accessory cells comprise a variety of macrophages, including those with phagocytic antigen-processing, antigen-presenting and non-specific effector functions.

Non-immunologically active **stromal cells** comprise the lymphatic and vascular endothelial cells, and fibroblasts, which elaborate the stromal reticular framework. Many of the endothelial cells are highly specialized for interaction with lymphoid cells.

Each lymph node is divided into several functional compartments

The lymph node is a bean-shaped organ with a fibrocollagenous capsule from which fibrous trabeculae extend into the node to form a supporting framework (Fig. 8.8).

The convex surface of the gland is penetrated by a number of afferent lymphatic vessels, which drain into the node, whereas at the hilum there is an efferent lymphatic vessel that transports lymph toward larger collecting lymphatic vessels. In turn these vessels drain into more proximal nodes or chains of nodes, before entering the blood via either the thoracic duct or the right lymphatic duct.

Lymph nodes contain three functional compartments (Fig. 8.9):
- A network of endothelial-lined **lymphatic sinuses** continuous with the lumina of the afferent and efferent lymphatic vessels
- A network of small blood vessels, where circulating lymphocytes enter the node
- A parenchymal compartment composed of superficial cortex, paracortex and medulla.

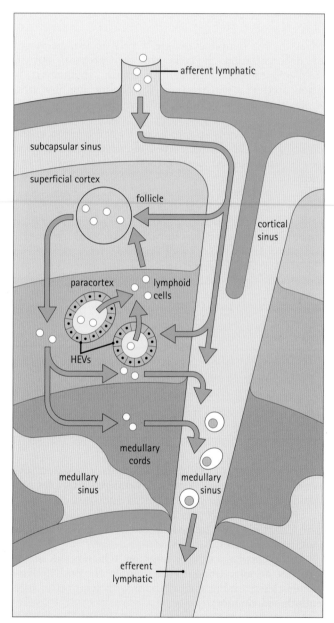

FIGURE 8.9 **Functional compartments of the lymph node.** Antigens, accessory cells and lymphocytes enter the lymph node via the afferent lymphatics, which drain into the subcapsular sinus and thence into the cortical sinuses. These antigens, accessory cells and lymphocytes may then enter the cortex or remain in the sinuses and leave the lymph node via the efferent lymphatic vessel. The majority of lymphocytes enter the node from the blood via the high endothelial venules (HEVs), which are lined by a special endothelium bearing lymphocyte-homing receptors.

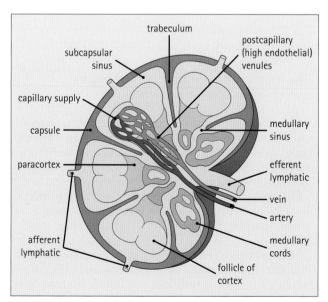

FIGURE 8.8 **Lymph node structure.** The bean-shaped lymph node has a hilum into which blood vessels enter, and from which efferent lymphatics emerge. It has an investing capsule. Afferent lymphatic vessels penetrate the convex surface of the gland and drain into the subcapsular and medullary sinus system. The lymphoid parenchyma is divided into cortex, paracortex and medulla. The most prominent structures in the cortex are the lymphoid follicles.

The structural integrity of the lymph node is provided by a framework of reticulin fibres (see p. 56), which are linked to the fibrous trabeculae. These fibres are most dense in the parenchymal compartment, although some do traverse the lymphatic compartment, where they are completely invested by endothelial cells.

Lymph node sinuses carry lymph throughout the nodal structure

Afferent lymphatics drain into a major subcapsular sinus running around the periphery of the lymph node. From this sinus, cortical sinuses pass down toward the medulla through the cortical cell mass.

Within the medulla, the dominant feature is a network of interconnected lymphatic channels called the medullary sinuses, which converge upon the efferent lymphatic vessel at the hilum.

Only the larger channels of the lymphatic compartment can be visualized by light microscopy. The cortical sinuses are generally difficult to see because of their highly convoluted shape and numerous fine extensions, which penetrate the cellular mass of the cortex.

The extremely thin and pale-staining endothelial lining cells of the sinuses are almost impossible to identify with ordinary staining methods.

The blood supply of lymph nodes is the main route of entry of lymphocytes into the node

The blood supply also provides the metabolic needs of the lymph node. One or more small arterial vessels enter the node via the hilum and then divide in the medulla into branches, which ramify into a capillary network corresponding to the cortical follicles and paracortex.

Within the paracortex, the postcapillary venules (see Chapter 9) have cuboidal endothelium-bearing specialized cell receptors (lymphocyte-homing receptors), which are recognized by circulating lymphocytes and facilitate the passage of lymphocytes from the blood and into the lymph node. The postcapillary venules are often described as **high endothelial venules (HEV)**.

The blood vessels of the superficial cortex and medullary cords are thought to be non-specialized and do not appear to allow the exit of lymphocytes. Small veins draining the node leave via the hilum.

The superficial cortex of the lymph node contains the densely staining spheroidal aggregations of lymphocytes (lymphoid follicles)

Some of the follicles (**primary follicles**) are of fairly uniform staining density; however, most of the follicles responding to antigen have less densely staining **germinal centres** and are described as **secondary follicles** (Fig. 8.10).

The lymphocyte population of the follicles consists predominantly of B cells, but there are smaller populations of Th cells, macrophages and accessory cells.

The main cells of the lymphoid follicles are B cells

B cells enter a lymph node via the HEV of the paracortex. Within a few hours, many have migrated to the

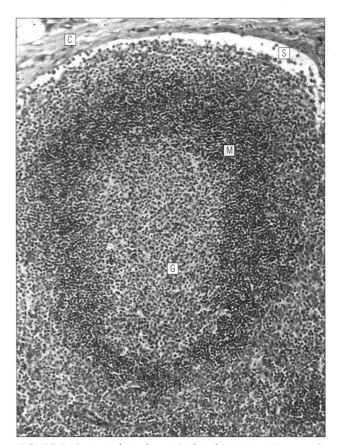

FIGURE 8.10 **Lymph node cortical architecture.** Micrograph showing the superficial cortex of the lymph node. The capsule (C) is composed of collagen, beneath which is the subcapsular sinus (S). A secondary follicle containing a germinal centre (G) with a mantle zone (M) is present in the underlying cortex.

superficial cortex. If activated, they proliferate and remain in the lymph node for an extended period as memory cells or plasma cells. In contrast, non-activated cells re-enter the general circulation within a matter of hours via the efferent lymph.

The primary follicles contain mainly naive B cells and some memory cells. The secondary follicles, in contrast, contain small naive B cells peripherally and activated B cells in their germinal centres.

It is possible to identify several stages in the maturation of B cells in the follicles (Fig. 8.11). Activated B cells proliferate and mature and thereby produce an expanded population of identical cells recognizing the same antigen.

The activated B cells in the germinal centre are collectively called **follicle centre cells**. They are characterized by open nuclei, and have more cytoplasm and are less densely packed than the smaller, more peripheral follicular B cells; this explains the lower staining intensity of the germinal centres.

The proliferation and differentiation of antibody-secreting plasma cells is thought to result from T cell–B cell interaction in the paracortex. The plasma cells then migrate directly to the medullary cords, where they are conveniently situated to secrete antibody into the efferent lymph.

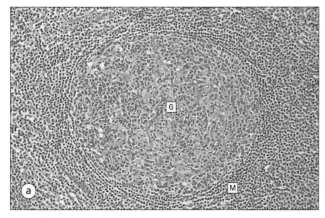

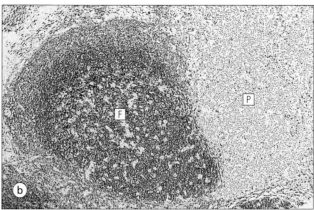

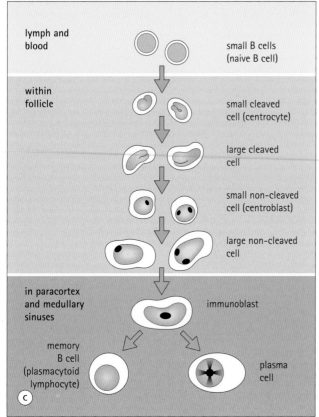

FIGURE 8.11 **Follicular B cells.** (a) Micrograph of an H&E-stained secondary lymphoid follicle, which consists mainly of B cells. Small naive B cells and a few T cells form the dark mantle zone (M), whereas the paler germinal centre (G) contains B cells in various stages of maturation. Accessory cells (see Fig. 8.12) are present, but are barely discernible at this magnification. (b) Micrograph of lymph node cortex stained to show B cells by an immunoperoxidase method. The follicle (F) is densely stained brown, being composed of B cells. The paracortex (P) is not stained, being composed of T cells. (c) The maturation of B cells from small naive cells to dividing cells responding to a specific antigen is associated with a distinct series of morphological changes. From the small lymphocyte, the cell changes first into a centrocyte with a cleft nucleus, and then into a centroblast. This cell enlarges, leaves the follicle and migrates to the paracortex and medullary sinuses as an immunoblast, ultimately transforming into a plasma cell or a memory B cell.

Accessory cells in the superficial cortex are involved in antigen processing

A variety of immunological accessory cells are found in the superficial cortex. These are derived from bone marrow and reach the lymph node via the afferent lymph. These cells all appear to play some role in antigen processing; this also applies to the accessory cells of the paracortex and medulla.

The main accessory cell types in the superficial cortex are:
- **Sinus macrophages**, highly phagocytic cells of the subcapsular and cortical sinuses
- **Veiled cells**, monocyte-derived cells so named because of their veiled appearance on scanning

electron microscopy; they are located mainly in the subcapsular sinuses
- **Tingible body macrophages**, so named because they contain cellular debris and are found within the germinal centres with an abundance of lysosomal enzymes
- **Marginal zone macrophages**, which constitute a morphologically diverse group of phagocytic cells located within the follicular interstitium immediately beneath the subcapsular sinus
- **Follicular dendritic cells**, which have numerous fine branching surface projections covered by electron-dense material.

Follicular dendritic cells retain antigen on their surface for many months. These cells present antigen directly to

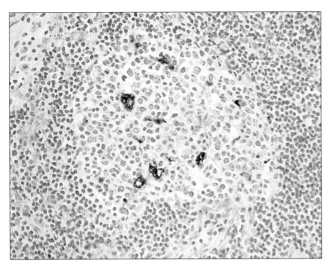

FIGURE 8.12 **Follicular accessory cells.** The follicular accessory cells are not easily distinguished in H&E sections, but can be stained by immunochemical techniques. This micrograph shows the tingible body macrophages stained brown by localizing a lysosomal enzyme, cathepsin D.

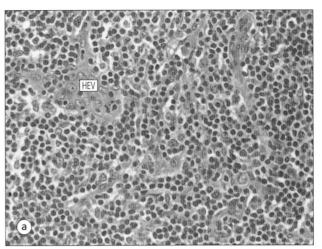

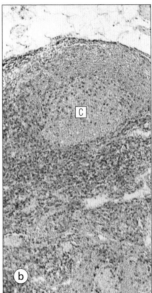

FIGURE 8.13 **Lymph node paracortex.** (a) Micrograph of lymph node paracortex showing sheets of T cells, which vary in morphology from small inactive cells to large cells representing activated proliferating T cells. The high endothelial venules (HEV) are prominent, but accessory cells are inconspicuous even at high magnification. (b) Micrograph of lymph node stained by an antibody technique that detects T cells. The paracortex stains brown (i.e. is T cell in nature), whereas the adjacent portion of cortical follicle (C) is not stained, being composed of B cells.

B cells and lack the class II MHC expression normally seen on other antigen-presenting cells.

These immunological accessory cells cannot be readily distinguished in H&E sections, but may be stained by immunochemical techniques for special macrophage markers (Fig. 8.12).

The main cells of the lymph node paracortex are T cells

The cell population of the paracortex consists of lymphocytes and accessory cells, which constantly move in and out of the region.

T cells dominate the paracortex (Fig. 8.13), entering the node from the blood via the HEV and leaving 6–18 hours later via the efferent lymphatic.

When activated, T cells enlarge to form lymphoblasts. These then proliferate to produce an expanded clone of activated T cells. In a T-cell-dominated immunological response, the paracortex may expand into the medulla, producing a so-called **paracortical reaction**. Activated T cells are then disseminated via the circulation to peripheral sites, where much of their activity occurs.

Accessory cells of the paracortex act as antigen-presenting cells

Interdigitating cells are prominent in the paracortex and are one form of 'dendritic APC', being so named because of their numerous cytoplasmic processes which interdigitate with those of other cells. These cytoplasmic processes also make numerous contacts with other cell types in the vicinity.

Macrophages are also found in the paracortex. Their cytoplasm is often observed packed with lipid (possibly engulfed cell membrane) and nuclear debris.

The lymph node medulla is composed of a series of sinuses separating cords of cells

The medulla of the lymph node contains mainly:
- Cell-rich medullary cords
- Wide medullary sinuses (separating the medullary cords) through which lymph percolates toward the hilum from the cortex
- Larger blood vessels and their supporting trabeculae.

As in the cortex, the interstitial compartment of the medulla is supported by a framework of reticulin fibres, a small number of which traverse the sinuses.

The medulla contains plasma cells and macrophages

The most common cells in medullary cords are plasma cells and their precursors. Plasma cells synthesize antibody, which is carried from the node to the general circulation via the efferent lymph. In addition, some mature plasma cells probably migrate from the node.

Classic macrophages are the main accessory cell type in the medulla. They are located in the sinuses and derive support from the traversing reticulin fibres.

Lymph entering the node is filtered and antigens are presented to lymphoid cells

Lymph draining into a lymph node via afferent lymphatics first enters the subcapsular sinus and then percolates through the cortical sinusoidal maze to drain into the medullary sinuses before leaving the node via the efferent lymphatics.

Some particulate matter is probably taken up from the lymph and disposed of by the phagocytic activity of the endothelial cells without evoking any immune response.

Antigens are phagocytosed and processed by various types of APC exposed to the lymph. They are then transferred via the APC cytoplasmic extensions to sites where they may be encountered by lymphocytes.

Lymphocytes entering a lymph node in the afferent lymph constitute less than 10% of all of the lymphocytes entering the node, except in the case of mesenteric nodes, where they may constitute up to 30%. The rest

CLINICAL EXAMPLE
SPREAD OF CANCER TO LYMPH NODES

Cancerous cells may break off from primary tumours and enter lymphatic vessels, from where they migrate to lymph nodes. Once in the node they adhere to and proliferate in the sinuses (Fig. 8.14).

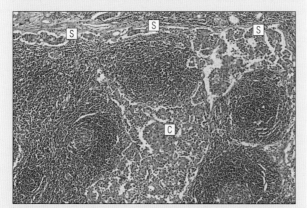

FIGURE 8.14 **Spread of cancer to lymph nodes.** Micrograph showing clumps of cancer cells from a carcinoma of the stomach in the subcapsular (S) and cortical (C) sinuses of a lymph node.

KEY FACTS
LYMPH NODES

- Function to allow interaction between antigen and lymphoid cells
- Main site for proliferation of lymphoid cells in an immune response
- Follicles are composed of B cells (follicle centre cells)
- Paracortex is composed of T cells
- Medulla contains plasma cells and macrophages
- Most lymphocytes enter the node from specialized high endothelial venules
- Antigen from tissues enters the node in lymph which circulates around a series of sinuses.

of the lymphocytes gain entry via the high endothelial venules.

Activated lymphocytes pass through the endothelium of the subcapsular sinus and enter the germinal centres of the cortical follicles.

Spleen

The spleen lies in the left upper abdomen and weighs around 150 g in the adult.

The two principal functions of the human spleen are:
- To mount a primary immune response to antigens in the blood
- To act as a filter to remove particulate matter and aged or abnormal red cells and platelets from the circulation.

The following description is specific to **human** spleen.

The spleen contains vascular sinusoids supported by a reticulin scaffold.

The spleen has a thin fibrocollagenous capsule from which short septa extend into the organ. These septa support an extensive meshwork of reticulin fibres that serve as a scaffold for the splenic parenchyma.

The reticulin framework is also attached to fibrocollagenous tissue associated with a branching arterial and venous network emanating from the splenic hilum. Such perivascular tissue does not form septa: it forms a sheath around the larger vessels.

Most of the spleen is composed of a vast array of sinusoids and vascular sinuses filled with blood (**red pulp**). A branching array of arteries (central arteries) associated with aggregates of lymphoid tissue is called **white pulp** (Fig. 8.15), and accounts for 5–20% of the total mass of the spleen.

The splenic red pulp is composed of cords of cells separated by sinusoids

The red pulp consists of loose support tissue supported by reticulin fibres with several functional areas:
- **Capillaries**, which terminate by draining into a fusiform-shaped macrophage-lined space, forming the ellipsoidal (sheathed) capillaries
- A **parenchyma** composed of stellate reticular support cells, which surrounds sponge-like cavities

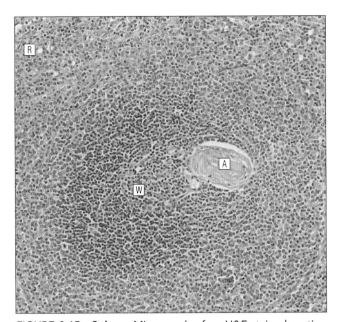

FIGURE 8.15 **Spleen.** Micrograph of an H&E-stained section of spleen. The white pulp (W) is seen as dense-staining aggregates of lymphoid cells adjacent to central arteries (A). The red pulp (R) is less densely stained as it has fewer nuclei, and at this magnification it is not possible to distinguish between the various sinuses and parenchymal components.

through which blood from the sheathed capillaries slowly percolates
- **Venous sinuses**, which run adjacent to columns of parenchymal tissue and drain blood that has filtered through the parenchyma, as well as blood that has come directly from the sheathed capillaries (Figs. 8.16, 8.18).

The sinuses are lined by flattened endothelial cells resting on a discontinuous basement membrane, which is interrupted by numerous narrow slits through which red cells squeeze. Phagocytic cells are closely associated with the walls of these sinuses.

The splenic white pulp is composed of lymphoid cells

The white pulp or splenic lymphoid masses are of two types: T cell and B cell. The functions of these two types of lymphoid tissue appear to be similar to those of the paracortex and superficial cortex of the lymph nodes.

White pulp T cells belong mainly to the Th subset and form irregular masses around the central arteries. The central arteries are generally located at one side of the T-cell area (Fig. 8.17).

At the periphery of the T-cell zone is a narrow mantle zone of small lymphocytes enclosed by a broader marginal zone, in which less densely packed larger lymphocytes and dendritic APC surround fine vascular channels with a reticulin scaffold.

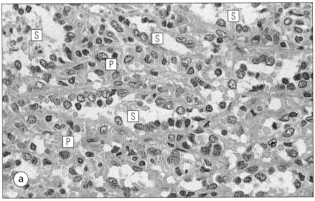

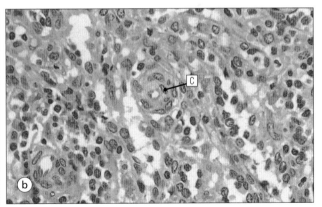

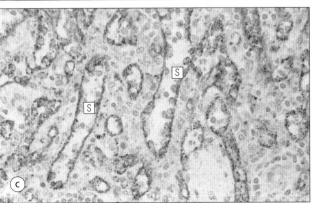

FIGURE 8.16 **Splenic red pulp.** (a) Micrograph of red pulp, which is composed of parenchymal areas (P), termed 'splenic cords', and sinusoids (S). The endothelial cells protrude into the sinuses. (b) Micrograph of an ellipsoidal sheathed capillary (C), seen here in cross-section. (c) Micrograph of splenic red pulp venous sinusoids, which have been immunostained for the lysosomal enzyme cathepsin-D. This technique highlights in brown the abundant network of phagocytic macrophages associated with the walls of the venous sinusoids (S).

White pulp B cells form follicles, which are usually located near an arteriole. In young people, many of the follicles have germinal centres; the proportion of such follicles diminishes with age.

In addition to these lymphoid areas associated with the central arteries, a significant number of B-cell, T-cell and plasma-cell aggregates are present in the splenic parenchyma.

The perilymphoid zones of the red pulp are adapted for antigen presentation

The zone of red pulp immediately surrounding the T and B lymphoid masses is composed of a sparse reticulin scaffold and anastomosing fine vascular channels surrounded by dendritic APC (marginal zone).

About 10% of blood entering the spleen is believed to pass into this perilymphoid parenchyma, from where it drains into the sinusoids or directly into the venous sinuses of the red pulp.

The function of the sinuses in the perilymphoid zones is not clearly understood, but they may be a means of enhancing the interaction of APC and splenic lymphoid immune responsive tissue with antigens that are blood-borne rather than tissue-based (e.g. circulating bacteria in septicaemia).

The splenic vasculature is arranged to filter blood through the red pulp

Central arteries run eccentrically in the white pulp of the spleen and lead to:
* Strands of arterioles and capillaries which supply the white pulp
* Arterioles and capillaries that run directly into a system of marginal zone fine vascular sinusoids (see Fig. 8.18).

ADVANCED CONCEPT
SPLENIC BLOOD CIRCULATION

Blood can be filtered by percolation through the parenchyma (splenic cords) and then into the sinusoids – **open** circulation – the main route of blood flow in the human spleen.

The **closed** circulation appears to be a minor component of human splenic blood flow. Blood from the perimarginal cavernous sinuses bypasses the slow route through the splenic parenchyma and enters the splenic venous sinus instead. This provides a system for blood to pass rapidly through the spleen without filtration. In humans, a small number of capillaries arising from the central arteries also open directly into the venous sinuses.

CLINICAL EXAMPLE
SPLENECTOMY

Removal of the spleen is necessary:

* When it is ruptured following abdominal trauma
* In some diseases, for example lymphomas
* As part of major surgery, for example removal of the stomach for cancer.

Effects of Splenectomy

The effects of removing the spleen highlight its main functions.

Changes in the Blood

The blood film (Fig. 8.17) from a patient who has had a splenectomy shows increased numbers of platelets and abnormal red cells with deformed shapes (poikilocytosis). In addition, aged red cells contain blue-staining particulate inclusions of nuclear material (Howell–Jolly bodies).

These nuclear remnants would normally be removed by percolation through the splenic cords and into the splenic sinuses.

Infection

Patients who have had a splenectomy are at risk of developing life-threatening bacterial septicaemia. The most common organism involved is *Streptococcus pneumoniae*. The spleen filters the blood and any blood-borne organisms are phagocytized by the macrophages in the splenic sinusoids. But in a person without a spleen, the organism can circulate in the blood and reproduce. It is therefore recommended that anyone undergoing a splenectomy should be immunized against *S. pneumoniae*.

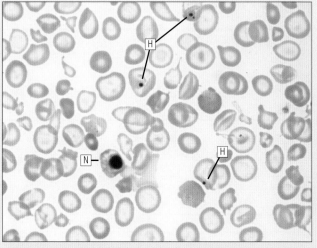

FIGURE 8.17 **Post-splenectomy blood film.** Micrograph of blood film from a patient following splenectomy. The red cells have bizarre shapes and in this field some of the cells contain small particulate dark-staining inclusions (Howell–Jolly bodies, arrows). A nucleated RBC is also present (arrowhead). (Image courtesy of Vishnu VB Reddy, MD Professor of Pathology University of Alabama at Birmingham.)

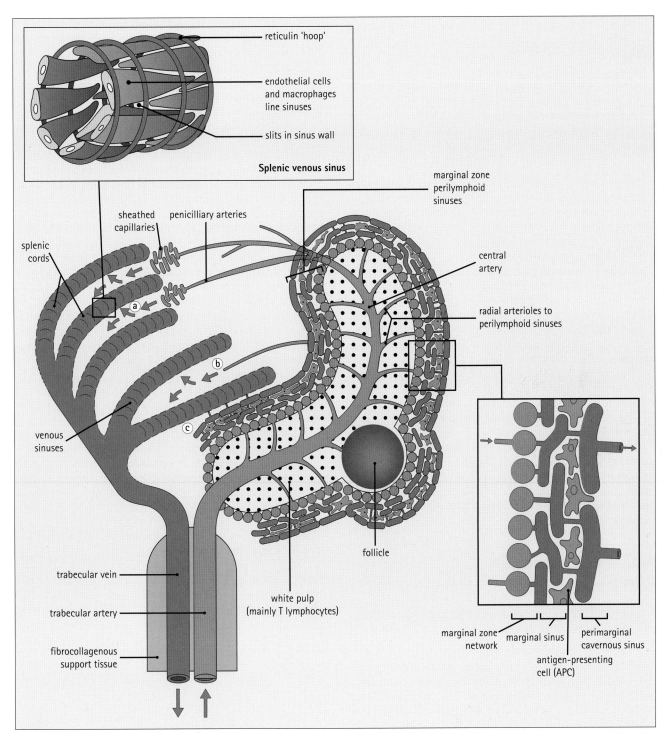

reticulin 'hoop'

endothelial cells
and macrophages
line sinuses

slits in sinus wall

Splenic venous sinus

marginal zone
perilymphoid
sinuses

sheathed
capillaries

penicilliary arteries

splenic
cords

central
artery

radial arterioles to
perilymphoid sinuses

venous
sinuses

follicle

white pulp
(mainly T lymphocytes)

trabecular vein

trabecular artery

fibrocollagenous
support tissue

marginal zone
network

marginal sinus

perimarginal
cavernous sinus

antigen-presenting
cell (APC)

FIGURE 8.18 **Vascular anatomy of the spleen.** The spleen has two main functions: it removes aged and effete red cells from the circulation, and it mounts an immune response to antigens, particularly bacteria, circulating in the blood. Blood enters the spleen in the splenic artery; this branches to form the trabecular arteries, which give rise to a series of central arteries surrounded by T cells of the white pulp. For red cells to be removed, blood passes along the central arteries and then enters the red pulp through a series of specialized vessels (penicilliary arteries and sheathed capillaries) to drain into the splenic parenchyma (splenic cords). The blood then percolates through spaces between the reticular cells forming the splenic cords, and squeezes through narrow slit spaces to enter the splenic venous sinuses. Normal red cells are deformable and survive this passage, but aged red cells have rigid membranes and are lysed. Fragments of destroyed red cells are removed by phagocytic cells along the sinus walls. Red cells leave the system via trabecular veins and enter the splenic vein. This pathway is the open circulation (a). A proportion of the splenic circulation enters small arterioles to reach a series of marginal sinuses, which run around the lymphoid sheaths. In this area, blood comes into contact with dendritic antigen-presenting cells, and foreign antigens can be trapped and presented to appropriate lymphoid cells. Most of the blood from the marginal sinuses around the lymphoid sheaths enters the red pulp and then drains into the venous sinuses (b) but a small proportion passes directly into the sinuses and forms what is termed the closed circulation (c).

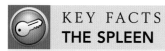

The marginal zone sinusoids are arranged concentrically around the white pulp in the perilymphoid zone. In human spleen, perfusion studies have defined three concentric systems:

- The marginal zone network
- The marginal sinuses
- The perimarginal cavernous sinus.

The central arteries terminate in a series of straight arterial vessels, traditionally called **penicilliary arteries**. These arteries are devoid of an investing layer of lymphoid cells and run in the red pulp. In turn, they give rise to arterioles and capillaries, which tend to leave the arterioles at right-angles.

The splenic capillaries of the red pulp have a standard endothelial cell structure, which terminates abruptly in a fusiform arrangement of mononuclear phagocytes. They are described as ellipsoid sheathed capillaries (see Fig. 8.16b).

Most of the sheathed capillaries drain into the splenic parenchyma proper, which consists of a sponge-like network of spaces between stellate reticular cells (splenic cords). A small proportion of the sheathed capillaries also drains directly into the perimarginal cavernous sinuses.

Mucosa-associated Lymphoid Tissue

Lymphoid cells may concentrate in mucosal surfaces to provide defence

In addition to the mass of the peripheral lymphoid tissue encapsulated in the lymph nodes and spleen, the body contains an equally large amount of non-encapsulated lymphoid tissue which is located in the walls of the gastrointestinal, respiratory and urogenital tracts.

This tissue is known as **mucosa-associated lymphoid tissue (MALT)** and takes the form of diffuse infiltrates or more discrete nodules; it provides immunological protection against invasion by pathogens via vulnerable exposed absorptive surfaces.

The **gut-associated lymphoid tissue (GALT)** includes:
- The palatine, lingual and pharyngeal tonsils (adenoids)
- Mucosal nodules in the oesophagus
- **Peyer's patches** in the small intestine (see Chapter 11)
- Lymphoid aggregations in the large intestine and appendix

- A vast number of lymphocytes and plasma cells scattered throughout the lamina propria of the small and large intestines.

The bronchus-associated lymphoid tissue (BALT) is located beneath the mucosa of the large respiratory passages (bronchi) and shows close structural similarities with other forms of MALT.

In large aggregations of MALT, which are seen mainly in the tonsils and Peyer's patches, the lymphoid tissue is arranged into follicles, which often contain germinal centres and are similar to those of the lymph nodes.

With immunohistochemical techniques, discrete B- and T-cell zones containing typical antigen-processing accessory cells can be identified and have functions analogous to those of the superficial cortex and paracortex of the lymph node, respectively. The T cells found in mucosal tissues are mainly of the TCR-1⁺ type.

The scattered lymphocytes in the lamina propria of the gut and respiratory tract include B cells, some of which mature into antibody-secreting plasma cells. All classes of antibody are produced, but IgA predominates.

IgA is secreted into the gut lumen in a form called 'secretory IgA', which is resistant to enzymatic digestion and provides protection against pathogens before they breach the tissues.

IgG and IgM are secreted into the lamina propria to deal with organisms eluding the surface protective mechanisms.

IgE mediates the release of histamine from mast cells, which are present in large numbers in the lamina propria.

The recirculation of lymphoid cells from mucosal-associated lymphoid tissues is to local lymph nodes, rather than to lymph nodes that drain non-mucosal tissues.

Peyer's patches are large aggregations of lymphoid tissue found in the small intestine

Peyer's patches number about 200 in humans. They extend through the lamina propria and submucosa, and often bulge into the gut lumen (Fig. 8.19). The overlying

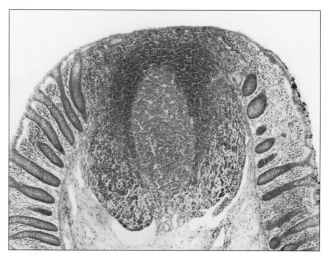

FIGURE 8.19 **A Peyer's patch composed of lymphoid cells, including a germinal centre, associated with the bowel mucosa.**

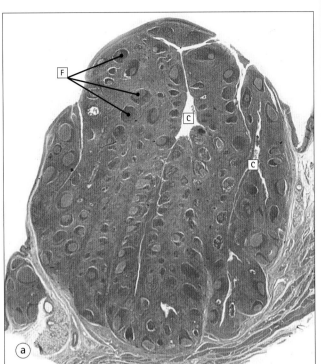

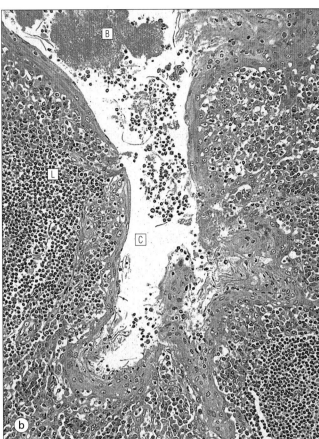

FIGURE 8.20   **Palatine tonsil.** (a) Low-power micrograph showing a typical tonsillar architecture with squamous epithelium folded into crypts (C) associated with dense lymphoid aggregates in which follicles are visible (F). (b) Medium-power micrograph of a tonsil showing a tonsillar crypt (C) lined by squamous epithelium and surrounded by tonsillar lymphoid tissue (L). The crypt contains colonies of oral commensal bacteria (B), which is a normal finding.

epithelium of a Peyer's patch (dome epithelium) is characterized by cuboidal, rather than tall columnar cells (see Fig. 11.26), and contains large numbers of intraepithelial lymphocytes. Goblet cells are absent.

Some of the epithelial cells exhibit numerous surface microfolds instead of the usual microvilli and have been designated **M cells**. These cells migrate from the mucosal crypts and function in the transfer of antigen between the lumen and the Peyer's patch.

Tonsils are lymphoid tissues in the oropharynx

Waldeyer's ring of pharyngeal lymphoid tissue comprises four groups of tonsillar tissue. The largest is the palatine tonsils, which contain 12–15 deep tonsillar crypts lined by stratified squamous epithelium (Fig. 8.20). These crypts frequently contain plugs of lymphocytes, bacteria and epithelial debris, which may become calcified.

The tonsils contain numerous lymphoid follicles with germinal centres, and the lymphoid tissue as a whole appears to have a similar cellular make-up to that of Peyer's patches. The epithelium overlying the tonsillar tissue contains T cells as well as dendritic APC. For other components of Waldeyer's ring, see page 167 and page 188.

Bronchus-associated lymphoid tissue is encountered in the lung

The lymphoid aggregates of the respiratory tract are similar to those of the gut (i.e. Peyer's patches), but are generally smaller. They are covered by similar antigen-sampling and transport M cells, as in the gut. There are no afferent lymphatics; however, efferent lymphatics drain lymph to the regional nodes.

Activated lymphocytes derived from the respiratory tract aggregations tend to home in specifically on the respiratory mucosa.

CLINICAL EXAMPLE
TUMOURS OF THE LYMPHOID SYSTEM

The main primary tumours of the lymphoid system are derived from lymphocytes and their precursors, and are termed lymphomas. The diseases usually begin in lymph nodes, which become enlarged and firm; it may be localized or may involve several lymph node groups. In addition, lymphoma may also involve the spleen, bone marrow or liver. The first lymphoma was described by Thomas Hodgkin and this specific type has subsequently been named 'Hodgkin's lymphoma'. Thus, the main categories of lymphoma are:

- Hodgkin's lymphoma, and (with the wit and intellectual rigour for which pathologists are renowned)
- Non-Hodgkin's lymphoma.

Accurate identification of the specific type of lymphoma is very important in management and prognosis, and immuno-cytochemical methods are used to identify whether the tumour cells are B lymphocytes or T lymphocytes (see Figs 8.11b, 8.13c). Histological assessment of the cytological and nuclear characteristics of the tumour cells allows them to be identified as mature forms ('low grade') or immature precursor forms ('high grade'). High-grade lymphomas behave in a more malignant manner but are highly sensitive to cytotoxic chemotherapy.

For online review questions, please visit https://studentconsult.inkling.com.

END OF CHAPTER REVIEW

True/False Answers to the MCQs, as Well as Case Answers, Can be Found in the Appendix in the Back of the Book.

1. Which of the following features are indicative of B lymphocytes?
   (a) Turn into plasma cells and secrete immunoglobulin
   (b) Are derived from cells which originate in the bone marrow
   (c) Are the main cell type in the paracortex of lymph nodes
   (d) Have receptors for antigen on their surface
   (e) Can be seen as small lymphocytes in peripheral blood

2. Which of the following features are present in T lymphocytes?
   (a) May be seen as large granular lymphocytes in peripheral blood
   (b) May express CD4 or CD8
   (c) Secrete antibodies as well as cytokines
   (d) May be divided into two main groups on the basis of expression of distinct types of T-cell receptors
   (e) Are the main cell responsible for the cell-mediated immune response

3. Which of the following is true of the thymus gland?
   (a) Is divided into red and white areas
   (b) Contains epithelial cells which interact with developing T cells
   (c) Contains structures called Hassall's corpuscles which are vessels wrapped by surrounding macrophagic cells
   (d) Undergoes involution after puberty
   (e) Becomes replaced by adipose tissue in adult life

4. In lymph nodes, which of the following features are present?
   (a) The germinal centres are found in the superficial cortex and are predominantly composed of B cells
   (b) The majority of lymphocytes gain entry via the high endothelial venules in the paracortex
   (c) Antigen-presenting cells are not found in germinal centres but are concentrated in the paracortex
   (d) Lymph enters the subcapsular sinus via afferent lymphatics
   (e) Plasma cells are mainly concentrated in the medullary sinuses

CASE 8.1   A BOY WITH BIG LYMPH NODES

A 12-year-old boy is admitted to hospital for investigation of enlarged lymph nodes in the neck. He had been complaining of being unwell for about 6 weeks and had lost weight. He had what his mother described as drenching sweating attacks at night that often woke him up. On examination, he had palpable enlarged lymph nodes in the neck.

Surgical excision of a lymph node was performed so that it could be looked at histologically. The reporting pathologist noted the following: 'There is expansion of germinal centres associated with extensive expansion of paracortical areas. There are multiple aggregates of epithelioid macrophages with multinucleate forms within the lymph node. These are surrounded by zones of activated T cells. The appearances are those of granulomatous inflammation. In the centre of many granulomas are areas of necrosis. These features suggest that tuberculous infection is the most likely cause'.

Q. Describe the anatomical and histological background to the case. Concentrate on describing the normal structure of a lymph node.

Chapter 9

Blood and Lymphatic Circulatory Systems and Heart

Introduction

The main transport systems are the circulatory systems, in which substances are dissolved or suspended in liquid and carried from one part of the body to another in a series of tubes (vessels). There are two main circulatory systems: the blood circulatory system and the lymphatic system.

The **blood circulatory system** is the main method of transporting oxygen, carbon dioxide, nutrients and metabolic breakdown products, cells of the immune and other defence systems, chemical messengers (hormones) and many other important substances (e.g. clotting factors). Transfer of transported substances from blood to tissue and vice versa occurs in the systemic and pulmonary **capillary systems** (Fig. 9.1). These tiny thin-walled vessels permit the passage of fluid, small and large molecules, dissolved gases and even cells across their walls in both directions. The circulatory network that transports blood to the capillaries is called the **arterial system**, and the network that carries blood away from the capillaries is called the **venous system**.

The **lymphatic circulatory system** drains extracellular fluid from the tissues, returning it to the blood circulatory system after passage through lymph nodes. This system is also involved in absorption of nutrients from the gut.

Blood Circulatory System

> **The two main blood circulatory systems are the systemic and pulmonary systems**

There are actually three types of blood circulatory system, two of which (systemic and pulmonary circulations) depend on a central pump, the heart, to push the blood around (Fig. 9.1). The third system is the portal system, discussed below.

The systemic circulation transfers oxygenated blood from a central pump (the heart) to all of the body tissues (systemic arterial system) and returns deoxygenated blood with a high carbon dioxide content from the tissues to the central pump (systemic venous system).

The pulmonary circulation transfers deoxygenated blood with a high carbon dioxide content from a central pump (the heart) to the lungs (pulmonary arterial system) and transfers reoxygenated blood from the lungs back to the central pump (pulmonary venous system).

The **portal systems** are specialized vascular channels that carry substances from one site to another, but do not depend on a central pump (see p. 152).

Systemic Blood Vessels

There are two main types of large blood vessel:
- **Arteries**, which carry blood away from the heart towards the capillary systems at relatively high pressure
- **Veins**, which carry blood back to the heart from the capillary systems at relatively low pressure.

The systemic arterial circulation is an extensive high-pressure system. The structure of its vessels reflects the high pressures to which they are subjected.

The output of the left ventricle is carried in large-diameter vessels with a high component of elastic tissue in their walls that smooths the systolic pressure wave. These are called the **large elastic arteries** (i.e. the aorta and its large branches, such as the carotid, subclavian and renal arteries).

Distal to these large elastic arteries are smaller vessels in which the artery walls become proportionately more muscular. These **muscular arteries** gradually decrease in size as they branch within tissues until they form **arterioles**. The arterioles then open into a system of very fine vessels termed **capillaries**.

From capillaries, blood moves into **venules** and then into **veins**, which become progressively larger as they approach the heart. The large veins carry blood at low pressure and hence have a small amount of muscle in their wall compared with arteries.

The pulmonary circulation has only to transfer blood a short distance from the right ventricle of the heart to the capillary systems of the lung, and from there back to the left atrium of the heart. Because the distances are short compared with those involved in the more complex systemic circulation, the pressures within the pulmonary circulation are much lower and the vessel walls are generally thinner. The detailed histology of the pulmonary vasculature is discussed in Chapter 10.

> **The larger blood vessels are composed of three layers which vary in prominence in different vessel types**

The walls of blood vessels are made up of three identifiable layers (tunica): **intima**, **media** and **adventitia**.

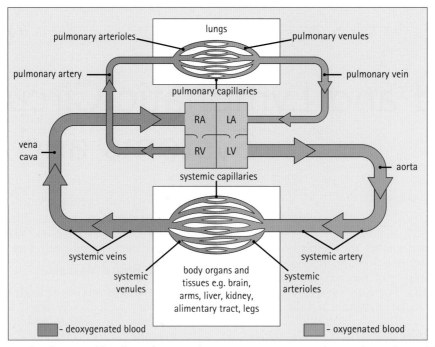

FIGURE 9.1 Systemic and pulmonary blood circulations. The main components and interrelationships of the systemic and pulmonary blood circulations. The heart is a four-chambered pump central to both systems. The direction of blood flow is indicated by arrows. Blood vessels that transport blood away from the heart are called 'arteries' (arterial systems) and those that take blood to the heart are called 'veins' (venous systems). The systemic venous and pulmonary arterial vessels carry deoxygenated blood; the pulmonary venous and systemic arterial vessels carry oxygenated blood. In organs and tissues other than the lung, the oxygenated blood gives up much of its oxygen and becomes deoxygenated; in the lungs deoxygenated blood is oxygenated. Gaseous exchange takes place in small, thin-walled vessels called 'capillaries'.

The tunica intima is composed of a lining layer of highly specialized multifunctional flattened epithelial cells termed **endothelium**. This sits on a basal lamina (the internal elastic lamina); beneath this is a very thin subendothelial layer of fibrocollagenous support tissue containing occasional contractile cells with some of the properties of smooth muscle cells but which are also capable of synthesizing collagen and elastin (like fibroblasts) and which also can have phagocytic properties (like histiocytes/macrophages). These cells are called **myointimal cells** and become very important in the development of the most common arterial disease, atherosclerosis (see p. 148).

The media is the middle layer in a blood vessel wall and is composed predominantly of smooth muscle reinforced by organized layers of elastic tissue, which form elastic laminae. The media is particularly prominent in arteries, being relatively indistinct in veins and virtually non-existent in very small vessels. In vessels that are close to the heart, receiving the full thrust of the systolic pressure wave, elastic tissue is very well developed, hence the term **elastic arteries**. In muscular arteries and arterioles, the elastic lamina separating the tunica media and the tunica adventitia is the **external elastic lamina**.

The tunica adventitia is the outer layer of blood vessels. It is composed largely of fibroblasts and collagen, but smooth muscle cells may be present, particularly in veins. The adventitia is often the most prominent layer in the walls of veins. Within the adventitia of vessels with thick walls are small blood vessels, the **vasa vasorum**, which send penetrating branches into the media to

supply it with blood. These are not seen in thinner vessels, which obtain their oxygen and nutrients by diffusion from the lumen. The adventitia also carries autonomic nerves which innervate the smooth muscle of the media.

The differences between the layers in the wall of a small artery and a small vein are illustrated in Figure 9.2. Although the smaller vessels progressively lose the media and adventitia, all blood vessels have a tunica intima lined internally by the flat endothelial cells. The smallest vessels, the capillaries, have only a layer of endothelial cells sitting on a basal lamina. The endothelial cells lining the entire blood circulatory system are vitally important cells, with many functions.

The endothelium is highly specialized, with endocrine, exocrine, cell adhesion, clotting and transport functions

The endothelium is composed of flattened cells with diverse functional roles. In routine histological sections, the cytoplasm of most endothelial cells is barely visible and only the small flattened nuclei are seen. Ultrastructurally, each cell can be seen to be anchored to the underlying basal lamina; individual cells are anchored together by adhesion junctions, including prominent tight junctions which prevent diffusion between cells. A prominent feature of endothelial cells is the presence of many pinocytotic vesicles, which are involved in the process of transport of substances from one side of the cell to the other. In small blood vessels of the nervous system, the endothelial cells express transport proteins, which are responsible for the active transport of all substances, for example glucose, into the brain. Ultrastructurally, endothelial cells also contain smooth and rough endoplasmic reticulum and free ribosomes, with occasional mitochondria and variable numbers of microfila-

ments. The characteristic cytoplasmic organelle of the endothelial cell is an electron-dense ovoid structure called the **Weibel–Palade body**, which are storage granules containing von Willebrand factor, P-selectin, and other vascular modulators. (Fig. 9.3b).

Endothelial cells are able to sense changes in blood pressure, oxygen tension and blood flow by as yet unknown mechanisms. In response to changes in local factors they respond by secreting substances which have powerful effects on the tone of vascular smooth muscle (endothelins, nitric oxide and prostacyclin, PGI2). Substances that cause relaxation of vascular smooth muscle increase local blood flow by causing vasodilation.

Endothelial cells are important for control of blood coagulation, and under normal circumstances the endothelial surface prevents blood clotting. This is done by high expression of factors that prevent blood clotting and low expression of factors that activate this process (Fig. 9.3a).

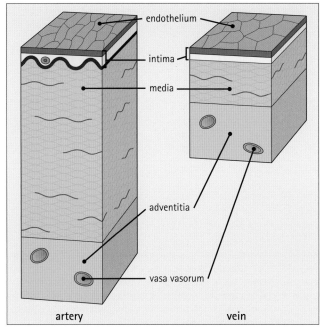

FIGURE 9.2 **General structure of blood vessel wall.** The wall of a blood vessel is divided into intima, media and adventitia. In an artery, the intima contains elastic lamina and myointimal cells. In an artery, the media is much more developed than in a vein of the same diameter.

KEY FACTS
ENDOTHELIUM

- Cells are bound together by junctional complexes and have many pinocytotic vesicles
- Cells have many functional roles despite their apparent structural simplicity
- Normally secretes factors which prevent blood clotting
- Normally secretes factors which maintain the tone of vascular smooth muscle
- Can be activated by cytokines to express cell adhesion molecules which allow white blood cells to stick.

Factor secreted by endothelium	Activities
prostacyclin	vasodilation, inhibits platelet aggregation
nitric oxide	vasodilation, inhibits platelet adhesion and aggregation
tissue plasminogen activator (tPA)	regulates fibrinolysis
thrombomodulin	anticoagulant activity
thromboplastin	promotes blood coagulation
platelet activating factor (PAF)	activation of platelets and neutrophils
von Willebrand factor	promotes platelet adhesion and activation of blood coagulation

(a)

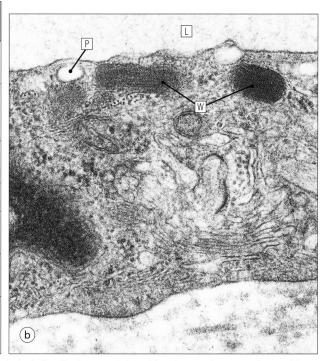

(b)

FIGURE 9.3 **Endothelial cells.** (a) Substances produced by endothelial cells that modulate blood coagulation and vasodilation. (b) High-power electron micrograph of part of an endothelial cell showing characteristic Weibel–Palade bodies (W) close to the surface contacting the vessel lumen (L). There are also pinocytotic vesicles (P), and smooth and rough endoplasmic reticulum.

Elastic arteries are characterized by multiple elastic laminae in the media

Elastic arteries are the largest arteries and receive the main output of the left ventricle: thus they are subjected to high systolic pressures of 120–160 mmHg. Furthermore, these large vessels are adapted to smooth out the surges in blood flow, as blood is impelled through them only during the systolic phase of the cardiac cycle. The elastic tissue in their walls provides the resilience to smooth out the pressure wave.

ADVANCED CONCEPT
ACTIVATED ENDOTHELIUM

The endothelium can adapt rapidly to changes in its environment. Under certain circumstances, especially in response to inflammation, the endothelium may become activated and change its function.

Endothelium may become activated by cytokines and develop specialization for emigration of lymphoid cells. The endothelial cells become cuboidal in shape and express surface adhesion molecules, which facilitate lymphocyte adhesion and migration. This type of endothelium is normally seen in the specialized venules in the lymph node paracortex (high endothelial venules).

Endothelium may become activated by cytokines and express cell adhesion molecules for neutrophils. This normally occurs after any form of tissue damage and allows neutrophils to migrate into local tissues in the process of acute inflammation. The substance P-selectin, a cell adhesion molecule, is stored in special vesicles (Weibel–Palade bodies) inside the endothelium (see Fig. 9.3b). With appropriate stimulation, these vesicles dock with the endothelial cell membrane. P-selectin is then available on the cell surface for neutrophil adhesion.

Endothelium is normally locally impermeable to substances in the blood. Under the effects of certain factors, for example histamine, endothelial cells lose attachment to each other and retract. This allows fluid and proteins to diffuse out into the local tissues, causing tissue swelling, termed **oedema**. This reorganization of cell–cell junctions is rapid and reversible and takes place in the space of a few minutes.

The intima of large elastic arteries is composed of endothelium with a thin layer of underlying fibrocollagenous tissue.

Elastic arteries have a thick, highly developed media of which elastic fibres are an important component. These are arranged in circumferential sheets between the layers of smooth muscle fibres throughout the thickness of the media. In the largest artery, the aorta, there are often 50 or more layers (Fig. 9.4).

The elastic fibres are arranged so that they run circumferentially rather than longitudinally in order to counteract the tendency of the vessel to overdistend during systole. Return of the elastic fibres from the stretched to the unstretched state during diastole maintains a diastolic pressure within the aorta and large arteries of about 60–80 mmHg. Interposed between

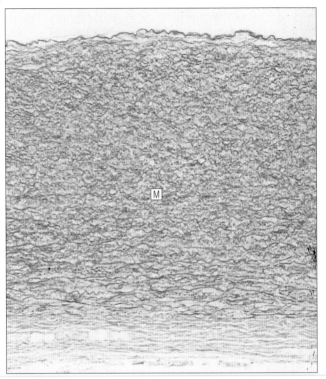

FIGURE 9.4 **Elastic artery.** Low-power view of elastic van Gieson-stained large elastic artery (aorta). The predominant layer is the media (M), which is composed of elastic fibres (black) arranged as concentric sheets and separated by smooth muscle fibres and collagen.

the elastic layers are smooth muscle cells and some collagen.

With age, and particularly in association with the common disease of the intima, atherosclerosis (see p. 148), the elastic fibres and smooth muscle fibres of the media of an elastic artery undergo degeneration and are replaced by non-elastic, non-contractile collagen. This loss of elasticity and contractility means that the artery is less capable of sustaining an intraluminal pressure during diastole, and the diastolic pressure falls. In the presence of an often increased systolic pressure, this is manifest clinically as a wide pulse pressure (i.e. difference between systolic and diastolic pressures). The most severe complication of the loss of elastic and smooth muscle fibres is the permanent pathological dilatation of the elastic artery (usually the aorta). This is called **aneurysm** formation (see 'Clinical Example' box, p. 148).

The adventitia of the large vessels carries vasa vasorum and nerves.

Muscular arteries have a media composed almost entirely of smooth muscle

The large elastic arteries gradually merge into muscular arteries by losing most of their medial elastic sheets, usually leaving only two layers, an internal elastic lamina and an external elastic lamina, at the junction of the media with, respectively, the intima and the adventitia. The general structure of a muscular artery is shown in Figure 9.5a.

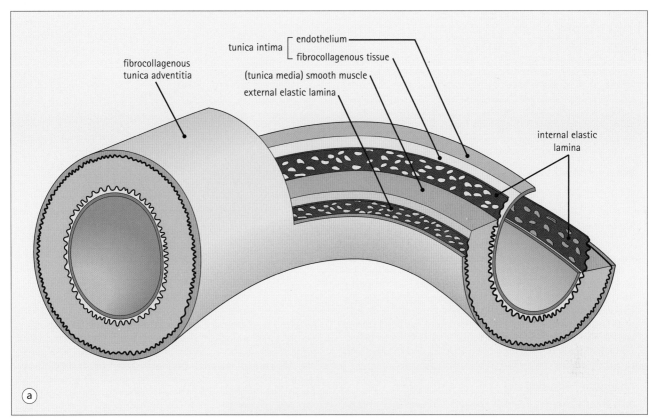

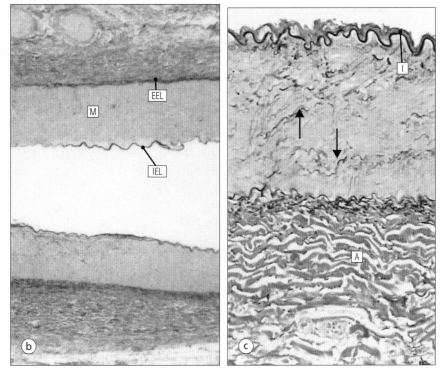

FIGURE 9.5 **Muscular artery.** (a) The most prominent layer of a muscular artery is the media. Composed of smooth muscle, it is bounded by an internal and an external elastic lamina. (b) Elastic van Gieson-stained longitudinal section through a muscular artery. The intima is scarcely visible, the predominant layer being the muscular media (M) situated between an internal elastic lamina (IEL) and an external elastic lamina (EEL), which are composed of condensed sheets of elastic fibres (black). The outer adventitia stains red, being composed largely of collagen. (c) Medium-power view of the same artery showing the intima (I) and the fine black-staining elastic fibres running through the muscular media (arrows). In this large muscular artery the collagenous adventitia (A) is thick.

In a muscular artery the media is composed almost entirely of smooth muscle. These arteries are therefore highly contractile, their degree of contraction or relaxation being controlled by the autonomic nervous system as well as by endothelium-derived vasoactive substances. A few fine elastic fibres are scattered among the smooth muscle cells, but are not organized into sheets. These are most numerous in the large muscular arteries, which are a direct continuation of the distal end of the elastic arteries (Fig. 9.5b,c).

Muscular arteries vary in size from about 1 cm in diameter close to their origin at the elastic arteries, to

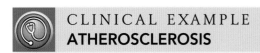

CLINICAL EXAMPLE
ATHEROSCLEROSIS

Atherosclerosis is a disease of the arteries which starts in the intima. It is characterized by infiltration of the intima by oxidized fatty acids, which accumulates in macrophages and myointimal cells, accompanied by increased deposition of collagen. Such intimal thickening forms a so-called 'atheromatous plaque'.

There are three common consequences of atheroma:

Impaired Blood Flow

Atheromatous change leads to a reduction in the size of the lumen of the vessel so that blood flow is decreased.

Thrombus Formation

Another complication of atherosclerosis is that it damages the smooth internal lining of endothelial cells, exposing circulating blood to the underlying intimal collagen. This can trigger coagulation to form a mass of blood clot, termed a 'thrombus', within the vessel. Thrombus further reduces the lumen of the vessel and may block it completely (Fig. 9.6), resulting in death of the tissue (infarction) supplied by the vessel. The myocardium is particularly vulnerable to infarction (see Fig. 9.24), as is the brain (stroke) and the feet and toes (gangrene).

Aneurysm Formation

As a plaque of atheroma enlarges, elastic fibres and smooth muscle are lost from the underlying media. In the large elastic arteries, such as the aorta, these specialized components become replaced by non-contractile, inelastic collagen and the vessel dilates to form an abnormally wide sac termed an 'aneurysm'. The danger of an aneurysm is that the vessel wall is greatly weakened and is prone to burst.

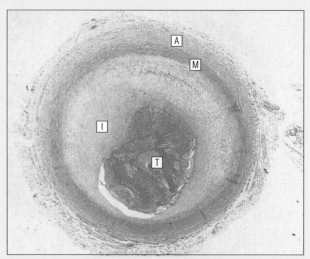

FIGURE 9.6 **Coronary artery atheroma and thrombosis.** Micrograph showing a transverse section from the coronary artery supplying the area of dead muscle shown in Figure 9.24. The lumen has been greatly reduced by thickening of the intimal layer (I) by atheroma. The media (M) and adventitia (A) are normal. The intimal thickening and irregularity have led to the formation of a thrombus (T), which has blocked the vessel lumen.

about 0.5 mm in diameter. In the larger arteries there may be 30 or more layers of smooth muscle cells, whereas in the smallest peripheral arteries there are only two or three layers. The smooth muscle cells are usually arranged circumferentially at right-angles to the long axis of the vessel.

The internal elastic lamina is commonly a distinct prominent layer, but the external elastic lamina is less well defined (see Fig. 9.5).

Arterioles are the smallest branches of the arterial tree

Arterioles vary in diameter, ranging from 30 μm to 400 μm (0.4 mm).

The intima of an arteriole is composed of endothelial cells lying on a basement membrane, with an underlying fine internal elastic lamina in the larger arterioles.

The arteriolar media is composed of one or two layers of smooth muscle cells (Fig. 9.7). As the arterioles become smaller, the continuous layers of smooth muscle become progressively discontinuous. In the smallest arterioles, the endothelial cells have basal processes, which pierce the basement membrane and make junctional contacts with the smooth muscle cells. The adventitia of arterioles is insignificant.

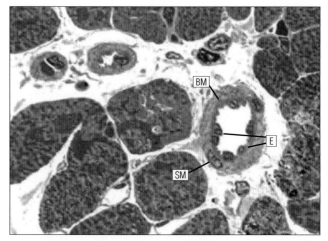

FIGURE 9.7 **Arteriole.** Micrograph of a thin epoxy resin toluidine blue-stained section of three arterioles showing basement membrane (BM) as a pale-staining membrane surrounded by a layer of smooth muscle cells (SM). The inner endothelial cells (E) in the larger vessel appear rather cuboidal because it has contracted during the biopsy process. Note that the three arterioles differ not only in size, but also with regard to the number of muscle cells.

Arterioles are very responsive to vasoactive stimuli and make a major contribution to vascular resistance.

KEY FACTS
ARTERIAL SYSTEM

- Large elastic arteries have a media composed of concentric layers of elastic and smooth muscle (for example aorta and subclavian arteries)
- Muscular arteries have a prominent media composed of smooth muscle which is bounded by internal and external elastic laminae (for example coronary arteries)
- Arterioles are the smallest part of the arterial tree and have three to four complete layers of smooth muscle in their media.

The microvasculature starts at the level of the arterioles

The microvasculature (Fig. 9.8) is composed of small-diameter blood vessels with partly permeable thin walls that permit the transfer of some blood components to the tissues and vice versa. Most of this exchange between blood and tissues occurs in the extensive capillary network, the smallest arterioles (metarterioles) emptying into the capillary system. The capillary networks drain into the first components of the venous system, the venules.

Capillaries are specialized for diffusion of substances across their wall

Capillaries are the smallest vessels of the blood circulatory system (5–10 μm in diameter) and form a complex interlinking network.

Capillaries have the thinnest walls of all blood vessels and are the major site of gaseous exchange, permitting the transfer of oxygen from blood to tissues, and carbon dioxide from tissues to blood. Fluids containing large molecules pass across the capillary wall in both directions.

The capillary wall (Fig. 9.9) is composed of endothelial cells, a basement membrane and occasional scattered contractile cells called 'pericytes'.

Capillaries may be of two types: continuous or fenestrated

Capillaries with **continuous** endothelium are the most common type, the endothelial cells forming a complete

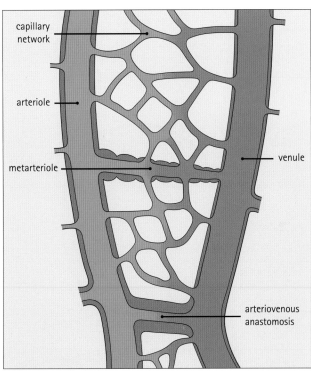

FIGURE 9.8 **Microvasculature.** Blood flows from arteriolar to venular vessels through a complex network of capillaries, arising either directly from the arteriole or from the smaller metarteriole. Opening of the arteriovenous anastomosis directs blood flow out of the capillary network.

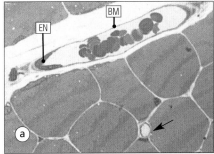
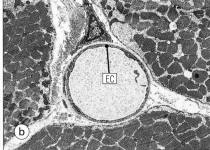
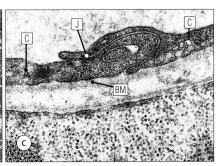

FIGURE 9.9 **Capillary.** (a) An epoxy resin section stained with toluidine blue of a capillary in longitudinal section. The wall is composed almost entirely of thin basement membrane (BM), the endothelial cytoplasm lining its internal surface not being visible at this magnification. An endothelial cell nucleus (EN) can be seen at one end. A similar but smaller capillary is seen in transverse section (arrow) between individual muscle fibres. (b) Electron micrograph of the capillary arrowed in (a). At this low magnification, the endothelial cytoplasm (EC) is just visible, but the basement membrane is indistinct. (c) High-power electron micrograph of part of the capillary wall showing the basement membrane (BM), endothelial cytoplasm (C) and anchoring junction (J) between the cytoplasm of adjacent endothelial cells.

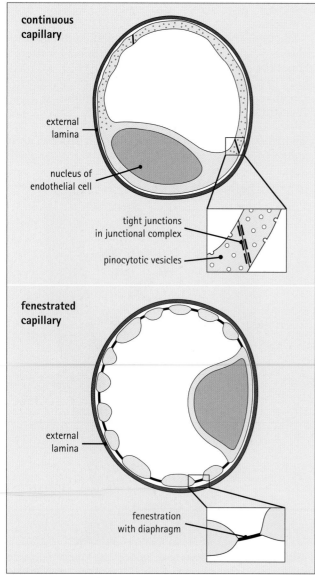

FIGURE 9.10 **Types of capillary.** There are two types of capillary: continuous and fenestrated. In continuous capillaries substances are transported across the wall by pinocytosis.

internal lining to the capillary with no intercellular or intracytoplasmic defects (Fig. 9.10).

Capillaries with **fenestrated** endothelium are seen most commonly in the gastrointestinal mucosa, endocrine glands and renal glomeruli (see Figs 15.8, 15.14). The endothelial cell cytoplasm is pierced by pores (fenestrations), which extend through its full thickness. In some fenestrations there is a thin diaphragm that is thinner than the cell membrane; its nature is uncertain.

Sinusoids are large-diameter channels with thin walls

Highly specialized vascular channels, called 'sinusoids', are seen in some organs, for example the liver (see Fig. 12.1) and spleen (see Fig. 8.16). They are endothelium-lined channels with a larger diameter than capillaries, and scanty, discontinuous or absent basement membrane.

The endothelial cells in sinusoids are commonly highly fenestrated, often with large pores, and there may be substantial gaps between the cells.

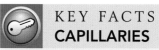

KEY FACTS
CAPILLARIES

- Receive blood from arterioles and metarterioles (see Fig. 9.8)
- Are composed of a single layer of endothelium attached to a basal lamina
- Most have a continuous layer of endothelial cells which are tightly attached (continuous type)
- Some have pores which allow free diffusion from the lumen to tissues (fenestrated type).

Blood from capillaries enters a system of venules

Capillaries drain into **postcapillary venules**, which are the smallest venules (10–25 μm in diameter). They resemble capillaries in structure, but have more pericytes (Fig. 9.11).

Postcapillary venules drain into **large collecting venules** 20–50 μm in diameter, in which the pericyte layer becomes continuous and surrounding collagen fibres appear.

As the collecting venules become larger bore the pericytes are progressively replaced by smooth muscle cells, which form a layer 1–2 cells thick, and a fibrocollagenous adventitia becomes identifiable; these are **muscular venules** and are 50–100 μm in diameter. Muscular venules drain into the smallest veins.

Veins have thin walls and carry blood at low pressure

Veins vary in size from less than 1 mm to 4 cm in diameter. In comparison with arteries of comparable external diameter, veins have a larger lumen and a relatively thinner wall, and are therefore commonly collapsed in histological sections unless infusion-fixed.

Although intimal, medial and adventitial layers are present in veins they are less clearly demarcated than in arteries, and it is often difficult to identify where one layer ends and another begins. Furthermore, there is considerable variation in vein wall structure according to location. The following description of veins of different sizes is therefore a generalization.

Small veins are a continuation of the muscular venules and have a similar wall structure, but are larger – up to 1 mm in diameter – with more clearly defined muscle cell and outer fibrocollagenous layers (Fig. 9.12a).

Medium-sized veins are 1–10 mm in diameter. They have an inner layer of endothelial cells on a basement membrane. This is separated by a narrow zone of collagen fibres from an indistinct condensation of elastic fibres producing a thin, discontinuous internal elastic lamina.

The inner layer is fairly consistent in structure, differing only in quantity of collagen and elastic fibres between

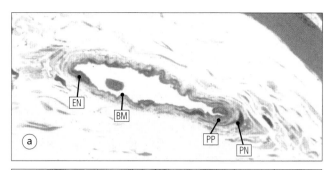

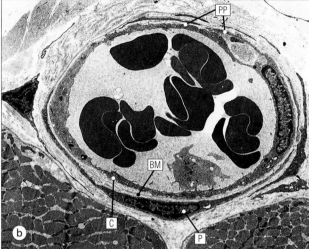

FIGURE 9.11 **Postcapillary venule.** (a) Toluidine blue-stained epoxy resin section of a partly collapsed postcapillary venule. The endothelial cell nucleus (EN) and basement membrane (BM) can be identified. There are a few pericyte processes (PP) and a pericyte nucleus (PN) in the wall, but the details are not clearly visible. (b) Electron micrograph of a postcapillary venule showing the endothelial cell cytoplasm (C), basement membrane (BM) and pericytes (P) more clearly. Note that the finer pericyte processes (PP) apparently intervene between layers of the basement membrane.

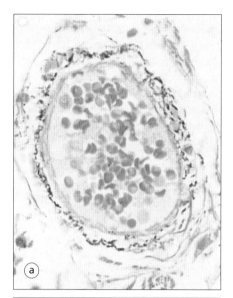

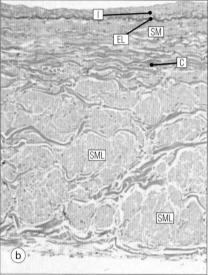

FIGURE 9.12 **Veins.** (a) Micrograph showing an elastic van Gieson (EVG)-stained small vein. The rather variable and irregular arrangement of smooth muscle (yellow), collagen (red) and elastic fibres (black) in its wall is evident. (b) Micrograph showing the wall of the largest vein in the body, the inferior vena cava. There is a distinct intima (I) and internal elastic lamina (EL), a layer of smooth muscle (yellow, SM) and an irregular layer of thick collagen (red, C). This collagen indicates the approximate beginning of the adventitial layer, the thickest layer in large veins, being expanded by the presence of large bundles of longitudinally running smooth muscle (SML) (EVG stain).

the endothelium and the condensation of elastic fibres. However, the outer layers – still called 'the media and adventitia', but often arbitrarily and with little justification – vary considerably in thickness, proportions of collagen, elastic fibres and smooth muscle, and in the orientation of the muscle fibres in particular.

Large veins have an inner (intimal) layer similar to that of medium-sized veins, but there are usually more collagen and elastic fibres between the endothelial basement membrane and the elastic lamina, which is generally discontinuous. External to the elastic lamina there is a layer of smooth muscle embedded in collagen, and outside this is a thick layer of collagen in which there are bundles of longitudinally oriented smooth muscle fibres. Some elastic fibres intermingle with the collagen (Fig. 9.12b).

Valves in large veins assist the flow of blood to the heart

Venous circulation of blood is maintained by the contraction of venous smooth muscle, supplemented to varying degrees by external pressure from the contraction of the surrounding skeletal muscle responsible for arm and leg movement. Such assistance from skeletal muscle contraction is particularly important for maintaining the venous circulation of the arms and legs.

The veins in the arms and legs, which carry blood against gravity, are equipped with valves to prevent blood flowing back down the vein. These valves are thin flaps of intima that project into the lumen, the free edges of the valve flaps pointing toward the heart; this allows blood to flow towards the heart, but prevents backflow. Incompetence of the valves in the veins of the legs causes varicose veins.

Valves are also present in other medium and large veins, their number varies depending on whether or not the vein is carrying blood against gravity.

Arteriovenous anastomoses allow blood to bypass capillary beds

In addition to the microvasculature (i.e. arterioles emptying into a capillary network, which drains into a venular system), there are additional vessels that bypass the capillary bed, allowing arterioles to communicate directly with venules; these are arteriovenous anastomoses (see Fig. 9.8).

At its arteriolar end, an arteriovenous anastomosis is thick-walled, mainly due to an abundant smooth muscle coat which is richly innervated. Contraction of the thick smooth muscle layer closes off the lumen of the anastomosis at its origin and diverts blood into the capillary bed; relaxation opens up the lumen, allowing blood to flow directly into a venule and thereby bypassing the capillary network.

Arteriovenous anastomoses are widespread, but are most common in the skin in certain regions such as the fingertips, lips, nose, ears and toes. They are thought to play an important role in the skin's thermoregulatory function (see Chapter 18). Closure of the anastomosis diverts blood into the extensive dermal capillary system and permits heat loss, and opening of the vessel closes the capillary bed and conserves heat.

In the fingertips, there is a highly specialized type of arteriovenous anastomosis, the glomus body, which has a prominent arterial end (Sucquet–Hoyer canal) connecting directly to the venular end. The canal is surrounded by modified smooth muscle cells (glomus cells), which are richly innervated by the autonomic nervous system.

Blood vessels have both efferent and afferent innervation

Blood vessels that can significantly alter their lumen size by contraction and relaxation of their smooth muscle fibres have a major supply of adrenergic sympathetic fibres, stimulation of which causes muscle contraction and vasoconstriction.

Some blood vessels in skeletal muscles also have a cholinergic sympathetic innervation capable of producing vasodilation.

In certain areas, blood vessels have an afferent innervation, which provides information about the luminal pressure (baroreceptive information) and blood gas (i.e. carbon dioxide and oxygen) levels (chemoreceptive information). These are mainly located in the carotid sinuses, and in the region of the aortic arch, pulmonary artery and large veins entering the heart.

Afferent fibres from the carotid sinus receptors travel in the glossopharyngeal nerve to the cardiorespiratory centres in the brain stem.

Portal Blood Systems

A portal system connects two capillary systems

Portal circulations are venous channels that connect one capillary system with another and do not depend on the central pumping action of the heart.

The nature of portal connecting vessels varies from site to site; for example, the vessels of the hepatic portal system (see Fig. 12.2), which connects capillaries in the intestine to the capillary-like sinusoids in the liver, are venous in nature, being small venules adjacent to the capillary beds, and medium and large-sized veins in between. In the other main portal system, between the hypothalamus and the posterior pituitary (see Fig. 14.3), the connecting vessels are large capillaries and venules.

Lymphatic Circulatory System

The lymphatic system carries fluid that drains from the intercellular space of tissues

The intercellular spaces of almost all tissues contain small endothelial-lined tubes, which are blind ending but otherwise identical in structure to blood capillaries. These are lymphatic capillaries and are permeable to fluids and dissolved molecules in the interstitial fluid.

In some areas, the lymphatic capillaries have a fenestrated endothelium and a discontinuous basement membrane, permitting the entry of larger molecules, such as large molecular weight proteins, triglycerides, etc. and also some cells, particularly cells of the immune system.

The lymphatic capillary network acts as a drainage system, removing surplus fluid (lymph) from tissue spaces. Lymph is normally a clear colourless fluid, but lymph draining the intestine during absorption is often milky in appearance because of its high lipid content. This is called 'chyle'.

The lymphatic capillaries merge to form thicker-walled vessels which resemble venules and medium-sized veins.

Lymph moves sluggishly from the capillary network into the larger lymphatic vessels; backflow is prevented by numerous flap-like valves similar to those in veins (Fig. 9.13).

On its way to the larger vein-like lymphatics from the smaller lymphatics, lymph passes through one or more lymph nodes. It enters the lymph node at its convex periphery and leaves it through one or two lymphatic vessels at the concave hilum (see Fig. 8.8). During this passage, any antigens in the lymph can be processed by the immune system. Activated lymphocytes, which are important to immune defence, are added to the lymph.

The larger lymphatic vessels have muscular walls and pump the lymph into the following two main lymphatic vessels:

- The thoracic duct, which empties lymph into the venous system at the junction of the left internal jugular and left subclavian veins

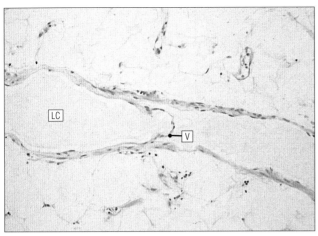

FIGURE 9.13 **Lymphatic capillary.** Micrograph showing a large lymphatic capillary (LC) containing pale pink-staining lymph. Note the delicate flap-like valves (V) controlling the direction of flow.

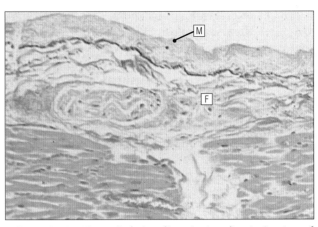

FIGURE 9.14 **Visceral pericardium (epicardium).** Section of thin epicardium showing a narrow layer of fibrocollagenous tissue (F) containing elastic fibres (black), covered by flat mesothelial cells (M) identical to those of the inner surface of the parietal pericardium (elastic van Gieson's stain.)

CLINICAL EXAMPLE
SPREAD OF CANCER BY LYMPHATICS

All lymphatic capillaries from a particular area drain into lymph nodes serving that area (regional lymph nodes). Such drainage is particularly important in the spread of cancer, as cancer cells can enter the lymphatic capillaries and be carried to other sites. Cancer cells may also be trapped in the regional lymph node, where they can multiply and produce secondary tumours at some distance from the site of the primary cancer (see Fig. 8.14).

For example, most cancers that originate in the breast may be carried in the lymph to the regional lymph nodes of the breast, most of which are in the subcutaneous tissue of the axilla. Careful palpation of the axillary lymph nodes to detect possible tumour nodules is therefore a vital part of the physical examination of any patient with suspected breast cancer.

- A more variable lymphatic vessel, the right main lymphatic duct, which empties into the junction between the right internal jugular and right subclavian veins.

Stem Cells and the Vasculature

Blood vessels have long been touted as sources for stem or progenitor cells in regenerating tissues. And blood vessels are known to serve as a niche for stem cells in various tissues. However, the definitive identification of vascular stem cells is not well accepted in the scientific community. Many investigators feel that haemangioblast progenitor cells do give rise to endothelium. And that stem cell antigen 1 (Sca-1) positive adventitial cells or pericytes in adult blood vessels do indeed have stem or progenitor cell potential. The integral role that blood vessels play in regenerative activities does suggest that blood vessel stem cells may play an important role in tissue regeneration, although additional research is needed.

The Heart

The heart is a muscular pump with four chambers. Two of these, the **atria**, receive blood from the systemic and pulmonary venous circulations, whereas the other two, the **ventricles**, pump blood into the systemic and pulmonary arterial circulations. In between the cardiac chambers and at the two outflow portals of the heart are the **heart valves**, which prevent backflow of blood.

The wall of the heart is composed of the epicardium, the myocardium and the endocardium

The three layers of the heart wall are:
- A very thin outer **epicardium** (visceral pericardium) covered with flat mesothelial cells to produce a smooth outer surface
- A middle **myocardium** making up the vast bulk of the heart wall and composed of specialized muscle (cardiac muscle), which is responsible for the pumping action of the heart
- A very thin, inner smooth lining, the **endocardium**, covered by endothelial cells in direct contact with the circulating blood.

The pericardium surrounds the heart and is lined by mesothelial cells

The heart is enclosed within the pericardial sac, which is composed of compact fibrocollagenous and elastic tissue and lined internally by a layer of flat mesothelial cells, termed the **parietal pericardium**. This smooth mesothelial layer reflects over the outer surface of the heart to form the **visceral pericardium** (Fig. 9.14), also termed the **epicardium**.

The pericardial cavity is the space between the parietal and visceral pericardial layers. It contains a small amount of serous fluid to lubricate the surfaces and permit friction-free movement of the heart within the cavity during its muscular contractions.

When the visceral or parietal pericardium sustains structural damage as a result of disease, the smooth lubricated surfaces are lost and the friction-free movement is impaired. This can be detected clinically by listening over the heart area with a stethoscope, and a scratching noise can be heard in time with each systolic heartbeat. This is called a **pericardial friction rub**, and indicates abnormal roughening of the pericardial surfaces. This commonly occurs when there has been a myocardial infarct (see 'Clinical Example' box, p. 161) and is an indication that the full thickness of the myocardium of the left ventricular wall has been damaged, from the inner endocardium to the outer pericardium.

The epicardium forms the outer covering of the heart and has an external layer of flat mesothelial cells. These cells lie on a stroma of fibrocollagenous support tissue, which contains elastic fibres, as well as the large arteries supplying blood to the heart wall and the larger venous tributaries carrying blood from the heart wall. The large arteries (coronary arteries) and veins are surrounded by adipose tissue, which expands the epicardium.

The coronary arteries originate from the first part of the aorta just above the aortic valve ring and pass over the surface of the heart in the epicardium, sending branches deep into the myocardium. This superficial location of the arteries is of great practical importance, as it permits surgical bypass grafting of blocked arteries.

The myocardium is composed of specialized striated muscle termed cardiac muscle

The bulk of the heart is myocardium, which is the contractile element composed of specialized striated muscle fibres called 'cardiac muscle' (see Fig. 5.10).

The amount of myocardium and the diameter of muscle fibres in the chambers of the heart vary according to the workload of the chamber (Fig. 9.15).

The left and right atria push blood into empty ventricles against minimal resistance during diastole, and therefore have a thin wall composed of cells of small diameter.

The right ventricle pushes blood out through the pulmonary valve and through the pulmonary arteries to the lungs (see Fig. 9.1). It therefore has a moderately thick muscle layer composed of fibres intermediate in diameter between atrial and left ventricular muscle cells.

The left ventricle pumps blood through the high-pressure systemic arterial system, and therefore has the thickest myocardium with the largest diameter muscle fibres (see Fig. 9.15b).

Because the myocardial muscle fibres of the left ventricle have the greatest workload (pumping blood throughout the body at a systolic pressure of 120 mmHg) they have the largest energy output and therefore the greatest oxygen requirements. If the oxygen supply is reduced, a common sequela of coronary artery disease, the muscle fibres become ischaemic and cannot function to their optimum ability. This produces the symptoms of **angina** and eventual **myocardial infarction** (see p. 161). The cardiac muscle fibres of the atria operate at much lower pressures, and therefore have lower oxygen

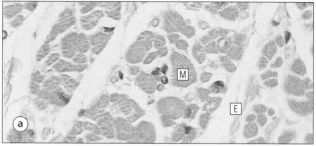

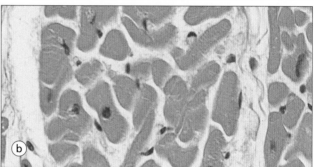

FIGURE 9.15 **Myocardium.** (a) Micrograph of left atrial myocardium in approximate transverse section. The myocardial fibres (M) form an interconnecting network separated by loose fibrocollagenous tissue (the endomysium, E). (b) Micrograph of left ventricular myocardium in approximate transverse section at the same magnification as (a). The general structure is the same as left atrial myocardium, but the fibres of the left ventricle are larger in diameter and have larger nuclei.

demands, and almost never become significantly ischaemic in coronary artery disease.

The outer surface of the myocardium beneath the pericardium is smooth, but the internal surface beneath the endocardium is raised into trabeculations, which are most marked in the ventricles. The trabeculations are covered by smooth endocardium and do not interfere with the smooth flow of the blood.

In both ventricles, raised mounds of cardiac muscle (papillary muscles) protrude into the ventricular lumina and point towards the atrioventricular valves. Papillary muscles are the site of attachment of chordae tendineae, narrow tendinous cords that tether the atrioventricular valve leaflets to the wall of the ventricle beneath them (see Figs 9.18a and 9.29b).

Cardiac muscle cells secrete atrial natriuretic hormone

Atrial myocardial fibres are smaller than those of the ventricles and contain small neuroendocrine granules, which are usually sparse and located close to the nucleus; they are most numerous in the right atrium. These granules secrete atrial natriuretic hormone when the atrial fibres are stretched excessively.

Atrial natriuretic hormone increases the excretion of water and sodium and potassium ions by the distal convoluted tubule of the kidney. It also decreases blood pressure by inhibiting renin secretion by the kidneys and aldosterone secretion by the adrenals (see Chapter 14).

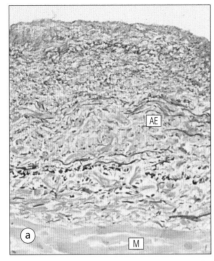

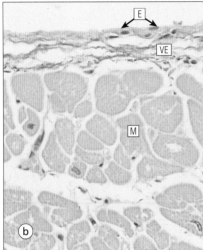

FIGURE 9.16 **Endocardium.** (a) Micrograph of elastic van Gieson (EVG)-stained right atrial endocardium (AE). The collagenous content stains red, elastic fibres stain black, myocardial muscle fibres (M) stain yellow. The nature of endocardial fibres is not apparent in a routine H&E-stained section. The atrial endocardium is much thicker than that which covers the ventricles. (b) Micrograph of EVG-stained left ventricular endocardium (VE) at the same magnification. It is a much thinner layer than in the atrium and contains much less elastic tissue; the muscle fibres (M) are large. The inner endothelial cell layer is always poorly preserved in postmortem material, as here (E).

The endocardium lines the chambers of the heart and varies in thickness in different areas

The internal lining of all four heart chambers is the 'endocardium', which is composed of three layers (Fig. 9.16):
- The layer in direct contact with the myocardium
- The middle layer
- The innermost layer.

The outermost layer is composed of irregularly arranged collagen fibres that merge with collagen surrounding adjacent cardiac muscle fibres. This layer may contain some Purkinje fibres, which are part of the impulse conducting system.

The middle layer is the thickest endocardial layer and is composed of more regularly arranged collagen fibres containing variable numbers of elastic fibres, which are compact and arranged in parallel in the deepest part of the layer. Occasional myofibroblasts are present.

The inner layer is composed of flat endothelial cells, which are continuous with the endothelial cells lining the vessels entering and emerging from the heart.

The endocardium is variable in thickness, being thickest in the atria and thinnest in the ventricles, particularly the left ventricle. The increased thickness is due almost entirely to a thicker fibroelastic middle layer (see Fig. 9.16). Localized areas of endocardial thickening (jet lesions) are common, particularly in the atria, and result from turbulent blood flow within the chamber.

The heart valves prevent blood flowing back into the heart chambers after emptying

During contraction of the ventricles (systole), blood is prevented from flowing back into the atria by two valves:
- The right atrioventricular (tricuspid) valve between the right atrium and right ventricle
- The left atrioventricular (bicuspid or mitral) valve between the left atrium and left ventricle.

Similarly, to prevent blood flowing back into the two ventricles at the end of their contraction, there are valves between the ventricles and the large vessels into which they empty:
- The pulmonary valve between the right ventricle and its outflow vessel, the pulmonary artery
- The aortic valve between the left ventricle and its outflow vessel, the aorta.

A central fibrocollagenous skeleton anchors the valves and chambers of the heart together

The heart has a fibrocollagenous skeleton, the main component being the **central fibrous body**, located at the level of the cardiac valves.

Extensions of the central fibrous body surround the heart valves to form the **valve rings**, which support the base of each valve. The valve rings on the left side of the heart surround the mitral and aortic valves and are thicker than those on the right side, which surround the tricuspid and pulmonary valves.

A short downward extension of the fibrocollagenous tissue of the aortic valve ring forms a fibrous septum between the right and left ventricles called the **membranous interventricular septum**. This is a minor component of the septum between the right and left ventricles, most of which is composed of cardiac muscle covered on both sides by endocardium. The membranous part is located high in the septal wall beneath the aortic valve.

The aortic and pulmonary valves have three cup-like cusps

The outflow valves of the right and left ventricles, the pulmonary and aortic valves, are composed of three cup-like cusps that fit closely together when closed. Because of their shape they are called 'semilunar valves'.

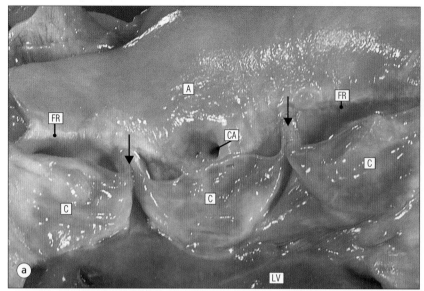

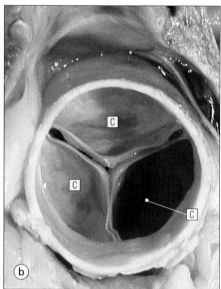

FIGURE 9.17 **Aortic valve.** (a) The opened aortic valve between the left ventricle (LV) and its large emptying artery, the aorta (A). The three cusps (C) of the valve, the commissures (arrows), the origin of one of the coronary arteries (CA) and the pale fibro-collagenous valve ring (FR) are clearly seen. (b) The closed aortic valve viewed from above. Note how closely the three cusps (C) fit together. The pressure of blood against the closed valve ensures coronary artery blood flow during diastole.

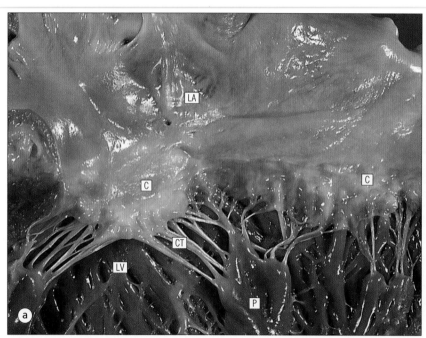

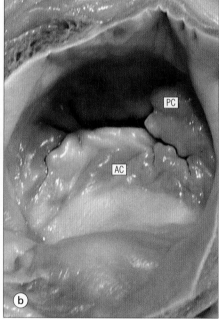

FIGURE 9.18 **Mitral valve.** (a) The opened left side of the heart to demonstrate the mitral valve between the left atrium (LA) and the left ventricle (LV). It has two cusps (C), the free edges of which are tethered to the papillary muscles (P) by thin chordae ten-dineae (CT). (b) The closed mitral valve viewed from above. There are two cusps, one anterior (AC) and one posterior (PC).

The base of each valve is attached to a fibrocollage-nous valve ring. The junctions between the cusps and are called 'commissures' (Fig. 9.17).

The mitral and tricuspid valves are attached to heart muscle by tendinous cords

The atrioventricular valves are thin flaps attached to their respective valve ring at the base, and tethered on their undersurface (ventricular surface) by the chordae tendineae (Fig. 9.18). This prevents eversion of the valve leaflets into the atrium during ventricular contraction.

A heart valve is composed of fibroelastic tissue and is covered by endothelium

The heart valves all have the same general structure with a dense fibrocollagenous central plate (the fibrosa), which is an extension of the fibrocollagenous tissue of

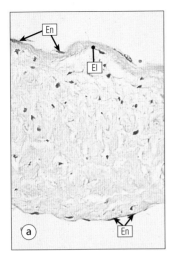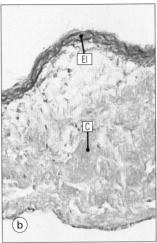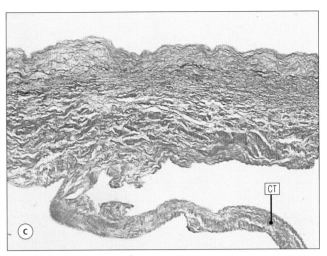

FIGURE 9.19 **Histology of heart valves.** (a) High-magnification micrograph of H&E-stained aortic valve. The bulk of the valve leaflet is composed of loose fibrocollagenous tissue with non-staining glycosaminoglycans between the collagen fibres. There is a dense area of elastic tissue (El) on the superior surface. The flat endocardial cells (En) can be seen clearly on both surfaces of the valve. (b) High-magnification micrograph of elastic van Gieson (EVG)-stained aortic valve. The dense elastic tissue (El) stains black and the collagen (C) stains red. (c) Micrograph of EVG-stained mitral valve close to its origin at the left atrioventricular valve ring. The leaflet is composed of red-staining collagen with some elastic fibres (black) running through it. The collagen is thickest, densest and most irregular on its inferior (ventricular) surface, where the chordae tendineae (CT) are attached. The chordae have a structure similar to that of tendon (see Fig. 13.9).

the central fibrous body and the fibrocollagenous valve ring. The fibrosa is covered on both surfaces by a layer of fibroelastic tissue, and is covered by outer layers of flat endothelial cells. The thickness of the layers varies between valves, and between sites within the same valve, and with age (Fig. 9.19).

There are minor modifications to this general structure in the atrioventricular valves. Much of the lower ventricular surface of the atrioventricular valves is roughened, the roughening marking the points of insertion of the chordae tendineae. The chordae are not inserted solely at the free edge of the leaflet: some attach further back and a few small chordae insert near the base. The chordae fibres merge with the collagenous fibres of the central fibrosa of the valve leaflet. The atrioventricular valves may also have a thin layer of muscle fibres, continuous with those of the atrial wall, on their upper surface.

In addition to the general histological structure of heart valves, the aortic valve shows prominent fibroelastic thickening at the sites of cusp apposition during valve closure. This is sometimes visible as white lines (linea alba) just below the free edge of the cusps, with a central nodule at the midpoint of each cusp, the nodule of Arantius (see Fig. 9.17). These are present but much less prominent on the pulmonary valve cusps because of the less forceful valve closure in the low-pressure pulmonary system.

The conducting system of the heart is composed of modified muscle fibres

The heart contracts involuntarily, at a rate of around 70 beats per minute. The rhythmic contractions of atria and ventricles do not depend on nerve stimulation, but result from impulses generated within the heart itself. However, the autonomic nervous system can control the rate of

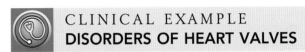

CLINICAL EXAMPLE
DISORDERS OF HEART VALVES

There are three important abnormalities of the heart valves, all most commonly affecting the structure of the valves of the left side of the heart.

Rheumatic Valve Disease

Heart valves are damaged during the acute stage of a childhood illness called 'rheumatic fever'. Healing of such damage results in progressive scarring of the valve leaflets and their elastic content is replaced by irregular masses of collagen scar. The valves therefore become more rigid. The leaflets may also partially fuse, which limits their ability to open (stenosis) or close (incompetence).

Calcific Valve Disease

Calcific valve disease mainly affects the aortic valve, particularly if it is congenitally abnormal with only two cusps (i.e. bicuspid). Over time, the valves become thickened and distorted by fibrous scarring and deposition of calcium nodules (Fig. 9.20). This renders the valve leaflets immobile and impairs blood flow from the left ventricle during systole, leading to heart failure.

Infective Valvitis

Heart valves may become colonized by bacteria or fungi, most commonly when the valve has been damaged previously, for example by rheumatic disease. The damaged valve becomes covered in thrombus (blood clot), in which organisms proliferate. This causes signs of infection, the valve may become eroded and badly damaged, and fragments of thrombus may break off and enter the systemic circulation, where they can block smaller systemic arteries.

Continued

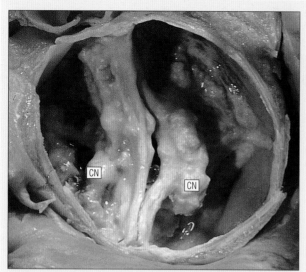

FIGURE 9.20 **Calcific valve disease.** A bicuspid aortic valve that has become thickened and distorted by fibrous scarring and calcium nodule (CN) deposition. Compare with a normal valve, Figure 9.17b.

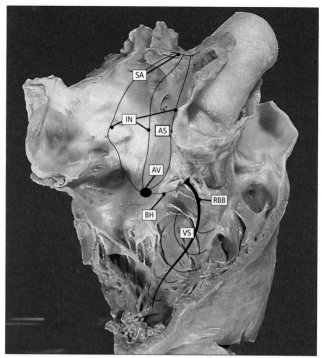

FIGURE 9.21 **Conducting system of the heart.** The opened right side of the heart trimmed to expose the septum between the two atria (AS) and the septum between the two ventricles (VS). The sinoatrial node (SA), internodal atrial muscle (IN), atrioventricular node (AV), bundle of His (BH) and right bundle branch (RBB), are indicated; the left bundle branch runs down on the left ventricular side of the interventricular septum.

heartbeat; stimulation of the parasympathetic (vagus) innervation slows the heart rate, and sympathetic stimulation increases it.

The conducting system of the heart is composed of muscle fibres, which are modified to act as transducers rather than contractile cells. The impulse for contraction is initiated at a small group of specialized cells called the **sinoatrial (SA) node**, which acts as a pacemaker and stimulates atrial contraction. The impulse passes through the atrium and arrives at another node, the **atrioventricular (AV) node**. This node then initiates the later contraction of the ventricles, the impulse passing down specialized bundles of cardiac muscle (the main bundle, the right and left bundle branches and the Purkinje fibres) to the farthest reaches of the ventricular muscle (Fig. 9.21).

Firing of the sinoatrial node regulates the cardiac rate

The SA node is located where the main vein from the upper part of the body (the superior vena cava) enters the right atrium (Fig. 9.22). Its position is constant, but the curved linear structure is so small that it is not visible to the naked eye, being only 1–1.5 cm long and only 0.1–0.15 cm wide on the outer surface of the vena caval–atrial junction, just beneath the pericardium.

The SA node is composed of an irregular meshwork of muscle fibres 3–4 μm in diameter. These are considerably smaller than normal atrial cardiac muscle fibres.

In contrast to normal cardiac muscle cells, SA muscle fibres do not have intercalated discs but connect with each other by desmosomes. They contain few myofibrils and lack an organized striation pattern.

The cells of the SA node are embedded in a bulky fibrocollagenous support tissue containing numerous

blood vessels, including a prominent central artery, the nodal artery. Numerous nerve fibres can be seen peripherally.

The impulse generated by the SA node passes quickly to the AV node, stimulating atrial contraction in the process.

The long-standing belief that the impulse travels to the AV node by diffuse radiation along all atrial muscle fibres is probably inaccurate, as specific bundles of atrial muscle (internodal atrial muscle), which preferentially conduct the impulse, have been identified. Three such specific bundles: the anterior, middle and posterior internodal tracts, have so far been described. These are histologically indistinguishable from other atrial fibres.

The atrioventricular node is composed of specialized muscle fibres

The AV node is located beneath the endocardium of the medial wall of the right atrium, just in front of the opening of the coronary sinus and immediately above the tricuspid valve ring. It is thus situated at the base of the interatrial septum, at the junction between atria and ventricles, and between the central fibrous body and endocardium.

Histologically, the AV node is composed of a network of small muscle fibres identical to those of the SA node, but less haphazardly arranged. As in the SA node, the

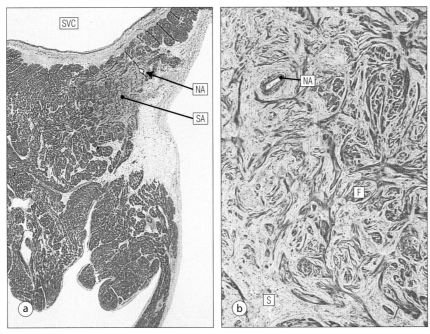

FIGURE 9.22 **Sinoatrial node.** (a) Micrograph showing the sinoatrial (SA) node situated in the atrial wall close to the entrance of the superior vena cava (SVC). The node is highlighted in this pentachrome stain by the pale blue-staining fibrocollagenous support tissue in which the cardiac pacemaker cells are embedded. Note the nodal artery (NA). (b) Medium-power micrograph showing the irregular whorled network of small nodal fibres (F) embedded in the bulky fibrocollagenous stroma (S). A small nodal artery (NA) is present.

fibres of the AV node are embedded in a fibrocollagenous stroma and have rich blood and nerve supplies.

The bundle of His, and the bundle branches arising from it, convey impulses to Purkinje fibres and the ventricles

The small fibres at the anterior end of the AV node are more regularly arranged and eventually become a distinct bundle of parallel fibres that forms the main bundle conducting the impulse from the AV node to the ventricles. This conducting bundle, the **bundle of His**, penetrates the collagen of the central fibrous body and then runs anteriorly for a short distance along the upper border of the muscle of the interventricular septum before dividing into right and left bundle branches.

The left bundle branch arises fan-like over a broad area as individual fibres, which leave the bundle of His; the remaining fibres form a distinct right bundle branch.

The left bundle branch fascicles run down beneath the endocardium of the left side of the interventricular septum in two main groups, a posterior group and a smaller anterior group.

The right bundle branch runs down beneath the endocardium of the right side of the interventricular septum as a single bundle.

The right and left bundle branches connect with a complex network of specialized conduction fibres, the **Purkinje fibres**, which are large muscle fibres with vacuolated cytoplasm owing to a high glycogen content, and scanty myofibrils. They lie in clusters of up to about six fibres (Fig. 9.23).

The Purkinje fibres, and other components of the conducting system, may be damaged during myocardial infarction (see 'Clinical Example' box, p. 161). Like the normal myocardial fibres they may degenerate and die as a result of lack of oxygen when the arterial supply is cut off. This leads to abnormal heart rhythms (**dysrhythmias**), two of which (asystole and ventricular fibrillation) are almost instantaneously fatal unless rapidly corrected. These are important and common causes of fatality within the first few minutes and hours after a coronary artery occlusion.

The heart has a rich vascular supply

Because of its constant contractile activity, the heart has enormous energy demands and therefore requires a substantial arterial supply. The left ventricle has the greatest oxygen demand and consequently, the best arterial supply. Thus, any interruption in the cardiac arterial supply affects the structure and function of the left ventricle in particular (see Fig. 9.24).

The heart is supplied by two coronary arteries that arise as direct side branches of the aorta, just above two of the cusps of the aortic valve (see Fig. 9.17a). These are the left and right coronary arteries. Histologically, the main coronary arteries are medium-sized muscular arteries (see Fig. 9.5). They run in the epicardium and send branches into the myocardium, with a fine capillary bed running around the individual cardiac muscle cells. The least well-perfused part of the left ventricular muscle is the zone just below the endocardium, the subendocardium. This tenuous perfusion combined with the

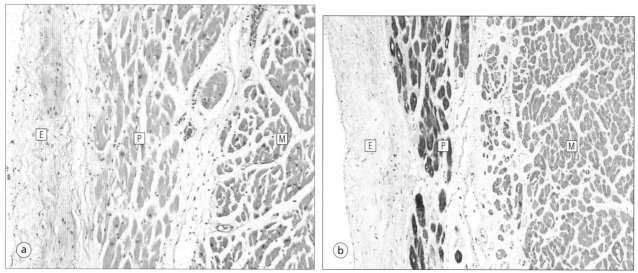

FIGURE 9.23 **Purkinje fibres.** (a) Micrograph showing the large pale-staining Purkinje fibres (P) lying just under the endocardium (E) lining the interventricular septum and separated from the myocardium (M) by a zone of loose fibrocollagenous tissue. (b) The Purkinje fibres can be distinguished from normal cardiac muscle by a higher glycogen content as detected by a periodic acid–Schiff (PAS) stain and by high levels of the normal muscle protein αβ-crystallin, as shown in this immunoperoxidase-stained preparation.

KEY FACTS
THE HEART

- Has a central fibrous core and is made up of epicardial, myocardial and endocardial layers
- Epicardium (pericardium) covers the outer surface of the heart, contains the main coronary artery branches and is covered externally by smooth mesothelium
- Myocardium is the contractile component of the heart and is composed of cardiac muscle cells which are striated and linked by intercalated discs
- The endocardium lines the internal surface of heart chambers and is covered by flat endothelial cells, which lie on a layer of fibroelastic tissue
- The conduction system is composed of muscle fibres modified for impulse conduction rather than contraction
- Valves have a central fibrous core covered by fibroelastic tissue with endothelium on their surfaces
- Atrial muscle cells secrete atrial natriuretic hormone
- The heart has a rich blood supply from two main coronary arteries (left and right), which arise as direct branches of the aorta just above the aortic valve ring.

increased wall stress during systole makes the subendocardial region of the ventricular wall the most susceptible to ischaemic injury.

Venous tributaries run with the major coronary arteries before draining into a large venous channel, the coronary sinus, which runs in the atrioventricular groove on the posterior aspect of the heart, before opening into the right atrium at the coronary sinus opening.

Stem Cells and the Heart

Despite the dogma regarding regenerative limitations of the heart, endogenous adult cardiac stem cells have been isolated in many species on the basis of positive Sca-1 and c-kit stem cell markers (Fig. 9.25). These human cardiac stem cells have been identified, isolated and shown to differentiate into cardiomyocytes, smooth muscle cells, or endothelial cells both in vitro and in vivo. These studies engender hope that stem cell methodologies can in the future be used to regenerate damaged heart tissues in clinical settings.

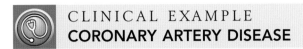

CLINICAL EXAMPLE
CORONARY ARTERY DISEASE

The most common and important disease of the heart is narrowing of the coronary arteries by atherosclerosis. This impairs the function of the left ventricle because it reduces the blood flow and hence the oxygen supply to cardiac muscle. The coronary arteries are particularly prone to this common disease, with two main consequences.

Angina

Slowly progressive reduction of the coronary artery lumen by atheroma reduces blood flow and impairs oxygenation of the left ventricular muscle, leading to a characteristic pattern of chest pain (angina), which is usually brought on by exertion (i.e. when the left ventricular muscle is working harder).

Myocardial Infarction

Complete obstruction of one of the coronary arteries or its branches (see Fig. 9.6) results in one area of the heart muscle being deprived of blood and therefore oxygen. Such affected heart muscle fibres die and are not replaced. This process is called 'myocardial infarction' (Fig. 9.24), colloquially known as a heart attack.

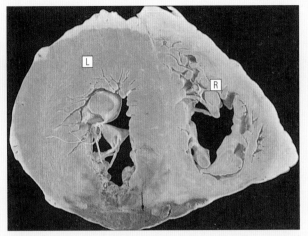

FIGURE 9.24 **Myocardial infarction.** A transverse slice across the left (L) and right (R) ventricles. The left ventricular myocardium is increased in thickness as a result of persistent high blood pressure (hypertension). The posterior part of the left ventricular wall and septum shows reddish-brown discolouration (arrow) due to infarction (i.e. death of tissue following sudden deprivation of oxygenated blood supply) resulting from occlusion of the right coronary artery. Blood has seeped into the dead myocardium and rupture of the heart is imminent.

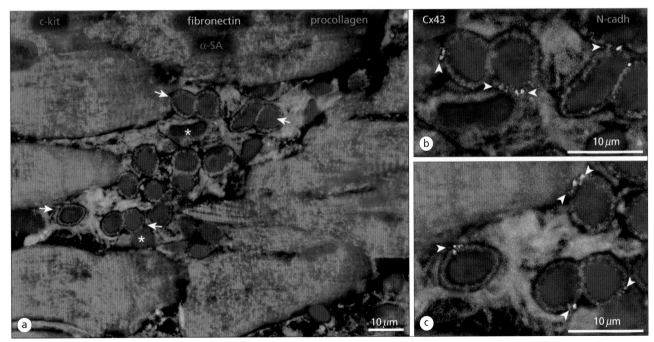

FIGURE 9.25 **Human Cardiac Stem Cells.** Cardiac niches in the human heart. Cluster of c-kit–positive cardiac stem cells (green). Arrows in A define the areas shown at higher magnification in B and C (magnification 1600X). Gap junctions (connexin 43, white; arrowheads) and adherens junctions (N-cadherin, magenta; arrowheads) are illustrated. Connexin 43 and N- cadherin are present between cardiac stem cells and myocytes (α-sarcomeric actin, red stain) and fibroblasts (procollagen, light blue; asterisks). (From: Human cardiac stem cells. Bearzi C, Rota M, Hosoda T, et al. Proc Natl Acad Sci U S A. 2007 Aug 28; 104(35):14068–73. Epub 2007 Aug 20. Copyright 2007 National Academy of Sciences, USA.)

PRACTICAL HISTOLOGY

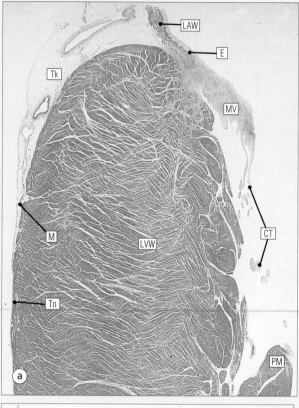

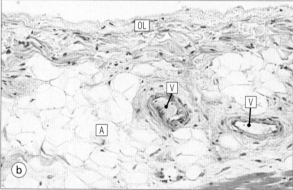

FIGURE 9.26 **Histology of the heart.** (a) Low-power micrograph showing part of the wall of the left atrium (LAW) and left ventricle (LVW). Part of the mitral valve (MV), papillary muscles (PM) and chordae tendineae (CT) are also shown. Note that the left atrial wall has a relatively thick endocardium (E), whereas the thin endocardium of the left ventricle cannot be discerned at this magnification. Thick (Tk), thin (Tn) and medium (M) pericardium can all be seen on the outer surface of the heart. (b) Medium-power view of medium thickness pericardium from the area labelled M in (a). The outer layer (OL) is mesothelium-covered collagenous and elastic tissue, beneath which is a narrow adipose tissue layer (A) containing blood vessels (V).

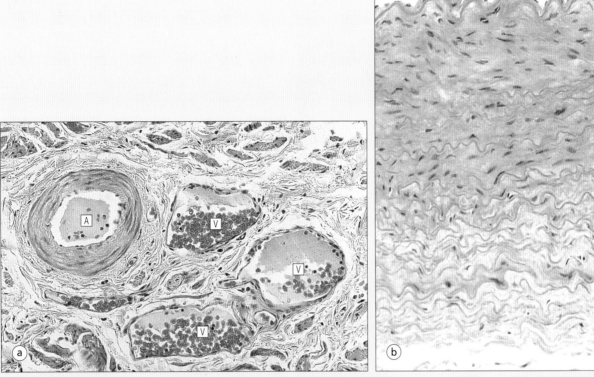

FIGURE 9.27 **Small and large arteries.** (a) This photomicrograph shows a small muscular artery (A) cut in transverse section, together with some distended thin-walled small veins (V). With the H&E stain the elastic lamina can be difficult to see; it is more clearly seen in a special stain for elastic tissue (see Fig. 9.5b,c). (b) Micrograph showing the H&E appearance of a typical large elastic artery in the systemic circulation, in this case the aorta, at high magnification. The media is composed of alternate layers of relatively indistinct smooth muscle fibres and laminae of intensely eosinophilic, slightly refractile, elastic tissue.

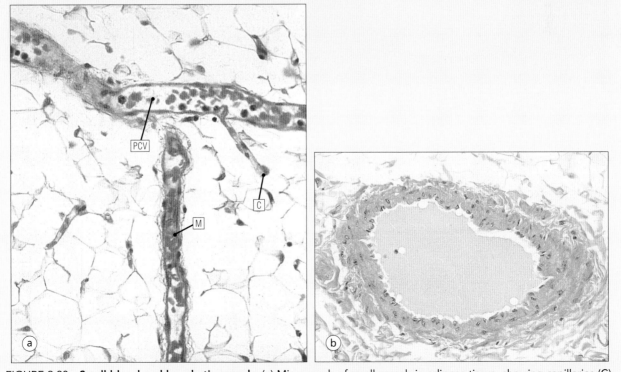

FIGURE 9.28 **Small blood and lymphatic vessels.** (a) Micrograph of small vessels in adipose tissue, showing capillaries (C). One capillary is opening into a postcapillary venule (PCV), into which a direct metarteriole (M) is also opening. (b) Micrograph of a large lymphatic vessel containing pink-staining lymph. Note that the muscle in the media merges into an indistinct adventitial layer. The nuclei of some of the endothelial cells are just visible.

PRACTICAL HISTOLOGY

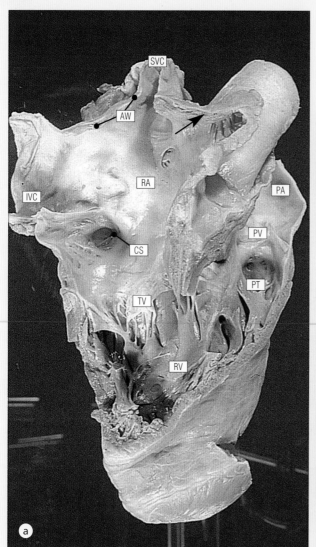

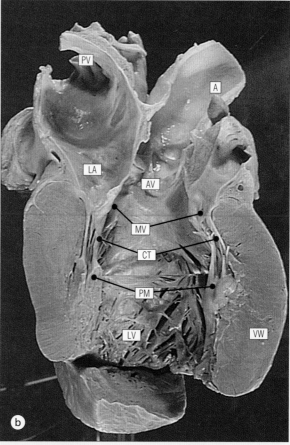

FIGURE 9.29 **Anatomy of the heart.** (a) Opened right side of the heart. In the right atrium (RA), note the opening of the superior vena cava (SVC), the inferior vena cava (IVC), the coronary sinus (CS) and the thin atrial wall (AW). The arrow marks the site of the sinoatrial node. In the right ventricle (RV), note the flaps of the right atrioventricular (tricuspid) valve (TV) separating the ventricle from the atrium, the pulmonary outflow tract (PT) with the pulmonary valve (PV) between it and the pulmonary artery trunk (PA). (b) Opened left side of the heart. Blood enters the left atrium (LA) through the pulmonary veins (PV), and leaves through the left atrioventricular (mitral, bicuspid) valve (MV) into the left ventricle (LV). In the left ventricle, note the thick muscular wall (VW), the papillary muscles (PM) and the chordae tendineae (CT), which link them to the leaflets of the mitral valve. Blood leaves the left ventricle through the aortic outflow tract and the aortic valve (AV) and enters the aorta (A).

For online review questions, please visit https://studentconsult.inkling.com.

END OF CHAPTER REVIEW

True/False Answers to the MCQs, as Well as Case Answers, Can be Found in the Appendix in the Back of the Book.

1. **Which of the following are true in the heart?**
   (a) The main coronary arteries run in the epicardium
   (b) Myocardial cells have central nuclei and are striated
   (c) The endocardium contains elastic tissue
   (d) The valves are composed of dense collagenous tissue and lack an endocardial covering
   (e) The pericardial sac is lined by mesothelial cells

2. **In the arterial system, which of the following features are present?**
   (a) Large elastic arteries that do not contain smooth muscle in their media
   (b) Muscular arteries that have both an internal and external elastic lamina
   (c) Muscular arteries that do not have an intimal layer
   (d) The tone of smooth muscle is regulated by factors secreted by the endothelium as well as innervation by the autonomic nervous system
   (e) Vasa vasorum supply blood to the walls of large arteries

3. **Which of the following is true regarding the cardiac conducting system?**
   (a) Cardiac contractions originate in the sinoatrial node
   (b) Internodal atrial muscle carries signals directly to the left and right bundle branches
   (c) Purkinje fibres are indistinguishable from adjacent myocardial cells
   (d) The atrioventricular node gives rise directly to the bundle of His
   (e) The atrioventricular node is the only part of the conducting system composed of neuronal tissue

4. **In the lymphatic circulatory system, which of the following are seen?**
   (a) Lymphatic capillaries take fluid from the extracellular space
   (b) The term 'chyle' is used to describe lipid-containing lymph draining from the intestines
   (c) Large lymphatic vessels have smooth muscle in their walls
   (d) Valves assist the flow of lymph
   (e) Lymph which goes to the lymph nodes returns to the venous system via a main lymphatic such as the thoracic duct

CASE 9.1   SUDDEN DEATH IN AN OBESE WOMAN

A 57-year-old obese woman collapses with acute breathlessness, becomes blue in the face and dies within a few minutes. According to her husband she had been unwell with flu for about 4 days, most of which time she had spent in bed. The family practitioner explains to the distraught husband that the death must be referred to the Coroner for the district, and that an autopsy will be necessary. He undertakes to meet the widower after the autopsy to explain to him the cause of death, and few days later the husband arrives with a Death Certificate issued by the Coroner, which states:

Cause of death   1(a)   Massive pulmonary
                                     thromboembolism
                              (b)   Deep vein thrombosis (Rt leg)

The family practitioner explains that a blood clot had formed in the veins deep in the muscles of the right calf and had probably enlarged over a few days. A piece of the blood clot had then broken off and passed into the main blood vessel of the lung which it had blocked off, leading to sudden death.

Q. Describe the structural and anatomical background to this case.

CASE 9.2   A MAN WITH CENTRAL CHEST PAIN

A 62-year-old cab driver is admitted to hospital as an emergency with a central crushing chest pain, persisting for 14 h. It came on while he was gardening but did not go away when he rested, nor overnight with complete bed rest. On examination, he was severely breathless, with white froth on his lips, cyanosed and in distress. He had a weak rapid pulse and was hypotensive (low blood pressure). The examining physician could hear widespread crepitations over both lung fields, and also could hear a scratching noise over the heart area in time with each systole; he explains to the attending students (of whom you are one) that this represents a pericardial friction rub. An ECG carried out in the Emergency Room (ER) shows changes that the physician explains as indicative of an anteroseptal myocardial infarction of the left ventricle.

After emergency treatment in ER, the patient is transferred to a coronary care unit, where his cardiac activity is continuously monitored and treatment is maintained.

He appears to be making a good recovery, but on the eighth day he suddenly collapses and dies. At postmortem his pericardial cavity is found to be greatly distended by blood.

Q. Describe the structural and anatomic background that explains this case. Include an explanation for the pericardial friction rub and the postmortem findings in the pericardium.

Chapter 10

Respiratory System

Introduction

The respiratory system transfers oxygen from the air into the blood, and carbon dioxide from the blood into the air

Blood oxygen is used for cellular respiratory processes that generate carbon dioxide as a by-product. The gaseous exchange occurs in the distal part of the respiratory tract, where air-containing cavities (alveolar sacs) are in intimate contact with thin-walled blood vessels. The proximal part of the respiratory tract (upper respiratory tract) forms a series of transport passages by which air passes between the atmosphere and the gas exchange areas of the alveolar sacs (Fig. 10.1). On its way to the alveolar air sacs, the air is cleaned (by removal of particulate matter) and moistened, and its temperature is approximately equated to body temperature.

In addition, the proximal part of the respiratory tract has specialized structures involved in the perception of smell and flavour (olfactory mucosa) and the production of sound (larynx).

Upper Respiratory Tract

Ciliated, mucin-secreting epithelium lines the upper airways

The architecture of the nasal cavity and paranasal sinuses provides a large surface area for warming and moistening inspired air, and for trapping particulate matter.

Air enters the respiratory system through the nostrils – the openings to the exterior at the front of the nasal cavity.

The external aspect of the nostrils is covered by skin, which extends for a short distance into the opening of the nostril (the vestibule) but then becomes a non-keratinizing squamous epithelium. Although occasional patches of stratified squamous epithelium persist, most of the nasal and paranasal sinus cavities are lined by a pseudostratified columnar epithelium, many of the columnar cells bearing numerous cilia. Scattered among these columnar cells are mucus-secreting (goblet) cells with microvilli on their luminal surface. This pattern, with minor variations, is seen throughout most of the air-conducting part of the respiratory tract, and is known as **respiratory-type epithelium** (Fig. 10.2).

The nasal and sinus submucosa is highly vascular and contains both mucous and serous glands

Beneath the nasal epithelium, the lamina propria contains many glands (Fig. 10.3) equipped with basal myoepithelial cells (see p. 82). Three main types of glands can be distinguished. Most are mucous glands, which secrete mucus to supplement that produced by the goblet cells in the lining epithelium. Some are serous cells containing basophilic granules (similar to those seen in the salivary glands, see p. 197), which produce small amounts of amylase. Lastly, there are serous cells containing eosinophilic granules (similar to those seen in the lacrimal glands), which produce lysozyme.

Inspired air is moistened by the secretions of the serous glands, and a sheet of mucus secreted by the goblet cells lies on the mucosal surface and traps any inhaled particulate contaminants. The mucus is then wafted backward (upward) by cilia toward the pharynx, where it is swallowed or expectorated.

The lamina propria also contains variable numbers of immune cells (see Chapter 8), which are mainly lymphocytes, plasma cells and macrophages, together with a few neutrophils and eosinophils. Eosinophils are particularly numerous in people who suffer from allergic rhinitis (hay fever).

A characteristic feature of the lamina propria is the presence of many blood vessels, which form an interconnecting network, the vessels being surrounded by a supporting stroma in which smooth muscle is prominent. This highly vascular submucosa makes a major contribution to the warming of inhaled air.

The paranasal sinuses are cavernous spaces in the maxillary, ethmoid, sphenoid and frontal bones of the face

Known, respectively, as the **maxillary, ethmoid, sphenoid** and **frontal** sinuses, each sinus communicates with the main nasal cavity through a series of orifices (Fig. 10.4a), and is lined by epithelium similar to that of the main nasal cavity. In addition to providing an increased surface area for the moistening and warming of inhaled air, the sinus cavities play a role in the nature of the sounds produced in speech and song.

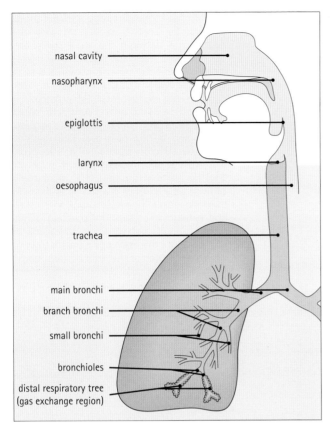

FIGURE 10.1 **Upper respiratory tract transport passages.** The part of the respiratory tract that transports air from the atmosphere to the distal respiratory tract, where gaseous exchange takes place.

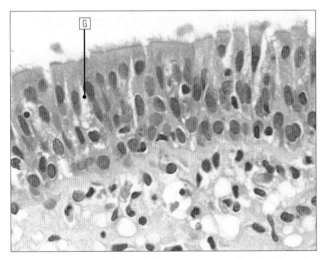

FIGURE 10.2 **Nasal epithelium.** Micrograph showing the characteristic ciliated columnar epithelium lining the nasal cavity. There are occasional scattered mucus-secreting goblet cells (G).

The nasopharynx is a posterior continuation of the nasal cavities and becomes the oropharynx at the levels of the soft palate

The nasopharynx, like most of the upper respiratory tract, is lined by columnar ciliated epithelium (Fig. 10.5)

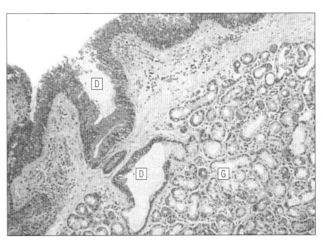

FIGURE 10.3 **Nasal lamina propria.** Micrograph showing sub-epithelial tissue of the nose. Numerous seromucous glands (G) discharge their secretions on to the epithelial surface through wide ducts (D).

containing occasional mucous-secreting goblet cells, but there are frequently patches of squamous epithelium, which arise by an adaptive process known as 'metaplasia' (see p. 175). The stratified squamous epithelium is normally non-keratinizing and increases in amount as you approach the oropharynx, and with increasing age. In this location, the presence of squamous epithelium is always indicative of disease, usually persistent insult to the original columnar epithelium.

In the nasopharyngeal submucosa, there is abundant **mucosa-associated lymphoid tissue (MALT)**, forming part of the so-called Waldeyer's ring of pharyngeal lymphoid tissue. This mucosa-associated lymphoid tissue samples inhaled antigenic material and prepares defence mechanisms against it (see Chapter 8). Most of the nasopharyngeal lymphoid tissue is diffuse within the submucosa, but larger nodular aggregates occur where the posterior wall of the nasopharynx meets its roof; these elevated areas of nasopharyngeal lymphoid tissue are called the **nasopharyngeal tonsils** or **adenoids**, and are covered by ciliated columnar epithelium which clefts down into the lymphoid tissue mass, increasing the surface area of contact between lymphoid tissue and epithelium. Mucus-secreting goblet cells are more numerous within these clefts than on the surface.

The **eustachian** or **auditory tubes** run from the middle ear cavities (see p. 385) down to the nasopharynx, opening into the lateral walls on either side; there is usually a small aggregation of lymphoid tissue in the nasopharyngeal submucosa where the eustachian tube opens into the nasopharynx, again part of the protective ring of mucosa-associated lymphoid tissue. The tube itself is lined by the same ciliated columnar epithelium, with mucous goblet cells, as the nasopharynx. The function of the tube is to ensure that the cavity of the middle ear (the tympanic cavity) is at atmospheric pressure, i.e. the same pressure as the air in the nasopharynx.

As with all upper respiratory tract epithelium, the eustachian tube epithelium initially reacts to injury by excessive secretion of mucus from the goblet cells in the

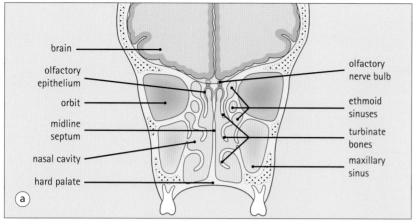

brain
olfactory epithelium
orbit
midline septum
nasal cavity
hard palate

olfactory nerve bulb
ethmoid sinuses
turbinate bones
maxillary sinus

(a)

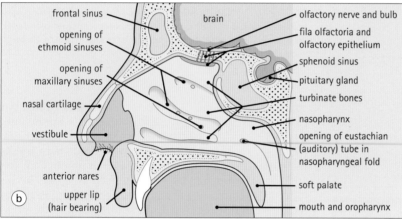

frontal sinus
opening of ethmoid sinuses
opening of maxillary sinuses
nasal cartilage
vestibule
anterior nares
upper lip (hair bearing)

brain

olfactory nerve and bulb
fila olfactoria and olfactory epithelium
sphenoid sinus
pituitary gland
turbinate bones
nasopharynx
opening of eustachian (auditory) tube in nasopharyngeal fold
soft palate
mouth and oropharynx

(b)

FIGURE 10.4 **Nasal cavity and paranasal sinuses.** (a) Coronal section showing the relationship between the nasal cavity and ethmoid and maxillary sinuses. The frontal (anterior) and sphenoid (posterior) sinuses are not shown in this plane of section. The surface area of the respiratory mucosa is increased by long curved turbinate bones arising from the lateral walls of the nasal cavity, and by the paranasal sinus system. Note the olfactory epithelium and its proximity to the olfactory nerves and bulbs. (b) Sagittal section showing the relationship between the nasal cavity, the anterior nares (nostrils), vestibule, nasopharynx and frontal and sphenoid sinuses. The opening of the frontal sinus is not shown in this plane of section. Note the openings beneath the two upper turbinates of the ethmoid and maxillary sinuses, and the opening in the nasopharyngeal fold of the eustachian tube from the middle ear.

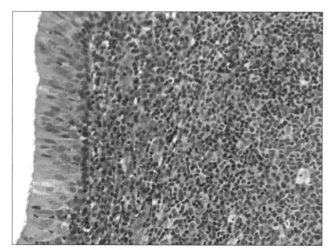

FIGURE 10.5 **Nasopharynx.** Micrograph showing tall, ciliated columnar epithelium, with abundant lymphoid tissue in the submucosa. In this young non-smoking adult, there is no squamous metaplasia of the epithelium.

middle ear. Viruses and bacteria can also gain access to the middle ear from an infected nasopharynx, causing middle ear infection (otitis media).

Olfactory mucosa is located in the roof of the nasal cavity

The olfactory mucosa, which senses smell and the more sophisticated aspects of taste, is located in the roof of the nasal cavity and extends a short way down the septum and lateral wall (see Fig. 10.4a).

Olfactory mucosa has a pseudostratified columnar epithelium composed of olfactory receptor cells, supporting (sustentacular) cells and basal cells. The disposition of these cells results in the pseudostratified appearance, as the nuclei of each type occupy different levels (Fig. 10.6a,b). Beneath the olfactory epithelium are small serous glands (of Bowman) with short ducts that penetrate the olfactory epithelium. Their secretion may act as the solvent in which odorous substances dissolve.

The olfactory epithelium is composed of basal, sustentacular and olfactory receptor cells

Basal cells. The nuclei closest to the basement membrane of olfactory epithelium belong to the small basal cells. These cells are not in contact with the lumen and form the stem cells from which new olfactory cells can

lining epithelium, with loss of cilia from the surface of the columnar epithelium cells. This excess of mucus, together with the reactive enlargement of the lymphoid tissue at the nasopharyngeal end of the eustachian tube, can lead to occlusion of the lumen of this narrow tube. This results in failure of the pressure equilibration function of the tube, with increased pressure and pain in the

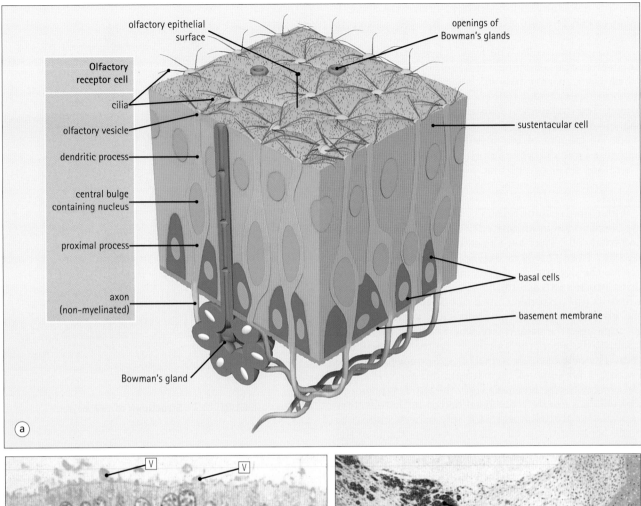

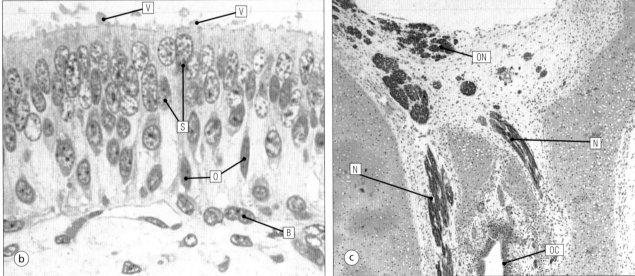

FIGURE 10.6 **Olfactory mucosa.** (a) This three-dimensional drawing shows the components of the olfactory mucosa, Bowman's glands and the nerves leaving the base of the olfactory epithelial cells on their way to the main olfactory nerve. (b) Micrograph of a 0.5 μm acrylic resin section of human olfactory mucosa from an 18-week-old fetus before the associated bone plates have fully calcified. The nuclei of the basal (B), olfactory (O) and sustentacular (S) cells can be identified. The olfactory vesicles (V) on the luminal surface are just discernible. Compare with (a). (c) Micrograph showing the nerve twigs (N) from the olfactory receptor cells (OC) fusing before passing upwards through the cribriform plate of the skull to join the olfactory nerve (ON), first cranial nerve, demonstrated using immunocytochemical method for neurofilament protein.

develop. Olfactory cells normally survive for about 1 month and regenerate after damage, the only neurons to do so.

Sustentacular cells. The nuclei closest to the lumen in olfactory epithelium belong to tall sustentacular cells, which have a narrow base in contact with the basement membrane, expanding to more bulky cytoplasm near the lumen. The oval nuclei of sustentacular cells lie close to the lumen, and the perinuclear cytoplasm contains a moderate amount of rough endoplasmic reticulum and numerous mitochondria, implying a synthetic function. There are small cytoplasmic accumulations of yellow-brown pigment and numerous microvilli on the luminal surface.

Olfactory receptor cells. The olfactory receptor cells are bipolar neurons insinuated between the sustentacular and basal cells. They have a central bulge containing the nucleus; from this area extend two cytoplasmic processes, the dendritic and proximal processes. The **dendritic process** extends to the surface of the epithelium, where its tip is expanded into a club-shaped prominence, the **olfactory vesicle**. This bears cilia, some of which protrude into the nasal cavity, whereas other lateral cilia insinuate between the microvilli of the sustentacular cells. The cilia have the typical 9 + 2 arrangement (see Fig. 3.17) for some of their length, but there is a long distal portion, which contains only the two central fibres. The cilia are inserted into basal bodies in the olfactory vesicle. The **proximal process** is very narrow and passes down between the basal cells and basal portions of the sustentacular cells to penetrate the basement membrane. It then joins other non-myelinated processes to form the so-called **fila olfactoria**, which ultimately form synaptic connections in the **olfactory bulb** (the first cranial nerve; see Figs 10.4 and Fig. 10.6c). The proximal processes are therefore regarded as axons.

Larynx

On its way to the trachea, air from the nasopharynx passes through the laryngeal region

The laryngeal region has a complex architecture to:
- Prevent inspired air entering the oesophagus
- Prevent ingested food and fluid entering the trachea
- Permit the production of complex sounds.

The laryngeal region therefore comprises:
- The **epiglottis**, which diverts inhaled air down through the larynx to the trachea and thence to the lung, at the same time preventing ingested food and fluid passing into the airways
- The **true vocal cords**, which are responsible for the production of sound by vibrating in a stream of forcibly expressed air, the nature of the sound being controlled by the vocalis muscle
- The **false vocal cords (vestibular or ventricular ligament)**, the **saccules** and **ventricles**, which modify the nature of the sounds produced by the vibrating true cords (Fig. 10.7).

Laryngeal architecture is maintained by a series of cartilaginous plates (mainly the thyroid, cricoid and

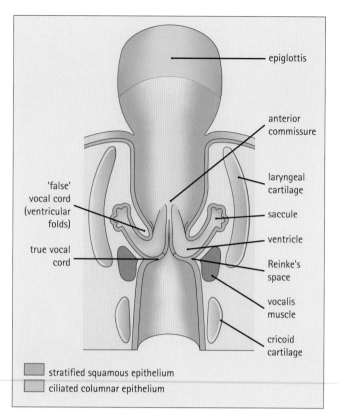

FIGURE 10.7 **Structures of the larynx.**

arytenoid cartilages). These are joined together by densely collagenous ligaments, and are mobilized by the action of small bands and sheets of striated muscle called the **intrinsic muscles of the larynx**.

The cartilages maintain the openness and shape of the airway, and move to prevent food inhalation during swallowing, which is also partly the responsibility of the epiglottis.

The epiglottis consists of a central sheet of elastic cartilage covered by mucosa on both sides

Movement of the epiglottis prevents ingested food and liquids passing into the trachea by covering the tracheal entrance during swallowing.

The anterior (lingual) surface is covered by stratified squamous epithelium continuous with that of the dorsal surface of the posterior part of the tongue.

The posterior surface, which faces the pharynx and larynx, is covered in its upper half by stratified squamous epithelium, and in its lower half by ciliated pseudostratified columnar epithelium. The lower half contains many seromucous glands, which penetrate deeply into the central elastic cartilage plate (Fig. 10.8).

The false and true vocal cords are folds of mucosa

Below the epiglottis, the laryngeal mucosa is everted into the laryngeal lumen to form two pairs of folds, an upper pair of false vocal cords and a lower pair of true vocal cords.

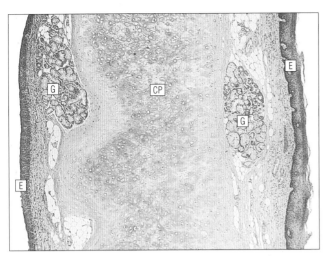

FIGURE 10.8 **Epiglottis.** Micrograph of epiglottis showing its central cartilaginous plate (CP) and seromucous glands (G), some of which split the cartilage, and the two types of epithelium (E) on its two faces.

Between these cords, an outpouching of laryngeal mucosa forms the **ventricle** (Fig. 10.9) and its upward extension, the **saccule**, on each side.

The areas where the ends of the true cords are attached to the anterior and posterior walls of the larynx are called the **anterior** and **posterior commissures**, respectively.

The **false cords** are covered by ciliated columnar epithelium (Fig. 10.9c), but islands of non-keratinizing stratified squamous epithelium are common in adults, becoming more extensive with increasing age.

Beneath the epithelium, a loose fibrocollagenous supporting stroma contains numerous blood and lymphatic vessels, as well as seromucinous glands and fibres of skeletal muscle from the thyroarytenoid muscle. Small islands of elastic cartilage and adipose tissue may also be found in adults, adipose tissue being most commonly seen in the elderly.

The **true cords** are covered by stratified squamous epithelium, which shows a rete ridge formation (see Chapter 18) on its free edge and inferior surface, although its upper surface is flat. The epithelium contains occasional melanocytes, but no significant melanin is formed. The immediate subepithelial support tissue (**Reinke's space**) contains loose fibrocollagenous tissue, which is virtually devoid of lymphatic vessels. This is an important factor in limiting or delaying the spread of cancers arising in the true vocal cords.

Beneath Reinke's space are the fibroelastic fibres of the vocal ligament, to which the skeletal muscle fibres of the vocalis part of the thyroarytenoid muscle are attached (Fig. 10.9c). There may be islands of elastic cartilage in the vocal ligament.

The **saccule and ventricle** are covered largely by respiratory-type ciliated columnar epithelium, and contain seromucous glands in their subepithelial tissue (Fig. 10.9d). In children, lymphoid aggregates are common, some with germinal centres.

The anterior and posterior commissures are covered with ciliated columnar epithelium, and their subepithe-lial zone consists of dense fibrocollagenous tissue containing seromucous glands. Lymphatics and blood vessels are common in both regions and are an important factor in the further spread of cancers of the vocal cords that invade locally to the commissures.

Phonation. The function of the larynx is to make noise for the purpose of communication. Air is forcibly expelled from the lungs and rushes upwards past the laryngeal structures, particularly through the gaps between the true and false vocal cords. The distance between the right and left true vocal cords, and the tension within the cords, can be finely controlled by will using the vocalis muscle, which occupies much of the bulk of the true cords. Forced passage of air past the cords causes them to vibrate, generating noise, the nature and pitch of which depends on the rate of cord vibration, the degree of tension within them and the intercord space.

The sounds generated by the true cord are greatly modified by a combination of many factors, including resonance produced by the generated sound waves passing the false cords and entering the ventricle and saccule, reverberation of the sound around the nasal and oral cavities, and the control imposed on the sound emitted by movements of tongue and lips.

KEY FACTS
NASAL CAVITY AND SINUSES

- Nose and sinuses are lined by pseudostratified, ciliated columnar epithelium with goblet cells
- Main function is to filter, warm and moisten inhaled air
- Sinus cavities and turbinate bones provide a large surface area
- Mucosa-associated lymphoid tissue (MALT) is present in the nasopharyngeal tonsil (adenoid)
- Nasopharynx communicates with the middle ear cavity through the auditory (eustachian) tube
- Roof of nasal cavity is the site of olfactory mucosa which includes bipolar olfactory neurons.

KEY FACTS
LARYNX

- Comprises epiglottis, false and true vocal cords, ventricles and sacculus
- The epiglottis prevents food and drink entering the respiratory tract
- Vibration of the true cords generates sound, the character of which is modified by false cords, ventricles and sacculus and further by mouth, tongue, nose, palate and lips
- Movement of true cords to create sound is under voluntary control, by the vocalis muscle
- Only the true cords and part of the epiglottis are covered by stratified squamous epithelium. All the other laryngeal structures are covered by ciliated columnar epithelium with mucus-secreting goblet cells.

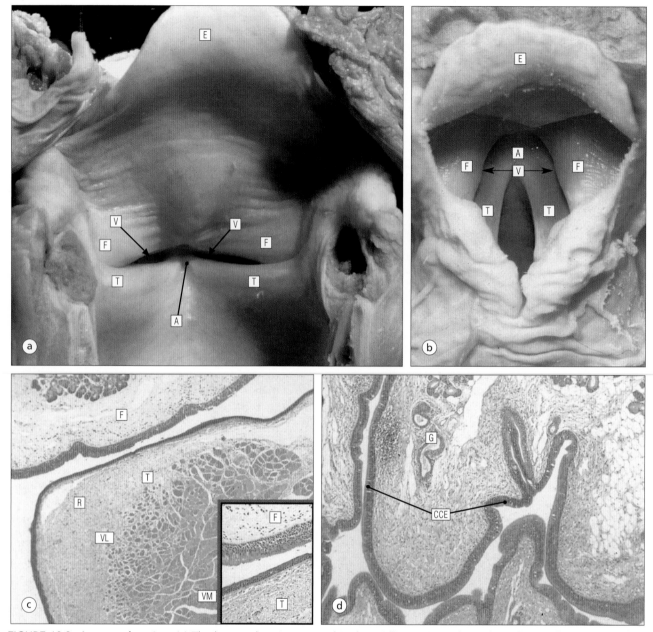

FIGURE 10.9 Laryngeal region. (a) The laryngeal region opened in the midline posteriorly to show the epiglottis (E), the false cords (F), the true cords (T) and the openings of the ventricles (V) between them. This view also shows the anterior commissure (A). (b) The vocal cords as seen from above when examined clinically with a laryngoscope. Note the epiglottis (E), false cords (F), true cords (T), the opening of the ventricles (V) and the anterior commissure (A), where the true vocal cords meet in the midline anteriorly. (c) Low-magnification micrograph showing the histology of the false (F) and true (T) cords. The false cord (F) is covered by ciliated columnar epithelium and contains seromucous glands. The true (T) cord is covered by non-keratinizing stratified squamous epithelium and contains Reinke's space (R), fibres of the vocal ligament (VL) and the skeletal muscle fibres of the vocalis muscle (VM). Inset: Micrograph showing the epithelia of the true and false cords at a higher magnification. (d) Micrograph of the saccule, which is lined by ciliated columnar epithelium (CCE) and is rich in seromucous glands (G).

The trachea is lined with respiratory mucosa and is braced with cartilage

Below the larynx, the airway continues as the trachea, which runs down into the thoracic cavity where it divides into two main bronchi, one to each lung.

The trachea is a tubular structure about 10 cm long and 2–3 cm in diameter which is rendered rigid and non-collapsible by a number – usually 15–20 – of incomplete circular rings of cartilage that occupy 70–80% of its circumference. Only a narrow strip of the posterior tracheal wall is deficient in cartilage; here the gap between the ends of each cartilage ring is bridged by a dense fibrocollagenous ligament rich in elastic fibres and bundles of smooth muscle (**trachealis** muscle), which permit some constriction of the tracheal lumen. The ligament linking the two cartilage ends prevents dilation (Fig. 10.10a).

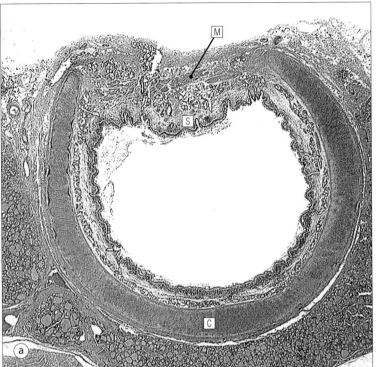

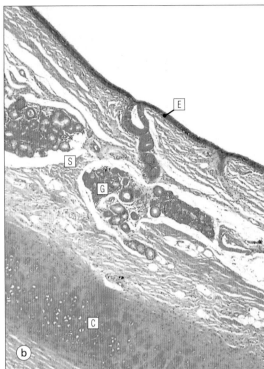

FIGURE 10.10 **Trachea.** (a) Micrograph showing a child's trachea with an incomplete cartilage hoop (C), the free ends of the cartilage being joined by a band of muscle (M). The submucosa (S) contains numerous seromucous glands, particularly where the cartilage is deficient. (b) Micrograph showing tracheal mucosa with ciliated respiratory epithelium (E) on its surface and seromucous glands (G) in the submucosa (S). The inner part of the tracheal cartilage ring (C) can be seen at the base of the micrograph.

The internal lining is a pseudostratified ciliated columnar epithelium containing scattered goblet cells. Subepithelial seromucous glands are particularly numerous in the posterior band devoid of cartilage (Fig. 10.10b).

The trachea bifurcates into two main bronchi, which further subdivide

The **main bronchi** are extrapulmonary and enter each lung with the pulmonary arteries at the lung hilum. They then divide into **lobar bronchi**, one of which supplies each of the two lobes of the left lung (**left upper lobe bronchus** and **lower lobe bronchus**) and three lobes of the right lung (**right upper lobe bronchus, middle lobe bronchus** and **lower lobe bronchus**).

Each of the five lobar bronchi divides into a variable number of **segmental bronchi** delivering air to one of the bronchopulmonary segments, where the bronchi divide for a further variable number of generations, eventually terminating in **bronchioles**.

Throughout their course, the bronchi have a similar structure to that of the trachea (Fig. 10.11), but there are variations. The basic structure comprises:

- A pseudostratified columnar ciliated epithelium
- Subepithelial fibrocollagenous tissue containing variable quantities of seromucous glands
- Variable amounts of smooth muscle, with elastic fibres arranged in longitudinal bands
- Variable amounts of partial cartilaginous ring.

Acute bronchitis, caused by viral or bacterial infection of the lining of the tracheobronchial tree, damages the

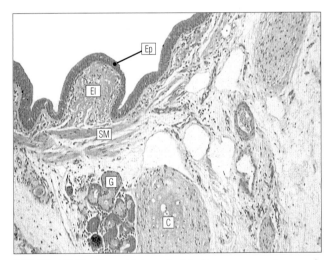

FIGURE 10.11 **Bronchial wall.** Medium-power micrograph showing a segment of the bronchial wall. Note the pseudostratified ciliated columnar epithelium (Ep), longitudinally running bands of elastin (El), bands of smooth muscle (SM), seromucous glands (G) and an isolated island of cartilage (C).

ciliated epithelium and permits the mucus to pass down (under the influence of gravity) into the distal portions of the respiratory tract. If the mucus contains inhaled pathogenic bacteria this may lead to **bronchopneumonia**, in which bacterial infection passes into the lungs through many small bronchioles. Because the direction of spread of infection is under the influence of gravity, the basal

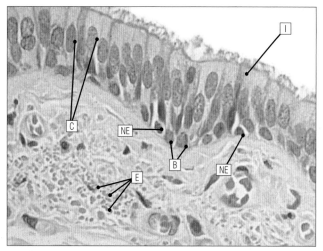

FIGURE 10.12 **Bronchial epithelium.** High-power micrograph of a thin acrylic resin section of the bronchial epithelium showing the various cell types present. Most of the cells are tall columnar ciliated cells (C) but scattered between them are occasional intermediate cells (I). Goblet cells are not seen in this section, but basal (B) and neuroendocrine (NE) cells are present on the basement membrane. Longitudinal elastic fibres (E) of the bronchial wall, here cut in transverse section, can also be seen.

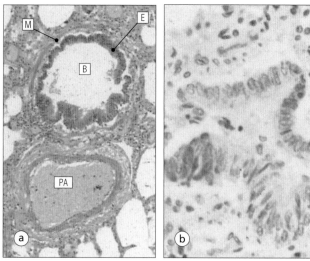

FIGURE 10.13 **Bronchiole.** (a) Micrograph of an H&E-stained section showing a bronchiole (B) close to a pulmonary artery (PA) branch. The wall is composed only of muscle (M), and its epithelium (E) is similar to bronchial epithelium. (b) Micrograph showing part of a bronchiole wall from a newborn stained by an immunoperoxidase method for bombesin, showing a so-called neuroepithelial body.

portions of the lower lobes of the lungs are most commonly affected (see lobar pneumonia, p. 176).

Several cell types make up the epithelial lining of the bronchial tree

The bronchial tree is lined by a ciliated columnar epithelium, which is pseudostratified in the larger bronchi and becomes less complex in smaller peripheral branches. The epithelium contains ciliated columnar cells, basal cells, intermediate cells, mucus-secreting goblet cells and neuroendocrine cells (Fig. 10.12).

Ciliated cells are columnar in most of the bronchial tree, but are shorter and almost cuboidal in the most peripheral branches. They have a basal nucleus, and lysosomes and numerous mitochondria in their supranuclear cytoplasm. The luminal surface of each cell bears about 200 cilia and some microvilli, each cilium being about 6 μm long.

Basal cells lie on the basement membrane and are small cells that are not in contact with the lumen. They are able to proliferate and differentiate into various respiratory cells during wound repair. Recent studies have also identified populations of c-kit positive human lung stem cells nested in niches in the distal airways. These cells are self-renewing, clonogenic and multipotent in vitro. Further research is needed to unlock their potential for regeneration of damaged lung tissue, so devastating to large numbers of pulmonary patients. **Goblet cells** are scattered between the ciliated cells and are most numerous in the main and lobar bronchi, becoming less common in the smaller branches. Their number increases in some chronic respiratory diseases.

Neuroendocrine cells are small round cells with dark-staining nuclei and clear cytoplasm, similar to those seen in the alimentary tract (see Fig. 11.41), and are located on the basement membrane. They are scattered throughout the tracheobronchial tree, but are most numerous in the smaller bronchi. Neuroendocrine cells possess cytoplasmic processes and contain characteristic neuroendocrine granules. They secrete hormones and active peptides, including bombesin and serotonin, and are most numerous in the fetal lung; they may be scattered in the basal layer of the surface epithelium or congregate in small clumps (Fig. 10.13b).

Neuroendocrine cells of the bronchial mucosa are the cells of origin of one of the most important and highly malignant tumours of the bronchus, **small cell undifferentiated carcinoma** (also called 'oat' cell carcinoma). Because they are neuroendocrine cells, some of these tumours secrete hormones or peptides, which can have significant metabolic effects, e.g. ACTH-like effects.

Smooth muscle, lymphoid tissue and seromucous glands are present in the wall of bronchi

The submucosa of the bronchial tree contains smooth muscle, seromucous glands and fibrocollagenous stroma with elastic fibres arranged in longitudinal bands.

In the main bronchi, the **smooth muscle** is largely confined posteriorly (as in the trachea), being attached to the ends of the incomplete cartilage rings, but in the intrapulmonary bronchi the muscle is submucosal and arranged in an irregular spiral with two components, one spiralling to the left, the other to the right. It persists in the airway walls down to the smallest branches (bronchioles, see p. 175), long after the cartilage component has disappeared.

Hypertrophy of the smooth muscle is an important component of some lung diseases (see 'Clinical Example', p. 180).

CLINICAL EXAMPLE
METAPLASIA IN THE UPPER RESPIRATORY TRACT

The function of the epithelial lining of the upper respiratory tract (from nose to the end of the respiratory bronchioles) is to moisten the passing inhaled air and to remove any inhaled particulate matter by entrapment in the mucous secretions, which are then wafted proximally by the action of cilia. However, the ciliated and mucous secreting epithelium that achieves this is, over a period of many years, subjected to a large number of insults, mainly chemical in the form of inhaled fumes from cigarettes, car exhausts, industrial chimneys, etc. It is also repeatedly damaged by low-grade viral and bacterial infections. After many such destructive insults, the specialized epithelium may be replaced by stratified squamous epithelium, which is not specialized to remove particulate material but is much more resistant to damage. This is an example of metaplasia, and is common in the epithelium of the upper respiratory tract. It has already been mentioned in the description of the nasopharynx (p. 167), but also occurs in the trachea and proximal parts of the bronchial tree, and is particularly common in cigarette smokers and people with recurrent bacterial bronchial infections.

Many examples of lung cancer originating in the bronchial tree are derived from areas of stratified squamous epithelium that have developed as a result of metaplasia. Hence, the tumours are squamous cell carcinoma, not adenocarcinomas derived from respiratory-type columnar epithelium. Similarly, almost all of the (much rarer) cancers that arise in the nasopharynx are squamous cell carcinomas arising in patches of metaplastic squamous epithelium.

The **submucosal bronchial glands** are seromucous glands, which empty into the lumen through short ducts. Other deeper glands with longer ducts are located between and beneath the cartilaginous plates. The serous component is thought to secrete lysozyme and glycoprotein.

The submucosal mucous glands of the tracheobronchial tree produce thin mucus which passes on to the mucosal surface and traps inhaled particulate matter and microorganisms. The cilia of the columnar epithelium constantly waft the thin sheet of mucus upwards to the throat, so that none of it (and none of the entrapped material) normally passes down into the lower parts of the respiratory tract. This is referred to as the 'mucociliary escalator'.

Myoepithelial cells (see p. 82) lie between the secretory and duct lining cells and their basement membrane, and some neuroendocrine cells are also present.

The bronchial wall contains mucosa-associated lymphoid tissue (MALT).

Lymphocytes and IgA-secreting plasma cells are closely associated with the bronchial glands and lymphoid aggregations are common, being most evident at bifurcations. The larger lymphoid aggregates occur in the proximal part of the bronchial tree and may have germinal centres.

Bronchi of all sizes contain some cartilage

The main extrapulmonary bronchi have regular incomplete cartilage rings like the trachea, but the intrapulmonary bronchi have an irregular, roughly circumferential arrangement of cartilage plates connected by dense fibrocollagenous bands.

As the bronchi branch and get smaller and more peripheral, the cartilage plates decrease in size and number and are mainly concentrated at bifurcations.

The bronchioles are the smallest part of the conducting airways

Bronchioles are distal airways located between the cartilage-walled bronchi and the site where the ciliated epithelium ceases.

The bronchioles branch repeatedly, and as they do so, reduce their luminal size. With the absence of cartilage, smooth muscle becomes the major component of their wall.

Bronchioles are lined by ciliated columnar epithelium without pseudostratification, and the cells become lower and near cuboidal in the small peripheral branches. Occasional goblet cells persist, as do small numbers of neuroendocrine cells (sometimes clustered to form so-called **neuroepithelial bodies**, see Fig. 10.13b) but there are no seromucous glands, and an additional cell type, the **Clara cell**, is found.

The Clara cell is not ciliated and is most numerous in the terminal bronchioles. It contains numerous mitochondria and abundant smooth endoplasmic reticulum near its rounded or dome-shaped luminal surface, which bulges above the level of adjacent ciliated cells; small electron-dense granules are also seen in the apical cytoplasm.

Clara cells secrete lipoproteins that prevent luminal adhesion should the airway collapse (Clara cell protein; CC10) and a 16 kilodalton protein (CC16) that has been

ADVANCED CONCEPT
CLARA CELLS

Contain:

- Many large mitochondria, abundant smooth ER and secretory granules
- Lipoprotein that prevents luminal adhesion and a 16 kilodalton protein (Clara cell protein; CC16).

Proposed functions include:

- Protection against deleterious effects of inhaled toxins and carcinogens
- Some role in surfactant production or elimination
- Possible stem cell, capable of producing other types of bronchiolar epithelial cell.

Some words of caution: There is marked species variation in the numbers and structure of Clara cells. Most of the research work has been carried out using rodents, in which the cells are numerous and distinct.

associated with the inflammatory and coagulation cascades. This protein is used as a marker for bronchoalveolar lavage fluid and as an indicator of lung injury (decreased CC16 indicates Clara cell injury).

The final bifurcations of the bronchiolar tree produce **terminal bronchioles**, which are the smallest bronchioles, concerned solely with air conduction.

Distal Respiratory Tract

Gaseous exchange occurs in the distal respiratory tract

The terminal bronchiole leads into the distal respiratory tree, which is concerned with gaseous exchange.

The first elements of this system are the respiratory bronchioles, which are lined by cuboidal ciliated epithelium. This merges with the flattened epithelium lining ill-defined conduits outlined by a spiral of smooth muscle (alveolar ducts). The walls of these ducts are composed largely of the openings of laterally disposed air sacs (alveoli). Each alveolar duct terminates in two or three alveolar sacs formed from the confluence of the openings of several alveoli (Fig. 10.14a).

Alveoli are air sacs that are the main site of gaseous exchange

Alveoli number 150–400 million in each normal healthy lung, and provide an enormous surface area (estimated at 70–80 m²) for gaseous exchange.

Each alveolus is a polygonal air space about 250 μm in diameter when normally inflated, with a thin wall which contains pulmonary capillaries and forms the air–blood barrier.

Most alveoli open into an alveolar sac or an alveolar duct, but a few open directly into a respiratory bronchiole. Pores (of Kohn), which are 1–12 μm in diameter, permit communication between adjacent alveoli (Fig. 10.14b).

The pores of Kohn provide direct communication from alveolus to alveolus, permitting rapid and even distribution of air throughout the lobe of the lung during inspiration. Unfortunately, some types of pathogenic bacteria can occasionally evade the protective mechanism of the mucociliary escalator in the trachea and bronchi, and quickly gain access to the alveolar air spaces, where they may proliferate and pass rapidly from alveolus to alveolus through the pores of Kohn until an entire lung lobe is infected. This is **lobar pneumonia** (see bronchopneumonia, p. 173).

The cellular components of the alveoli include type 1 and type 2 pneumocytes, which lie on the alveolar basement membrane, and alveolar macrophages.

Type 1 pneumocytes are very thin cells which allow gaseous diffusion

Type 1 pneumocytes represent about 40% of the alveolar cell population but form 90% of the surface area lining the alveolar sacs and alveoli.

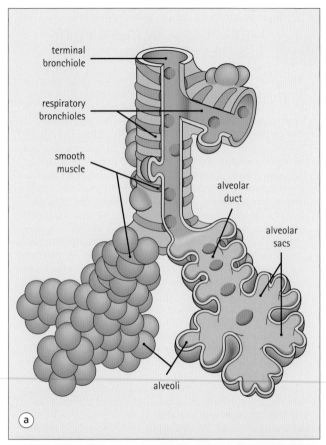

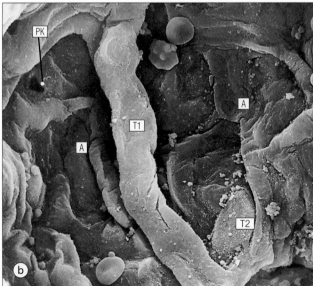

FIGURE 10.14 **Distal respiratory tree.** (a) The relationships between the terminal bronchiole, respiratory bronchiole, alveolar ducts, alveolar sacs and alveoli. The brown bands are smooth muscle. (b) Low-power scanning electron micrograph of an alveolar sac looking into two of the alveoli (A) that open into it. The two alveoli are separated by a wall, which is covered by type 1 pneumocyte cytoplasm (T1). On the left is a pore of Kohn (PK), and a round type 2 pneumocyte (T2) can be seen in the right alveolus.

Type 1 pneumocytes are attenuated flat cells with greatly flattened nuclei, and are joined together by occluding or tight junctions (see p. 37). They contain scanty mitochondria and organelles, and their cytoplasm provides a very thin covering to the alveolar basement membrane, its thinness contributing to the efficiency of the air–blood barrier.

Type 2 pneumocytes secrete surfactant

Type 2 pneumocytes represent 60% of the alveolar cell population numerically, but occupy only 5–10% of the alveolar surface area.

Unlike the thin, flat type 1 cells, type 2 pneumocytes are rounded cells which are commonly located in obtuse angles in the polygonal alveolus (Fig. 10.15a). Their nuclei are round and dark-staining, and their cytoplasm is rich in mitochondria and both rough and smooth endoplasmic reticulum. They also contain electron-dense vesicles and large spherical bodies of variably lamellated material, which is composed of phospholipid, protein and glycosaminoglycans, and forms the basis of pulmonary surfactant. The granular surfactant material is extruded from the lamellar bodies through their microvillus luminal surfaces (Fig. 10.15).

When the alveolar epithelium is exposed to certain toxic agents, particularly if there is extensive destruction of the sensitive type 1 pneumocytes, type 2 pneumocytes increase in size and number; it is believed that

ADVANCED CONCEPT
SURFACTANT AND THE TYPE 2 PNEUMOCYTE

The main function of type 2 pneumocytes is the production of pulmonary surfactant:

- Surfactant is a complex mixture of phospholipids (mainly dipalmitoyl phosphatidylcholine), carbohydrates (glycosaminoglycans) and proteins (including SP-A, SP-B, SP-C and SP-D)
- When released from the type 2 pneumocyte, surfactant produces a monolayer lining the internal alveolar surface, with a lower aqueous phase and a superficial lipid phase
- Surfactant acts like a detergent by reducing alveolar surface tension, preventing collapse of alveoli during expiration and facilitating expansion during inspiration
- Type 2 pneumocytes and surfactant are first detectable at about 28 weeks' gestation, after which time premature babies are theoretically capable of respiratory survival
- Between 28 weeks and term, amounts of surfactant may be inadequate, and exogenous surfactant can be insufflated into the immature lungs of these premature infants
- Surfactant deficiency leads to alveolar collapse, with type 1 pneumocyte damage leading to infantile respiratory distress syndrome, also referred to as hyaline membrane disease.

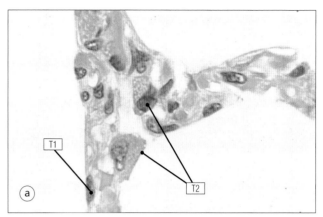

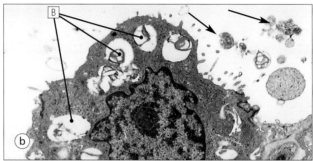

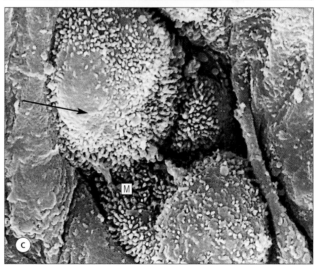

FIGURE 10.15 **Type 2 pneumocyte and surfactant.** (a) An H&E-stained thin acrylic resin section showing the confluence of the alveolar walls of three adjacent alveoli. In the angles are rounded cells with vacuolated cytoplasm; these are type 2 pneumocytes (T2). The nucleus of a type 1 pneumocyte (T1) is also seen. (b) Electron micrograph showing an active type 2 pneumocyte. The cell is round and has a convex luminal face, which is covered with microvilli. The most obvious intracytoplasmic organelles are large membrane-bound spherical bodies (B) containing lamellated lipoprotein material, which represents the surfactant substance. These can often be seen discharging their contents on to the luminal surface (arrows). (c) Scanning electron micrograph of two type 2 pneumocytes. Note the microvilli (M), and small amounts of granular material (arrow), which is recently disgorged surfactant.

some type 2 cells can act as precursor cells for type 1 pneumocytes.

Alveolar macrophages phagocytose inhaled bacteria and particulate matter

Normally alveolar macrophages lie on top of the alveolar lining cells and are also seen apparently free in the alveolar space, often containing phagocytosed material, particularly inhaled carbon particles.

Alveolar macrophages patrol the alveolar air spaces and the interalveolar septa (interstitium, Fig. 10.16), passing freely between the two. They phagocytose inhaled debris (e.g. fine dust, including carbon), and are an important defence mechanism against inhaled bacteria. They also remove excess surfactant and secrete a large number of agents, including enzymes, such as lysozyme, collagenases, elastases and acid hydrolases.

After phagocytosis, macrophages may enter the respiratory and terminal bronchioles, where they either pass

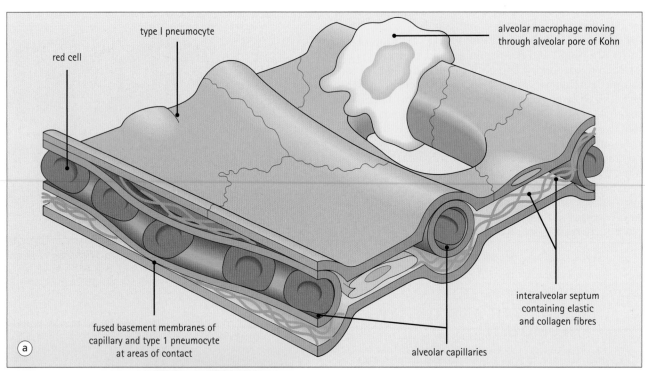

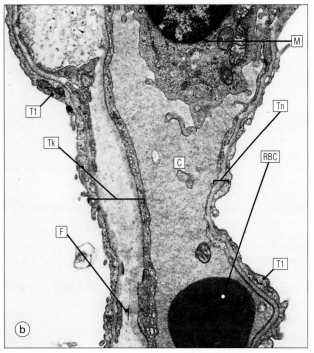

FIGURE 10.16 **Interalveolar septum and air–blood barrier.** (a) The interalveolar septum showing the pulmonary capillaries coursing through the alveolar wall, sometimes in close contact with one wall, then the other. (b) Transmission electron micrograph through the alveolar wall. It is largely occupied by a capillary (C) containing a red blood cell (RBC) and a monocyte (M). The monocyte will leave the capillary and ultimately enter the alveolar lumen to become an alveolar macrophage. Note the thin (Tn) and the thick (Tk) parts of the alveolar wall. Both sides of the alveolar wall are covered by a thin layer of type 1 pneumocyte cytoplasm (T1). In the thick part, between type 1 pneumocyte cytoplasm and the capillary wall, there are collagen and elastic fibres (F).

into lymphatic vessels and become transported to regional lymph nodes, or they adhere to the ciliated mucus-coated epithelium, which is the first step on the mucociliary escalator. This eventually carries them up to the trachea and main bronchi, from which they are cleared in the mucus by coughing. Alternatively, the macrophages may remain in the interstitium.

Elastic tissue is an important functional component of the alveolar wall

Elastin has remarkable properties of stretch and recoil (see p. 59) and has three important functions in the alveolar walls. First, it allows the lungs to stretch to accommodate the inhaled air. Then, having thus stored energy, it allows air to be expelled from the alveoli by recoiling. Finally, it acts as a spring, tethering the soft-walled bronchioles, which contain no cartilage, to the lung parenchyma and indirectly to the pleura, thus preventing bronchiolar and alveolar collapse during exhalation.

Gaseous exchange occurs across the air–blood barrier in the alveoli

Oxygen diffuses from the alveolar cavity into the blood in the alveolar capillaries to become linked to red cell haemoglobin, and carbon dioxide diffuses from blood into the alveolar air. Each capillary is closely apposed to two alveolar cavities, and is therefore located in the interalveolar septum or interstitium. Where the capillary contacts the alveolar wall, its basement membrane appears to fuse with that of the alveolar wall (see Fig. 10.16).

When the pressure in the pulmonary capillaries is increased, the fluid component of the blood, particularly water, can pass out of the capillary lumen into the alveolar lumen, so that the alveoli become filled with water (plus solutes and low molecular weight proteins). When this is extensive, there is no room for air to enter the alveoli and the patient becomes extremely breathless and shows severe cyanosis because gaseous exchange is greatly reduced. This is the basis of **acute pulmonary oedema**, as may occur when the left side of the heart fails to empty and pressure builds up in the pulmonary veins draining into the left atrium; this increased pulmonary venous pressure is reflected back into the extensive pulmonary capillary system. This is the structural and physiological basis of **acute congestive left heart failure**.

Parts of the interalveolar septum not occupied by the capillary contain fine collagen and elastic fibres together with some fibroblasts and macrophages.

Thus, in some places the capillary is in direct contact with the alveolar wall (thin part) but in others is separated from it by cells and fibres (thick part). The thin part is the site of gas exchange and the thick part is where liquids can move between the air spaces and the interstitium.

Macrophages move freely from alveolus to alveolus through the pores of Kohn. Both sides of the interalveolar septum are covered by a thin layer of type 1 pneumocyte cytoplasm (see Fig. 10.16).

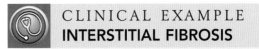

CLINICAL EXAMPLE
INTERSTITIAL FIBROSIS

In some lung diseases, the fibroblasts in the interalveolar septa increase in number and secrete excess collagen and elastin. This results in fibrocollagenous thickening of the septa (interstitial fibrosis).

Interstitial fibrosis increases the rigidity of the lung and limits expansion, but most importantly, impairs gaseous exchange because of the accumulation of collagen fibres between the capillary and alveolar walls, which impairs gas diffusion.

Pulmonary Vasculature

The lungs have a dual blood supply and venous drainage

Blood to the lungs is provided by the pulmonary and bronchial arteries and veins.

The more important of the two systems physiologically is the pulmonary vascular system, as this is the capillary component of the system and is the site of gaseous exchange. The bronchial system provides oxygenated blood to the larger components of the bronchial tree (see p. 182).

The pulmonary arteries supply the lung with relatively deoxygenated blood from the right side of the heart. This venous blood has supplied the body's tissues with oxygen and collected carbon dioxide (see Fig. 9.1).

The pulmonary arteries enter each of the lungs at the hilum and closely follow the course of the adjacent bronchus and its branches, dividing more or less with the bronchi. The vessels culminate in the extensive intimate **pulmonary capillary** network within the interalveolar septae (see Fig. 10.16). The capillary network empties its reoxygenated blood into **pulmonary venules and veins**, which eventually convey the blood to the left side of the heart for distribution to other organs.

Since the pulmonary arterial and venous system is a low-pressure system (i.e. pulmonary artery systolic pressure is 25 mmHg, whereas systemic arterial systolic pressure is 110–135 mmHg), the structure of its vessels differs considerably from those of the systemic circulation (see Chapter 9).

The proximal pulmonary artery branches are elastic arteries

From their origin at the pulmonary valve ring to the intrapulmonary branches at the level where the bronchi lose their cartilage plates to become bronchioles, the pulmonary arteries are elastic arteries.

These arteries have three main components (Fig. 10.18):

- A narrow intima composed of a single layer of endothelium lying on a narrow layer of scanty collagen fibres and myofibroblasts

CLINICAL EXAMPLE
CHRONIC OBSTRUCTIVE AIRWAYS DISEASE

The most common lung disease in the Western world is chronic obstructive airways disease, which is characterized by difficulty in getting air into and out of the distal respiratory tree.

There are three main disease processes causing chronic obstructive airways disease: asthma, chronic bronchitis and emphysema. These conditions may be present alone or in combination.

Asthma

Asthma is caused by a combination of bronchoconstriction and excessive production of particularly viscid mucus, both of which obstruct the airways.

Chronic Bronchitis

In chronic bronchitis, the bronchial walls are thickened by a combination of muscle layer thickening and an increase in number and size of the mucous glands. This correlates with excessive mucus, which is expectorated in this condition.

Emphysema

Emphysema is characterized by destruction of the walls of the alveolar ducts, sacs and alveoli, with permanent dilatation of air spaces (Fig. 10.17). This leads to loss of the elastic support for the bronchioles and results in their collapse, particularly during exhalation, and air trapping, as air is unable to pass the obstructed lumen.

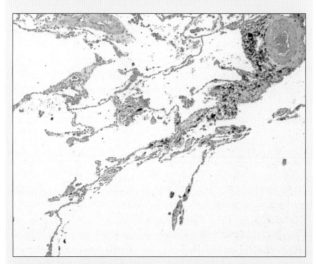

FIGURE 10.17 **Emphysema.** Micrograph of lung from patient with severe emphysema, showing extensive destruction of the alveolar walls.

- A media composed of many layers of elastic fibres, which are irregular and fragmented in the pulmonary trunk and main pulmonary arteries, but more regular and intact in the peripheral branches. Between the elastic fibres are smooth muscle cells and some collagen

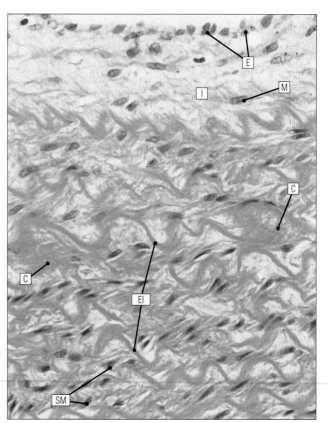

FIGURE 10.18 **Elastic pulmonary artery.** Micrograph of an elastic pulmonary artery from a child. Note the endothelium (E), the scanty myofibroblasts (M) in the narrow intima (I), the thick media composed of fairly regularly organized alternating lamellae of elastic fibres (El) and intervening smooth muscle cells (SM) and collagen (C). The elastic is easily seen in this H&E section because the lamellae are so thick.

- Elastic laminae composed of longitudinally running fibres that form flat, interlinked strands of varying breadths. This particular orientation is probably an adaptation to counteract the stretching forces during lung expansion. In the aorta, which is exposed to circumferential stretch during systole, the elastic fibres are circumferential.

The distal pulmonary arteries are muscular arteries

At about the bronchial/bronchiolar junction, the medial elastic laminae largely disappear and the arteries become muscular.

These arteries continue to follow the bronchioles as far as the terminal and respiratory bronchioles, but also give off supernumerary arteries as side branches.

The media of the muscular pulmonary artery is composed largely of circularly orientated smooth muscle (Fig. 10.19a) and occasional collagen and elastic fibres. The organized laminated elastic tissue is confined to distinct internal elastic laminae (see Chapter 9).

Continuous branching of the muscular pulmonary arteries produces progressively smaller vessels with

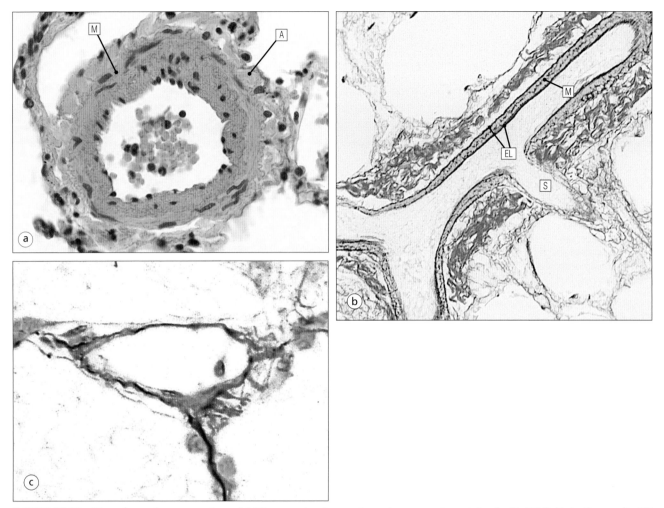

FIGURE 10.19 **Muscular pulmonary artery.** (a) Micrograph of muscular pulmonary artery stained with H&E. Note the media (M) and adventitia (A). (b) Micrograph of a smaller muscular pulmonary artery stained by the elastic van Gieson method to show the media (M) lying between two distinct dark-staining elastic laminae (EL). In addition to giving off a lateral supernumerary branch (S), this artery is bifurcating into two vessels with less well-formed arterial walls. (c) Micrograph showing a small pulmonary arteriole. This is a thin-walled vessel resembling a small pulmonary artery from which the muscular media between the two elastic laminae has disappeared. Transitional vessels with only an occasional remnant of the spirally arranged muscular media can sometimes be identified.

narrower bores and thinner walls, because of diminishing smooth muscle in the media (Fig. 10.19b). The muscle layer becomes discontinuous and finally disappears, the vessel then being called a 'pulmonary arteriole' (Fig. 10.19c).

Arterioles are difficult to distinguish from venules. The alveolar capillaries are discussed in Figure 10.16.

Pulmonary veins drain into the left atrium

Oxygenated blood from the alveolar capillaries enters small venules, then large venules, small veins, large veins and finally the main pulmonary veins, which empty into the left atrium.

The small venules are composed of a thin intima lying on a narrow zone of collagen and elastic fibres. These small tributaries fuse to form larger venules, which run in the fibrocollagenous septa and are associated with increasing numbers of myofibroblasts and smooth muscle cells in the media (Fig. 10.20).

Larger veins have a distinct media with a variably continuous internal elastic lamina and irregularly arranged smooth muscle fibres.

The largest pulmonary veins have a media in which elastic fibres are irregularly interspersed with collagen and smooth muscle fibres, rather than being confined to clearly defined elastic laminae.

Pulmonary vasculature varies considerably at the extremes of age

Before birth, the pulmonary vasculature is barely perfused because of the bypass through the patent foramen ovale and ductus arteriosus. Thus, the muscular pulmonary arteries have a small lumen, large endothelial cells and a thick media. In addition, there are small bundles

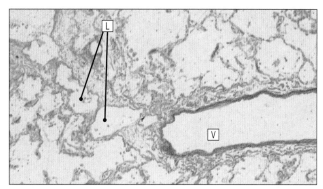

FIGURE 10.20 **Pulmonary vein.** Pulmonary veins (V) are thin-walled vessels that run in the fibrocollagenous septa with pulmonary lymphatics (L). Small venules resemble pulmonary arterioles, but the larger veins contain collagen and elastic fibres, as well as smooth muscle, outside the basement membrane. The smooth muscle cells and elastic fibres are haphazardly arranged, but in large pulmonary veins, the elastic fibres may form an interrupted or continuous elastic lamina. There are no valves in pulmonary veins of any size.

of longitudinally running smooth muscle fibres in the intima.

These features change progressively to the adult pattern in the first few weeks of life, and new supernumerary arteries develop.

In old age, the veins and muscular pulmonary arteries thicken as a result of irregular fibrocollagenous thickening of the intima.

The bronchial arteries are direct lateral branches of the thoracic aorta

The bronchial arteries provide a secondary blood supply, which perfuses each lung at systemic arterial pressure to provide it with oxygenated blood.

The bronchial arteries follow the course of the bronchial tree and its branches to the level of the respiratory bronchioles, where they anastomose with the pulmonary artery branches. They also communicate with the pulmonary arterial system by capillary anastomoses in the bronchial submucosa.

In children, the bronchial arteries are histologically similar to other systemic muscular arteries (see Chapter 9). They have a muscular media and a distinct internal elastic lamina, but no cohesive external elastic lamina (Fig. 10.21a).

In adults, the bronchial arteries develop smooth muscle, arranged longitudinally in small bundles within the intima. These are particularly prominent in some forms of chronic lung disease, but are found from about 20 years of age in normal, healthy individuals (Fig. 10.21b).

The bronchial veins drain into the azygos and hemiazygos veins

There are numerous anastomoses between the bronchial and pulmonary veins, the bronchial veins running, with the bronchial arteries, in the adventitia of the airways.

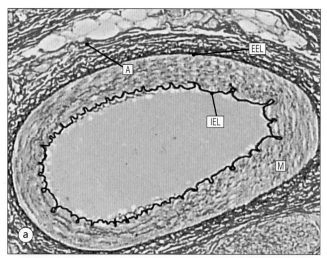

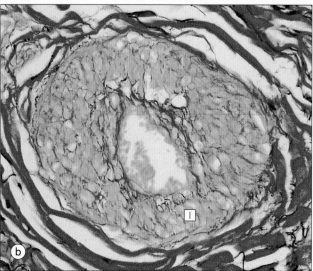

FIGURE 10.21 **Bronchial artery.** (a) Low-magnification micrograph of a bronchial artery from a 2-year-old child stained by the elastic van Gieson method to show its muscular media (M) between the internal and external layers of elastic lamina (IEL) and (EEL). Elastic fibres appear black under the microscope. It is very similar to a normal systemic muscular artery and has a fibrocollagenous adventitial layer (A). (b) High-magnification micrograph of a bronchial artery from a healthy 50-year-old man stained by the EVG method. It shows marked thickening of the intima (I) by longitudinal smooth muscle cells (yellow).

There are no lymphatic vessels from the alveolar air sacs and interalveolar septa

Any fluid in the air spaces is absorbed into the thick part of the alveolar wall. This fluid diffuses proximally in the interstitium until it enters small lymphatics at about the level of the respiratory bronchioles. The small lymphatics merge to form larger vessels that follow the bronchial tree proximally as far as the lung hilum, draining into a series of peribronchial lymph nodes on the way.

Another system of lymphatics runs in the visceral pleura and fibrocollagenous septa that divide the lung parenchyma into discrete lobules; these peripheral pleural lymphatics drain directly into the pleural space.

Pleura

The pleurae are the linings of the thoracic cavity

The lungs are contained within the thoracic cavity, which is capable of increasing and decreasing in size by intercostal muscle relaxation and contraction. The internal lining of the thoracic cavity and the outer surface of the contained lungs are smooth, low-friction surfaces bathed with a small quantity of lubricating fluid. These surfaces are the pleurae. The outer surface of the lung is the visceral pleura, which is composed of five ill-defined layers:

- An outer layer of flat, mesothelial cells
- A narrow zone of loose, fibrocollagenous tissue, with no identifiable basement membrane between it and the mesothelium
- An irregular, external elastic layer
- An interstitial layer of loose, fibrocollagenous stroma containing lymphatics, blood vessels and nerves, together with some smooth muscle fibres
- An ill-defined internal elastic layer containing short lengths of elastic fibre, some of which merge with those of the interalveolar septa of the most peripheral alveolar groups.

These layers vary markedly from site to site (Fig. 10.22) but are particularly irregular in the region of a fibrocollagenous, interlobular septum, where the ill-

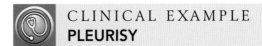

CLINICAL EXAMPLE
PLEURISY

When the normally smooth and slippery surfaces of the visceral and parietal pleura become abnormally roughened, they scrape against each other roughly, instead of sliding smoothly and effortlessly. This scraping can be heard through a stethoscope (pleural friction rub) as a scratching noise in time with inspiration and expiration. The pleura contains sensory nerves, so the condition is painful, the pain being most obvious when big inspiratory or expiratory movements are made, particularly from coughing. This condition is called pleurisy and occurs when the pleura is damaged by inflammation, particularly with bacterial infection of the lungs, where the infection spreads out to the pleural surface. Because of the pain on breathing, patients with pleurisy have shallow breathing and are loath to cough.

defined elastic networks of the pleura often fuse into a single layer before extending partway into the septum.

Parietal pleura forms the internal lining of the thoracic cavity. Merging with the visceral pleura at the hilum of each lung, it has a similar structure but is usually simpler, with only one layer of elastic fibres.

Parietal pleura sits on a layer of adipose tissue, beneath which is a layer of dense fibrocollagenous tissue, which is, in turn, continuous with the periosteum of the ribs and the perimysium of the intercostal muscles.

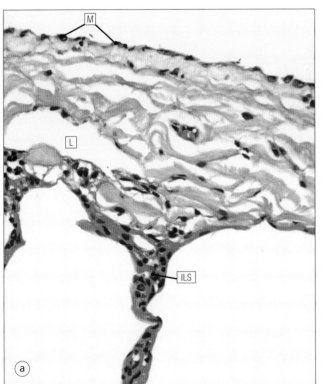

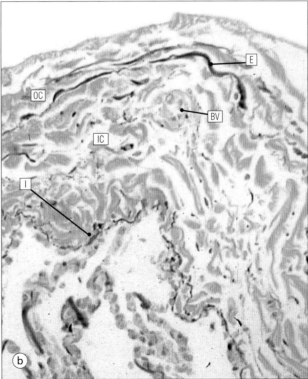

FIGURE 10.22 **Visceral pleura.** (a) Visceral pleura (stained H&E) showing some of the flat outer mesothelial cells (M), and the insertion of an interlobular septum (ILS) containing a lymphatic vessel (L) on its way to draining into the pleural cavity. Blood vessels and collagen fibres can be seen in the pleura. (b) The elastic van Gieson stain (elastic black, collagen red) reveals the ill-defined layered structure. The irregular external elastic layer (E) and ill-defined fragmented finer internal elastic layer (I) can be seen, as can the outer (OC) and interstitial (IC) collagenous layers, the latter containing blood vessels (BV).

PRACTICAL HISTOLOGY

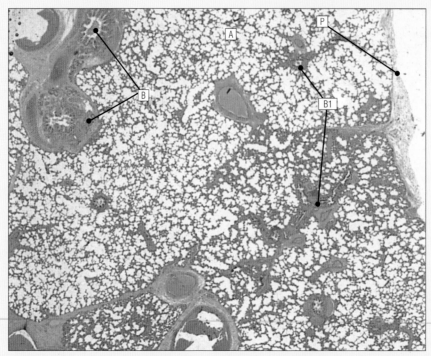

FIGURE 10.23 **Lung architecture.** Low-power micrograph showing the general architecture of the lung of a child. Bronchi (B), bronchioles (B1), the alveolar network (A) and the outer covering of pleura (P) are indicated.

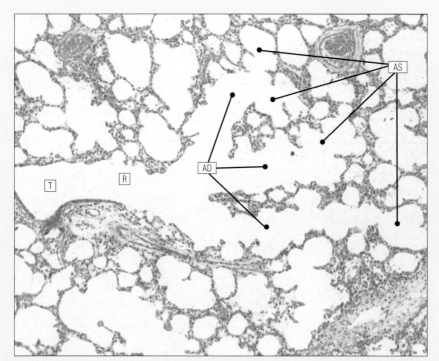

FIGURE 10.24 **Distal air passages.** Micrograph showing a terminal bronchiole (T) giving off a respiratory bronchiole (R), which has divided into three alveolar ducts (AD) with alveoli opening into them. They terminate in the alveolar sacs (AS), into which a number of alveoli open directly.

For online review questions, please visit
https://studentconsult.inkling.com.

? END OF CHAPTER REVIEW

True/False Answers to the MCQs, as Well as Case Answers, Can be Found in the Appendix in the Back of the Book.

1. Which of the following features are seen in the true vocal cords of the larynx?
   (a) Are covered by ciliated columnar epithelium
   (b) Are rich in lymphatics
   (c) Are rich in capillaries
   (d) Contain fibres of the vocal ligament
   (e) Contain fibres of the vocalis muscle

2. Arrange the following components of the respiratory tract in correct anatomical order moving from proximal to distal?
   (a) Alveolar duct
   (b) Terminal bronchiole
   (c) Alveolus
   (d) Respiratory bronchiole
   (e) Alveolar sacs

3. Which of the following features are seen in Type 1 pneumocytes?
   (a) Are more numerous than type 2
   (b) Are joined to each other by tight junctions
   (c) Are rich in mitochondria
   (d) Have prominent surface microvilli
   (e) Are very resistant to inhaled toxins

4. Which of the following features are seen in Type 2 pneumocytes?
   (a) Have surface microvilli
   (b) Are flat attenuated cells
   (c) Are stem cells which can produce new type 1 and type 2 pneumocytes
   (d) Can become detached to act as intra-alveolar macrophages
   (e) Contain multilamellate bodies in their cytoplasm

CASE 10.1   A CASE OF ANOSMIA

A 24-year-old man was involved in a drunken fracas outside a nightclub, during which he was thrown to the floor and banged his head on a concrete slab. He was admitted to hospital unconscious with profuse nosebleeds, and investigations showed a crack fracture of the base of the skull in the anterior cranial fossa. For 2 h, watery fluid also passed down the nose, and tests showed characteristics of cerebrospinal fluid. He was treated conservatively, recovered consciousness and made a good recovery. His only long-term impairment was total anosmia (loss of sense of smell).

Q. Describe the structural background to this case.

CASE 10.2   A CASE OF HOARSE VOICE

A 69-year-old man is referred to an otorhinolaryngologist because of progressive loss of voice for 3 weeks, getting worse daily. On direct laryngoscopic examination, the surgeon finds a small warty malignant tumour growing on the free edge of the left true vocal cord. It does not seem to have spread anteriorly or posteriorly to the commissures. Biopsy shows a carcinoma, a malignant tumour of the epithelium, originating from the epithelium covering the true cord.

Q. Describe the structural background to this case. Explain why the lack of involvement of commissures is important, and speculate whether this man's prognosis would have been better if the tumour had originated in the false cords instead of the true cords.

CASE 10.3   A CASE OF DETERIORATING CHEST INFECTION

A 78-year-old woman, a resident in a care home, became ill during an influenza epidemic, with fever, malaise, runny nose, sore throat and a cough. Whereas the other members of the care home who had also contracted influenza showed evidence of improvement after 5 or 6 days, this lady did not improve, becoming increasingly short of breath and cerebrally disorientated. She is admitted to hospital, where physical examination indicates that the bases of both lung fields are solid, with little or no air entry. Urgent chest X-ray confirms that there is consolidation of the lungs in the basal parts of the lower lobes, indicating pneumonia.

Q. Describe the structural background to this case. Explain how infecting organisms can spread through the lung.

Chapter 11

Alimentary Tract

Introduction

The alimentary tract is best considered as a muscular tube lined internally by an epithelium that varies in structure according to specialized functions required at particular sites along its length; with a few local variations, the structure of the musculature is similar throughout.

The function of the alimentary tract is to take in raw food material and to fragment it into small portions. These are then acted upon by a series of secretions, mainly enzymes, which convert the large molecules into smaller molecules, thus permitting their absorption into the blood and lymph circulation.

The small molecules are mainly amino acids, small peptides, carbohydrates, sugars and lipids, which are transported by the blood and lymph mainly to the liver, where they are used as the building blocks in the synthesis of essential proteins, carbohydrates and lipids.

The alimentary tract can be divided into three functional components, with an additional auxiliary gland system

The three functional components are the **oral cavity**, the **simple transport** passages and the **digestive tract** (Fig. 11.1).

The **oral cavity** is the area where food is ingested, broken up into smaller fragments by the action of the teeth, and softened by secretions in the form of saliva from the salivary gland. The food material is moved around in the oral cavity by movement of the jaws and tongue to facilitate fragmentation. The moistened and fragmented bolus of food is then transferred by deglutition (swallowing) to the first of the simple passages, the oesophagus.

The **simple transport passages** have no function other than to act as a contractile conduit to pass semisolid material from one area to another. The first simple transport passage is the pharynx, through which food from the mouth passes into the oesophagus which then transfers the moistened food bolus to the first part of the digestive tract, the stomach, before major digestion begins. The oesophagus is long, and the food bolus is forced along it by smooth muscle action in peristalsis, under involuntary nervous control. The other simple transport passage is the anal canal at the end of the digestive tract. This transports semisolid undigested waste material (faeces) from the end of the digestive tract to the exterior. The initial stimulus to transport is involuntary as a result of increasing distension of the rectum, but the timing of the evacuation of faeces can (usually) be controlled by voluntary (skeletal) muscle in an external sphincter. For semisolid material to pass easily through these simple transport passages, it is important that it is lubricated by mucus. For movement through the oesophagus, the mucus is incorporated into the food bolus in the mouth, having been secreted by mucous glands. In the anus, the faeces are lubricated by mucus secreted by the goblet cells in the colonic epithelium.

The **digestive tract** proper comprises the stomach, the small intestine and large intestine (colon and rectum). The stomach acts as a reservoir where the ingested fragmented food is held up by a sphincter until the acid and enzymatic secretions of the stomach mucosa have broken up the fragmented food into a semiliquid slurry (chyme), which then passes through the sphincter into the small intestine. Here, the process of digestion is continued by a combination of enzymes and other chemicals secreted by the small intestine itself and by the auxiliary glands, the liver and pancreas, the secretions of which enter the small intestine via ducts. In addition to this digestion function, the main function of the small intestine is absorption of the breakdown products of food digestion. The liquid food residue passes from the small intestine into the large intestine, where the majority of the fluid content is reabsorbed until the waste material is converted into semisolid waste material, lubricated for easy passage through the anal canal by mucus secreted by goblet cells in the colon and rectum.

All the components of the alimentary tract are structurally specialized to carry out their specific functions.

The **auxiliary gland systems** contributing to the function of the alimentary tract are the salivary glands, the liver and the pancreas, all of which pass their secretions into the main alimentary tract through ducts. The salivary glands are discussed on page 197, the pancreas on page 214, and the liver, which has many important functions other than those associated with digestion, merits a chapter of its own (Chapter 12).

Oral Cavity and its Contents

The oral cavity is lined throughout by stratified squamous epithelium but contains many highly specialized structures

The mouth is lined by stratified squamous epithelium, the underlying submucosa containing varying numbers of

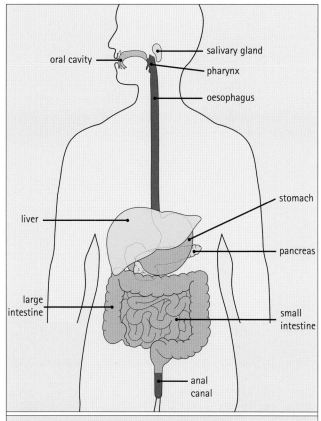

Three functional compartments		
	oral cavity	ingestion and fragmentation of food
	simple passages	transport of food or its residues without significant modification (oesophagus and anus)
	digestive tract	secretes enzymes induced in breakdown of food; absorbs molecules produced (stomach, small and large bowel)

Auxiliary gland system		
	secretory organs	located outside digestive tract and produce secretions which enter the gut via long ducts (salivary glands, pancreas, liver)

FIGURE 11.1 **The alimentary tract.**

salivary glands, which can secrete both a serous and a mucous fluid. Skeletal muscle fibres are common in the deeper layers and are responsible for altering the size and shape of the cavity and for moving food; skeletal muscle fibres form the bulk of the tongue, and are also numerous and important in the cheeks.

In some areas, the deep tissues of the oral cavity consist of bone, either simple plates of bone (as in the hard palate) or modified bone (teeth). The immovable hard palate produces a rigid structure against which the tongue can move, and the teeth, which are embedded in bony supports (the mandibles and maxillae), are the main tools for fragmenting ingested food.

The lips are covered by squamous epithelium and contain glands and underlying muscle

The oral orifice is bounded by the lips, the external aspects of which are covered by hair-bearing skin with sebaceous glands and eccrine sweat ducts. Between the hair-bearing outer surface and the moist, fluid-bathed inner surface, there is a transitional zone known as the vermilion because of its pinkish-red appearance. Here, the epithelium is non-keratinizing stratified squamous with a prominent rete ridge system (see Chapter 18) and the papillae between the epithelial downgrowths contain prominent blood vessels, which are responsible for the pinkish-red colour.

The inner surface of the lips is lined by a non-keratinizing stratified squamous epithelium with a less well-developed rete ridge system, and small clumps of salivary tissue disgorge their secretions on to its surface through short ducts. In addition, occasional sebaceous glands (Fordyce's spots), which are particularly common near the angles of the mouth, open directly on to the mucosal surface, rather than into a hair follicle as in the skin.

In the deeper parts of the lips, bundles of striated muscle fibres (orbicularis oris muscle) are arranged mainly in a concentric manner around the oral orifice. This muscle is responsible, among other things, for opening and closing the oral orifice.

The cheeks are lined internally by squamous epithelium and contain glands and deep muscle

The cheeks are lined by thick non-keratinizing squamous epithelium, the cells of which are often rich in glycogen. Areas of keratinization are common, usually as a result of chronic friction from ill-fitting dentures or from persistent cheek biting. The submucosa contains minor salivary glands (buccal glands) and occasional sebaceous glands (Fordyce's spots), whereas the deep tissues contain the skeletal muscle fibres of the cheek muscles (buccinator).

The palate is rich in salivary gland tissue (palatine salivary glands)

The surface epithelium of the palate is non-keratinizing, stratified squamous epithelium with, in the hard palate, a prominent rete ridge pattern, which reflects the frictional shearing stresses this area is subjected to by food during mastication. Beneath the salivary gland tissue the submucosa is firmly tethered to the periosteum of the palatal bone plate. The oral surface of the soft palate is similarly covered with non-keratinizing stratified squamous epithelium, which extends on to its free posterior edge, where there is a transition to the ciliated columnar epithelium covering the nasal surface.

The floor of the mouth contains salivary glands

The floor of the mouth is covered by thin non-keratinized stratified squamous epithelium, which is continuous with that of the ventral surface of the tongue.

The floor of the mouth is also rich in salivary gland tissue, with many minor salivary glands in the floor of the mouth (minor sublingual glands) and larger glands situated on either side of the midline frenulum of the ventral surface of the tongue (major sublingual glands, see p. 197).

The tongue is muscular and covered in squamous epithelium

The tongue is a highly muscular organ that protrudes upwards and forwards into the oral cavity from its floor. The ventral surface of the tongue is covered by thin non-keratinizing stratified squamous epithelium, continuous with that of the floor of the mouth. In contrast, the dorsal surface, which is commonly in contact with the hard palate during feeding, talking and at rest, is covered with a thick keratinizing stratified squamous epithelium, which shows considerable specialization.

The upper surface of the tongue is divided into two main zones

The dorsal surface of the tongue is divided into an anterior two-thirds and a posterior one-third. The two parts are separated by a V-shaped line of 6–10 dome-shaped protrusions, the 'circumvallate papillae' (Fig. 11.2). Circumvallate papillae appear as flattened domes, the bases of which are depressed below the dorsal surface.

Each circumvallate papilla is surrounded by a narrow, moat-like channel, in the epithelium of which are numerous taste buds. These taste buds are thought to detect bitter taste. Small salivary glands discharge their secretions into the channels (Fig. 11.3).

The posterior third of the tongue is characterized by the presence of lymphoid tissue

Low smooth dome-shaped elevations of the covering epithelium of the posterior third of the tongue are due to lymphoid tissue (the lingual tonsillar tissue) in the submucosa (Fig. 11.4). This lymphoid tissue is part of the mucosa-associated lymphoid tissue system (MALT, see p. 140) protecting (with the palatine tonsils and the pharyngeal adenoids) the oral portal of entry.

Lymphocytes are numerous within the overlying non-keratinizing stratified squamous epithelium, which extends down into the lymphoid tissue as narrow clefts. Small salivary glands open into the bottom of the narrow clefts, becoming more prominent and numerous near the line of circumvallate papillae.

The surface epithelium of the anterior two-thirds of the tongue is raised in a series of elevations called papillae

The three types of papillae in man are circumvallate (described above), filiform and fungiform.

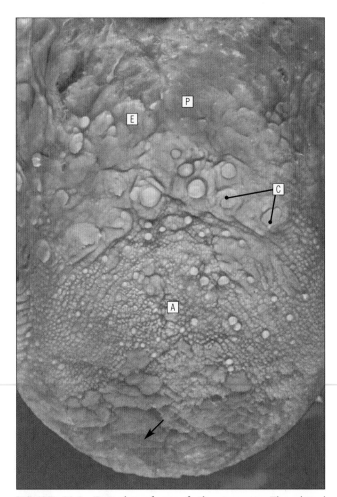

FIGURE 11.2 **Dorsal surface of the tongue.** The dorsal surface of the tongue can be divided into a posterior third (P) with smooth, dome-shaped elevations (E), and an anterior two-thirds (A) by a V-shaped line of circumvallate papillae (C). The surface of the anterior two-thirds is roughened by the presence of small filiform and fungiform papillae and by a surface keratin layer. In places the surface keratin may become thick and stained by food (coated tongue, arrow), particularly in the elderly (as here), and the coating may contain numerous bacterial colonies.

Filiform papillae are the most numerous papillae and are found all over the dorsum of the anterior two-thirds of the tongue. They are tall, narrow and pointed (Fig. 11.5) and are keratinized, particularly at their tips. Filiform papillae contain no identifiable taste buds.

Fungiform papillae (see Fig. 11.5) are scattered apparently randomly among the filiform papillae on the dorsal surface of the tongue, and have a mushroom shape. Taste buds are present in their covering epithelium, those at the anterior tip of the tongue detecting sweet taste, and those just behind the tip and some way along the lateral borders detecting salty taste.

Taste buds are specialized sensory organs located in the epithelium of the tongue

Each taste bud occupies the full thickness of the epithelium and comprises pale-staining spindle-shaped cells in

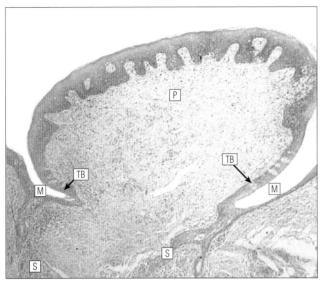

FIGURE 11.3 **Circumvallate papilla.** The circumvallate papilla (P) is surrounded by a moat (M), into the bottom of which empty prominent salivary glands (S). Taste buds (TB) are particularly numerous in the walls of the moat.

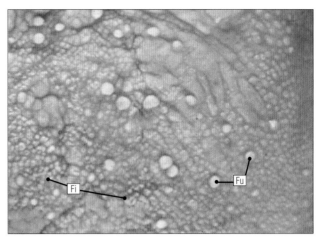

FIGURE 11.5 **Fungiform and filiform papillae.** Part of the dorsal surface of the anterior two-thirds of the tongue showing the gross appearance of the mushroom-like fungiform papillae (Fu) and the smaller filiform papillae (Fi).

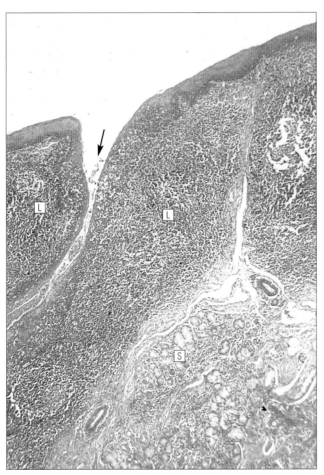

FIGURE 11.4 **Posterior third of the tongue.** Posterior third of the tongue showing lymphoid tissue (L), cleft-like invaginations of the epithelium (arrow) and salivary glands (S) opening into the depths of the clefts.

an oval cluster (Fig. 11.6). The luminal surfaces of the cells open into a small defect in the epithelium, the taste pore, and each cell bears a number of microvilli. Ultrastructurally, some of the spindle-shaped cells have synaptic vesicles and are associated with small afferent nerve fibres; these are the taste receptor cells. Other cells with more electron-dense cytoplasm and scanty secretory granules near the luminal surface are thought to act mainly as supporting sustentacular cells, but may also secrete glycosaminoglycans into the taste pore.

There are also cells resembling the taste receptor cells but lacking the synaptic vesicles and afferent nerve connections. The turnover of these cells is rapid (every 10–14 days), so there is a population of small rounded stem cells at the base of each taste bud from which the other cell types derive.

The taste buds of the dorsal tongue detect only acid, sweet, bitter and salty, and provide early warning that food may be unpalatable. Appreciation of more subtle flavours depends on the smell receptors in the nose (see p. 168).

KEY FACTS
ANTERIOR TWO-THIRDS OF THE TONGUE

- Covered by stratified squamous epithelium, thin on ventral surface, thick and papilliform on dorsal surface
- Filiform, fungiform and circumvallate papillae on anterior two-thirds; the latter demarcate anterior and posterior parts of the tongue
- Taste buds are present on circumvallate and fungiform papillae
- Consists of striated muscle with small amount of adipose tissue
- Salivary tissue in submucosa, mainly near circumvallate papillae.

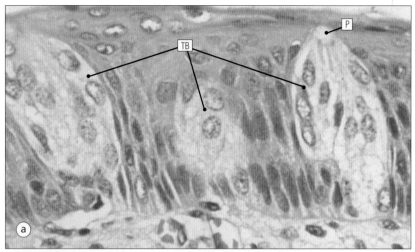

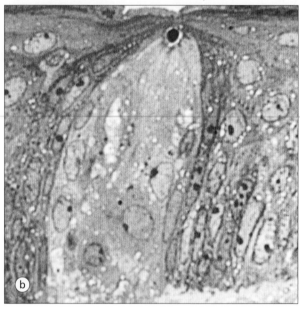

FIGURE 11.6 **Taste buds in circumvallate papilla.** (a) This thin acrylic resin section, stained with H&E, is from a circumvallate papilla of a surgically removed human tongue from an elderly man. It shows the oval taste buds (TB), which occupy the full thickness of the epithelium. The luminal aspect of the spindle-shaped cells opens on to the surface at the taste pore, the beginning of which is shown here (P). (b) An epoxy-resin section (0.5 μm thick) of a single taste bud, stained with toluidine blue to show the taste receptor cells with a mixture of spherical and spindle-shaped nuclei. A small bead of dark-staining glycosaminoglycan material is present in the taste pore.

KEY FACTS
POSTERIOR THIRD OF TONGUE

- Covered by smooth, non-papillate stratified squamous epithelium
- Submucosa contains lymphoid aggregates (MALT), forming part of Waldeyer's ring
- Bulk is muscle and adipose tissue, with some salivary tissue in submucosa and muscle, mainly near circumvallate papillae.

Skeletal muscle in the tongue is arranged in many directions

The musculature of the tongue comprises a complex pattern of skeletal muscle fibres. These fibres run in bands longitudinally, vertically, transversely and obliquely, with a variable amount of adipose tissue in between (Fig. 11.7).

This arrangement gives the tongue great mobility to manipulate food around the mouth for efficient fragmentation, and for moving fragmented food backwards prior to swallowing; it also provides the fine control of tongue movement that is essential for speech.

Abundant islands of salivary tissue are present in the submucosa between the muscular core of the tongue and the surface epithelium in the region of the junction between the posterior one-third and the anterior two-thirds. Some of the deeper salivary gland collections extend down into the superficial parts of the muscular zone.

Teeth

Introduction

The main task of the oral cavity, the fragmentation of large food masses, is performed by the teeth, which are hard, heavily mineralized structures embedded in the raised alveolar ridges of the maxilla and mandible.

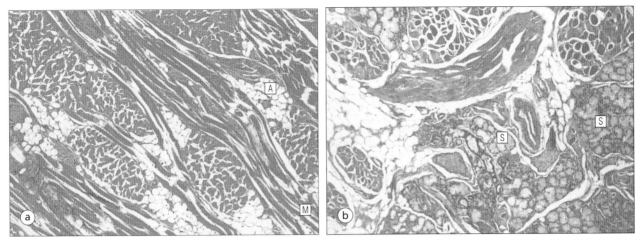

FIGURE 11.7 **Musculature of the tongue.** (a) In the anterior two-thirds of the tongue, the striated muscle bundles (M) are tightly packed with relatively little intervening adipose tissue (A). Note that the muscle bundles run in many directions. In the bulkier, less mobile posterior third of the tongue, the adipose tissue is more abundant. (b) Collections of salivary glands (S) are numerous in the submucosa and muscular core of the posterior tongue, particularly close to the junction between the posterior one-third and anterior two-thirds.

Teeth are arranged so that the free surface of those embedded in the mandible (lower teeth) oppose and contact those in the maxilla (upper teeth), allowing food material to be trapped between them.

The anterior teeth (incisor and canine teeth) have narrow, chisel-shaped or pointed free edges for chopping food into medium-sized pieces, whereas the posterior teeth (premolars and molars) have broader, flatter, free surfaces for grinding medium-sized food pieces into smaller fragments.

The mandible is joined to the body of the skull by the temporomandibular joint, which permits the mandible to slide backwards and forwards, and from side to side, thus aiding the grinding of food between the broad surfaces of the opposing molar teeth.

Each tooth can be divided into two anatomical components: the crown and the root

The tooth is divided into two structural regions:
- The crown protrudes into the oral cavity
- The root is embedded in the bone of the mandible or maxilla.

The junction between the crown and the root is called 'the neck'. The mature tooth has five components: the central pulp cavity, dentine, enamel, cementum and periodontal ligament (Fig. 11.8).

The centre of each tooth comprises the pulp, which contains nutrient vessels and nerves

The pulp cavity is the soft central core of the tooth and contains collagen and fibroblasts embedded in an acellular matrix. The cavity approximates in shape that of the tooth as a whole and its acellular matrix is composed of glycosaminoglycans.

Through the pulp cavity run the blood vessels that nourish the odontoblasts (see below) and the nerve twigs that provide dental sensation. These vessels and nerves enter and leave through a small **apical foramen** at the tip of the root.

The pulp cavity is narrow throughout most of the root (the **root canal**), but is expanded in the neck and crown (the **pulp chamber**). Its outer surface is lined by odontoblasts, which continually produce dentine. As dentine is progressively laid down, the pulp cavity diminishes in size.

Dentinogenesis and Odontoblasts

The specialized mineralized matrix of the tooth is called dentine and is secreted by odontoblasts

Dentine is composed of mineral salts and organic material. The mineral salts are calcium salts in the form of crystalline hydroxyapatite (about 70–80%) arranged as long, hollow parallel tubules, the **dentinal tubules**. Within these, run the organic material in the form of fine cytoplasmic processes of the odontoblasts, and the type I collagen fibres and glycosaminoglycans that they produce (about 20–30%).

Dentine is initially laid down by odontoblasts as a glycosaminoglycan matrix in which collagen fibres are linearly arranged. This non-mineralized predentine is synthesized by odontoblasts located at the outer limits of the pulp cavity (Fig. 11.9).

In man, the odontoblast cytoplasmic processes extend only 25–50% of the full length of the dentinal tubule, thus dentine close to the dentine–enamel border appears to contain empty tubules. In life, these empty tubules may contain fluid, which is lost during tissue processing.

As odontoblasts progressively synthesize new predentine at the inner surface of the pulp cavity (Figs 11.9, 11.10), the cavity slowly decreases in size throughout life.

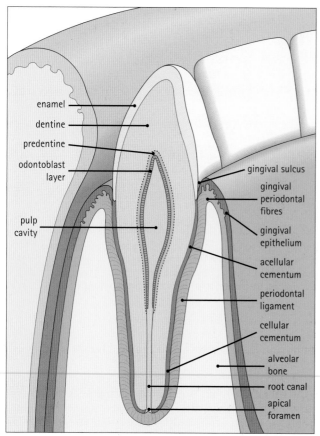

FIGURE 11.8 **Mature incisor tooth.** The central pulp cavity, the outer layer of which contains cells (odontoblasts) that produce the specialized extracellular matrix components of the teeth, is surrounded by dentine, a relatively acellular mineralized material forming the bulk of each tooth. The dentine of the crown of the tooth is covered by enamel, a heavily mineralized material forming a resistant outer coat. At the neck of the tooth, enamel is continuous with cementum. This is a bone-like material forming an outer coat to the dentine in the root. Cementum is linked to the alveolar bone of the mandible or maxilla by the periodontal ligament, which is composed of tightly packed collagen fibres embedded at one end into the cementum of the tooth and at the other end into the bone forming the tooth socket.

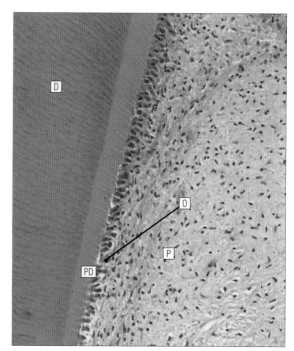

FIGURE 11.9 **Dentine, predentine and odontoblasts.** Micrograph showing pulp cavity (P) lined externally by a layer of odontoblasts (O), external to which is a pale staining band of predentine (PD). The outer layer is mineralized dentine (D), in which the pattern of dentinal tubules can be seen.

Ameloblasts and Enamel Formation

Enamel is the hardest material in the body

Enamel is composed almost entirely of the mineral hydroxyapatite $(Ca_{10}(PO_4)_6(OH)_2)$, which is arranged in tightly packed hexagonal enamel rods or prisms (Fig. 11.12) about $4\,\mu m$ in diameter, although some may measure up to $8\,\mu m$.

Each enamel rod extends through the full thickness of the enamel. The small interstices between adjacent rods are occupied by hydroxyapatite crystals. A small amount of organic matrix (protein and polysaccharide) represents the remnants of the matrix synthesized and excreted by the enamel-producing cells, 'the ameloblasts', prior to mineralization of the enamel.

Enamel is formed during tooth development by the ameloblasts

Ameloblasts degenerate when the tooth erupts, after which time the enamel cannot be replaced by new synthesis. In the developing tooth (see Fig. 11.17), the functioning ameloblast is a tall, narrow cell, with its base attached to the cells of the stratum intermedium (Fig. 11.13). The nucleus is located basally and basal cytoplasm contains abundant mitochondria. The supranuclear cytoplasm contains a large, active Golgi complex and abundant rough endoplasmic reticulum, together with microtubules, which are predominantly

Dentinogenesis commences with the formation of predentine by odontoblasts

In predentine, randomly scattered collagen fibres (type I collagen) produced by the odontoblasts are embedded in an extracellular matrix of phosphoprotein and glycosaminoglycans (mainly chondroitin-6-sulfate).

Mineralization is initiated by the discharge of the matrix vacuoles from the odontoblast process and its branches running through the predentine layer.

Some time after its formation, predentine becomes mineralized at its border with previously mineralized dentine; close to this predentine–dentine border the collagen fibres of predentine become more numerous and tightly packed. The dentine lining the dentinal tubules (peritubular dentine) is particularly compact and heavily mineralized (Fig. 11.11).

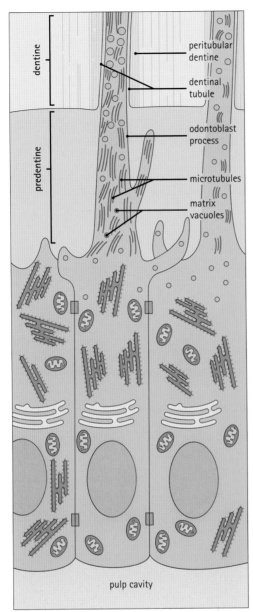

FIGURE 11.10 **Odontoblasts and dentinogenesis.** The functioning odontoblast is a tall, narrow cell, the base of which contacts cells and fibres of the pulp cavity (mainly fibroblasts and collagen). Its nucleus is basal and its cytoplasm is rich in mitochondria and rough endoplasmic reticulum. It has a large supranuclear Golgi complex. At the apex of the cell the cytoplasm is drawn out into a long odontoblast process which runs through the predentine and dentine layers in the dentinal tubule, while small side branches penetrate the predentine. The cytoplasm of the odontoblast process and its branches contains numerous microtubules as well as small matrix vacuoles, which contain Ca^{2+} and PO_4^- ions. The matrix vacuoles play a key role in the mineralization of the dentinal matrix. The mechanism is almost identical to that whereby matrix vesicles from osteoblasts produce mineralization of osteoid matrix to produce bone mineralization (see Fig. 13.20).

longitudinally arranged, and secretory vacuoles which become larger and more numerous near the upper pole.

At the upper pole, the cell elongates into a single large Tomes' process, and forms a fringe of smaller processes around its neck. The Tomes' process contains

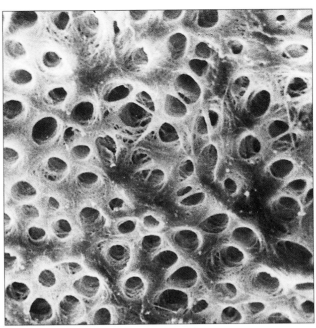

FIGURE 11.11 **Dentinal tubules.** Scanning electron micrograph of dentine at a point well distant from the predentine layer. The mineral material contains regular empty dentinal tubules because the cytoplasmic processes of the odontoblasts extend only a short way into the tubules. Note the more compact dentine lining the tubules.

numerous microtubules and large numbers of secretory vacuoles.

The rough endoplasmic reticulum synthesizes various proteins and glycoproteins (including amelogenin and enamelin), which form the organic matrix of enamel (pre-enamel) and are packaged by the Golgi complex into secretory vacuoles. These then move into the Tomes' process and the small neck processes, discharging their contents on to the surface.

Mineralization of the matrix proteins by hydroxyapatite occurs almost instantaneously, producing small enamel crystallites and, with progressive mineralization, the enamel rods or prisms.

The compact structured enamel prisms are probably derived from the surface of the main Tomes' process, whereas the small amount of less compact interprism enamel, which has a larger organic matrix component, is probably derived from the small neck processes.

Enamel covers the dentine only in the region of the exposed crown (Fig. 11.14); in the root, the dentine is covered by cementum (see Figs 11.8, 11.15).

Cementum and Periodontal Ligament

Cementum is a bone-like tissue; it is calcified and contains collagen

A thin layer of cementum covers the root of the tooth, being thin, compact and acellular (acellular cementum) over the upper region, but thicker and containing lacunae

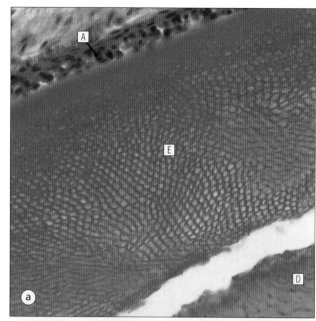

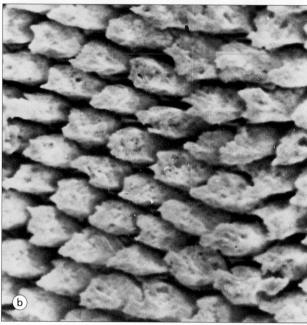

FIGURE 11.12 **Enamel.** (a) H&E-stained section of early forming enamel (E) being produced by a layer of ameloblasts (A). The enamel shows a distinctive pattern owing to the arrangement of enamel prisms and abuts the dentine (D). (b) Scanning electron micrograph showing the characteristic arrangement of tightly packed enamel prisms or rods.

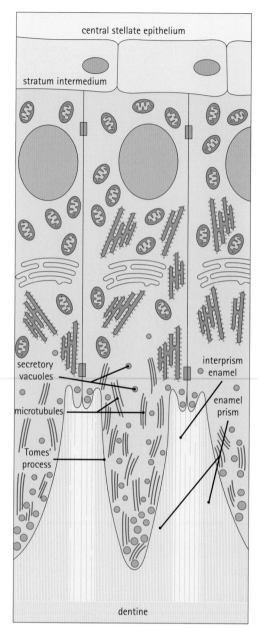

FIGURE 11.13 **Ameloblasts and enamel formation.** The functioning ameloblast is a tall, narrow cell, with its base attached to the cells of the stratum intermedium. The Tomes' process at the upper pole is rich in secretory vacuoles containing organic matrix proteins and numerous microtubules. Each Tomes' process has small associated cytoplasmic processes around it; these also produce some enamel, but the main enamel prisms are produced by the Tomes' process.

and cementocytes (cellular cementum) lower down (see Fig. 11.15).

Cementocytes resemble osteocytes (see Chapter 13) and remain viable throughout life, being nourished through canaliculi which link the lacunae. They can become activated to produce new cementum when required.

In addition to the cementocytes, which are scattered throughout the cellular cementum, there is a layer of cells called 'cementoblasts', which are similar to the actively synthetic osteoblasts of bone (see Fig. 13.17).

Cementoblasts lie against the surface of the periodontal ligament and probably produce most new cementum by appositional deposition.

The periodontal ligament is a suspensory ligament tethering the tooth in the bony alveolar socket of the mandible or maxilla

The periodontal ligament is composed of dense collagen and fibrocytes, with the fibres running across the gap between the cementum of the tooth and the bone of the

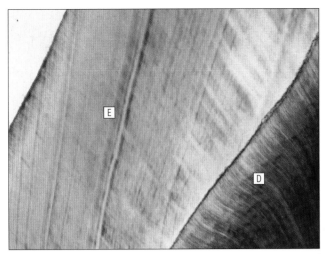

FIGURE 11.14 **Formed enamel.** Unstained ground section of a mature human tooth showing the characteristic patterns of enamel (E) and dentine (D); the tightly packed dentinal tubules are clearly seen. The linearity of the compact parallel enamel prisms runs from the dentinal–enamel interface in straight lines to the surface. The coarse, slightly curved, oblique lines seen in this photomicrograph are an artifact produced by the grinding process used to make this section.

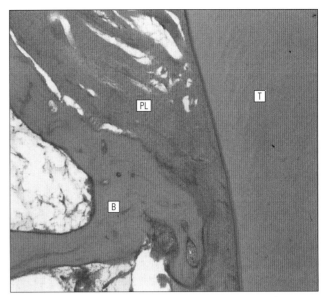

FIGURE 11.16 **Periodontal ligament.** H&E-stained section showing the relationship between the tooth (T), bony socket (B) and the fibrous periodontal ligament (PL) at the neck of the tooth.

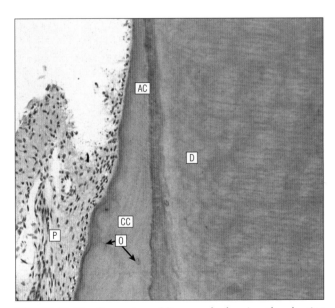

FIGURE 11.15 **Cementum.** Micrograph showing the dentine (D), cementum and fibrous periodontal ligament (P) of the root of a tooth at the junction between the narrow compact acellular cementum (AC) and the broader cellular cementum (CC), in which osteocyte-like nuclei can be seen (O).

fibres of the periodontal ligament become the gingival periodontal fibres and blend with the submucosa of the gingivae.

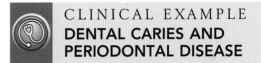

CLINICAL EXAMPLE
DENTAL CARIES AND PERIODONTAL DISEASE

The most common disorders of teeth are:

- Abnormal tooth eruption, leading to malalignment of teeth
- Dental caries
- Periodontal disease.

Dental caries results when bacterial plaque produces acid, which dissolves the calcium hydroxyapatite of the enamel. Such focal decalcification may progress until the erosion involves the deeper dentine, from where the acids and bacteria can advance more rapidly down the dentinal tubules to the pulp cavity, causing tooth pain.

Continued bacterial damage can produce a tooth abscess in the soft pulp.

Destruction of the pulp cavity and its contained blood vessels leads to death of the odontoblast layer and eventual death of the tooth.

Periodontal disease is caused by the accumulation of bacterial plaque (calcified food and bacterial debris) in the gingival sulcus. This excites inflammation in the adjacent gum which gradually forces the gingiva away from the tooth, widening and damaging the gingival sulcus; deep periodontal pockets form in which food particles and bacteria become trapped. Bacterial proliferation then leads to further inflammation of the gum (gingivitis) and the periodontal ligament (periodontitis).

Persistent periodontitis destroys the periodontal ligament and the tooth becomes loose in its socket.

alveolar socket (Fig. 11.16). As the collagen fibres are embedded in a ground substance, this ligament also acts as a shock-absorber, as well as permitting limited movement of the tooth within the bony socket.

At its cemental and alveolar limits, some of the collagen fibres are inserted into the cementum and bone. The alveolar bone at the inner margin of the socket is composed of woven bone rather than compact lamellar bone. Above the upper limit of the alveolar bone, the

Tooth Development

Teeth develop from both ectoderm and mesoderm

Teeth develop from both ectoderm and from mesenchyme of mesodermal origin, the ectodermal component being the enamel derived from the enamel organ and the mesenchyme producing the rest of the tooth.

The enamel organ originates as a cellular downgrowth of the oral epithelium, initially in the form of a cap-shaped epithelial tooth bud connected to the overlying oral epithelium by the dental lamina. Beneath the epithelial tooth bud, a condensation of mesenchyme contributes to the rest of the tooth.

The stages in tooth formation are summarized in Figure 11.17.

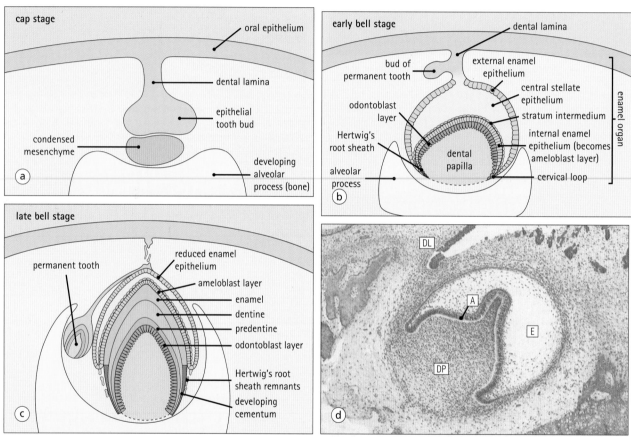

FIGURE 11.17 **Tooth development.** (a) Early stage of tooth formation from both ectodermal (epithelial) and mesenchymal components. (b) The cells of the epithelial tooth bud develop into the enamel organ, differentiating into a bell-shaped structure with a central core of loosely arranged stellate cells (stellate epithelium) and a peripheral layer of cuboidal or low columnar epithelium. The outer cell layer of the convex surface is the external enamel epithelium, and that of the concave surface the internal enamel epithelium. The internal enamel epithelium differentiates into an outer layer of tall columnar ameloblasts (see Fig. 11.13) and a two- to three-cell thick inner layer called the 'stratum intermedium'. Where the external and internal enamel epithelium meet is called the 'cervical loop'. An extension downward of cells of the external enamel epithelium forms the so-called 'Hertwig's root sheath', which defines the final size of the tooth root, being later replaced by the cementum. In the concavity of the enamel organ the mesenchyme continues to condense to form the dental papilla, and a row of odontoblasts develops at its junction with the enamel organ, in contact with the ameloblast layer. In deciduous teeth, like the incisor shown here, the permanent tooth arises from a side-growth from the dental lamina. (c) Odontoblasts begin to produce predentine and this stimulates the production of enamel by the ameloblasts. Calcification of the predentine and pre-enamel begins almost immediately, and dentine and enamel continue to be laid down until the form of the tooth is complete. The dental papilla becomes enclosed by dentine to form the dental pulp. The non-ameloblast components of the enamel organ become much reduced and eventually atrophy. When enamel formation is complete, the ameloblasts degenerate to form a thin layer of irregular cells, which ultimately disappear when the tooth erupts. The cells of Hertwig's root sheath begin to degenerate as the cementum is deposited by cementoblasts on the surface of the dentine of the tooth root. Partial development of the permanent tooth continues alongside the deciduous tooth in the same manner. (d) Micrograph of a resin section of a developing tooth at the early bell stage, showing the enamel organ (E), including the ameloblast layer (A), the dental papilla (DP) and the degenerating dental lamina (DL).

The Gums

The gingiva (gum) is the portion of oral mucosa covering the alveolar bone ridge surrounding the tooth

The gingival mucosa is continuous with the alveolar mucosa covering the rest of the bone. A small sulcus lies between the tooth and the bulk of the gingiva.

The sulcal epithelium is thin stratified squamous, whereas that on the outer surface of the gingiva is thick and keratinized, with a prominent rete ridge pattern.

The submucosa in the region of the gingival sulcus is commonly infiltrated by chronic inflammatory cells and also contains gingival periodontal fibres, which are an extension of the upper limit of the periodontal ligament.

Salivary Glands

There are three main salivary glands and many minor glands

The mouth receives secretions from salivary gland tissue located both inside and outside the mouth. These glands may contain mucus-secreting cells, serous cells or a mixture of both. The serous glands secrete a watery solution containing enzymes (e.g. amylase, lysozyme), IgA secretory piece and lactoferrin, an iron-binding compound.

The largest salivary glands are located outside the mouth and transfer their secretions into the oral cavity by long ducts; smaller glands, sited mainly in the submucosa of the oral lining, are less well-defined and empty their secretions into the mouth by short ducts.

The main salivary glands are the submandibular, the parotid and the large sublingual glands.

The submandibular salivary gland secretes a mixed serous/mucous product

The submandibular glands are roughly ovoid in shape and are situated on either side of the neck just below the mandible. Their ducts open into the floor of the mouth, one on each side of the frenulum of the tongue.

The submandibular glands are typical mixed glands containing both serous and mucous elements, with serous elements predominating.

The secretory acini are composed mainly of epithelial cells, which are responsible for the serous secretion, and are plump cells filled with prominent, purplish-staining zymogen granules.

The mucus-secreting cells are pale-staining with abundant clear cytoplasm, and often form blind-ending tubules, the blind end bearing a demilune or crescent of zymogen-rich serous cells (Fig. 11.18).

The secretory acini empty into intercalated ducts, which are lined by cuboidal or low columnar epithelium and merge to form intralobular ducts. These are characterized by tall columnar epithelium, which stains pale pink and shows a characteristic striated pattern (see Fig.

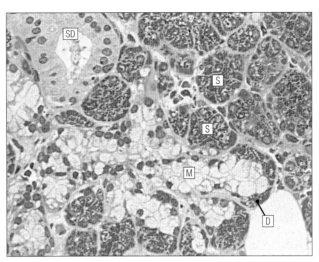

FIGURE 11.18 **Submandibular salivary gland.** The submandibular salivary gland has both a mucous and a serous component. The serous component (S) contains numerous large zymogen granules, whereas the mucous component (M) is often arranged in duct-like structures, the ends of which are capped by the so-called 'serous demilunes' (D). A striated duct (SD) shows the characteristic features of an ion exchange epithelium.

3.23) of basal cytoplasm. Hence, intralobular ducts are commonly called 'striated ducts'.

Intralobular duct epithelium is biochemically active and modifies the concentration and content of the fluids produced by the secretory acini.

The intralobular striated ducts fuse to form larger interlobular ducts which are lined by a non-striated, often pseudostratified, epithelium. Interlobular ducts then join to form the major ducts, some of which (particularly the main submandibular duct) may have a ciliated epithelium.

There is a network of myoepithelial cells between the epithelium and the basement membrane of the acini and much of the ductular system, contraction of the myoepithelial cells squeezing the secretion toward the major ducts.

The parotid salivary glands secrete a serous product

The parotid glands are situated below and in front of the pinna on each side of the face. They are flat and well encapsulated and the facial nerve runs through them, dividing them into superficial and deep portions. Their long ducts open into the oral cavity opposite the second upper molar tooth on each side.

The parotids are composed entirely of serous glands rich in zymogen granules, with a variable amount of adipose tissue in the interstitium between parotid lobules (Fig. 11.19).

The sublingual glands secrete a mainly mucous product

The large sublingual glands are located in the floor of the mouth, one on either side of the frenulum of the tongue.

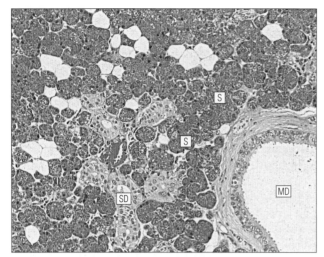

FIGURE 11.19 **Parotid salivary gland.** The parotid salivary gland is composed entirely of granular serous cells (S), with variable amounts of intervening adipose tissue. Note the cluster of small ducts (SD) and part of a major duct (MD).

Their short ducts open into the mouth near to, or with, the submandibular ducts. These glands are composed predominantly of mucous cells.

There are numerous smaller groups of salivary gland tissue

The oral cavity contains a large amount of salivary gland tissue scattered diffusely in the submucosa.
The most important are:
- Lingual glands in the submucosa and muscle layers of the dorsal surface of the tongue (see Fig. 11.7b)
- Minor sublingual glands close to the larger major sublingual glands (other tongue glands are found on the inferior surface of the tip of the tongue and on its lateral borders)
- Labial glands on the inner surface of the lips
- Palatine glands in the submucosa of the soft and hard palates
- Tonsillar glands in the mucosa associated with the palatine and pharyngeal tonsils
- Buccal glands in the submucosa lining the cheeks.

The labial, sublingual, minor lingual and buccal glands are composed predominantly of mucous cells, but some serous cells may be present. The palatine and lateral lingual glands are entirely mucus secreting.

Transport Passages

The pharynx, oesophagus and anal canal are comparatively simple transport tubes through which ingested food is transmitted by peristalsis without undergoing significant metabolic change. They are muscular tubes lined internally by stratified squamous epithelium and some mucous glands which provide lubricating mucus.

The pharynx is divided into oropharynx and nasopharynx

The pharynx is located at the back of the mouth and transfers partly fragmented food from the oral cavity into the upper end of the oesophagus. It also connects the nasal system of air chambers and the upper end of the trachea. The opening of the mouth into the pharynx is the **oropharynx**, and the nasal opening is the **nasopharynx**. The eustachian tube from the middle ear (see Chapter 10, p. 167) opens into the pharynx on each side.

The oropharynx and pharynx proper are lined by largely non-keratinizing stratified squamous epithelium. The nasopharynx is mainly lined by ciliated columnar epithelium but stratified squamous epithelium occurs at its lower end where it joins the oropharynx.

The submucosa of the pharynx is well endowed with lymphoid tissue

There is a particularly prominent aggregation of lymphoid tissue in the nasopharynx, forming the pharyngeal tonsil (adenoids). At the junction between the mouth and pharynx, in the oropharynx, are large lymphoid tonsillar masses in the gap between the glossopalatine and pharyngopalatine arches on each side. These are the palatine tonsils. The tonsils are discussed on pages 141 and 167.

Oesophagus

Introduction

The oesophagus lies between the pharynx and the stomach. It transports food in an undigested but fragmented form to the stomach, where digestion begins. It is about 25 cm long, originating from the pharynx at the level of the cricoid cartilage and extending down the posterior mediastinum in the midline to the level of the diaphragm; it penetrates the left crus of the diaphragm before opening into the stomach at the oesophagogastric junction.

The oesophagus is lined by squamous epithelium, which lies over a lamina propria and a muscularis mucosae

The oesophageal mucosa is composed of non-keratinizing stratified squamous epithelium, lamina propria and muscularis mucosae (Fig. 11.20). The basal zone of the epithelium may be several cell layers thick and consists of cuboidal or rectangular cells with dark nuclei and purple-staining cytoplasm, in which there is no glycogen. Scattered in this layer are occasional melanocytes and neuroendocrine cells.

Above the basal zone, the epithelial cells are larger and may be rich in glycogen, gradually becoming more flattened as the lumen is approached (Fig. 11.21).

The average epithelial thickness is 500–800 μm, but this is difficult to measure accurately because the lower border is irregular and tongues of lamina propria extend

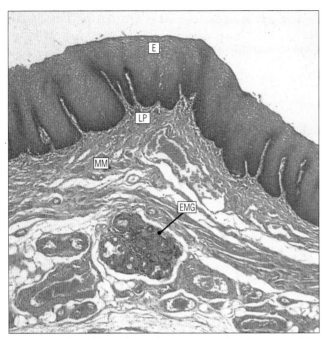

FIGURE 11.20 **Oesophageal mucosa and submucosa.** The oesophagus is lined by non-keratinizing stratified squamous epithelium (E), beneath which is a thick lamina propria (LP) and muscularis mucosae (MM). The submucosa contains abundant vessels and nerves together with oesophageal mucous glands (EMG), which are characteristically surrounded by lymphocytic infiltrate.

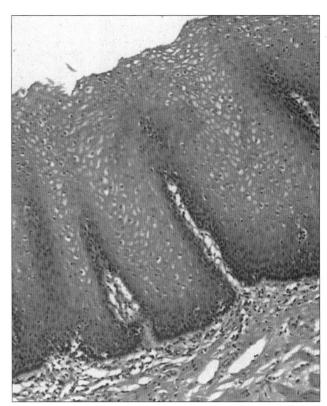

FIGURE 11.21 **Oesophageal epithelium.** At high magnification, the oesophageal squamous epithelium contains some pale-staining cells distended with glycogen; its lower border is irregular.

up toward the luminal surface, giving an appearance similar to the rete ridge arrangement in the epidermis of the skin (see Chapter 18).

The oesophageal lamina propria consists of loosely arranged collagen fibres and fibroblasts embedded in an acellular glycosaminoglycan matrix, with a normal scattering of lymphocytes and eosinophils, as well as occasional mast cells and plasma cells.

The muscularis mucosae is of variable thickness, being particularly thick at the lower end where it approaches the oesophagogastric junction. In the upper oesophagus, the fibres appear to be arranged haphazardly, but in the lower third, there are continuous sheets of longitudinal and circular smooth muscle.

The submucosa of the oesophagus contains mucous glands, lymphoid tissue, nerves and blood vessels

The submucosa of the oesophagus is broad and contains mucous glands (see Fig. 11.20) that secrete acid mucins. Each gland has 2–5 lobes, which drain into a short duct lined by stratified columnar epithelium, the duct penetrating the muscularis mucosae, lamina propria and epithelial layer to open into the lumen. Lymphocytes, plasma cells and eosinophils are particularly common around the glands and their ducts (see Fig. 11.20). Aggregations of lymphoid cells forming small follicles are common in the oesophageal submucosa near the squamous/columnar epithelial junction.

Oesophageal submucosa is also particularly rich in blood vessels, lymphatics, nerves and ganglion cells.

The muscle of the oesophagus contains both striated and smooth types

The muscularis proper of the oesophagus varies along its length, although it is generally arranged in discrete circular and longitudinal layers. In the upper third of the oesophagus the layers are composed almost entirely of striated muscle, but a gradual transition to smooth muscle occurs in the middle third, where both striated and smooth muscle fibres are found together. The muscle layers in the lower third are composed entirely of smooth muscle and are continuous with the smooth muscle layers of the stomach.

The oesophagogastric junction is an important site of pathological abnormality

Unlike the rest of the oesophagus, which is lined by stratified squamous epithelium, the short length (1–1.5 cm long) of oesophagus below the diaphragm is lined by columnar epithelium similar to that of the cardiac region of the stomach; this is the oesophagogastric (squamous/columnar) junction (Fig. 11.22). Disease results from exposure of the squamous epithelium of the lower oesophagus to acid and digestive enzymes from the stomach (Fig. 11.23).

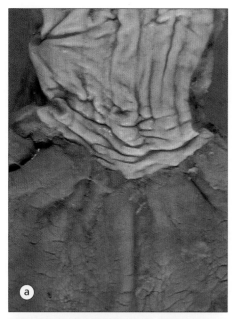

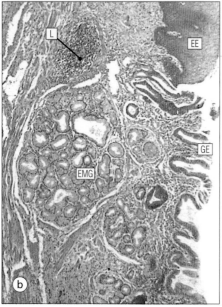

FIGURE 11.22 **Oesophagogastric junction.** (a) Macroscopic appearance of the junction between the oesophagus and stomach. Most of the oesophagus is lined by a stratified squamous epithelium (pale), whereas the stomach epithelium appears brown. (b) H&E section of the squamous/columnar junction in the region of the oesophagogastric junction showing the abrupt transition between oesophageal squamous epithelium (EE) and columnar gastric epithelium (GE). In the region of the junction, lymphoid aggregates (L) and oesophageal mucous glands (EMG) are particularly prominent.

KEY FACTS
OESOPHAGUS

- Lined by non-keratinizing stratified squamous epithelium
- Submucosa contains mucous glands, lymphoid aggregates, and prominent blood vessels, particularly at lower end
- Muscle is striated type in upper third, smooth muscle in lower third, and both in middle third
- Lower oesophagus is an important site of common diseases, particularly ulceration, stricture and cancer.

CLINICAL EXAMPLE
OESOPHAGEAL ULCERATION AND BARRETT'S OESOPHAGUS

The squamous epithelium of the oesophagus is protected from exposure to gastric acid by:

- The anatomical arrangement of the oesophagogastric junction
- The small oesophagogastric muscular sphincter, which in most cases prevents reflux of gastric contents into the lower oesophagus.

However, the system is not foolproof, and reflux of acid gastric secretions may occur into the lower oesophagus causing inflammation and pain. Under the constant irritating effect of reflux of acidic gastric secretions, the epithelium in the lower oesophagus changes its form from stratified squamous epithelium to a gastric type of glandular epithelium. This condition is called 'Barrett's oesophagus', and is an example of epithelial metaplasia (see p. 175).

The islands of columnar epithelium in Barrett's oesophagus are particularly prone to ulceration and inflammation (Fig. 11.23) and are also predisposed to the development of one type of oesophageal cancer.

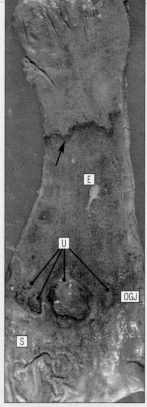

FIGURE 11.23 **Barrett's oesophagus.** The lower half of the oesophagus (E) and the upper part of the stomach (S). Compare with Figure 11.22a. At the oesophagogastric junction (OGJ) are four ulcers (U), which lie in inflamed metaplastic glandular (columnar) mucosa that extends up as far as the arrow. Above the arrow, there is normal oesophageal stratified squamous epithelium, which shows yellowish discolouration as a result of repeated vomiting. Healing of such ulcers can lead to scarring of the lower end of the oesophagus, and thereby narrowing of its lumen (i.e. an oesophageal stricture), so that swallowing becomes almost impossible.

Anal Canal

The anal canal is a muscular conduit transporting faeces for elimination

The anal canal transports the residue of ingested food after it has been digested and most of its water content has been extracted (i.e. faeces) from the rectum to the exterior in the process known as defecation.

Anatomically, the anal canal is a tube 3–4 cm long (Fig. 11.24), the diameter of which is controlled by two sphincter systems.

The internal anal sphincter is composed of smooth muscle and is a localized thickening of the circular muscle of the lower rectum. It is under autonomic control and responds to distension of the rectal reservoir.

The external anal sphincter is composed of skeletal striated muscle and is continuous with the fascia and muscles of the pelvic floor. It is under voluntary control.

The anal canal is mainly lined by stratified squamous epithelium

At its upper end, the anal canal is lined by columnar epithelium identical to that of the rectum. This changes to a non-keratinizing stratified squamous type at the level of the pectinate (or dentate) line, which marks the site of the anal membrane of the fetus (i.e. the junction of gut endoderm and the ectodermal invagination of the proctodeal pit).

The pectinate line is a line of small crescentic valve-like mucosal extrusions, with small vertical folds, the anal columns, arising from their junctions.

Small branched tubular glands, the anal glands, open into the anal canal just above the pectinate line, and another set of glands, the prominent apocrine glands of the perianal skin, lie at the lower end of the anal canal (circumanal glands).

Two prominent venous plexuses are associated with the anal canal

The internal haemorrhoidal plexus lies in the submucosa of the upper end of the canal above the level of the pectinate line.

The external haemorrhoidal plexus lies in the submucosa at the lower end in the region of the junction between anal canal and perianal skin.

The internal haemorrhoidal plexus is particularly prone to become greatly enlarged as a result of chronic congestion secondary to raised intrapelvic pressure, such as may occur during pregnancy and repeated excessive straining to defecate due to constipation. This enlargement causes the veins to bulge into the anal canal and even to become so large that they protrude outside the anal orifice. Here, they are subject to trauma and inflammation and may become extremely painful. These protrusions are called '**haemorrhoids**' or 'piles', and when they protrude from the anal orifice, 'prolapsed piles'.

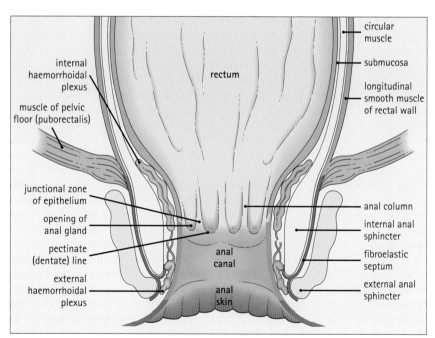

FIGURE 11.24 **Anal canal.** The anal canal showing the epithelial linings of the rectum (columnar), anal canal (non-keratinizing stratified squamous) and anal skin (keratinizing epidermis rich in hair follicles, eccrine and apocrine glands). There is a variable junctional zone of epithelium at the pectinate line. The internal sphincter is a continuation of the circular smooth muscle layer of the rectum, and the external sphincter is composed of skeletal muscle under voluntary control. The rectal longitudinal muscle loses its fibres at the level of the puborectalis muscle of the pelvic floor and continues as a fibroelastic septum between the internal and external sphincters. Note the positions of the internal and external haemorrhoidal plexuses; haemorrhoids (piles) result from enlargement of the internal haemorrhoidal plexus.

Digestive Tract

The digestive tract is the site of several processes:
- Major digestion of food material (some digestion begins in the mouth as a result of salivary secretion of diastase)
- Absorption of the end products of digestion
- Absorption of ingested fluids and reabsorption of secreted fluids.

The digestive tract comprises the stomach, small intestine (i.e. duodenum, jejunum and ileum) and large intestine (i.e. caecum, appendix, colon and rectum). Its basic structure is shown in Figure 11.25.

The digestive mucosa, composed of lining epithelium, lamina propria and muscularis mucosae, is the most variable component of the digestive tract and usually contains a mixture of epithelial cell types, both absorptive and secretory. The epithelium is supported by a variable layer, the lamina propria, which is composed of supporting cells and their products (including collagen). Within the lamina propria are small blood vessels, lymphatics, nerve fibres and cells belonging to the immune and defence systems (see Chapter 8), particularly macrophages and lymphocytes. The deep aspect of the lamina propria rests on a usually thin muscle layer, the muscularis mucosae.

The surface area of the digestive passages is increased by the formation of folds and glands

The efficiency of absorptive and secretory processes is improved by increasing the surface area of contact between the epithelial cells and the lumen. This is achieved by:
- Intrusions or folding of the lining epithelium into the lumen (i.e. villi or plicae)
- Inversions of the epithelium to form tubular structures, the lumina of which communicate with the main lumen
- Formation of complex glands within or exterior to the tract wall.

Examples of these structural modifications will be discussed in relation to specific areas of the digestive tract.

The submucosal layer contains vessels, nerves and a specialized nerve plexus

The submucosa lies between the mucosa and the main muscle layer of the digestive tract wall. It is composed of fibroblasts, collagen and acellular matrix, and contains blood vessels, lymphatics and nerves, which supply or

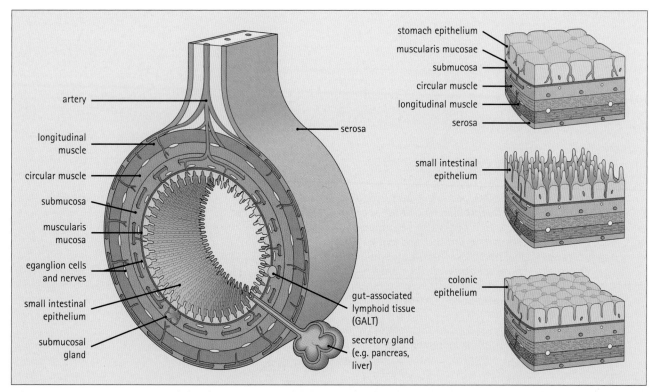

FIGURE 11.25 **Basic structure of the digestive tract.** The digestive tract is a muscular tube lined internally by specialized epithelium which, for most of its length, has a combined secretory and absorptive function. Three patterns of epithelial structure (stomach, small intestine and colon) are shown in this diagram. Externally, the tract has an outer layer of flat mesothelium, where it runs through the peritoneal cavity. Various secretory organs, which are derived embryologically as outgrowths of the putative alimentary tract, lie partly or completely outside it. These organs (e.g. pancreas and liver) produce secretions which are vital for the tract to function normally; they are transferred to the digestive tract lumen by one or more ducts.

drain their smaller equivalents in the lamina propria of the mucosa.

In addition, the submucosa contains clumps of ganglion cells associated with the autonomic nerve supply of the tract, and in some areas contains lymphoid aggregates and follicles, which are part of the gut-associated lymphoid tissue (GALT) (see below).

The smooth muscle in the bowel wall is arranged in distinct layers which are each oriented in different directions

The musculature of the alimentary tract is responsible for moving the luminal contents gradually along the tract from mouth to anus. It therefore extends beyond the digestive part of the tract into the transport passages (i.e. the oropharynx, oesophagus and the anal canal). Movement is achieved by peristalsis, whereby a wave of contraction moves distally, forcing the luminal contents onward into the relaxed segment ahead.

There are two layers of smooth muscle throughout most of the digestive tract and a third layer in the stomach (see below). Traditionally identified as an outer longitudinal layer and an inner circular layer, they are in fact arranged spirally, with the inner circular layer being a compact spiral and the outer longitudinal layer being a more elongated helix (i.e. a similar arrangement to that of the smooth muscle of the ureter; see Fig. 15.34).

Between the two main smooth muscle layers of the digestive tract are small blood and lymphatic vessels, together with the nerves and ganglion cells of the autonomic nervous system.

The basic pattern of two muscle layers that extend into the transport passages of the alimentary tract, proximally into the oesophagus and distally into the anal canal, is modified by the presence of some skeletal muscle.

Localized thickenings of muscle in the bowel wall act as valves and are called sphincters

In some areas, the basic muscle pattern is also modified by a localized increase in the circular muscle to act as a sphincter. Sphincter contraction occludes the lumen and thus prevents the passage of the luminal contents.

The pyloric sphincter is the most important sphincter and is located at the junction between the stomach and duodenum. By contracting, it delays stomach emptying, thereby permitting continued food breakdown in the stomach.

The oesophagogastric sphincter is located between the lower oesophagus and proximal stomach; it normally prevents reflux of gastric contents into the oesophagus.

The ileocaecal valve is situated between the terminal ileum and caecum; it delays the discharge of ileal contents into the caecum.

The internal anal sphincter, sited at the upper end of the anal canal, retains faecal waste material in the rectum until controlled defecation is possible.

The outer coat of the bowel wall is called the adventitia, being covered in some parts by peritoneum

The adventitia is the outer coat of the digestive tract and surrounds the external layer of muscle. It is composed of loosely arranged fibroblasts and collagen embedded in matrix, with variable numbers of adipocytes.

The adventitia contains large blood and lymphatic vessels and nerves, the major arterial supply and venous drainage of the tract wall passing through it.

Some of the digestive tract is retroperitoneal but most is within the peritoneal cavity, and here the outer surface of the adventitia over much of its circumference is covered by a layer of flattened epithelium, the mesothelium (visceral peritoneum). This is identical to and continuous with the mesothelium lining the peritoneal cavity internally and covering the mesenteric attachment of the alimentary tract to the posterior abdominal wall (parietal peritoneum).

Adventitia covered by mesothelium (i.e. adventitia of the stomach, most of the small intestine and the large intestine) is commonly called the **serosa**. Where adventitia is not covered by a mesothelium (i.e. adventitia of part of the duodenum and some of the colon), it merges with adjacent tissues.

Immunological defence against antigens ingested in the digestive tract is provided by the gut-associated lymphoid tissue (GALT)

Throughout the digestive tract, the lamina propria contains cells of the immune system (see Chapter 8), including lymphocytes, plasma cells and macrophages. In addition to these cells, there are individual intraepithelial lymphocytes (see Fig. 11.26).

The lymphoid cells are commonly arranged as large follicles, often with germinal centres, and are partly located in the mucosa and partly in submucosa, thus splitting the muscularis mucosae. In the ileum, the follicles aggregate to form substantial nodules called 'Peyer's patches' (see p. 140).

Although lymphoid follicles and Peyer's patches contain both B and T lymphocytes, the diffuse, nonfollicular infiltrate in the lamina propria is composed largely of T lymphocytes.

The mucosal epithelial cells that overlie the lymphoid follicles and Peyer's patches differ from the usual epithelial cells in both structure and function, and are called 'M cells' (Fig. 11.26). They are cuboidal or flat rather than tall columnar, and have luminal microfolds rather than tall microvilli.

M cells are believed to take up antigenic macromolecules from the intestinal lumen, incorporating them into endocytotic vesicles and then transporting them to the lateral intercellular space in the region of an intraepithelial lymphocyte.

The gut has both intrinsic and extrinsic innervation

The intrinsic innervation is collections of nerves and ganglion cells in the submucosa, which form an interconnected network called the 'submucosal (Meissner's) plexus' (Fig. 11.27a), whereas collections of nerves and ganglion cells between the inner circular and outer longitudinal components of the muscularis proper form a network called the 'myenteric (Auerbach's) plexus' (Fig. 11.27b).

The extrinsic system comprises an autonomic input from parasympathetic (stimulatory) and sympathetic (inhibitory) abdominal plexuses that modulates the activity of the intrinsic innervation of the gut. In addition, sensory nerves derived from neurons in cranial and spinal nuclei terminate in the bowel as tendril-like sensory endings.

The afferent autonomic impulses mediate visceral reflexes and sensations such as hunger and rectal fullness.

The viscera are insensitive to pain, any painful sensations resulting from excessive contraction or distension of the bowel muscle, or from the sensory nerves in the peritoneum.

Stomach

From the oesophagus, food enters the stomach, which is a dilated portion of the digestive tract where fragmented food is retained, while it is macerated and partially digested. At the lower end of the stomach the pyloric sphincter (see Fig. 11.33) prevents the passage of food until it is converted into a thick semiliquid paste or pulp (chyme).

There are three layers of muscle in the stomach wall

The muscular wall of the stomach differs from the standard digestive tract pattern by the presence of a third layer of oblique muscle fibres. These lie internal to the circular layer and assist in the complex churning action necessary to mix food thoroughly with the secretions of the gastric mucosa.

The stomach muscle layers are thick. When contracted, they decrease the stomach capacity and the mucosa is thrown up into longitudinal folds called 'rugae', which are most prominent on the convexity of the stomach (the greater curvature). This is the state of the stomach when it is empty; when it is full, the musculature relaxes and thins and the rugae stretch flat as the stomach distends.

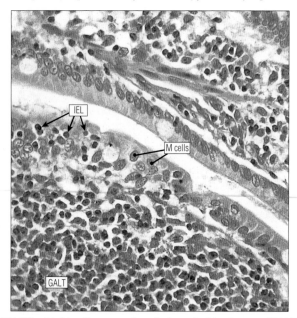

FIGURE 11.26 **Gut-associated lymphoid tissue (GALT).** Micrograph showing the typical arrangement of a nodule of gut-associated lymphoid tissue (GALT) in the lamina propria. The epithelial cells (M cells), closely associated with the lymphoid aggregate, are cuboidal and show no cytoplasmic specialization such as mucin droplet formation. Note the intraepithelial lymphocytes (IEL).

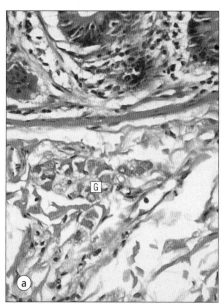
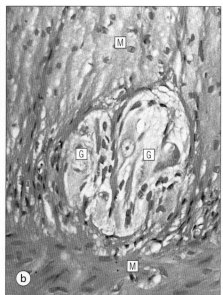

FIGURE 11.27 **Intrinsic innervation.** (a) High-power micrograph showing a cluster of ganglion cells (G) in the small bowel submucosa (Meissner's plexus). (b) High-power micrograph showing clusters of ganglion cells (G) between the two muscle layers (M) of the muscularis proper (myenteric or Auerbach's plexus).

The stomach is ideally equipped for its role as a reservoir by its distensibility, the presence of the pyloric sphincter and the mechanisms preventing reflux at its upper end.

The gastric epithelium secretes hydrochloric acid, digestive enzymes and mucus. It also contains a population of hormone-secreting cells

Food is converted into chyme by the secretions of the gastric mucosa into the lumen.

These are:
- A dilute solution of hydrochloric acid (approximately 0.16 N)
- Solutions of proteolytic enzymes, mainly pepsin
- Small amounts of other enzymes (e.g. rennin and gastric lipase)
- Mucins, mainly in the form of neutral mucins.

The major functions of the gastric epithelium are the secretion of acid and digestive enzymes. It also secretes mucus to lubricate ingested food and to protect itself from the corrosive effects of the acid and enzymes. The surface area of the stomach epithelium is increased by downgrowths that form glands.

The secretions are produced by three main cell types. In addition, there is a population of endocrine cells and a population of stem cells from which the other cell types are derived. The cell types are:
- Mucous cells
- Acid-producing cells (oxyntic or parietal cells)
- Enzyme-producing cells (chief cells or peptic cells)
- Stem cells
- Enteroendocrine cells.

Gastric mucous cells are of two types: surface mucous cells and neck mucous cells

Surface mucous cells (Fig. 11.28) are tall and columnar with basal nuclei and clear-staining luminal cytoplasm distended by numerous small mucin vacuoles, which are discharged into the stomach lumen by exocytosis. The cells also have prominent endoplasmic reticulum, and the Golgi complex is located above the nucleus.

The luminal surface of surface mucous cells shows scanty short microvilli with a surface glycocalyx, and junctional complexes join adjacent cells near the luminal surface.

The lateral borders of the cells are often separated by a considerable intercellular gap, which is traversed by cytoplasmic protrusions of the lateral walls; this separation disappears as the apical surface is neared, where the binding of adjacent cells is very tight. Surface mucous cells are also thought to produce blood group substances.

Neck mucous cells are smaller and less regular in shape than surface mucous cells, mainly because they are compressed and distorted by adjacent cells. They have a basal nucleus and finely granular cytoplasm owing to the presence of small mucin vacuoles which are considerably smaller than those in the surface mucous cells.

The vacuoles are distributed throughout the cytoplasm and are not aggregated near the luminal surface as

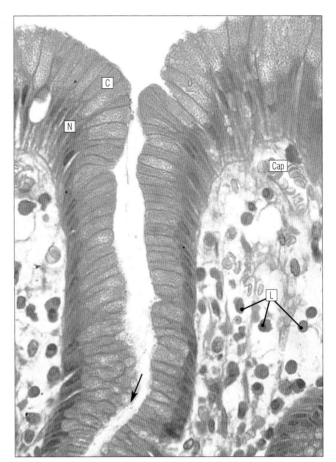

FIGURE 11.28 **Gastric mucous cells.** In this high-power micrograph, the gastric surface mucous cells have basal nuclei (N) and bulky luminal cytoplasm (C) filled with pale-staining mucus. As the neck region is approached (arrow), the cells (neck mucous cells) are smaller and contain less mucus. Note the prominent capillaries (Cap) and lymphoid cells (L) in the lamina propria.

they are in the surface mucous cells. By light microscopy it is not always apparent that neck mucous cells contain mucin, and a PAS stain is often necessary to highlight it.

The acid-producing cells of the stomach are called parietal cells

The acid-producing cells are large pyramidal cells with central nuclei and pale eosinophilic cytoplasm. The cytoplasm often appears vacuolated, particularly around the nucleus. The cell attachment to the basement membrane is broad, but their luminal aspect is narrow, being compressed between adjacent cells. Despite this, these cells have a vast luminal surface area as a result of deep microvilli-lined invaginations producing so-called 'canaliculi' (Fig. 11.29).

In the cytoplasm close to the canaliculi are clusters of round or oval vesicles that have clear centres and distinct membrane borders and which are thought to be involved in the transfer of substances from the cytoplasm to the lumen of the canalicular system. The rest of the cytoplasm is packed with round or oval mitochondria with closely packed cristae. This high concentration of

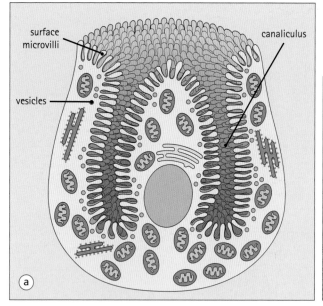

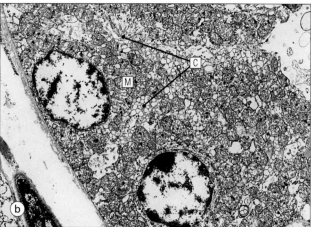

FIGURE 11.29 **Acid-producing cells.** (a) The acid-producing cell has an intricate system of invaginations (canaliculi) lined by microvilli, which produce the perinuclear vacuolated appearance seen on light microscopy. The rest of the cytoplasm is packed with mitochondria, particularly at the cell periphery. A small Golgi and some rough endoplasmic reticulum are also present, with vesicles close to the canaliculi. (b) Electron micrograph showing the intricate canalicular system (C) of an acid-producing cell; the cytoplasm is largely occupied by tightly packed mitochondria (M).

mitochondria is responsible for the eosinophilia of the cell cytoplasm, particularly at the periphery. A small Golgi and some rough endoplasmic reticulum are also present.

Parietal cells also produce intrinsic factor, the glycoprotein that avidly binds to vitamin B_{12} to render it absorbable by the digestive tract.

Chief cells secrete the enzyme pepsin

The enzyme-producing cells of the stomach are also known as chief or peptic cells. They have large basal nuclei and contain eosinophilic refractile cytoplasmic granules and a rich rough endoplasmic reticulum (Figs 11.30, 11.31); they therefore resemble the exocrine cells of the pancreas (see p. 215).

ADVANCED CONCEPT
ACID-PRODUCING CELLS

The acid-producing cells have abundant carbonic anhydrase, which is thought to play a vital role in generating H^+ ions for the production of hydrochloric acid (HCl).

Carbon dioxide (CO_2) diffuses across the basement membrane from blood capillaries into the cell, where it links with water molecules (a reaction catalysed by carbonic anhydrase) to produce carbonic acid (H_2CO_3); this instantly dissociates into an H^+ ion and an HCO_3^- ion. The latter passes back into the blood, whereas the H^+ is pumped into the lumen of a canaliculus. Chloride ions (Cl^-) are actively transported across the cell into the canaliculus from the capillaries in the lamina propria.

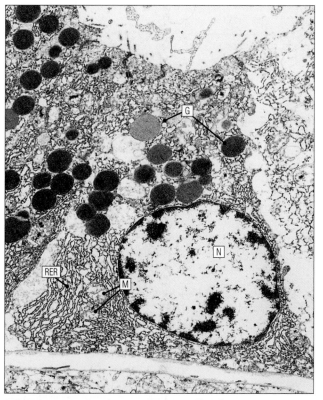

FIGURE 11.30 **Enzyme-producing cells.** Electron micrograph of an enzyme-producing cell showing its large basal nucleus (N), abundant mitochondria (M), abundant rough endoplasmic reticulum (RER), and the grey-staining spherical granules (G), which contain pepsinogen and are responsible for the eosinophilic granular appearance of these cells in H&E-stained sections (see also Fig. 11.31).

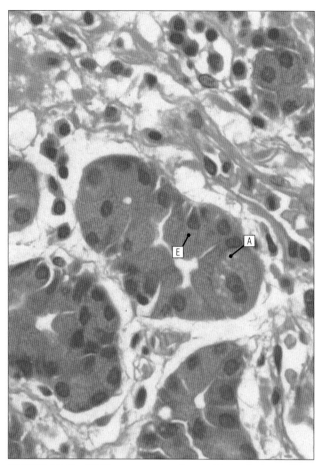

FIGURE 11.31 **H&E appearance of an acid-producing cell (A) from the body of the stomach.** Note the enzyme-producing cells (E).

The granules contain the inactive enzyme precursor pepsinogen, which is disgorged into the gastric lumen, where it is converted by gastric acid into the active proteolytic enzyme pepsin.

Pepsin is a potent enzyme, breaking down large protein molecules into small peptides and converting almost all of the structural proteins into soluble small molecular weight substances; it is largely responsible for the conversion of solid food particles to fluid chyme.

Endocrine cells in the gastric mucosa secrete a variety of hormones

Enteroendocrine cells (see Chapter 14) of the stomach are small and round and are situated on the epithelial basement membrane. In H&E paraffin sections, they have a round, central dark-staining nucleus and a rim of clear cytoplasm (Fig. 11.32a).

Ultrastructurally the cytoplasm contains membrane-bound neurosecretory granules, the shape, size, number and electron density varying according to the substance secreted.

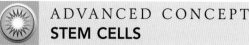

ADVANCED CONCEPT
STEM CELLS

The epithelial cells of the gastric mucosa are formed from stem cells. Stem cells are the precursor cells of all epithelial cells of the gastric mucosa. They are small cells with oval basal nuclei and show no cytoplasmic specialization when completely undifferentiated, but are capable of differentiating into mucous, acid-producing, enzyme-producing or endocrine cells.

Normally present in very small numbers in humans, they increase in number and activity when the gastric epithelium is continually damaged, for example in chronic irritation of the gastric mucosa (i.e. chronic gastritis). A surge of stem cell activity enables an ulcerated area of the stomach to be rapidly re-epithelialized. Such regeneration is an important final step in the healing of a stomach ulcer.

Immunocytochemical methods demonstrate that:
- Endocrine cells storing and secreting serotonin, somatostatin (Fig. 11.32b) and a vasointestinal polypeptide-like (VIP) substance are present in the cardiac, body and antral regions
- Cells secreting gastrin and a bombesin-like peptide are concentrated in the pyloric mucosa, where gastrin-secreting cells are concentrated mainly in the neck region, with rare scattered cells in the depths of the glands.

The gastric mucosa can be divided into three histological zones: a superficial zone, a neck zone and a deep zone

There are three zonal divisions of the gastric mucosa. The superficial zone is composed of a layer of surface mucous cells with downgrowths which are variously called 'foveolae', pits or crypts.

The mucous cells lining the pits are not as tall and columnar as those on the surface; they also contain less mucin.

The superficial zone is roughly constant in its content and structure throughout the stomach.

The neck zone between the superficial and deep zones is narrow and composed largely of immature stem cells mixed with some neck mucous cells. The immature stem cells proliferate and migrate upwards to replenish the predominantly mucous cells of the superficial zone, and downwards to replenish the cell types in the glands of the deep zone.

The deep zone is composed of glands, the bases of which lie close to or in the muscularis mucosae, whereas the upper ends open into the bases of the superficial zone pits.

The structure of the deep zone varies, there being three main histological patterns that delineate three main areas of the stomach: the cardia, the body and the pylorus (Figs 11.33, 11.34).

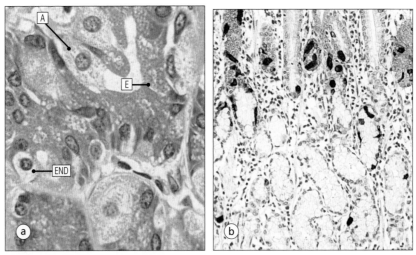

FIGURE 11.32 **Gastric endocrine cells.** (a) Micrograph of the base of glands in the body of the stomach showing the H&E appearance of gastric enteroendocrine cells (END). They are small with pale cytoplasm and a small, dark-staining central nucleus. Acid-producing (A) and enzyme-producing (E) cells are also evident. (b) Micrograph of an immunoperoxidase-stained section of stomach showing the distribution of somatostatin-secreting endocrine cells in the pyloric gastric mucosa. The cells are numerous in the neck region, with a few scattered cells in the deep glands.

 KEY FACTS
STOMACH

- There are three layers of smooth muscle in the wall
- Mucosa is divided into cardia, body and pyloric regions
- Parietal cells are specialized to produce acid and also secrete intrinsic factor
- Chief cells secrete the enzyme pepsin as an inactive precursor, pepsinogen
- Endocrine cells in the mucosa secrete gastrin, bombesin, somatostatin and VIP.

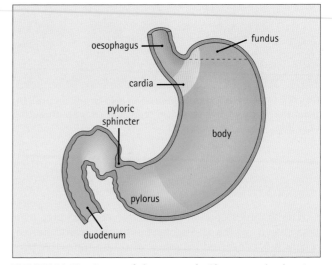

FIGURE 11.33 **Areas of the stomach.** The stomach, showing the three histologically distinguishable areas. The cardia extends from the squamous/columnar junction at the lower end of the oesophagus for a variable distance into the upper stomach, usually 2–3 cm down the lesser curve; cardiac mucosa may also extend part-way into the fundus, which is an anatomic rather than a histological feature. Pyloric mucosa lines a roughly conical area in the lower third of the stomach, starting about halfway down the lesser curve. The area is very variable and tends to begin higher on the lesser curve in women. Body mucosa occupies the rest of the stomach, including most of the anatomical fundus. The transition between the various mucosal patterns is commonly gradual, with a narrow junctional zone showing features of both.

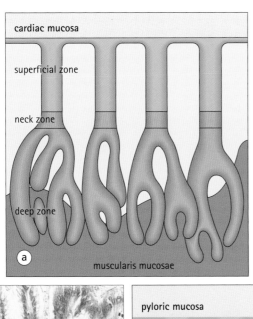

cardiac mucosa

superficial zone

neck zone

deep zone

muscularis mucosae

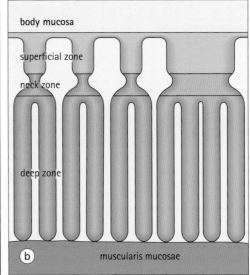

body mucosa

superficial zone

neck zone

deep zone

muscularis mucosae

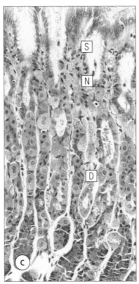

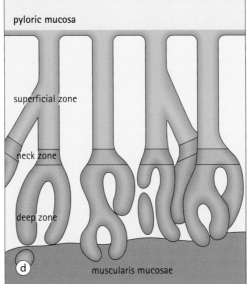

pyloric mucosa

superficial zone

neck zone

deep zone

muscularis mucosae

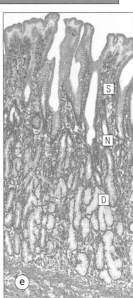

FIGURE 11.34 **Gastric mucosa.** (a) Cardiac mucosa. The superficial and deep zones of the cardiac mucosa are about equal in thickness. The surface and crypt epithelium is composed of mucous cells, and the deep zone is composed of tubular and branched glands lined by mucous cells, with scattered endocrine and acid-producing cells becoming more numerous near the junction with the body mucosa. Some of the more complex glands are coiled. The muscularis mucosae is thick and irregular, and often sends bundles of fibres towards the surface, interdigitating with the glands. The histological appearance of cardiac mucosa is shown in Figures 11.22b and 11.49. (b) Body mucosa. The superficial zone of the body mucosa accounts for only 25% or less of the mucosal thickness. Most pits open directly and singly on to the surface, but some fuse before opening, to form a wider crevice. The deep zone is composed of tightly packed long straight tubular glands that end blindly at the muscularis mucosae. At their upper ends the glands open into the bases of the crypts through a variably constricted neck region. The glands may open into single or larger fused crypts. The superficial zone is covered by surface mucous cells, with neck mucous cells covering the deeper parts of the pits. At the neck region, neck mucosa cells are mixed with stem cells. The glands are composed of acid-producing cells, enzyme-producing cells, neck mucous cells and scattered endocrine cells. (c) Body mucosa. H&E section of body mucosa showing the superficial zone (S) composed of mucus-secreting cells, a narrow neck zone (N) containing mainly stem cells and neck mucous cells, and the deep zone (D), largely composed of acid-producing and enzyme-producing cells. (d) Pyloric mucosa. The superficial zone of the pyloric region occupies slightly more than 50% of the mucosal thickness, and the crypts are often branched. The deep zone is composed of tortuous single or branched glands extending down to the muscularis mucosae. The cell content of the superficial and neck zones is the same as in the cardiac and body mucosa. The glands are lined by mucous cells, but scattered acid-producing cells and numerous endocrine cells are also present. Acid-producing cells become more numerous close to the pyloric sphincter. (e) Pyloric mucosa. H&E section of pyloric mucosa showing the superficial zone (S) occupying about 50% of the mucosal thickness. The narrow neck (N) and substantial deep (D) zones are composed of mucous cells, which form branching glands in the deep zone.

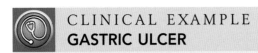

CLINICAL EXAMPLE
GASTRIC ULCER

The stomach normally contains an acid solution, but is protected from the damaging effects of the acid by various mechanisms, including the presence of a thin layer of mucus over the surface of the epithelial cells.

In some circumstances, particularly in association with *Helicobacter pylori* infection, these protective mechanisms break down and the acidic gastric contents damage the mucosa. The resulting death of epithelial cells and lamina propria leads to the formation of a shallow ulcer. Continued exposure of such an unprotected area leads to the formation of a deep ulcer (chronic gastric ulcer), which can extend through the submucosa and the muscle layers (Fig. 11.35) and takes a long time to heal.

If an ulcer penetrates the full thickness of the stomach wall, the wall may perforate and the gastric contents can then pour into the peritoneal cavity, causing peritonitis and often death.

Treatment of gastric ulcer is based on removing or decreasing the levels of gastric acid either by neutralizing them (e.g. with oral alkalis) or by decreasing the amount of gastric acid produced by blocking its secretion by the acid-producing cells (e.g. using H_2 antagonists and proton pump inhibition).

Because gastric acid also enters the first part of the duodenum, this area may also be subject to ulceration (duodenal ulcer), as may the lower oesophagus if reflux of gastric acid occurs (see Fig. 11.23).

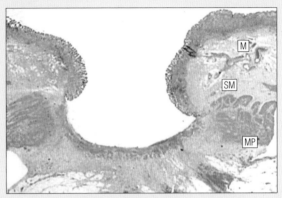

FIGURE 11.35 **Chronic gastric ulcer.** Micrograph of an H&E section through a chronic gastric ulcer, which has extended through the mucosa (M), submucosa (SM) and muscularis propria (MP).

Small Intestine

Introduction

When the pyloric sphincter opens, partially digested food (chyme) empties from the stomach into the small intestine, which is the main site for the absorption of amino acids, sugars, fats, and some larger molecules produced by digestion. The small intestine also secretes enzymes to complete the digestive processes begun in the stomach. It begins at the pylorus, the distal limit of the stomach, and ends at the ileocaecal valve, the proximal limit of the large intestine. At autopsy, when the longitudinal muscle is relaxed, the small intestine usually measures about 6 m, but in life it measures only about 3 m long. It is divided into three sections (duodenum, jejunum and ileum), although the transitions from one to the other are not precise.

The duodenum is the proximal 20–25 cm of small intestine and is entirely retroperitoneal. It has the shape of a letter C, with the head of the pancreas fitting into its concave edge. The bile and pancreatic ducts open into the duodenum in this concavity.

The jejunum begins where the duodenum emerges from behind the peritoneum and extends to an ill-defined junction with the ileum.

The ileum extends from the jejunum to the ileocaecal valve.

The small bowel has several modifications to increase its surface area

As the major absorptive site, the small intestine shows architectural modifications to its mucosa and submucosa to increase its surface area.

The mucosa and submucosa are thrown up into a large number of folds or plicae arranged circularly around the lumen. These are most prominent in the jejunum (Fig. 11.36a) and are absent from the distal end of the small intestine.

The surface of the plicae is further arranged into villi, which protrude into the intestinal lumen (Figs 11.36b,c; 11.37). Tubular glands or crypts extend down from the base of the villi to the muscularis mucosae. The small intestine has the standard arrangement of musculature (i.e. an external layer of longitudinal muscle and an inner circular layer) and a substantial submucosa in which GALT (see p. 203) is particularly prominent.

CLINICAL EXAMPLE
GLUTEN ENTEROPATHY (COELIAC DISEASE)

The absorptive function of the jejunum depends on the integrity of the villi. If enough villi are damaged, food material cannot be absorbed, leading to weight loss, diarrhoea, etc.

One important cause of extensive loss of villi is coeliac disease, due to allergy to the wheat protein, gluten. The resulting immune-mediated inflammation leads to flattening of the jejunal surface with extensive loss of villi (Fig. 11.38).

Gluten enteropathy commonly presents in babies and young children, with failure to thrive and to gain normal height and weight for their age.

(Continued on next page)

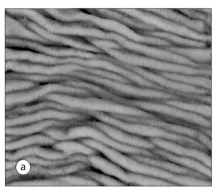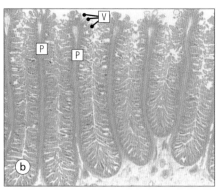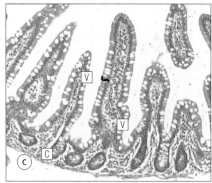

FIGURE 11.36 **Small intestine – general architecture.** (a) Macroscopic view of small intestinal mucosal surface showing tightly packed circumferential mucosal folds or plicae. (b) Low-power micrograph of the plicae (P) showing their complex mucosal surface, which is composed of large villi (V). (c) Micrograph showing the villi (V) protruding into the small intestinal lumen; note the crypts (C) between their bases.

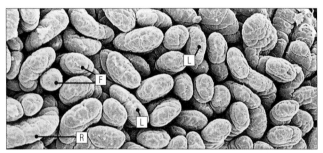

FIGURE 11.37 In two dimensions, the villi appear to have the same structure, but in three dimensions their structure can be seen to correspond to one of three main patterns: they are either finger-like (F), leaf-like (L) or ridge-like (R), as shown in this scanning electron micrograph. There are also occasional intermediate forms. The proportions of these patterns vary from site to site and also with age. In babies and young children, the villi of the duodenum and proximal jejunum are almost entirely leaf or ridge-like, finger-like villi appearing with age. The adult pattern is present by 10–15 years.

> The villi usually assume their normal structure when wheat and its products are excluded from the diet (i.e. a gluten-free diet), and the malabsorptive state subsequently improves.

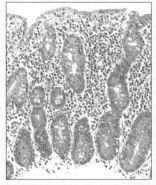

FIGURE 11.38 **Gluten enteropathy (coeliac disease).** Micrograph of villous damage resulting from gluten sensitivity. The jejunal mucosal surface is flattened owing to extensive loss of villi. Compare with Figure 11.36c.

There are three functional zones of small intestinal epithelium

The small intestinal epithelium can be divided into three functional zones. These are the villi, the crypts and the neck zone, where villi and crypts merge. (The features of the villi are discussed with Figure 11.39, and crypt structure is illustrated in Figures 11.40 and 11.41.)

The cells of the epithelium are enterocytes, mucous cells, Paneth cells, endocrine cells and stem cells, and their numbers and distribution vary in the different zones of the epithelium.

Enterocytes are the main cell in the villi and are absorptive in function

Enterocytes are tall columnar cells with round or oval nuclei in the lower third of the cell.

The luminal surface of enterocytes is highly specialized; each cell bears 2000–3000 tightly packed, tall microvilli, which are coated by a glycoprotein, the glycocalyx (see Fig. 11.39c). This is composed of fine filamentous extensions of the microvillus cell membrane.

The glycocalyx contains a number of enzymes (brush border enzymes, e.g. lactase, sucrase, peptidases, lipases and alkaline phosphatase), which are important in digestion and transport (see Fig. 11.39e).

Beneath the microvillus surface, the enterocyte cytoplasm contains lysosomes and smooth endoplasmic reticulum and paired centrioles in the terminal web region (see Fig. 3.15). Nearer the nucleus, the cell is rich in rough endoplasmic reticulum and mitochondria and there is a prominent Golgi. Between the nucleus and the basement membrane are mitochondria and many ribosomes and polyribosomes. The lateral walls of enterocytes show complex interdigitations, and are the sites of Na^+ and K^+ ATPase activity. The lateral walls are separated from the microvillus surface by desmosomes and tight junctions (see Fig. 3.7).

The ultrastructural features of the enterocyte are linked to its absorptive function, and therefore many of the features and mechanisms are common to other active absorptive cells, such as those of the proximal

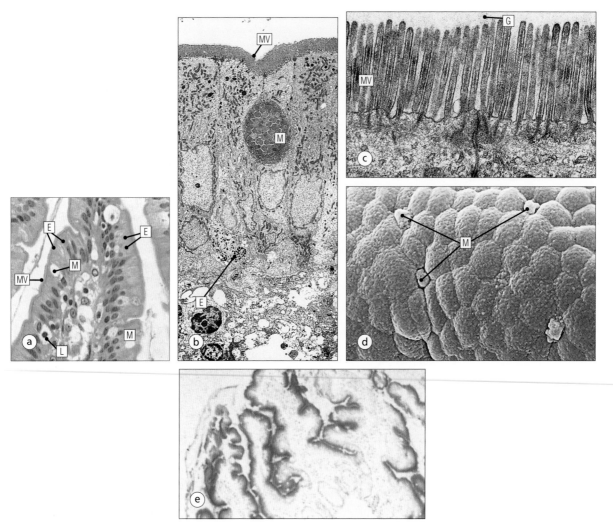

FIGURE 11.39 **Small intestine villus.** (a) Thin acrylic resin stained with H&E, showing a single villus, which is covered by tall enterocytes (E) bearing a prominent microvillus brush border (MV). Scattered among the enterocytes are occasional mucous cells (M) and intraepithelial lymphocytes (L). The stromal core contains small capillaries and lymphatics (not shown) and a number of lymphocytes, plasma cells and macrophages. (b) Electron micrograph of a row of enterocytes. Note the microvillus border (MV), part of a mucous cell (M) and the endocrine cell with basal granules (E). (c) Electron micrograph of microvillus brush border (MV) at high magnification. The glycocalyx (G) can be seen as a faint greyish haze on the surface of the microvilli. (d) Scanning electron micrograph of part of the villus surface. Note the tightly packed enterocytes, the microvilli of which are partly obscured by the layer of glycocalyx. Mucous cells discharging their mucus (M) are clearly seen. (e) Histochemical preparation of small intestine showing the distribution of the enzyme lactase (blue staining), which is localized to the luminal surface of the enterocytes. Like many other cell-bound enzymes responsible for food breakdown in the small intestine, the enzyme molecules reside in the glycocalyx.

convoluted tubule cell of the kidney. These absorptive mechanisms are illustrated and discussed in Chapter 15.

Mucous (goblet) cells are mainly found in the upper two-thirds of the crypts

Occasional mucous cells are scattered among the enterocytes of the villi (see Figs 11.39a,b).

Mucous cells contain globules of mucin in their luminal cytoplasm, the mucin being discharged on to the surface when the cytoplasm is fully expanded by mucin granules. The scanty basal cytoplasm is rich in rough endoplasmic reticulum.

Mucous cells are least frequent in the duodenum, and increase in number in the jejunum and ileum, being most numerous in the terminal ileum close to the caecum.

Paneth cells are found in the lower third of the crypts

Paneth cells have basal nuclei and prominent large eosinophilic granules in their luminal cytoplasm (Fig. 11.40). Ultrastructurally, these granules are spherical and electron dense, the remaining cytoplasm being rich in rough endoplasmic reticulum; these are features of a protein-secreting cell (see Fig. 3.20).

Paneth cells contain substances called 'defensins', which are secreted and protect against infection.

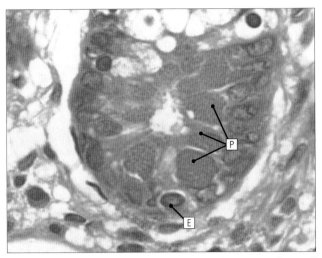

FIGURE 11.40 **Paneth cells.** Micrograph of the base of a small intestinal crypt from a paraffin section showing numerous Paneth cells (P) containing large numbers of bright red granules. A small endocrine cell (E) with ill-defined fine basal eosinophilic granules can also be seen.

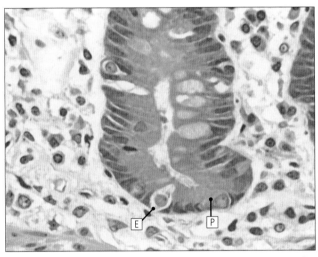

FIGURE 11.41 **Endocrine cell.** Micrograph of the base of a small intestinal crypt showing a typical pale-staining enteroendocrine cell (E). In this thin acrylic resin section, the Paneth cell (P) granules are difficult to see.

Endocrine cells are located mainly in the lower third of the crypts, but are also seen higher up in the villi

Endocrine cells in the small bowel resemble those seen in the stomach (see Fig. 11.32), being roughly triangular in shape, the broad base being in contact with the basement membrane, the narrow apex reaching the lumen. Their nuclei are spherical and their cytoplasm pale staining (Fig. 11.41).

Ultrastructurally, the cytoplasm contains neuroendocrine granules, and the luminal surface bears microvilli.

Small intestinal endocrine cells secrete a number of hormones and peptides, including serotonin (5HT), enteroglucagon, somatostatin, secretin, gastrin, motilin and vasoactive intestinal peptide (VIP).

Stem cells are found in the lower third of the crypts

The replication of stem cells replenishes the stock of the other cells, including the Paneth and endocrine cells. Most replication is to replace the mucous cells and enterocytes of the villi, as these cells have a rapid turnover, being shed from the tips of the villi about 5 days after production.

Before developing into the mature form of the two cell types, the stem cells differentiate into intermediate cells, which show some features of both mucous cells and enterocytes. This process appears to involve the Wnt signalling pathway. These cells occupy much of the upper two-thirds of the crypts.

Stem cells and intermediate cells are particularly numerous when there is increased cell loss from the villi, which is a common feature of many diseases affecting the small intestine; the crypts increase in length and show increased numbers of cells in mitosis (i.e. crypt or gland hyperplasia).

The lamina propria of the small intestine is most clearly seen in the core of the villi, but also surrounds and supports the gland crypts

The lamina propria of the small bowel is composed of collagen, reticulin fibres, fibroblasts and glycosaminoglycan matrix, through which run blood capillaries, lymphatics and nerves. It contains some smooth muscle fibres.

The blood vessels and lymphatics are particularly prominent in the villi, a central lymphatic (lacteal) running vertically down the centre of the core of each villus.

The lamina propria also contains lymphocytes, plasma cells, eosinophils, macrophages and mast cells.

The **lymphocytes** are largely T lymphocytes (approximately 70% T-helper and 30% T-suppressor; see Chapter 8); most of the **plasma cells** produce IgA. Lymphocytes are also present in the villous epithelium, usually in a basal position between the lateral intercellular spaces and, like those in the lamina propria, they are also T lymphocytes, but the subset pattern is different, about 80% being T-suppressor, the rest being T-helper types.

Eosinophils are common in the lamina propria throughout the digestive tract.

Macrophages are found mainly beneath the basement membrane in the upper reaches of the villi. They are thought to engulf particulate antigens and to ingest soluble antigens before presenting them to T lymphocytes.

Mast cells are seen mainly in the crypt region.

The submucosa of the small bowel contains vessels, lymphoid tissue and nerves

The small intestinal submucosa contains lymphatics, blood vessels and the submucosal plexus of nerves and ganglion cells. In addition, it contains part of the larger lymphoid aggregates of the GALT, which cross the muscularis mucosae.

In the first part of the duodenum, the submucosa contains mucus-secreting Brunner's glands.

KEY FACTS
SMALL BOWEL

- Characterized by a mucosa raised into finger-like villi which contain abundant blood vessels and lymphatics
- Lined by columnar epithelium with goblet cells
- Glycocalyx of surface epithelium has enzymes, e.g. lactase and alkaline phosphatase
- Duodenum is associated with submucosal mucous glands (Brunner's glands)
- Contains mucosal endocrine cells which secrete gut hormones
- Has two layers of muscularis propria separated by a myenteric nerve plexus.

The small intestine has regional specializations in duodenum, jejunum and ileum

The duodenum differs from the rest of the small intestine as follows:

- It is entirely retroperitoneal
- Its villous pattern contains a high proportion of leaf and ridge forms (see Fig. 11.37)
- It contains prominent mucus-secreting submucosal glands (Brunner's glands, Fig. 11.42), which penetrate and split the muscularis mucosae so that some acini are located within the lamina propria of the mucosa
- It receives secretions of glands located outside the digestive tract through long ducts; these glands are

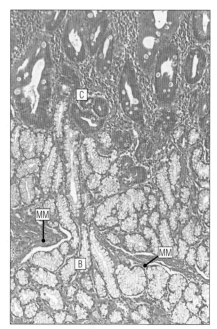

FIGURE 11.42 **Brunner's glands.** The first part of the duodenum is characterized by the presence of large, fluid-secreting mucous glands called 'Brunner's glands' (B), which empty into the neck of the crypts (C). The Brunner's glands are partly located in the lower mucosa, but pass through the muscularis mucosae (MM) into the submucosa.

the liver (see Chapter 12) and the exocrine component of the pancreas.

Brunner's glands are similar to the submucosal glands of the pyloric region of the stomach, being composed of mucous cells lining short ducts that open into the bases or sides of the crypts of the mucosa. Brunner's glands secrete an alkaline mucoid material (pH 8.0–9.5), which may protect the duodenal mucosa from the acid chyme, bringing its pH towards the level at which the pancreatic enzymes are most effective.

Brunner's glands are also thought to secrete urogastrone, a peptide that inhibits acid secretion by the stomach. Endocrine cells can be demonstrated in these glands immunocytochemically.

The **jejunum** is the main absorptive site of the digestive tract and shows not only the greatest development of plical folds (see Fig. 11.36a), but also the most complex villous system, with finger-like villi being predominant.

The **ileum** is characterized by the greatest development of GALT. The lymphoid cells aggregate into large nodules (Peyer's patches), which expand the lamina propria of the mucosa, split the muscularis mucosae and extend into the submucosa.

Exocrine Pancreas

The exocrine pancreas is a glandular organ which secretes into the gut via a main duct system

The pancreas is a long, thin tapering structure extending from its head, which occupies the space formed by the concavity of the duodenum, to its tail, which is situated in the left hypochondrium near the hilum of the spleen.

The main pancreatic duct joins the distal end of the bile duct to open into the lumen of the duodenum at a small raised mound, the **ampulla of Vater**.

The pancreas has a thin, ill-defined fibrocollagenous capsule, from which narrow irregular septae penetrate it, dividing it into lobules. Each lobule is composed of roughly spherical clusters (acini) of secretory exocrine cells (Fig. 11.43). Each acinus has an individual intra-acinar duct, which drains into progressively larger ducts.

Pancreatic exocrine cells are protein-secreting cells

The acini are composed of protein-secreting cells (pancreatic acinar cells), which have a broad base and narrow apical surface, covered by a few short microvilli.

The cells are rich in rough endoplasmic reticulum, which is concentrated mainly in the lower half of the cell, and is responsible for their cytoplasmic basophilia. The upper half of the cell, close to the lumen, contains variable numbers of eosinophilic zymogen granules, which contain the pre-enzymes synthesized by the cell (see Fig. 11.43a). Some cells contain large numbers of these granules, whereas others, which contain few or none, are thought to have recently disgorged their

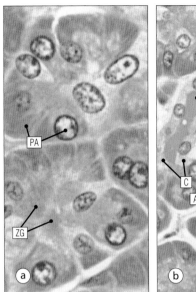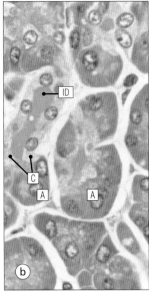

FIGURE 11.43 **Exocrine pancreas.** (a) Acini with acinar cells (PA) and eosinophilic zymogen granules (ZG) close to the lumen. (b) Part of the ductal system with centroacinar cells (C) arising from the acini (A) as the intra-acinar component of the intercalated duct (ID).

granules by exocytosis into the acinar lumen. It is thought that the pre-enzymes are synthesized by the rough endoplasmic reticulum and then transferred to the Golgi, which packages them into granules.

The pancreatic acinar cells produce and secrete the precursors of a wide range of enzymes

The secretions of pancreatic exocrine cells are involved in the breakdown of food in the lumen of the duodenum, and include proteolytic enzymes (particularly trypsinogen, chymotrypsinogen, procarboxypeptidases A and B and proelastase) and lipolytic enzymes (pro-phospholipase and pro-lipase). The pancreas also secretes amylase, cholesterol esterase and ribonucleases.

Activation of the proenzymes occurs only in the duodenal cavity, with the conversion of trypsinogen to active trypsin by an enterokinase located in the duodenal brush border triggering a cascade of reactions, in which the inactive precursors are converted to active enzymes.

Pancreatic secretion is alkaline owing to the selective secretion of bicarbonate ions, which is thought to be performed by the ductal system rather than by the acinar cells.

The control of pancreatic secretions is mainly mediated through hormones, the most important being secretin and cholecystokinin (pancreozymin).

Secretin stimulates the formation of the bicarbonate-rich fluid. Cholecystokinin is thought to stimulate the acinar cells to release their enzymes. Secretin and cholecystokinin are produced by the endocrine cells of the digestive tract mucosa, in response to the entry of acidic gastric contents into the duodenum.

Pancreatic secretions run in a ramified ductal system which merges into a main pancreatic duct

The pancreatic ductal system begins in the acinus. Pale-staining centroacinar cells represent the intra-acinar component of the intercalated duct, are lined by a simple monolayer of cuboidal epithelium and form a complex network (see Fig. 11.43b).

The intercalated ducts from individual acini fuse to form larger interlobular ducts, which run in the fibrocollagenous septa between the ill-defined pancreatic lobules and are lined by columnar epithelium.

Interlobular ducts join the main pancreatic ducts, which run longitudinally from the tail of the pancreas to its head and empty into the duodenal lumen at the ampulla of Vater. The main pancreatic ducts are lined by tall columnar epithelium containing a number of mucin-secreting goblet cells.

Large Intestine

The large intestine modifies the fluid content of faeces as it passes for elimination

The large intestine comprises the:
* Caecum
* Ascending, transverse and descending colons
* Sigmoid colon
* Rectum.

The structure of the large intestine is fairly constant throughout, although there are regional variations, particularly between the caecum and the rectum.

The main function of the large intestine is to convert the liquid small intestinal contents to solid indigestible waste material, faeces. This is achieved by extensive reabsorption of water and soluble salts from the bowel content, until it is semisolid. With increasing solidity, mucin is required to lubricate its passage along the bowel. The **appendix** is a small appendage arising from the caecum.

The large intestinal epithelium is specialized for mucus secretion, salt and water absorption

The epithelial component of the mucosa of the large bowel is a mixture of absorptive cells and mucous cells. These are arranged as simple, straight, non-branching tubular downgrowths extending from the surface to the muscularis mucosae. The cell types present are columnar cells, mucous cells, stem cells and endocrine cells (Fig. 11.44).

Other epithelial cells are found adjacent to the lymphoid aggregates in the lamina propria and are tightly packed cuboidal or columnar epithelial cells, which have relatively high nucleus to cytoplasm ratio and do not contain mucin. These cells are similar to the M cells associated with the lymphoid tissue in the small intestine.

Columnar cells are the most numerous type of epithelial cell in the large intestine. They are narrow slender cells and appear to be in a minority because they are

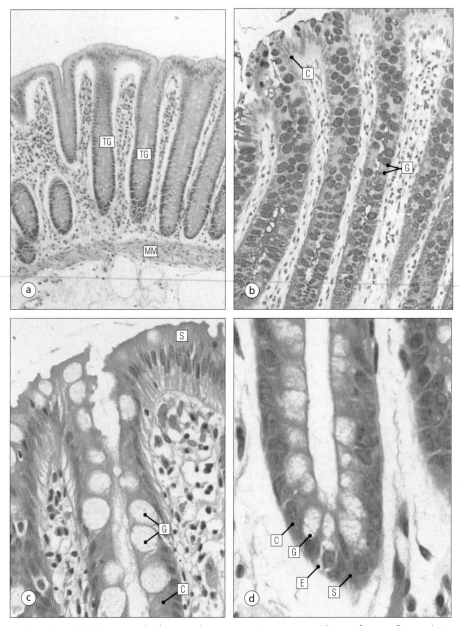

FIGURE 11.44 **Large intestine.** (a) Micrograph showing large intestine mucosa. The surface is flat and simple straight tubular glands (TG) extend down to the muscularis mucosae (MM). (b) The glands are lined by two populations of cells, the most numerous but less obvious being compressed tall columnar cells (C). The more easily seen cells are the mucous cells (mucus-secreting goblet cells, G), here stained blue by Alcian blue. (c) High-power micrograph showing both columnar cells (C) and goblet cells (G) in the upper part of the tubular gland, whereas the surface cells (S) are mainly columnar and contain little mucin. (d) At the bases of the glands, the cell population is a combination of uncommitted stem cells (S), goblet cells (G), columnar cells (C) and occasional small pale-staining endocrine cells (E).

compressed between the much larger mucous (goblet) cells. Their luminal surfaces have a microvillus brush border and there is evidence that they can produce and secrete a neutral polysaccharide, possibly glycocalyx material.

Columnar cells carry out the salt and water absorptive function of the colon. They lack brush border enzymes and so play no part in digestive breakdown, but have prominent lateral intercellular spaces, which suggests active fluid transport. Furthermore, they are well equipped with Na$^+$ and K$^+$ ATPases in the lateral cell membranes.

Mucous cells possess large numbers of mucin granules, which produce the bulging rounded cytoplasm responsible for their synonym, **goblet cells**. The mucin vacuoles are larger in the sigmoid colon and rectum than in the caecum and ascending colon, and there appears to be a difference in the type of mucin secreted. Mucin from the colon and rectum is highly sulfated; that from the caecum and ascending colon is less sulfated, and contains sialic acid radicals.

As the goblet cells approach the surface of the large intestine, they begin to discharge their mucus and continue to migrate upwards to form part of the surface epithelium, which is mainly composed of columnar cells.

Stem cells are the precursors of other cell types

Stem cells form all of the specialized cells of the large bowel mucosa. They are located at the bases of the tubular glands and can develop into either mucous or columnar cells or into large intestinal endocrine cells.

Although the main function of the stem cells is to maintain the cell populations of the colonic tubular glands during normal wear and tear and cell turnover, they are also vital in the rapid replacement of cells damaged by disease. When only the epithelial cells of the colonic tubular glands are destroyed, the stem cells restock them and the appearance of the glands is as before, i.e. straight tubular glands. When the damage is more severe and persistent, there is also destruction of the support cell and stromal architecture of the lamina propria supporting the glands; in this case, the stem cells produce new epithelial cells, but the glands so formed are architecturally distorted, often being short and branched instead of long, straight and a single tube. Also, the proportions of the various cell types in the regenerated glands may be abnormal, reduction in the number of mucin-secreting goblet cells being the most common. Histological identification of these changes in a colonic biopsy is an indication of an episode of severe mucosal damage in the past, for example in chronic ulcerative colitis (see p. 219).

Endocrine cells are comparatively few in number in the large bowel and are scattered among the other cells

In the large bowel, endocrine cells are mainly in the lower half of each tubular downgrowth and have a broad base, narrowing to a small luminal surface covered with microvilli. Their neuroendocrine granules are situated basal to the nucleus and can sometimes be seen as small eosinophilic dots in H&E paraffin sections.

Immunocytochemical methods have shown that these cells contain a number of substances related to their endocrine function, including chromogranin, substance P, somatostatin and glucagon.

The large intestinal lamina propria consists of collagen, reticulin and fibroblasts embedded in a glycosaminoglycan matrix

There is a layer of compact collagen immediately beneath the basement membrane of the surface epithelium.

The cell content of the lamina propria includes lymphocytes and scattered eosinophils, the lymphocytes being mainly T cells. Also present are small lymphoid follicles (part of the GALT, see p. 203), the larger of which breach the muscularis mucosae and extend into the submucosa. Cells containing PAS-positive granules, known as **muciphages**, are a common finding, particularly in the rectum.

The muscularis mucosae consists of a two-layered smooth muscle arrangement

The muscularis mucosae of the large bowel has an inner circular and an outer longitudinal layer, but this distinction is usually only clear in abnormally thickened muscle layers. Elastic fibres are also present.

The muscularis mucosae is penetrated by fine nerve twigs from the submucosal plexus, these nerves continuing vertically into the lamina propria. The innervation of the colon is particularly important in the diagnosis of Hirschsprung's disease (see Fig. 11.47).

The muscularis propria is responsible for the main propulsive forces in the bowel wall

The muscularis propria of the large intestine consists of an inner circular muscle layer and an outer longitudinal layer, which is not continuous, being concentrated into three bands, the **taeniae coli**. These muscle layers are responsible for propulsion of the gut contents by peristalsis.

 KEY FACTS
LARGE BOWEL

- Mucosa specialized for water and salt absorption and mucus secretion
- Mucosa characterized by long straight tubular glands of columnar epithelium containing goblet cells and absorptive cells
- Two layers to muscularis propria with intervening myenteric nerve plexus. Outer longitudinal muscle arranged as narrow bands (taeniae coli).

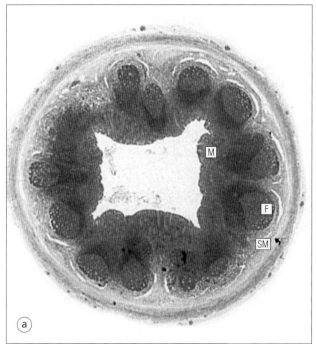
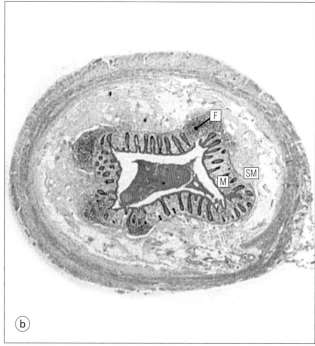

FIGURE 11.45 **Appendix.** (a) Transverse section of the appendix from a 10-year-old child. It is lined by large-bowel type mucosa (M), in which there are large lymphoid follicles (F) extending into the submucosa (SM). (b) Transverse section of appendix from a 36-year-old man at the same magnification as in (a). Note the relative reduction in size and the virtual disappearance of the lymphoid follicles (F). Mucosa (M); submucosa (SM).

Appendix

The appendix has the same basic structure as the large bowel

The appendix is a small, blind-ending tubular diverticulum arising from the caecum. It is normally 5–10 cm long and about 0.8 cm in diameter. Both measurements vary from person to person, but its diameter decreases with increasing age, being at its greatest at 7–20 years of age.

The wall of the appendix is composed of a muscularis propria, which has an outer longitudinal and an inner circular component like the rest of the digestive tract. The submucosa contains blood vessels, nerves and variable amounts of lymphoid tissue.

In children, the lamina propria and the submucosa contain abundant lymphoid tissue with prominent follicle formation (Fig. 11.45a). This is not present at birth, but progressively populates the appendix over the first 10 years of life, thereafter progressively disappearing, so that the normal adult appendix shows only traces of this tissue (Fig. 11.45b).

In children, this abundant lymphoid tissue can increase in bulk in response to a transient generalized viral infection or infection localized to the bowel. The lumen may become blocked off by inspissated feculent material, which can solidify excessively to become hard (a faecolith). This can obstruct the drainage of the distal part of the appendix, and the stasis of the secretions in the blocked-off distal end predisposes to bacterial infection. This is the basis of the common surgical emergency in children of acute appendicitis.

As the lymphoid tissue atrophies in the adult, the submucosa becomes progressively more collagenous, and in the elderly, the mucosa itself may become more fibrotic, particularly near the tip.

The mucosal epithelium of the appendix is colonic in nature

The mucosa of the appendix is composed of straight tubular glands containing tall columnar absorptive cells, mucin-secreting goblet cells and some enteroendocrine cells, which are mainly found in the bases of the glands. Enteroendocrine cells are also found in the submucosa, closely related to nerves and ganglion cells, particularly near the closed tip of the appendix.

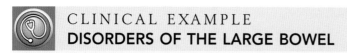

CLINICAL EXAMPLE
DISORDERS OF THE LARGE BOWEL

The colon and rectum are subject to a number of disorders, many of which are transient and the result of dietary indiscretion, for example following the ingestion of large quantities of beer! The three most important diseases of long duration in adults are:

- Cancer of the large bowel epithelium
- Diverticular disease, in which increased pressure in the bowel lumen forces mucosa through the muscle layers
- Ulcerative colitis, which is a severe ulcerating disease of the colonic mucosa.

Ulcerative Colitis

The cause of ulcerative colitis is not known, but large bowel mucosa is lost over an extensive area, with ulceration and destruction of the absorptive epithelium (Fig. 11.46).

This mucosal damage impairs water resorption from the colonic contents, and thus the normal solid faeces are replaced by large quantities of watery diarrhoea, which is similar in content and texture to the contents of the ileum. Destruction of the mucosa also leads to bleeding, so the watery diarrhoea is often mixed with blood.

Hirschsprung's Disease

In infants and children, the most important disease of the large bowel is Hirschsprung's disease, in which defecation is not possible because a segment of the lower rectum is completely devoid of ganglion cells in the submucosa and muscularis layers. Normal innervation is described on page 204 and illustrated in Figure 11.27.

The affected segment of bowel is narrowed and the child's abdomen distends with unpassed faeces, fatal perforation occurring if it is not treated.

Although the abnormality primarily affects the lower rectum, the aganglionic segment may be extensive, involving much of the distal colon.

Diagnosis is confirmed by rectal biopsy, establishing that submucosal ganglion cells are absent. A characteristic feature is hypertrophy of preganglionic nerve twigs in the muscularis mucosae, submucosa and lamina propria (Fig. 11.47).

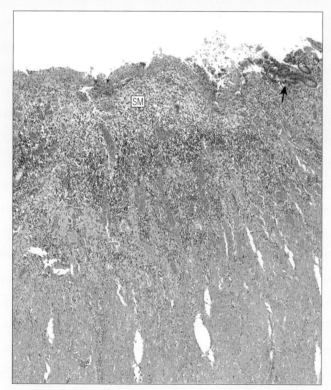

FIGURE 11.46 **Ulcerative colitis.** Micrograph of wall of sigmoid colon from a patient with ulcerative colitis. Note the complete destruction of the mucosa and some submucosa (SM) with infiltration of inflammatory cells (small blue cells). Only a few scattered remnants of absorptive and mucus-secreting epithelium remain (arrow).

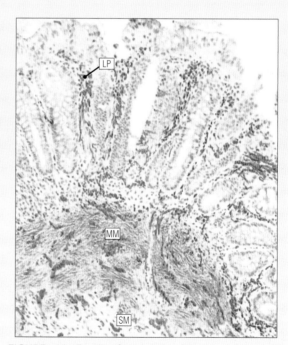

FIGURE 11.47 **Hirschsprung's disease.** Micrograph showing prominent nerve twigs in the lamina propria (LP), muscularis mucosae (MM) and submucosa (SM). This rectal biopsy from a child with Hirschsprung's disease has been stained by the cholinesterase enzyme histochemical technique.

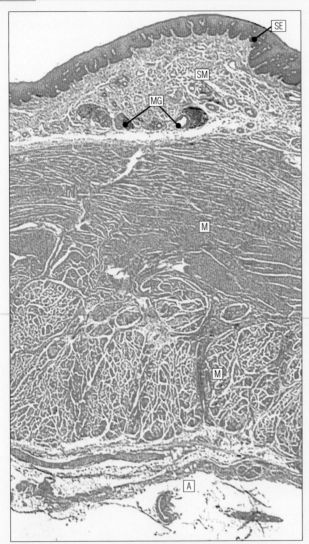

FIGURE 11.48 **Oesophagus.** This low-power micrograph shows the squamous epithelium (SE) of the lower third of the oesophagus and the submucosa (SM), containing oesophageal mucous glands (MG) surrounded by a prominent lymphocytic infiltrate. At this level of the oesophagus, the muscle layers (M) are composed entirely of smooth muscle. Higher in the oesophagus, there is a moderate amount of striated muscle. The outer adventitial layer (A) contains adipose tissue and a number of nerves and blood vessels.

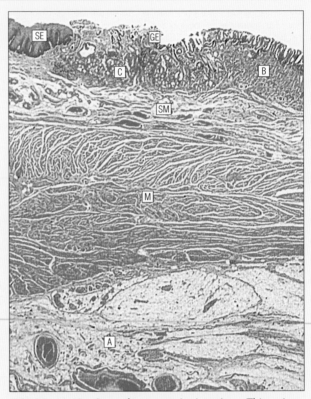

FIGURE 11.49 **Oesophagogastric junction.** This micrograph shows the junction between the squamous epithelium (SE) of the lower oesophagus and the glandular epithelium (GE) of the stomach. Two patterns of gastric mucosa can be seen, that closest to the oesophageal squamous epithelium being cardiac type (C, see also Fig. 11.34a), which in this case forms a narrow zone before gastric mucosa of body-type (B, see also Figs 11.34b,c). In this region, the submucosa (SM) is highly vascular, as is the adventitial layer (A). The separation of the muscle layers (M) into circular and longitudinal layers becomes indistinct in the oesophagogastric area.

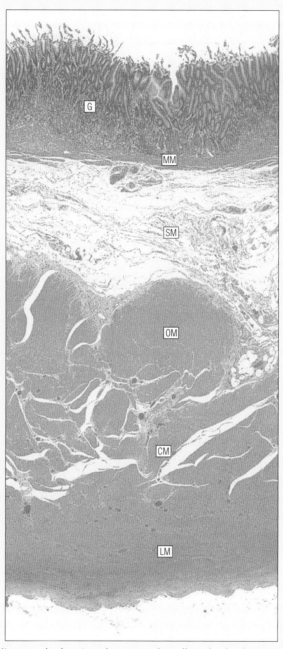

FIGURE 11.50 **Stomach wall.** Micrograph showing the stomach wall in the body region. The body mucosa is thick and composed largely of glands (G, see also Fig. 11.34). The distinct muscularis mucosae (MM) can be seen separating the epithelium from a loose-textured submucosa (SM). The three muscle layers frequently seen in the stomach are evident. There is an inner oblique (OM) layer, a middle circular (CM) layer and an outer longitudinal (LM) layer. The stomach lies within the peritoneal cavity and its outer coat is therefore a serosal layer covered by mesothelial cells.

PRACTICAL HISTOLOGY

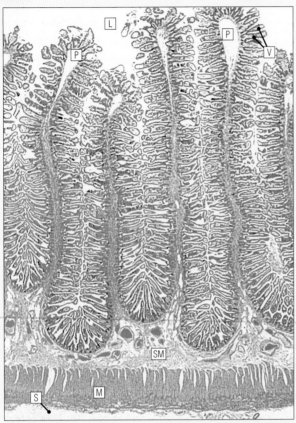

FIGURE 11.51 **Small intestine.** This low-power micrograph from the first part of the jejunum shows the characteristic structure of the small intestinal wall. The mucosal layer is thrown up into high folds (plicae P, see also Fig. 11.36a), the surfaces of which are modified to form numerous villi (V, see also Fig. 11.37). This modification enormously increases the surface area of epithelium exposed to small intestinal contents in the lumen (L). The submucosa (SM) is highly vascular and the double muscle layer (M) can be seen. The outer surface is covered by serosa (S). The pattern of extensive plication becomes progressively less marked in the lower reaches of the small intestine.

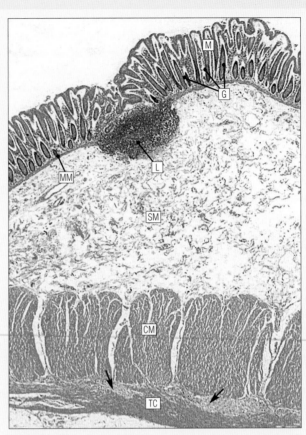

FIGURE 11.52 **Colon.** Micrograph showing the colon with its flat surfaced mucosa (M) composed of simple tubular glands (G, see also Fig. 11.44). There is a distinct muscularis mucosae (MM), which in this micrograph is breached in one area by a lymphoid aggregate (L) that lies partly in the mucosa and partly in the submucosa. This lymphoid aggregate is part of the GALT. The submucosa (SM) is loose and fibrocollagenous, allowing movement of the mucosa on the muscle layer. The muscle layer is composed mainly of circular muscle (CM), but there is a narrow discontinuous longitudinal muscle forming the taeniae coli (TC). There is a prominent collection of ganglia and nerves between the two muscle layers (arrows, see also Fig. 11.27).

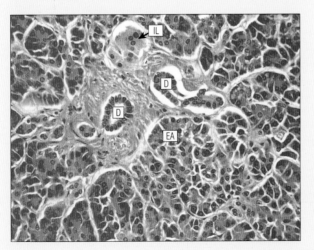

FIGURE 11.53 **Pancreas.** Low-power micrograph showing the pancreas with its duct systems (D), which drain the secretions of the exocrine acini (EA, see also Fig. 11.43) into the main pancreatic duct prior to discharge into the duodenum. Most of the pancreatic tissue shown here is composed of tightly packed exocrine acini, the details of which are not visible at this low magnification. A small islet of Langerhans (IL), the endocrine component of the pancreas (see Chapter 14), is also present in this field.

For online review questions, please visit
https://studentconsult.inkling.com.

END OF CHAPTER REVIEW

True/False Answers to the MCQs, as Well as Case Answers, Can be Found in the Appendix in the Back of the Book.

1. **Which of the following features are true of the oral cavity?**
   (a) The surface of the anterior two-thirds of the tongue is raised in a series of elevations called 'papillae'
   (b) Taste buds are found around the base of circumvallate papillae and in fungiform papillae
   (c) The tongue muscle is composed of complex interlaced pattern of non-striated smooth muscle fibres
   (d) The periodontal ligaments tether the teeth in the alveolar sockets of the mandible or maxilla
   (e) The floor of the mouth is lined by non-keratinized stratified squamous epithelium

2. **Which of the following features are present in salivary glands?**
   (a) Secretion of a watery solution which contains amylase and lysozyme
   (b) The submandibular glands have a mixed population of serous and mucous cells
   (c) The parotid glands are composed of mucus-secreting cells
   (d) Contain striated ducts which are lined by ion-pumping cells
   (e) Are found on the inner surface of the lips and in the submucosa of the dorsal tongue

3. **In the stomach, which of the following features are present?**
   (a) Acid is produced by chief (peptic) cells
   (b) Enzyme-producing cells secrete pepsinogen
   (c) The mucosa in the body is characterized by long, straight, tubular glands containing acid-producing, enzyme-producing, mucin-producing and neuroendocrine cells
   (d) The mucosa in the pylorus has relatively few acid-producing cells compared to the body region
   (e) Enteroendocrine cells secreting gastrin are concentrated in the cardiac region

4. **Which of the following features are present in the small bowel?**
   (a) Villi are seen macroscopically as large folds arranged circularly around the lumen
   (b) Enterocytes have a well-developed microvillus surface which forms the brush border
   (c) Paneth cells are seen as large, vacuolated, pale-staining cells and are found mainly in the neck region of intestinal crypts
   (d) Brunner's glands are serous in type and are found in the duodenum
   (e) All mucosal epithelial cells are derived from common specialized stem cells located in the crypts

CASE 11.1 AN OBESE MAN WITH HEARTBURN

An obese man of 56, a heavy smoker, is seen by his family practitioner because of severe intermittent pain in the centre of his lower chest. It is particularly bad at night when he first goes to bed and lies down. His doctor takes a full history and makes a diagnosis of gastro-oesophageal reflux disease (GORD); he prescribes antacids and recommends weight loss and stopping smoking. However, the patient returns 2 weeks later saying that his symptoms have not improved, and is anxious that he may have angina, a work colleague of his age having recently collapsed and died at work from a myocardial infarct. The doctor suspects non-compliance with his advice, but under duress, refers the patient to hospital for advice and investigation. At hospital, the patient gives exactly the same history. Investigation shows no evidence of myocardial ischaemia. An endoscopy shows inflammation and ulceration at the lower end of the oesophagus.

> **Q. Describe the structural and anatomical background to this case. Explain the differences between the normal lining epithelium of the oesophagus and that lining the upper part of the stomach.**

CASE 11.2 A YOUNG MAN WITH PERSISTENT SEVERE DIARRHOEA

A 26-year-old man is referred urgently to the hospital by his family practitioner because of severe, bloody diarrhoea, present for 3 days. He had been passing about 10–15 very liquid bloodstained stools per day, and was particularly distressed by the extreme urgency of defecation with little or no warning, leading to embarrassing incontinence.

On examination, he was anxious and distressed, with a fever (38.5°C) and a rapid pulse rate (105/min). He complained of lower abdominal discomfort but did not have a distended abdomen, and gave no history of vomiting or recent foreign travel. Full blood count showed anaemia (9.8 g/dL) with some hypochromic microcytic red cells, polychromatic red cells and increased platelet count; his ESR was 45 mm/h. A stool sample was sent to microbiology for urgent direct microscopy and culture, and he was admitted for further urgent investigation and treatment. Sigmoidoscopy showed redness of the large bowel mucosa and a biopsy was taken; this showed superficial ulceration of the large bowel mucosa with loss of surface epithelium associated with infiltration by neutrophils, indicating focal acute inflammation. No infective condition was identified.

A diagnosis of ulcerative colitis is made and further management is planned.

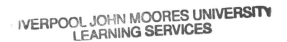

Q. Describe the structural and anatomical background to this case. What clinical effects can be explained by loss of the bowel surface epithelium through ulceration?

CASE 11.3 A WOMAN WITH ABDOMINAL DISCOMFORT, DIARRHOEA AND WEIGHT LOSS

A 32-year-old woman is referred to hospital by her family practitioner because of almost constant abdominal discomfort, sometimes with more severe pain, and frequent diarrhoea. She also complained of feeling generally unwell and had become excessively tired over the previous few months, and had lost considerable weight, despite an almost normal appetite. On examination, she was pale and thin, with a slightly bloated abdomen, which was somewhat tender on palpation. On more detailed questioning about her diarrhoea, she stated that there was no bleeding, and the stools were not often fluid, but very soft and pale, with a tendency to float and difficult to flush away. The physician recognized this as a description of steatorrhoea. Full blood count showed that she had a moderate iron deficiency anaemia but with a normal platelet count, suggesting that there had been no recent blood loss. A barium meal and small bowel follow-through showed mild dilation of the small bowel but no major structural abnormality. She underwent a jejunal biopsy, and the pathologist's report said that the changes were suggestive of gluten enteropathy (coeliac disease), with loss of the normal villous pattern and replacement of the small bowel by a flattened epithelium.

Q. Describe the structural, functional and anatomical background to this case. Describe the likely clinical and functional consequences of losing the small bowel villous pattern.

Chapter 12

Liver

Introduction

The liver acts as a vast biosynthetic chemical factory, synthesizing large complex molecules from substances brought to it in the blood, particularly substances recently absorbed by the intestine and transported by a portal blood system.

The liver has a wide range of functions, which accounts for its complex structure

All of the biochemical functions of the liver are carried out by the epithelial parenchymal cells of the liver, the hepatocytes, and are dependent on close interrelationships between:
- The vasculature (hepatic artery and portal vein branches, sinusoids and central veins)
- The hepatocytes
- The bile drainage systems (the canaliculi and intrahepatic bile ducts, Fig. 12.1).

Bile synthesis and secretion. The liver produces bile, which is an alkaline secretion containing water, ions, phospholipids, bile pigments (mainly bilirubin glucuronide) and bile acids (glycocholic and taurocholic).

Excretion of bilirubin. Bilirubin is produced in the spleen from the breakdown of the haem component of haemoglobin. In the liver the bilirubin is conjugated with glucuronic acid, and the conjugate (bilirubin glucuronide) is excreted in the bile and thence the faeces.

Protein metabolism. The liver is centrally involved in protein metabolism. It brings about deamination of amino acids; it produces urea from circulating ammonia; it also interconverts amino acids and produces the so-called non-essential amino acids. The liver synthesizes many proteins, including most of the plasma proteins such as albumin, blood clotting factors, such as fibrinogen, and prothrombin.

The profile of proteins secreted by the liver can be influenced by cytokines circulating in the blood. In patients with inflammatory disorders, circulating cytokines can increase the concentration of several liver-produced proteins in the blood, such as fibrinogen, transferrin and serum-amyloid A protein. The production of some other proteins is downregulated, for example albumin. This is called an 'acute-phase response'.

Carbohydrate metabolism. Lipids and amino acids are converted into glucose in the liver by gluconeogenesis. The liver makes and stores glycogen, as well as forming intermediary compounds in carbohydrate metabolism.

Lipid metabolism. The liver is involved in synthesis of cholesterol, lipoproteins and phospholipids. It synthesizes fat from other precursors. It also oxidizes fatty acids to provide energy.

Storage. The liver acts as a store for vitamins A, D and B_{12}. It stores iron as ferritin.

Conjugation and elimination of metabolites and toxins. The smooth endoplasmic reticulum of the liver possesses large numbers of enzymes that break down or conjugate metabolites or toxic substances (e.g. alcohol, barbiturates, etc.). Certain hormones are eliminated by the liver.

Liver Vasculature

The liver receives blood from two vessels, the hepatic artery and the hepatic portal vein

The liver receives blood from two sources:
- The hepatic artery perfuses the liver with oxygenated blood from the coeliac axis branches of the aorta
- The hepatic portal vein carries blood from the digestive tract and spleen to the liver, the blood from the digestive tract being rich in amino acids, lipids and carbohydrates absorbed from the bowel, and that from the spleen being rich in haemoglobin breakdown products.

In the liver, the two input circulations (hepatic artery and hepatic portal vein) discharge their blood into a common network of anastomosing small vascular channels, the sinusoids (Fig. 12.2). The terminal parts of the hepatic portal and arterial systems run together in a connective tissue framework called **portal tracts**, which also contain bile ductules.

After entering the liver at the porta hepatis, the portal vein divides within the liver into progressively smaller branches (interlobar, segmental and interlobular branches), which then branch further, eventually forming an extensive anastomosing network of terminal portal venules. Lateral side branches (inlet venules) of the terminal portal venules empty blood into the sinusoids, where it blends with blood from the terminal hepatic artery branches.

The hepatic artery divides into successively smaller branches, the terminal elements running with the terminal branches of the hepatic portal vein before emptying into the hepatic sinusoids by short side branches (the arteriosinusoidal branches). A peribiliary plexus of small

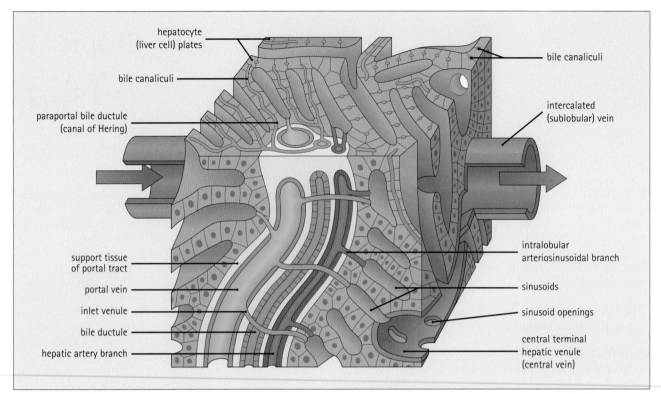

FIGURE 12.1 **Architecture of the liver.** Hepatocytes (liver cells) are arranged as interconnecting sheets of cells that surround sinusoids containing blood supplied by small side branches of the hepatic artery and portal vein. Sinusoidal blood drains into a central terminal hepatic venule, each of which empties into an intercalated (sublobular) vein. Bile produced by hepatocytes enters narrow canaliculi, which drain into small bile ducts running with the hepatic artery and portal vein branches. Larger bile ducts and branches of the hepatic artery and portal vein are surrounded by collagenous tissue to form portal tracts.

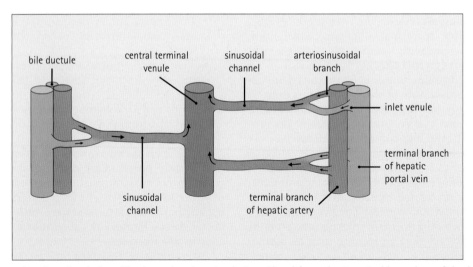

FIGURE 12.2 **Hepatic microcirculation.** The hepatic microcirculation. Blood from the terminal branches of the hepatic artery and the portal vein enters the sinusoidal system via small side branches, the arteriosinusoidal branch and inlet venule, respectively. It then passes along the sinusoid lumina towards the terminal hepatic venule (central vein). Although highly simplified here, in reality the sinusoidal system is an interconnecting system of capillary-like channels in close contact with the functioning liver cells (hepatocytes).

arterial branches supplies oxygenated blood into the large intrahepatic bile ducts before draining into the sinusoids, where it blends with blood from the portal venous system.

The sinusoids are surrounded on all sides by hepatocytes. In this way, blood flowing through the liver is exposed to a massive surface area of liver cells.

Hepatic sinusoids are the highly specialized liver capillary equivalents

The hepatic sinusoids permeate the whole of the liver. They are lined by a thin, discontinuous, highly fenestrated endothelium, which is closely related externally to plates and cords of hepatocytes (Fig. 12.3), albeit separated

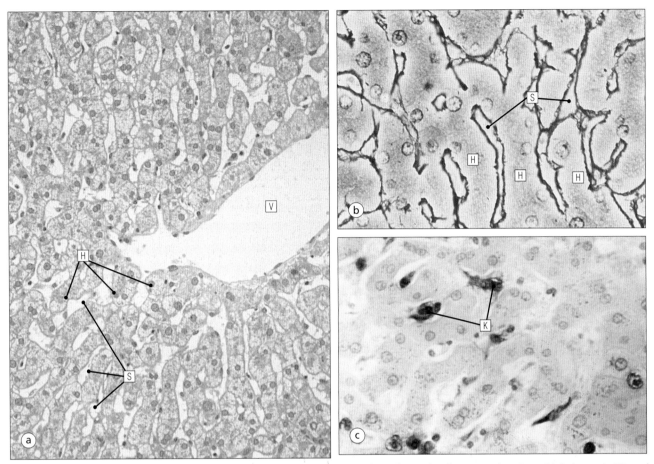

FIGURE 12.3 **Hepatic sinusoids.** (a) High-power micrograph showing the relationship between the sinusoidal channels (S) and the cuboidal hepatocytes (H). Note the terminal hepatic venule, V. (b) Micrograph of liver stained to demonstrate reticulin fibres (black), which run in the space of Disse between the hepatocyte surface and the endothelial cells lining the sinusoid (see also Fig. 12.5c,d). This method delineates the outline of the sinusoid (S) and the hepatocyte columns (H) and is used in the histological diagnosis of liver disease on small cores of liver tissue obtained by needle biopsy (see also Fig. 1.1). (c) Immunoperoxidase preparation (showing lysozyme) identifying scattered phagocytic Kupffer cells (K) in the sinusoid lining.

from them by a space. This perisinusoidal space of Disse is the main site where material is transferred between the blood-filled sinusoids and hepatocytes. This transfer is in both directions, with some material being taken up by hepatocytes as well as being secreted.

The hepatic sinusoids are partly lined by phagocytic cells (**Kupffer cells**), which are a form of macrophage and are derived from circulating blood monocytes.

Blood leaving the sinusoids enters the central venules of the liver lobules

Blood which has passed through the functioning liver parenchyma enters terminal hepatic venules (central veins of the lobules; discussed later on p. 231), which in turn unite to form intercalated veins; these then fuse to form larger hepatic vein branches. Hepatic veins are devoid of valves and open separately into the inferior vena cava as it passes through the liver on its way to the right atrium.

Lymphatic fluid drains from the liver to the thoracic duct

The liver produces a large volume of lymph. Fluid drains from the space of Disse into the portal tracts, in which it travels in fine channels. These lymphatic channels increase in size as the branches of the portal tracts merge towards the hepatic hilum. Finally, lymph drains into the thoracic duct. Such is the extent of lymph production by the liver that it comprises about half of the total lymph flow in the body under resting conditions.

Hepatocytes

The main functional cell of the liver is the hepatocyte

Hepatocytes (liver cells), which are intimately associated with the network of blood vessels (sinusoids), are polarized polyhedral cells with three identifiable types of surface (see below). As would be expected in cells that are so metabolically active, their cytoplasm is packed with a wide range of organelles.

The nuclei are large, spherical and central, and contain scattered clumps of chromatin and prominent nucleoli. Many cells are binucleate, and nuclei are frequently polyploid; progressively more tetraploid nuclei develop with age.

The Golgi is large and active, or small and multiple, and is mainly seen near the nucleus, with an extension lying close to the canalicular surface.

The vesicles and tubules of the abundant smooth and rough endoplasmic reticulum are continuous with the Golgi. There are numerous free ribosomes in the cytosol, as well as large glycogen deposits and some lipid droplets, the glycogen often being closely related to the smooth endoplasmic reticulum.

Lysosomes (see p. 24) of various sizes are numerous, some containing lipofuscin and lamellated lipoprotein. They are particularly large and numerous near the canalicular surface.

Peroxisomes (see p. 25) usually number 200–300 per cell.

Mitochondria are also abundant, numbering more than 1000 per cell, and are randomly scattered. This vast mitochondrial component gives the hepatocyte cytoplasm its eosinophilic granular appearance in H&E-stained paraffin sections.

Hepatocytes have three important surfaces

The hepatocyte surfaces are important because they are involved in the transfer of substances between hepatocyte, blood vessels and bile canaliculi.

The three types of surface are sinusoidal, canalicular and intercellular (Figs 12.4, 12.5).

KEY FACTS
HEPATOCYTES

- Metabolically highly active and rich in cytoplasmic organelles
- High energy requirement with numerous mitochondria
- Much of the cell surface is related to sinusoids where exchange of materials with blood takes place
- Part of the surface is in contact with bile canaliculi, where bile excreted from hepatocytes enters the biliary drainage system.

Sinusoidal surfaces are separated from the sinusoidal vessel by the space of Disse

Sinusoidal surfaces account for approximately 70% of the total hepatocyte surface. They are covered by short

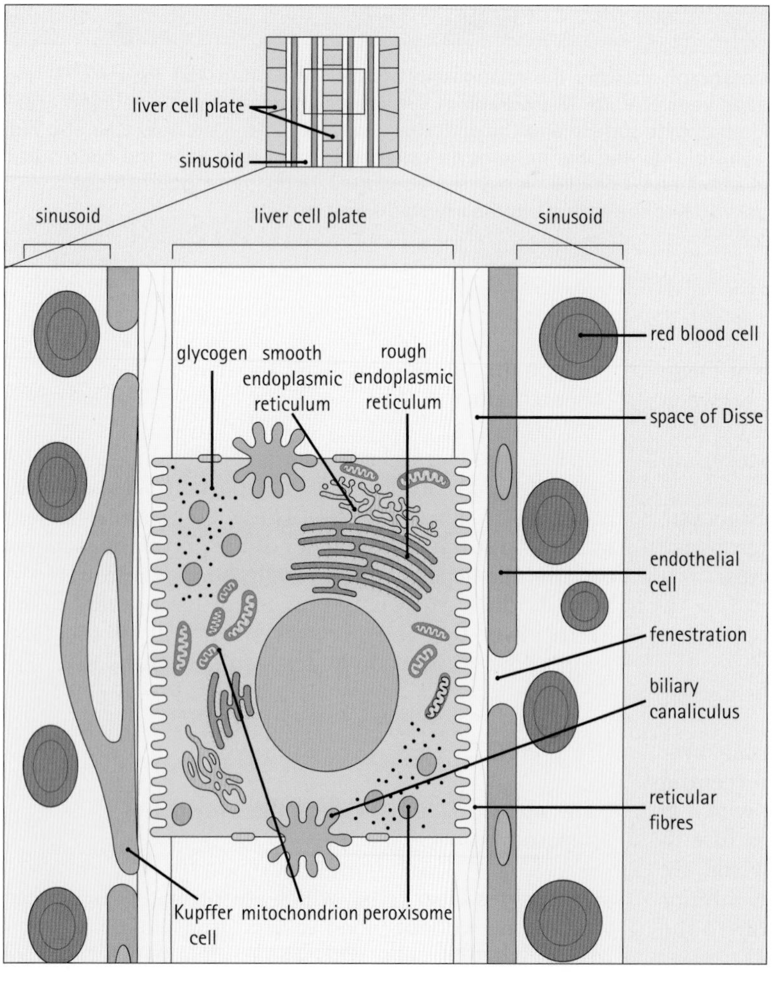

FIGURE 12.4 **Hepatocyte.** Hepatocytes are epithelial cells linked together by epithelial junctions. They have three types of cell surface, but in this two-dimensional diagram, only two of the three hepatocyte surfaces are shown, one that faces the sinusoid with a microvillar surface and one that forms a biliary canaliculus. Each hepatocyte contains abundant rough endoplasmic reticulum and smooth endoplasmic reticulum, reflecting biosynthetic roles. Mitochondria and peroxisomes are numerous. Glycogen is stored within the cytosol. The space of Disse separates the hepatocytes from a discontinuous layer of endothelial cells lining the sinusoids. Phagocytic Kupffer cells also line the sinusoids (not shown).

liver cell plate

sinusoid

sinusoid

liver cell plate

sinusoid

glycogen

smooth endoplasmic reticulum

rough endoplasmic reticulum

red blood cell

space of Disse

endothelial cell

fenestration

biliary canaliculus

reticular fibres

Kupffer cell

mitochondrion

peroxisome

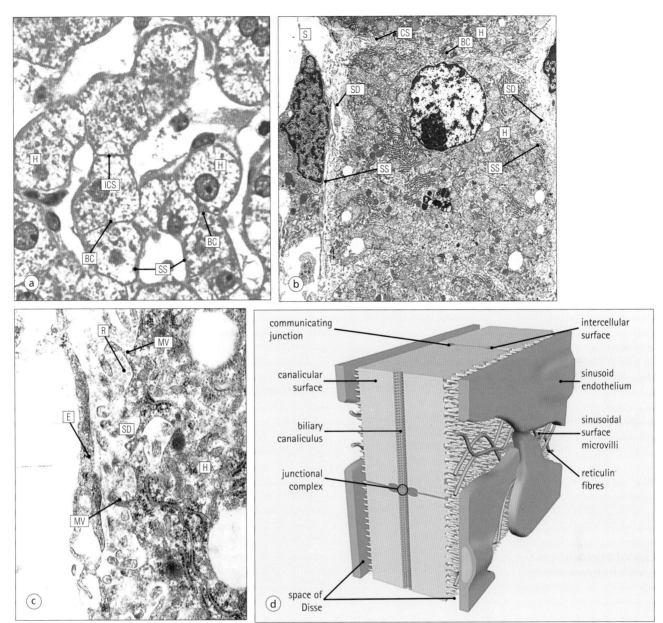

FIGURE 12.5 **Hepatocyte.** (a) Micrograph of a thin acrylic resin H&E-stained section of hepatocytes (H), which are roughly cuboidal and have a pale granular eosinophilic cytoplasm, much of the pallor being due to the presence of glycogen. The nuclei are central with a distinct nuclear membrane and prominent nucleoli. Some of the hepatocyte surface lines the sinusoidal channel (i.e. sinusoidal surface, SS), whereas other surfaces are in contact with adjacent hepatocyte (i.e. intercellular surfaces, ICS), some of the adjacent hepatocyte surfaces having bile canaliculi (BC) running between them. Details of the canaliculi cannot be distinguished by light microscopy. (b) Low-power electron micrograph showing some of the cytoplasm of two adjacent hepatocytes (H), joined by their canalicular surfaces (CS) in which a bile canaliculus (BC) can be seen. The other surfaces of the hepatocyte are the sinusoidal surfaces (SS) bordering the sinusoid lumen (S). The space between the hepatocyte surface and the sinusoid is the space of Disse (SD). (c) Medium-power electron micrograph showing the space of Disse (SD) between the sinusoidal surface of the hepatocyte (H) and the endothelial cell (E) lining the sinusoid. A number of irregular microvilli (MV) protrude into the space of Disse from the hepatocyte surface. The microvilli are much less regular in humans than in rodents. Some of the support fibres of the reticulin network (R) can be seen. (d) The space of Disse lying between the hepatocyte and the discontinuous endothelium lining the sinusoid. The space contains microvillus processes from the hepatocyte surface and collagenous reticulin fibres, which form a supportive mesh.

microvilli, which protrude into the space of Disse. Between the bases of the microvilli are coated pits (see Fig. 2.5), which are involved in endocytosis.

The sinusoidal surface is the site where material is transferred between the sinusoids and the hepatocyte.

Canalicular surfaces are the surfaces across which bile drains from the hepatocytes into the canaliculi

These account for approximately 15% of the hepatocyte surface and are closely apposed, except at the site of a canaliculus, which is a tube formed by the exact opposition of two shallow gutters on the surface of adjacent hepatocytes.

Canaliculi are about 0.5–2.5 μm in diameter, being smaller close to the terminal hepatic venule, and are lined by irregular microvilli arising from the canalicular surfaces of the hepatocytes.

Hepatocyte cytoplasm close to the canaliculi is rich in actin filaments, which are possibly capable of influencing the diameter of the canaliculus and thus the rate of flow.

The cell membrane around the canalicular lumen is rich in alkaline phosphatase and adenosine triphosphatase, and the canalicular lumen is isolated from the rest of the canalicular surface by junctional complexes (Fig. 12.6b).

The intercellular surfaces are the surfaces between adjacent hepatocytes that are not in contact with sinusoids or canaliculi

Intercellular surfaces account for about 15% of the hepatocyte surface. They are comparatively simple, but specialized for cell attachment and cell-to-cell communication via communicating junctions (see Fig. 3.14).

Hepatocyte Stem Cells and Liver Regeneration

The unique ability of the liver to regenerate itself has fascinated scientists for eons and has made it the prototype for mammalian organ regeneration. There are two main forms of regeneration in the liver in response to different types of liver injury. At the frontline of defence are mature, normally quiescent adult hepatocytes that proliferate and regenerate the liver after the majority of liver injuries due to drugs, toxins, resection, or acute viral diseases. The second layer of defence lies in the reserve progenitor cell population, which is also a quiescent compartment in the liver, but is activated when injury is severe, or when the mature hepatocytes can no longer regenerate the liver due to senescence or arrest. Studies of liver resections in man have demonstrated restoration of the residual liver size in 3–6 months.

Functional Organization of Hepatocytes

Hepatocytes have different metabolic profiles depending on how close they are to portal tracts

All hepatocytes are not equal, having different metabolic profiles depending on their distance from portal tracts.

Hepatocytes close to the portal tracts are exposed to blood that contains the highest oxygen concentration and contain enzymes involved in oxidative reactions. These cells make and store glycogen and produce and secrete proteins.

Hepatocytes furthest away from the portal tracts – those adjacent to the central venules – are most distant from the oxygenated arterial blood supply. These hepatocytes have little capacity for oxidative activities and contain many esterases, being involved in conjugating and detoxifying reactions.

Hepatocytes in between these extremes have intermediate metabolic properties.

These different metabolic profiles partly explain why different sets of hepatocytes are susceptible to different disease processes, especially responses to certain toxins.

The microanatomy of the liver has been described in two ways, termed the lobular and acinar concepts, respectively.

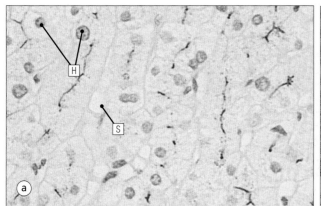 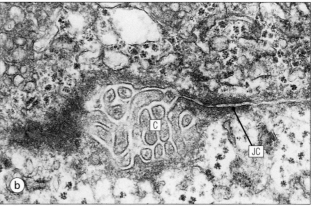

FIGURE 12.6 **Bile canaliculi.** (a) Micrograph showing bile canaliculi highlighted by an immunoperoxidase method for CEA, which shows the canaliculi as brown lines or dots, depending on whether they have been sectioned longitudinally or transversely. The nuclei and outlines of hepatocytes (H) can be seen, as can an occasional sinusoid (S). (b) Electron micrograph of the canalicular surface of two apposed hepatocytes. Note the canaliculus (C) filled with microvilli and the junctional complexes (JC) separating the canalicular lumen from the rest of the apposed hepatocyte.

The liver can be functionally divided into structures termed lobules

The components of the liver (i.e. the hepatocytes, terminal hepatic venules, portal triads and sinusoids) are arranged in a fairly constant pattern, which has been described as lobular (Fig. 12.7). The classic lobule is a roughly hexagonal structure in cross-section, being composed of:

- A central terminal hepatic venule, into which drains a converging series of sinusoidal channels like the spokes of a bicycle wheel

- Interconnecting plates of hepatocytes which surround sinusoidal channels and run between the central terminal hepatic venule and the periphery of the lobule
- Peripherally arranged portal tracts, each containing terminal branches of the hepatic artery and portal vein and a small tributary of the bile duct.

Thus, a ring of portal tracts forms the outer limit of each classic lobule.

The channels within each portal tract are surrounded by a small amount of fibrocollagenous tissue, and in some

FIGURE 12.7 **Hepatic architecture: lobule and acinus.** (a) The architecture of the liver and the relationship between the vessels and ducts in the portal tract, the sinusoids and the central veins. The lobular (orange) and acinar (green) concepts (see also Fig. 12.13b) are overdrawn. (b) Low-power micrograph showing the general liver architecture. Note the central terminal hepatic venules (CV), portal tracts (PT) and interconnecting cords of hepatocytes. The concepts of the hepatic lobule (L) and hepatic acinus (A), discussed on page 232, are overdrawn.

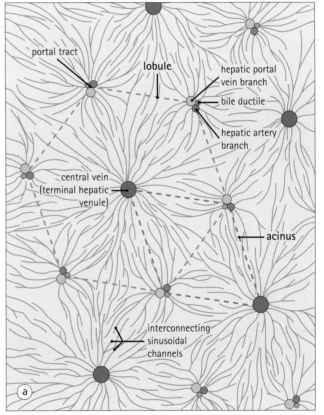

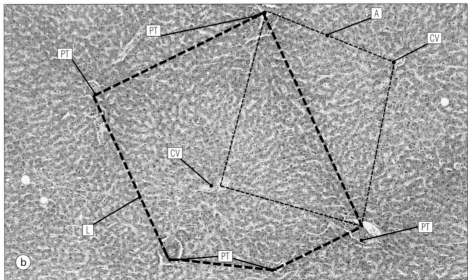

animals, particularly the pig, fibrocollagenous septa extend from one portal triad to another, clearly outlining the limits of each lobule. In humans, however, these fibrous septa are absent and so the lobule is less clearly defined.

In the lobule, three main zones of hepatocytes are identified, termed centrilobular, periportal and mid zones. Most of the nomenclature used in the descriptions of disease processes (e.g. centrilobular necrosis) is based on the lobular concept.

The outer layer of periportal hepatocytes adjacent to the portal tract is called the 'limiting plate'; it is the first group of hepatocytes to be damaged in inflammatory liver disorders that primarily involve the portal tracts.

The liver can also be functionally divided into structures called acini

The lobule concept has stood the test of time; however, it has also been proposed that the structure of the liver is best considered in terms of another structural unit, the acinus (see Fig. 12.7). The proposal is based on observations made on injection studies of the microcirculation of the liver; the acinus concept is based on the volume of liver receiving its blood supply from a single terminal branch of the hepatic artery contained within a portal tract. In this structural unit, the periphery of the acinus is the central vein, whereas the centre is the portal tract. In the acinar model, hepatocytes are divided into three zones:

Zone I: those hepatocytes closest to the portal tract which synthesize glycogen and proteins

Zone II: hepatocytes between zones I and III

Zone III: those hepatocytes adjacent to the central venule which contain esterases and conjugating enzymes.

The architectural arrangement of the liver remains immutable. The lobular and acinar concepts are simply two different ways of looking at the structure. In man, neither lobules nor acini have a clearly visible outline in histological sections.

CLINICAL EXAMPLE
CIRRHOSIS

Many slowly progressive diseases destroy hepatocytes and lead to distortion of liver architecture, particularly the relationships between the sinusoids, the portal venous system and the bile ducts.

Death of hepatocytes is followed by scarring, and, although hepatocytes can regenerate and produce a new population of cells, their connections with the portal system and the biliary drainage are destroyed. This pattern of liver disorder, known as cirrhosis (Fig. 12.8), is a common cause of chronic liver failure.

Cirrhosis is characterized by:

- Continuing death of hepatocytes
- Collapse of normal architecture
- Increased production of fibrocollagenous tissue, leading to irregular scarring
- Attempted regeneration of surviving hepatocytes, which form irregular nodules and have abnormal relationships with the microvasculature and bile drainage system. Regenerating hepatocytes are able to continue some synthetic functions but eventually fail to keep pace with normal demands, and the symptoms of liver failure begin to manifest themselves.

Cirrhosis produces chronic liver failure and symptoms appear progressively over a period of some years, usually culminating fatally in coma or as a result of the complications of portal hypertension.

Portal Hypertension

In cirrhosis, the sinusoidal connections between the portal venous system and the draining central terminal hepatic venules and hepatic veins are blocked or destroyed.

Portal venous blood cannot therefore flow through its normal channels (i.e. through sinusoids into central terminal hepatic venules). Thus, the blood pressure in the portal venous system increases considerably and causes portal hypertension.

One escape route for portal venous blood is via anastomoses with the systemic venous system; these are normally closed when portal pressure is low, but open when portal pressure rises.

When these anastomotic channels are distended with blood, they are called varices.

One of the sites of such an anastomosis is at the lower end of the oesophagus, which is unfortunate as the distended submucosal blood vessels (oesophageal varices) bulge into the lumen of the oesophagus and are easily eroded by gastric acid, resulting in torrential haemorrhage.

Bleeding from oesophageal varices is a severe complication of portal hypertension and cirrhosis and may be fatal.

Cirrhosis and portal hypertension most commonly follow persisting hepatocyte destruction due to alcohol toxicity, some forms of viral infection and autoimmune liver disease.

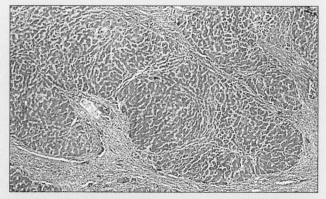

FIGURE 12.8 **Cirrhosis.** (Masson trichrome stain) Micrograph of cirrhotic liver. Compare with Figure 12.14 and note the fibrous scarring (blue), which has distorted the normal architecture. There are nodules of regenerating liver cells but their connections with the vascular supply and bile drainage system are destroyed. Masson trichrome stain has been used here.

Intrahepatic Biliary Tree

Bile produced by hepatocytes passes into bile canaliculi

The bile canaliculi carry the bile back to the portal tracts (i.e. in the opposite direction to the blood).

As the canaliculi approach the bile ductules (Fig. 12.9a) in the portal tracts, they open into short passages lined by small cuboidal cells (the canals of Hering). From here, bile flows into the bile ductules in the portal tract.

Bile ductules anastomose freely, fuse and increase in size to form larger ducts, the 'trabecular ducts' (Fig. 12.9b).

Many of these ducts fuse to form large intrahepatic ducts, which converge near the liver hilum into the main hepatic ducts (see p. 234).

Bile formed in the liver is passed into the gut through the extrahepatic bile ducts

The small tributaries of the intrahepatic biliary tree fuse to become increasingly larger channels, eventually fusing to become two large ducts, the right and left lobar bile ducts. These join at the hilum of the liver to form the common hepatic duct, which is the first part of the extrahepatic bile duct system (Fig. 12.10).

About 3–4 cm after leaving the liver, the common hepatic duct receives the cystic duct (a small duct from the gallbladder) and becomes the common bile duct.

The common bile duct is about 6–7 cm long and opens into the duodenum at the ampulla of Vater, having passed through the head of the pancreas and combined with the pancreatic duct.

KEY FACTS
BILIARY SYSTEM

- Bile produced by hepatocytes from breakdown products of haemoglobin
- Bile passes from canalicular surface of hepatocytes → bile canaliculi → bile ductules in portal tracts → trabecular ducts → intrahepatic bile ducts → lobar ducts → common hepatic duct
- Bile concentrated in gallbladder by extraction of water by absorptive epithelium, then stored
- Concentrated bile expelled from gallbladder by contraction of its smooth muscle wall into common bile duct, thence into duodenal lumen.

Gallbladder

Introduction

The gallbladder is an ovoid sac with a muscular wall and is capable of moderate distension. It concentrates and stores bile, receiving dilute watery bile from the common hepatic duct and emptying thick, concentrated, variably mucoid bile into the common bile duct.

Bile is transported in and out of the gallbladder through a short duct, the cystic duct. This duct contains a spirally arranged outgrowth of mucosa, which forms the spiral valve of Heister.

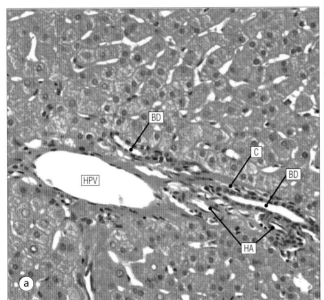

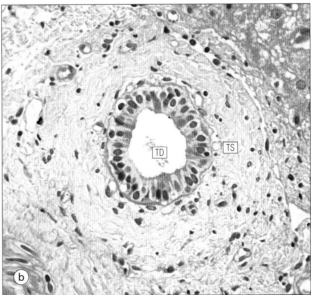

FIGURE 12.9 **Intrahepatic bile ducts.** (a) Micrograph showing a small bile ductule (BD) in the portal tract. It has a simple structure with low cuboidal epithelium and a narrow surrounding zone of collagen (C) and some smooth muscle fibres. A terminal branch of the hepatic portal vein (HPV) and hepatic artery (HA) are also present in the tract. (b) Micrograph of a transverse section of a trabecular duct (TD), which is larger than a bile ductule, with a larger lumen and a well-formed wall. It is surrounded by dense fibrocollagenous tissue of the trabecular septum (TS) in which it runs.

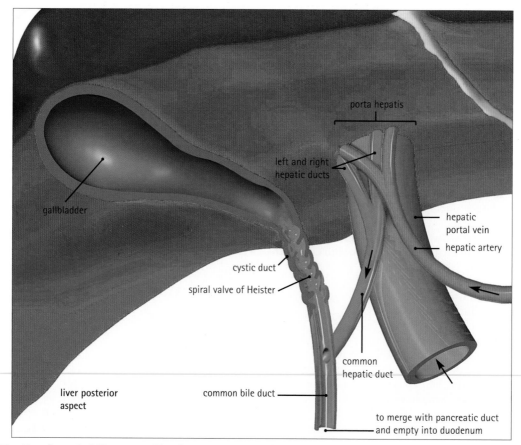

FIGURE 12.10 **Extrahepatic biliary tree.** The drainage system, whereby bile leaves the liver, is stored and concentrated in the gallbladder, and eventually enters the duodenum. The right and left hepatic ducts emerge from the posterior aspect of the liver at the porta hepatis and join to form the common hepatic duct. A side branch of this duct (the cystic duct) conducts bile into and out of the gallbladder. The common hepatic duct then continues as the common bile duct, passing through the head of the pancreas, where it merges with the pancreatic duct before entering the duodenum.

The gallbladder has a muscular wall

The gallbladder wall has a mucosa which comprises an absorptive epithelium resting on a highly vascular lamina propria. There is no muscularis mucosa. The muscle layer is normally thin and apparently haphazardly arranged but with a tendency to be circumferential. There is an outer dense fibrous layer, which is partly covered by peritoneal serosa, but partly loosely binds one aspect of the gallbladder to the underside of the liver.

The gallbladder mucosa is covered by tall columnar epithelial cells specialized for absorption

The lining cells have numerous microvilli on their luminal surfaces and complex interdigitations of their lateral walls (Fig. 12.11). These differently specialized surfaces are separated by junctional complexes (see Fig. 3.13).

Gallbladder epithelial cells are adapted for salt and water absorption, and have abundant basal and apical mitochondria, and Na^+ and K^+ transport ATPases in their lateral walls.

Na^+ and Cl^- ions are actively pumped out of the cell cytoplasm into the lateral intercellular space to produce an osmotic gradient between it and the gallbladder lumen. Water is therefore drawn into the space from the lumen and then enters the abundant capillary network in the lamina propria.

This mechanism is similar to that employed by the proximal convoluted tubule epithelial cell in the kidney to absorb water and ions (see Chapter 15).

Gallbladder epithelium is thrown up into folds or plicae, which flatten when the gallbladder is distended.

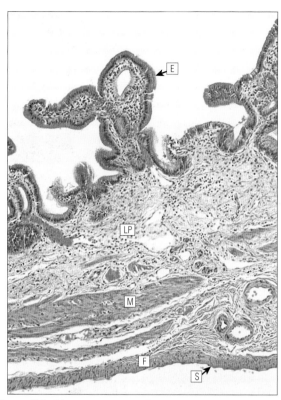

FIGURE 12.11 **Gallbladder wall.** The gallbladder receives bile from the liver through the common hepatic duct, via the cystic duct. The bile is concentrated (by absorption of water) and stored in the gallbladder until required, when it is squirted out into the common bile duct by contraction of the gallbladder wall to eventually pass into the duodenum. The gallbladder has an internal lining of absorptive epithelial cells (E) (see Fig 12.12), thrown into folds to increase the surface area for absorption. The lamina propria (LP) contains prominent blood vessels and a scattering of lymphocytes and plasma cells. The smooth muscle layers (M) are thin in a healthy gallbladder but become thickened if there is any obstruction to bile outflow (see Fig. 12.12). There is an outer layer of compact fibrous tissue (F), which has a serosal (S) surface over part of the gallbladder surface. Where the gallbladder wall lies against the underside of the liver, this fibrous layer loosely merges with the fibrous tissue of the liver capsule, though they can be easily separated by blunt dissection during surgical removal of the gallbladder (cholecystectomy).

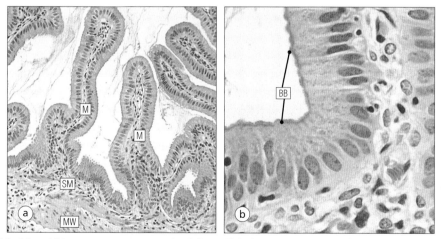

FIGURE 12.12 **Gallbladder.** (a) Low-power micrograph of the gallbladder showing the mucosa (M) with its ridged mucosal folds, the submucosa (SM) and the muscular wall (MW). (b) High-power micrograph of gallbladder epithelium. The cells are tall and columnar with basal nuclei and a luminal surface bearing microvilli. The microvilli are discernible as a faint brush border (BB).

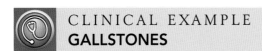

CLINICAL EXAMPLE
GALLSTONES

Gallstones (i.e. stones or calculi in the gallbladder or biliary tree) form when solid concretions of bile act as a nidus for calcium salt deposition. Small gallstones are asymptomatic; larger gallstones can cause obstructive jaundice or cholecystitis.

Obstructive Jaundice

Obstructive jaundice results from the blockage of a bile duct, for example by a gallstone that has passed out of the gallbladder and become impacted in the common bile duct on its way to the duodenum.

Blockage of the bile duct impedes the flow of bile into the duodenum. This results in:

- Damming of bile in the proximal biliary tree, intrahepatic bile ducts and eventually bile canaliculi
- Passage of retained canalicular bile into the hepatic sinusoids and thence into the bloodstream, producing jaundice
- Impaired intestinal breakdown of fat owing to lack of the emulsifying bile acids normally present in bile
- Pale faeces, the normal faecal colour being due to the presence of bile and its breakdown products.

Cholecystitis

Gallstones may become impacted in the cystic duct (Fig. 12.13a) and obstruct the flow of bile at this point. This has the following consequences, which are the basic features of so-called 'chronic cholecystitis' (Fig. 12.13b):

- The gallbladder contracts more strongly to try to overcome the obstruction, and consequently its musculature thickens
- Resulting high pressure within the gallbladder lumen pushes pouches of mucosa into the muscle layers (Rokitansky–Aschoff sinuses)
- Stasis of bile within the gallbladder predisposes to infection, and episodes of pain and fever are common.

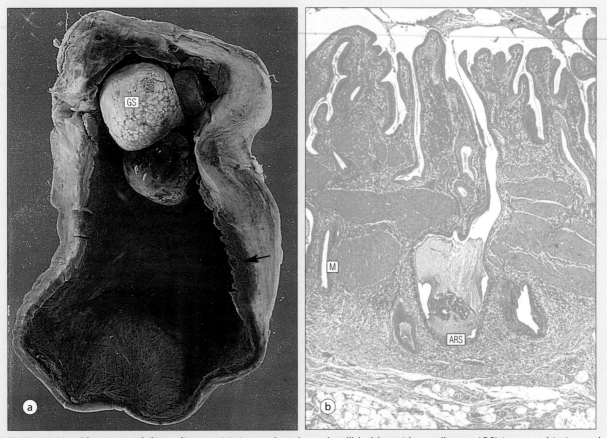

FIGURE 12.13 **Obstructive biliary disease.** (a) A greatly enlarged gallbladder with a gallstone (GS) impacted in its neck, close to the cystic duct. Obstruction of bile drainage has led to bile stasis and consequent infection, producing red inflamed mucosa (arrow). (b) Micrograph of a chronically obstructed gallbladder. The muscle layer (M) is thickened by hypertrophy and a pouch of epithelium-lined mucosa (Rokitansky–Aschoff sinus, ARS) has bulged through it. Compare with Figure 12.12a.

PRACTICAL HISTOLOGY

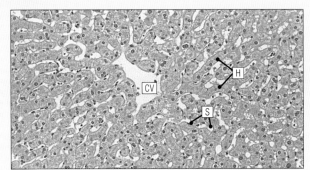

FIGURE 12.14 **Liver sinusoids and hepatocytes.** Micrograph showing sinusoidal channels (S) passing between interconnecting columns of hepatocytes (H) on their way to the central terminal hepatic venule (CV).

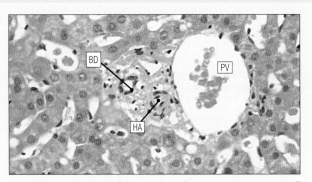

FIGURE 12.15 **Portal tract.** Portal tracts contain a small bile ductule (BD), a terminal branch of the hepatic artery (HA), and a component of the distal part of the hepatic portal venous system (PV). All are contained within a fibro-collagenous supporting stroma.

CLINICAL EXAMPLE
LIVER FAILURE

Liver disease can affect any of its functions, though when large numbers of hepatocytes are damaged, all of the functions tend to be disturbed.

Failure of Synthetic Functions

The liver fails to produce important proteins, such as albumin and the various protein clotting factors.

The reduced synthesis of albumin leads to a reduced oncotic pressure of the blood, which results in oedema and accumulation of watery fluid in the peritoneal cavity (ascites).

Failure of clotting factor synthesis leads to spontaneous bleeding.

Failure of Detoxification Functions

The liver fails to convert metabolic waste products into innocuous substances. Toxic substances therefore circulate in the blood and cause a number of symptoms, including confusion, altered consciousness and eventually hepatic coma, which is rapidly fatal.

Failure of Bile Secretion

Failure of adequate bile secretion into the alimentary tract leads to retention of bile in the liver, with some of the components of the retained bile entering the blood and producing yellowing discolouration of the blood plasma and tissues (i.e. jaundice).

Chronic Hepatic Failure

If hepatocyte damage is slowly progressive, the abnormalities outlined above develop insidiously over a period of years. This is called 'chronic hepatic failure' and is most commonly associated with cirrhosis (see Fig. 12.8).

Acute Hepatic Failure

If the liver disease is severe and of sudden onset, the metabolic abnormalities appear suddenly. This is acute hepatic failure, and is most commonly associated with some acute virus infections (e.g. hepatitis B virus infection) or exposure to liver toxins (e.g. paracetamol/acetamidophenol). In either case, acute hepatic failure results from the widespread death of liver cells.

CLINICAL EXAMPLE
TUMOURS OF THE LIVER AND BILIARY TREE

The commonest tumour to involve the liver is metastatic disease, as a result of spread of tumour from another primary site. Tumours of the gastrointestinal system commonly spread by the portal venous system to the liver, for example carcinoma of the colon or carcinoma of the stomach. Metastasis to the liver by bloodstream spread is also common from carcinoma of the lung and carcinoma of the breast.

Primary malignant tumours of the liver can be derived from hepatocytes (hepatocellular carcinomas). This type of tumour is predisposed by the presence of cirrhosis and by infection by hepatitis B or C virus.

Tumours derived from the biliary tree are uncommon. When they do occur, they are generally adenocarcinomas, as they are derived from the glandular epithelium that normally lines the biliary tract.

For online review questions, please visit https://studentconsult.inkling.com.

END OF CHAPTER REVIEW

True/False Answers to the MCQs, as Well as Case Answers, can be Found in the Appendix in the Back of the Book.

1. **Which of the following is true for the blood entering the liver through the hepatic portal vein?**
   (a) Is highly oxygenated
   (b) Contains material absorbed from food in the small intestine
   (c) Contains haemoglobin breakdown products from the spleen
   (d) Enters the hepatic sinusoids
   (e) Contains formed bile for metabolic breakdown by hepatocytes

2. **Which of the following features is indicative of the lobular concept of the liver?**
   (a) The terminal branch of the portal vein is at the centre of the lobule
   (b) The portal tracts are located at the periphery of the lobule
   (c) Blood passes from the periphery to the centre of the lobule
   (d) Bile passes from the hepatocytes to the centre of the lobule
   (e) The hepatocytes of the limiting plate are at the periphery of the lobule

3. **Which of the following features is true of bile?**
   (a) Is a product of haemoglobin breakdown in the liver
   (b) Is stored and concentrated in the gallbladder
   (c) Accumulates in the liver and blood when the common bile duct is blocked
   (d) Passes into the duodenum at the duodenal papilla (ampulla of Vater)
   (e) Is acidic and augments the effects of gastric acid in digestion

4. **Which of the following features are seen in hepatocytes?**
   (a) Are rich in peroxisomes
   (b) Have a canalicular surface which is involved in bile secretion
   (c) Are separated from the sinusoid endothelium by the space of Disse
   (d) Contain glycogen
   (e) Rest on a reticulin scaffold

CASE 12.1 A MAN WITH A BAD LIVER

A 62-year-old man is admitted to hospital having been found collapsed in the street. He is unresponsive and smells of alcohol. On examination, he is found to be hypoglycaemic and glucose is administered. His abdomen is distended and it is felt that he has ascites. He also has oedema of the ankles. His spleen appears enlarged on palpation.

Blood tests show an elevated bilirubin level and a low serum albumin.

Q. How do all these clinical findings relate to the normal structure and function of the liver? What pattern of liver disease is suggested by this case?

Chapter 13

Musculoskeletal System

Introduction

The musculoskeletal system, which provides mechanical support and permits movement, is composed of skeletal muscle, tendons, bones, joints and ligaments.

Skeletal muscles act as contractile levers, and are connected to bone by **tendons**. **Bones** act as rigid levers, articulating with other bones through **joints**, which are kept in relationship by **ligaments**.

A special characteristic of muscle, tendons and joints is the possession of a rich sensory nerve supply, which detects the position of the body and the velocity of movement. The integration of this sensory information by the central nervous system is vital for the musculoskeletal system to function normally.

The main functional attribute of bone is its specialized extracellular matrix, which is hardened by the deposition of calcium enabling it to function as a rigid lever.

The rigid, hard character of bone belies its importance as a metabolic reservoir of mineral salts and the fact that it is in a constant state of dynamic remodelling.

Skeletal Muscle

Skeletal muscle is responsible for voluntary movement

The histological characteristics of skeletal muscle cells and the structural basis of muscle contraction are described on pages 71–76.

Individual muscle cells are arranged into large groups to form anatomically distinct muscles. These are characterized by:

- An orderly alignment of the constituent cells to generate a directional force following contraction
- Anchorage to other structures by highly organized fibrocollagenous support tissues
- A rich blood supply reflecting high metabolic demands
- Innervation and control by specialized neurons (motor neurons) that terminate on muscle cells at specialized nerve endings (motor endplates)
- Incorporation of specially adapted skeletal muscle cells into structures called spindles, to act as sensors of muscle stretch.

Embryologically, muscle fibres develop from mesenchymal tissues

In embryogenesis, skeletal muscle develops from primitive mesenchymal tissues of the mesoderm. Small spindle-shaped or strap-shaped cells with a single nucleus and abundant pink-staining cytoplasm develop from primitive mesenchymal cells. These are skeletal muscle cell precursors, the rhabdomyoblasts (Fig. 13.1). Numerous individual rhabdomyoblasts then fuse to form multinucleate muscle fibres, the cells enlarging in size when they become connected to the nervous system and receive motor stimulation.

Residual cells with the function of rhabdomyoblasts (i.e. capable of differentiating further into functional striated muscle cells) persist in adult skeletal muscle as **satellite cells** (see Fig. 13.6). Following muscle damage and loss of fibres, these cells proliferate and may produce new muscle cells.

A muscle is composed of many muscle fibres

A mature muscle fibre is composed of large numbers of myofibrils bounded by a cell membrane termed 'the sarcolemma' (see Figs 5.2, 13.2).

Each skeletal muscle cell is typically extremely long (up to 10 cm in length), and it is therefore more usual to use the term 'skeletal muscle fibre' rather than cell.

Many muscle fibres are arranged together to form a muscle (Fig. 13.3). Despite being elongated, individual muscle cells do not extend the full length of a muscle but are arranged in overlapping bundles, the force of contraction being transmitted through the arrangement of the support tissues.

Different muscles are characterized by different physiological and metabolic properties

The physiological and metabolic properties of individual skeletal muscles are determined by differences in the structure of their constituent muscle fibres.

In both animals and man, it has been possible to define several subtypes of muscle fibre by macroscopic, physiological, biochemical and histochemical criteria, but there are marked interspecies variations.

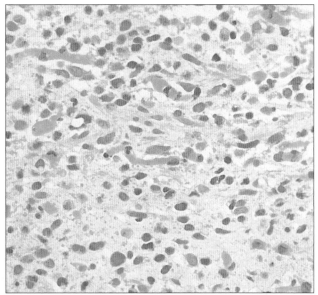

FIGURE 13.1 **Development of skeletal muscle.** This photomicrograph shows elongated rhabdomyoblasts, with abundant pink-staining cytoplasm, developing in primitive mesenchyme in human embryonic tissue.

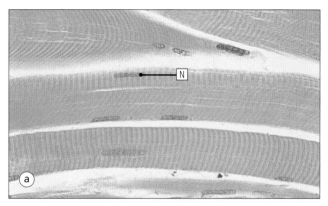

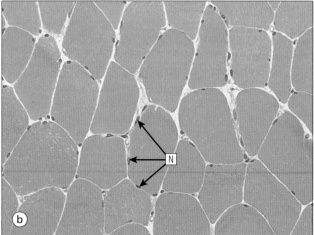

FIGURE 13.2 **Skeletal muscle fibres.** (a) Micrograph of skeletal muscle fibres in a longitudinal section showing prominent cross-striations. The dark bands are termed 'A bands' (anisotropic, i.e. birefringent in polarized light), and the light bands are termed 'I bands' (isotropic, i.e. no interference with polarized light). These bands correspond to the arrangement of thick and thin filaments in myofibrils (see Fig. 5.2). Nuclei (N) appear as elongated structures just beneath the cell membrane, and each fibre contains many nuclei. (b) Micrograph of skeletal muscle fibres in a transverse frozen section showing roughly hexagonal profiles with flattened sides where they are compressed by adjacent fibres. Nuclei (N) appear as small circular profiles at the periphery of each fibre. Individual myofibrils are generally not identifiable by light microscopy.

Histochemical staining for specific enzymes delineates several types of fibres and is a useful method for analysing muscle. Two main types of fibres are identified (types 1 and 2), and type 2 fibres can be subdivided into types 2A, 2B and 2C (Fig. 13.4). Type 2C fibres are thought to be a primitive form of type 2 fibre and, with appropriate innervation, are probably capable of developing into 2A or 2B fibres. Such histochemical staining is used routinely in the study of muscle pathology and allows the histological diagnosis of certain muscle diseases.

Histochemical staining can also be correlated with other functional and biochemical attributes of muscle (Fig. 13.4c).

Not all muscles have the same proportions of type 1 and type 2 fibres. In general, muscles with a role in maintaining posture (e.g. calf muscles) have a high proportion of type 1 fibres, whereas muscles used for short bursts of power have abundant type 2 fibres.

Different individuals are genetically endowed with variable proportions of muscle fibre types in defined muscles, and this may limit athletic prowess at a particular sport; training does not affect the proportion of fibres in any given muscle, but does influence their size.

Muscle has a rich blood supply because of the high energy demands of contraction

Large arteries penetrate the epimysium and divide into small branches that run in the perimysial support tissues, forming perimysial arteries and veins. These branches terminate in a vast capillary network, which runs in the endomysium. Each muscle fibre is served by several capillary vessels.

Normal adult skeletal muscle cells do not undergo cell division

Any increased demands placed on a muscle, for example by weight training, result in increased muscle size because the cells themselves increase in size (i.e. hypertrophy).

It is possible, however, for skeletal muscle cells to regrow because the pool of inactive stem cells in adult muscle called 'satellite cells' can be stimulated to divide following damage. These cells are not discernible by light

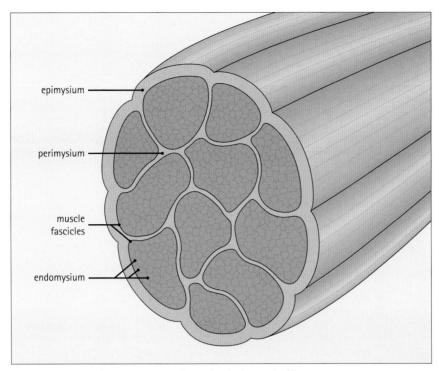

FIGURE 13.3 **Organization of muscle fibres into muscle.** Individual muscle fibres (see Fig. 5.1) are surrounded by endomysium, which is composed of sheets of external lamina identical to basement membrane (see p. 60). Endomysium secures the muscle fibres to each other and contains both capillary blood vessels and individual nerve axons (see Chapter 6). Clusters of muscle fibres are held together by fine sheets of fibrocollagenous support tissue (perimysium) to form fascicles. Blood vessels, lymphatic vessels and nerves run in the endomysial support tissues. An anatomically defined muscle is composed of many fascicles, which are surrounded externally by a thick layer of fibrocollagenous support tissue, the epimysium.

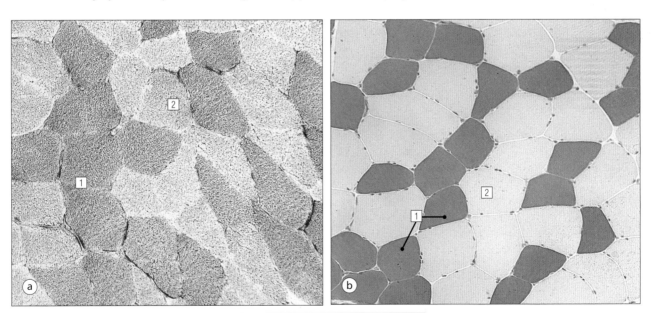

Fibre type	Metabolism	Contractile behaviour
1	oxidative	slow twitch
2A	oxidative and glycolytic	fast twitch, fatigue resistant
2B	glycolytic	fast twitch, fatigue sensitive

FIGURE 13.4 **Fibre types.** (a) Micrograph of a transverse frozen section of muscle stained by an enzyme histochemical method to demonstrate NADH transferase, which indicates oxidative capacity. Two different subtypes of fibre are evident. Type 1 fibres (1) show a high level of activity and stain darkly, whereas type 2 fibres (2) are paler because of their lower level of activity. (b) Micrograph of muscle stained for one form of myofibrillar ATPase at pH 4.2. This technique also delineates two fibre types. Type 1 fibres stain darkly, having a high level of activity, whereas type 2 fibres have a low level of activity and stain lightly. Note that the type 1 and 2 fibres are arranged in a haphazard or check pattern. (c) Table detailing the physiological features of different fibre types.

CLINICAL EXAMPLE
DISEASES OF MUSCLE

Several diseases of muscle have been attributed to specific metabolic or structural abnormalities (Fig. 13.5a).

Duchenne muscular dystrophy is the most common inherited muscle disease and characteristically affects male children. Such individuals become unable to stand unaided in early childhood and develop progressive muscle weakness, becoming wheelchair-bound by their mid-teens and typically dying in early adult life.

The abnormality in Duchenne muscular dystrophy is due to a defect in the gene coding for a protein termed 'dystrophin' (Fig. 13.5b). This protein links the actin cytoskeleton of muscle to the external lamina; its absence leads to abnormal muscle fibre fragility.

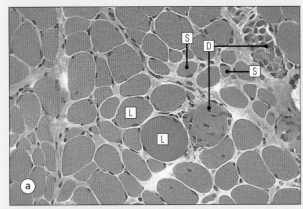
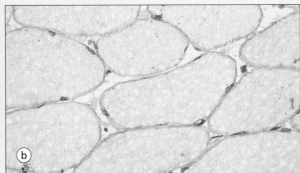

FIGURE 13.5 **Diseases of muscle.** (a) Micrograph of frozen section of skeletal muscle from a child showing the typical appearance of dystrophy, which is a congenital primary disorder of muscle. There is marked variation in fibre size, with some large fibres (L) and some abnormally small fibres (S). Some fibres are dead (D) and are being removed by phagocytic cells. (b) Micrograph of normal skeletal muscle stained by an immunocytochemical method for dystrophin (which stains brown), showing its localization in the sarcolemma. In Duchenne muscular dystrophy, this protein is absent.

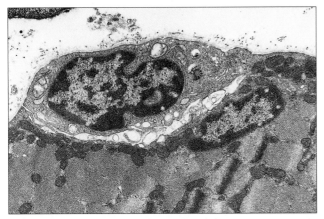

FIGURE 13.6 **Satellite cells.** Electron micrograph showing a satellite cell. These cells, small and spindle-shaped, are found immediately beneath the external lamina of a muscle fibre and act as stem cells in adult muscle.

microscopy, but may be seen ultrastructurally (Fig. 13.6). They are infrequent and appear as small spindle-shaped cells lying just beneath the external lamina of a muscle fibre.

Fibres that have regenerated in adult life following damage to a muscle can be detected histologically because they commonly contain centrally placed nuclei, rather than the peripheral nuclei typical of normal fibres.

Muscle contains stretch receptors

Although there are no pain receptors in skeletal muscle, there are receptors sensitive to stretch, which function as part of a feedback system to maintain normal muscle tone (i.e. the spinal stretch reflex arc).

Sensory fibres that provide information on the tension of skeletal muscle arise from two sources:
- Encapsulated nerve endings responding to stretch in the tendon associated with a muscle
- Spiral nerve endings (sensory afferent fibres) sensing stretch and tension of specialized muscle fibres contained in a special sense organ in muscle called the muscle spindle (Fig. 13.7).

The muscle spindle sensory mechanism maintains normal tone and muscle coordination.

Motor nerves to muscle terminate in motor endplates

Large nerves, containing both motor and sensory axons, enter muscles by penetrating the epimysium and branch to form small nerves, which run in the perimysium.

Perimysial nerves contain axons to fulfil both motor and sensory functions. The motor axons destined to innervate skeletal muscle (α efferent fibres) enter the endomysium as nerve twigs and branch to innervate several fibres.

At the end of each twig, the axon becomes modified to form a motor endplate, and it is this that activates skeletal muscle contraction (Fig. 13.8).

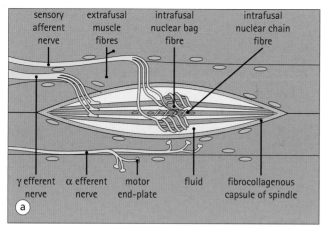
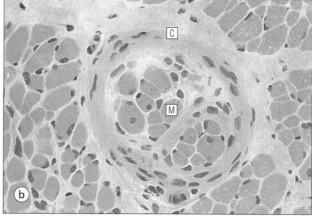

FIGURE 13.7 Sensory innervation of skeletal muscle. (a) The sensory innervation of muscle, which arises from two sources: encapsulated nerve endings in the tendons respond to stretch, and spiral nerve endings in muscle spindles sense stretch and tension. The muscle spindle is composed of a fusiform capsule of fibrocollagenous tissue (continuous with the perimysium) surrounding a group of 8–15 thin muscle fibres. These fibres are termed 'intrafusal fibres' to distinguish them from normal skeletal muscle fibres (extrafusal fibres). Two types of intrafusal fibres can be distinguished: those with a fusiform shape and a central aggregate of nuclei (nuclear bag fibres), and those of uniform width with dispersed nuclei (nuclear chain fibres). Specialized motor nerve fibres (gamma (γ) efferent fibres) innervate the intrafusal fibres and adjust their length according to the state of stretch of the muscle, which is detected by spiral nerve endings. The spiral nerve endings are wrapped around the intrafusal fibres and form special sensory afferent fibres running back to the spinal cord. (b) Micrograph of frozen section from a child's muscle showing a muscle spindle, identified by its circular fibrocollagenous capsule (C) and its content of intrafusal muscle fibres (M).

Activation of the motor axon causes the release of acetylcholine from its storage granules by exocytosis. Acetylcholine then diffuses across the gap between the axon and muscle fibre and interacts with specific membrane receptors to cause depolarization of the muscle fibre, which initiates contraction (see p. 73).

The activity of secreted acetylcholine is rapidly curtailed by the activity of an enzyme called 'acetylcholinesterase', which is bound to the basement membrane investing the junctional folds.

In addition to nerve fibres controlling voluntary movement, specialized motor axons (γ efferent fibres) innervate fibres in the muscle spindle.

CLINICAL EXAMPLE
MYASTHENIA GRAVIS

Myasthenia gravis is a disease caused by the formation of antibodies to the acetylcholine receptor on the sarcolemma in the junctional folds of the motor endplates. The antibodies bind to the acetylcholine receptors and thereby prevent released acetylcholine from interacting with the receptors and causing depolarization.

Affected individuals develop tremendous muscle weakness manifest by fatiguability, inability to lift the arms, failure to maintain an upright posture of the head, and drooping of the eyelids.

Treatment is by the administration of drugs (anticholinesterases) that inhibit the action of the enzyme acetylcholinesterase. This potentiates the action of released acetylcholine and allows it to bind to receptors not blocked by antibody.

Myasthenia gravis is an autoimmune disease.

Muscle Attachments

In order to transmit the force of contraction, the cell surface at the end of the muscle fibres is adapted for attachment to highly organized fibrocollagenous support tissues, which anchor the muscle to other structures.

Such anchorage may be provided by:
- Anatomically distinct tendons
- Broad areas of anchorage to a bony surface
- Broad areas of anchorage to sheets of fibrocollagenous support tissue (fascia) which run between muscles.

Tendons attach some muscles to bone

Muscles are connected to bone by dense compact collagenous tissue called 'tendinous tissue', which may be in the form of short sheets attaching to bone over a large area, often linear, or long cylindrical structures which connect some muscles to the bones of hands and fingers, and feet and toes. The largest and most distinct of the cylindrical type of tendons is the Achilles tendon, which connects the substantial muscle masses of the back of the calf with the bones at the back of the foot, involved in flexion and extension of the foot. A series of long cylindrical tendons run through the hands to the fingers.

Tendinous tissue is composed of tightly packed, longitudinally running collagen fibres, with the elongated flattened muscle nuclei of inactive fibrocytes scattered between them (Fig. 13.9). In tendon, these fibrocytes are sometimes called 'tenocytes' or 'tendinocytes'.

Tendinous tissue is relatively acellular and has both low oxygen/nutrient requirements and a very limited blood supply. Because of this poor vascularity, tendons that have been damaged by trauma (usually due to acute

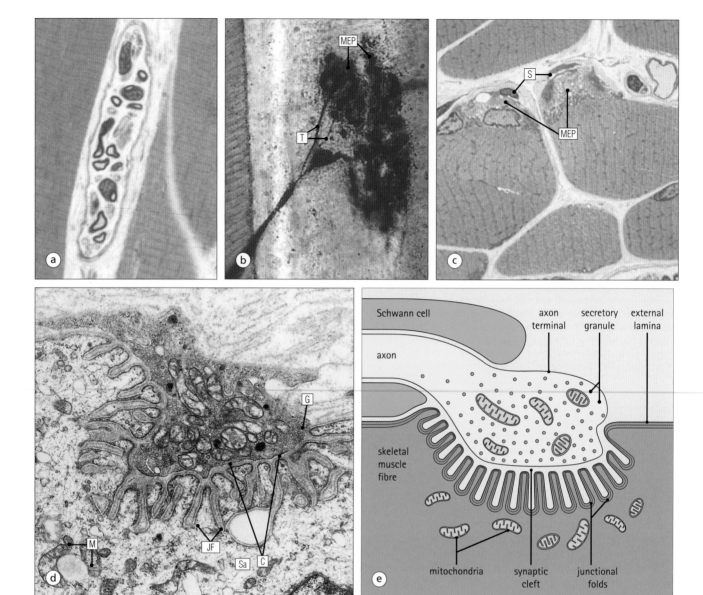

FIGURE 13.8 **Motor innervation of skeletal muscle.** (a) A thin resin section of skeletal muscle stained with toluidine blue showing a small perimysial nerve, which contains both motor (efferent) and sensory (afferent) fibres. (b) A methylene blue-stained teased preparation of muscle showing several nerve twigs (T) branching from a single axon to innervate muscle fibres. There is a bulbous swelling (the motor endplate, MEP) at the end of each twig at the site of connection with the muscle. The group of fibres innervated by a single axon is a motor unit. (c) Micrograph of a thin resin section of skeletal muscle stained with toluidine blue to show the motor endplate (MEP). The axon terminates in a dome-shaped swelling of the nerve terminal in direct apposition to the cell membrane of the muscle fibre, to form the MEP. This is invested by a layer of Schwann cell cytoplasm (S). (d) Electron micrograph of a motor endplate showing the cell membrane of the muscle fibre thrown into a series of deep folds (junctional folds, JF) beneath which the sarcoplasm (Sa) contains numerous mitochondria (M). In the terminal swelling of the motor axon, neurosecretory granules (G), containing the transmitter substance acetylcholine, and mitochondria are abundant. The terminal swelling of the axon is separated from the muscle cell membrane by a gap of 30–50 nm (the synaptic cleft, C), which includes the external lamina of the muscle. (e) The motor endplate. The sarcoplasmic membrane in the region of the motor endplate contains specialized receptors which, when activated by acetylcholine, permit muscle cell membrane depolarization.

overstretching, particularly in sporting injuries) are extremely slow to heal, e.g. Achilles tendon rupture, extensor tendonitis in the elbow ('tennis elbow').

Tendons attach to skeletal muscles at specialized structures called myotendinous junctions

The collagen fibres of tendons are firmly tethered to the muscle fibres of skeletal muscles at specialized areas called **myotendinous insertions** or **junctions** (Fig. 13.10).

At these sites, individual muscle fibres develop a complex interdigitating surface, which is tightly anchored to the collagen fibres of the intramuscular portion of the end of the tendon.

Many tendons lie within fibrocollagenous tendon sheaths

Where the long cylindrical type of tendon has to run over the surface of bone it must be protected from damage

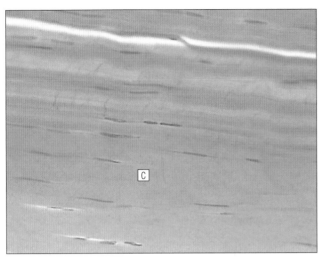

FIGURE 13.9 **Tendon.** Micrograph of tendon showing highly organized regular bundles of collagen (C) with a few interspersed fibrocytes.

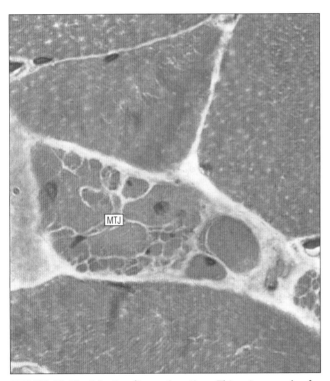

FIGURE 13.10 **Myotendinous junction.** This micrograph of a myotendinous junction (MTJ), shows apparent splitting of the rounded contour of a muscle fibre to form several small rounded structures separated by fibrocollagenous tissue. Such splitting of the terminal portion of the fibre increases the surface area available for anchorage to support tissues and thus contributes to the mechanical strength of insertion.

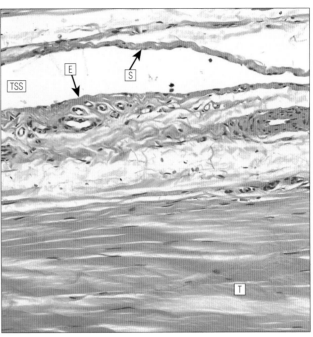

FIGURE 13.11 **Tendon sheath.** This long flexor tendon (T) from the finger has an epitendineum (E) coated by flat mesothelial cells on its outer surface. A thin fibrous tendon sheath (S) has a similar layer of flat mesothelial cells on its inner surface. The tendon sheath space (TSS) contains thin lubricating fluid secreted by the mesothelial cells.

due to repeated friction. An example is the long flexor tendons of the hand running to the fingers. This protection from friction damage is achieved by the tendon having a thin outer fibrous capsule sometimes called the **epitendineum**, coated on its outer surface by flat mesothelial cells, which are synovial in type and secrete small amounts of lubricating fluid similar to that which lubricates synovial joints (see p. 260). Such tendons are surrounded by a thin collagenous sheath which is lined internally by similar synovial-type mesothelial cells, also secreting lubricating fluid. This structure is called the **tendon sheath**, and the synovium related to the epitendineum and the tendon sheath is called **tenosynovium**. Thus, the tendon can slide effortlessly and without friction within a lubricated sheath (Fig. 13.11).

Despite these preventive measures, repeated overuse of some tendons (particularly in the hands) can lead to structural damage to both epitendineum and tendon sheath, which is manifest as a painful condition localized to the affected tendon ('tendonitis'). Various forms of tendonitis, particularly those affecting the hands and arms, are often regarded as components of so-called 'repetitive strain injury'.

Tendon is attached to bone by fibres which pass through the periosteum and penetrate into the bone

At the attachment to bone, the type I collagen fibres of a tendon merge with the type I collagen of the periosteum and send fibres that penetrate into the bone (Fig. 13.12). These are called Sharpey's fibres.

The original tendon collagen is probably incorporated into bone when the periosteum makes new bone, initially in bone development in intrauterine life, and is continually reinforced in periods of high periosteal activity during bone growth in childhood.

Maintenance of the tendon at the site of the bone attachment is the responsibility of the collagen-synthesizing fibroblasts of the periosteum. These cells

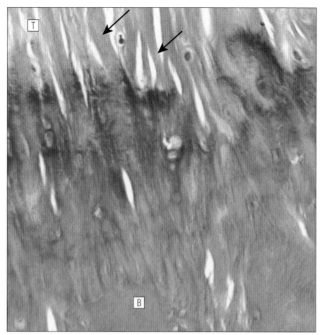

FIGURE 13.12 **Tendon insertion into bone.** Collagen fibres (arrows) from tendon (T) insert obliquely into bone (B). These are called 'Sharpey's fibres'. Other tendon collagen fibres merge with collagen fibres of the periosteum.

have the capacity to convert into chondroprogenitor cells (chondroblast precursors) or osteoprogenitor cells (osteoblast precursors, see Fig. 13.16). For this reason, the tendon close to its attachment to the bone may contain small islands of cartilage or bone.

Other important structures in the musculoskeletal system have a structure similar to that of tendon

Ligaments join one bone to another (see Fig. 13.29). Like tendons, they are composed of tightly packed collagen fibres running predominantly in the same direction, but less regularly than in long cylindrical tendons, with inactive elongated fibrocytes lying between the collagen bundles. In some areas there is a need for the ligaments to have elasticity, for example in the prominent and extensive ligaments that help to bind the bones of the vertebral column together (e.g. ligamentum flavum). In such areas the ligament contains abundant elastic fibres which also run, regularly spaced, parallel with the collagen fibres; these are sometimes called **elastic ligaments**.

Aponeuroses are flat sheets, often extensive, of tendon-like compact fibrocollagenous tissue, which may connect muscle to muscle (e.g. in the anterior abdominal wall), muscle to bone at an insertion, or muscle to long cylindrical types of tendon. Thus, many aponeuroses can be considered to be part of the tendinous system. Because the muscle fibres are attached to an aponeurosis in different directions, the component collagen of the aponeurosis is arranged in layers that run in different directions. Large aponeuroses are found in the palms and soles.

Bone

Introduction

Bone is a highly specialized support tissue which is characterized by its rigidity and hardness. Its four main functions are to provide **mechanical support** (e.g. ribs), to permit **locomotion** (e.g. long bones), to provide **protection** (e.g. skull) and to act as a **metabolic reservoir** of mineral salts.

Bone is composed of:
- Support cells (osteoblasts and osteocytes)
- A non-mineral matrix of collagen and glycosaminoglycans (osteoid)
- Inorganic mineral salts deposited within the matrix
- Remodelling cells (osteoclasts).

Bone contains a specialized extracellular matrix material called osteoid

Osteoid is a collagenous support tissue of type I collagen embedded in a glycosaminoglycan gel containing specific glycoproteins (e.g. osteocalcin) that strongly bind calcium. Deposition of mineral salts in the osteoid gives bone its characteristic rigidity and functional strength.

Osteoid is synthesized by specialized support cells called 'osteoblasts', which have the same collagen synthesis capacity as fibroblasts (see p. 63). Formed calcified bone can be eroded by osteoclasts, modified multinucleate phagocytic cells belonging to the monocyte/macrophage family (see p. 128).

Coordinated activity of osteoclasts (eroding formed bone) and osteoblasts (synthesized new osteoid) is important in maintaining bone structure, and any structural modifications necessary to meet increased or altered demands. This is called 'bone remodelling'.

Bone is constantly being remodelled

Bone is a dynamic tissue, being continually formed and destroyed under the control of hormonal and physical factors. This constant activity permits the process of modelling (i.e. modification of the bone architecture to meet physical stresses).

Bone turnover is normally low in adults, but in babies and children it is high to allow the growth and active remodelling required to cope with new demands, for example with the onset of walking.

In the adult, bone turnover can increase from its normal basal level to meet any increased demand, for example to increase bone bulk necessary for coping with increased physical activity, e.g. running, jumping and climbing in sporting activities, and in the repair of bone fracture. In addition, increased bone turnover and remodelling can be the result of pathological processes, for example following the excessive secretion of parathyroid hormone by overactive parathyroid glands or a parathyroid tumour (see pp. 273-274). Another example is Paget's disease (see below and p. 255 in the 'Clinical Example' box). In these cases, the bone remodelling is chaotic and random, and not related to the need to counter physical stress; thus the

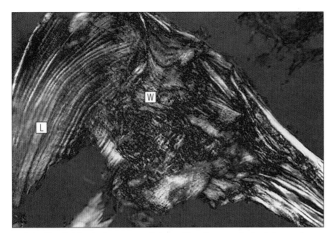

FIGURE 13.13 **Woven and lamellar bone.** Polarizing micrograph of repairing bone showing both recently formed woven bone (W) at the centre and original lamellar bone (L) on either side. Note the haphazard arrangement of the collagen fibres in the woven bone and the regular parallel arrangement in the lamellar bone.

bone architecture is seriously damaged, and symptoms such as pain and predisposition to fracture ensue.

Bone modelling is discussed in greater detail later.

The two main patterns of bone are called woven and lamellar

Two types of bone can be identified according to the pattern of collagen forming the osteoid:
- **Woven** bone is characterized by haphazard organization of collagen fibres and is mechanically weak
- **Lamellar** bone is characterized by a regular parallel alignment of collagen into sheets (lamellae) and is mechanically strong (Fig. 13.13).

Woven bone is produced when osteoblasts produce osteoid rapidly; the collagen fibres are deposited in an irregular, loosely intertwined pattern. This occurs initially in all fetal bones (see Fig. 13.25), but in this case, the resulting woven bone is gradually replaced by remodelling and the deposition of more resilient lamellar bone.

In adults, woven bone is created when there is very rapid new bone formation, as occurs in the repair of a fracture or in Paget's disease (see Fig. 13.24). Following a fracture woven bone is remodelled and lamellar bone is deposited, but in Paget's disease the woven bone persists and leads to mechanical weakness and bone deformity. Virtually all bone in the healthy adult is lamellar.

Bones have a dense outer cortex and an inner trabecular region

Most bones have a basic architecture composed of:
- An outer cortical or compact zone
- An inner trabecular or spongy zone.

Cortical bone forms a rigid outer shell that resists deformation, whereas the inner trabecular meshwork provides strength by acting as a complex system of

KEY FACTS
OSTEOID

- Is a specialized form of type I collagen embedded in a glycosaminoglycan gel
- The supporting gel contains specific proteins, e.g. osteocalcin, which have affinity for calcium
- Is synthesized and secreted by osteoblasts, which also orchestrate deposition of mineral salts
- May be deposited by osteoblasts in regular parallel sheets (lamellar) or haphazardly (woven)
- Healthy bone formed from lamellar osteoid is strong and efficient
- Bone formed from woven osteoid is comparatively weak, bulky and inefficient, and is usually pathological, resulting from fracture or Paget's disease.

CLINICAL EXAMPLE
ABNORMALITIES OF BONE ARCHITECTURE

Abnormal bone architecture may result from:

- Damage both to cortical and trabecular bone due to fracture
- Decreased cortical and trabecular bone due to osteoporosis
- Destruction of trabecular bone due to cancer
- Maldevelopment of bone
- Metabolic bone disease (see 'Clinical Example' boxes, pp. 254-255).

Osteoporosis

In old age, both cortical and trabecular bone become thinned (osteoporosis, see Fig. 13.23) and are therefore more fragile and more prone to fracture. Fracture of the neck of the femur is common in the elderly. Osteoporosis may also develop following disuse, for example in the leg bones of a wheelchair-bound person.

There is evidence that hormonal disturbances may induce osteoporosis in postmenopausal women.

Bone Involvement in Cancer

The bone marrow is a common site of spread of some forms of cancer, particularly cancers that originate in the breast (see Fig. 18.31), bronchus, prostate, thyroid and kidney. Proliferation of tumour cells frequently destroys the trabecular bone, and thus leads to an increased tendency to bone fracture (pathological fracture), an important complication of widespread cancer.

Maldevelopment

There are a number of diseases arising from impaired bone formation during embryological development. Many of these are incompatible with survival and such children commonly die in utero or shortly after birth. The most common maldevelopment of bone that is compatible with life is achondroplasia, resulting in a form of dwarfism characterized by a normal-sized trunk but short limb bones.

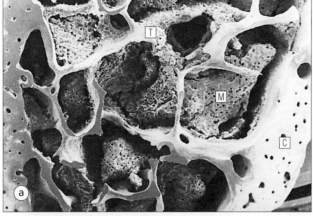

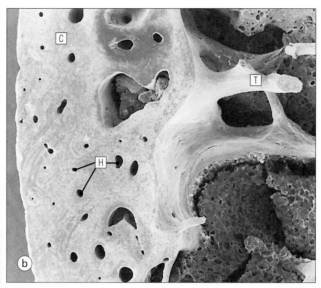

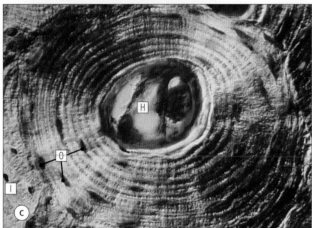

FIGURE 13.14 **Bone architecture: cortical and trabecular bone.** (a) Low-power scanning electron micrograph showing the architecture of bone (cortical and trabecular) and its relationship to bone marrow (see Chapter 7). The cortical bone (C) is dense and forms a compact outer shell which is bridged by narrow, delicate plates of trabecular bone (T). The spaces between the trabecular bone are occupied by yellow marrow (adipose tissue) or haemopoietic red marrow. Here the marrow (M) has retracted from the bone during tissue preparation. (b) Medium-power scanning electron micrograph showing more detail of cortical (C) and trabecular bone (T). The outlines of a number of Haversian systems (H) of various sizes, each with a central canal, can be seen. (c) Polarizing micrograph of a single osteon (Haversian system). A central Haversian canal (H) is surrounded by concentric layers of lamellar bone, which contains a number of dark black spaces marking the sites of osteocytes (O). Outside the Haversian system are less regularly arranged interstitial bone lamellae (I), which act as packing between adjacent Haversian systems.

internal struts. The spaces between the trabecular meshwork are occupied by bone marrow (see Chapter 7).

In bones with a substantial weight-bearing function the trabecular pattern is arranged to provide maximum resistance to the physical stresses to which that bone is normally subjected.

The specialized support cells of the bone reside either on its surfaces or within small spaces in formed bone termed 'lacunae'.

The details of normal bone architecture are shown in Figures 13.14 and 13.15.

Bone Cells

Four main types of cell maintain bone

Cells concerned with the production, maintenance and modelling of the osteoid are:
- Osteoprogenitor cells
- Osteoblasts
- Osteocytes
- Osteoclasts.

Osteoprogenitor cells are the stem cells of bone and form osteoblasts

Osteoprogenitor cells are derived from primitive mesenchymal cells. They form a population of stem cells that can differentiate into the more specialized bone-forming cells (i.e. osteoblasts and osteocytes).

In mature bone in which there is no active new bone formation or remodelling, the osteoprogenitor cells become flattened spindle cells closely applied to the bone surface, when they are sometimes called 'inactive osteoblasts'.

In actively growing bone, however, for example in fetal bone or in a period of high turnover in adult bone, these cells are much larger and more numerous, containing plump oval nuclei and more abundant spindle-shaped cytoplasm (Fig. 13.16), converting to cuboidal active osteoblasts.

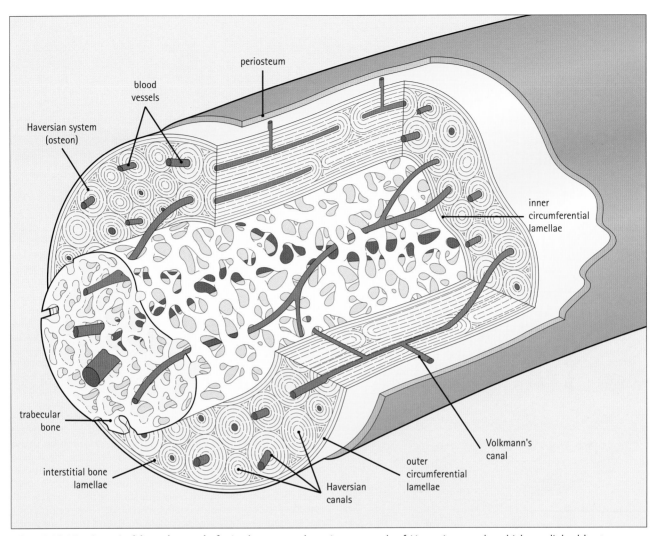

FIGURE 13.15 **A typical long bone shaft.** In the cortex there is a network of Haversian canals, which are linked by transverse Volkmann's canals. The canals contain blood vessels and some nerves. Each Haversian canal is surrounded by concentric layers of lamellar bone. These layers contain concentrically arranged rings of osteocytes, each lying in its small lacuna and communicating with osteocytes in its own and adjacent layers through cytoplasmic processes lying in narrow canaliculi. The Haversian canal and its concentric bone and osteocyte system is called a Haversian system or osteon. The interior of each Haversian canal is lined by flat osteoprogenitor cells or inactive osteoblasts, as are the inner surface of the cortical bone plate and the outer surfaces of the bone trabeculae. This layer, called the endosteum, provides a source of new osteoblasts necessary for new bone formation if remodelling is needed. Cortical remodelling in the Haversian canals is common. The Haversian canal systems, interspersed with irregularly arranged interstitial bone lamellae which act as packing, occupy the bulk of the cortex; inner and outer circumferential bone lamellae separate the Haversian systems from the endosteum and the outer surface of the bone, the fibrocollagenous periosteum. The strong, dense cortical bone encloses the medullary cavity comprising bone marrow and an interconnecting network of trabecular bone, providing strength with lightness.

FIGURE 13.16 **Osteoprogenitor cells.** Micrograph of toluidine blue-stained epoxy resin section showing numerous plump spindle-shaped osteoprogenitor (Op) cells in the developing skull bone of a 15-week human fetus. Derived from primitive mesenchymal cells, they are transformed into osteoblasts (Ob), which are larger and more cuboidal. The osteoblasts have begun to deposit osteoid collagen (C).

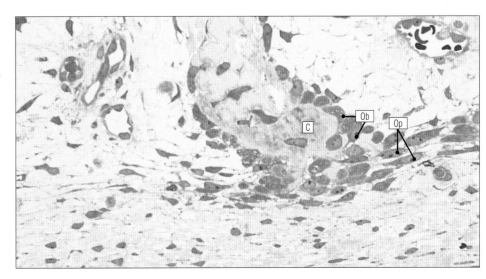

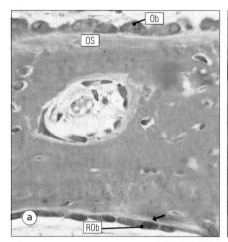

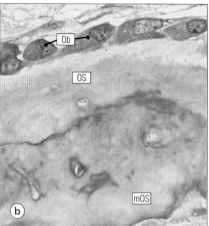

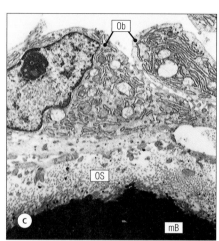

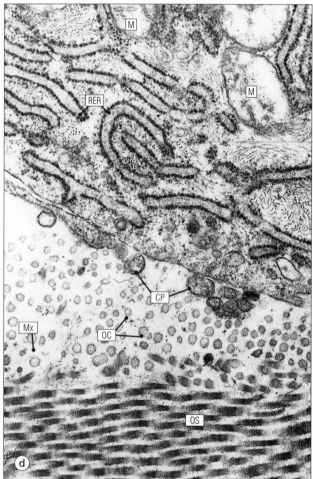

FIGURE 13.17 **Osteoblasts.** (a) Micrograph of an acrylic resin section of actively growing fetal bone stained by Goldner's method, which distinguishes mineralized bone (turquoise) from unmineralized osteoid. Note the zone of unmineralized newly formed osteoid (OS) adjacent to the row of actively synthesizing osteoblasts (Ob) on one side of the trabeculum. On the other side, a layer of now-flattened osteoblasts has entered an inactive resting phase (ROb) and its recently formed osteoid is now almost fully mineralized (arrow). (b) Micrograph of a toluidine blue-stained thin epoxy resin section of actively growing bone, with a row of cuboidal osteoblasts (Ob) actively synthesizing and secreting organic matrix (osteoid, OS); the cells have bulky baso-philic cytoplasm owing to their protein-synthesizing rough endo-plasmic reticulum. Some of the osteoid is lightly mineralized (mOS). (c) Low-power electron micrograph showing an osteo-blast (Ob) at the face of newly forming bone. Note the zone of unmineralized osteoid (OS), which has recently formed between the active osteoblast and the older mineralized bone (mB). (d) High-power electron micrograph showing the characteristic cytoplasmic features of an active osteoblast. The cytoplasm is rich in rough endoplasmic reticulum (RER) and there are promi-nent mitochondria (M); the collagenic protein precursors and glycosaminoglycans are synthesized in the RER and then pack-aged in the Golgi prior to transfer to the cell surface in secretory vesicles. The cell surface shows numerous cytoplasmic processes (CP), particularly on the face in contact with existing osteoid (OS). The secretory vesicles discharge their contents from this surface to form identifiable osteoid collagen fibres (OC) embed-ded in an electron-lucent matrix (Mx) of glycosaminoglycans and proteoglycans. The formation and secretion of collagen is described on page 56.

Osteoblasts synthesize the organic component of the bone matrix (osteoid)

Osteoid consists of type I collagen, glycosaminoglycans and proteoglycans.

When fully active, osteoblasts are cuboidal or polygo-nal cells. They have basophilic cytoplasm, which reflects the abundance of rough endoplasmic reticulum in their cytoplasm, resulting from their role as active protein-synthesizing and -secreting cells. For details of osteoblast structure and function, see Figures 13.17 and 13.20.

Osteocytes are inactive osteoblasts trapped in mineralized bone

When osteoblasts have completed a burst of osteoid-producing activity, most return to an inactive state, becoming flattened and spindle-shaped and closely applied to the now-inactive bone surface. Some

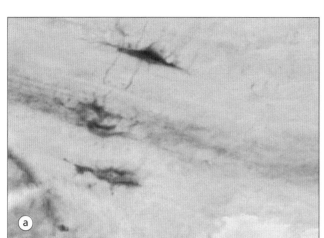
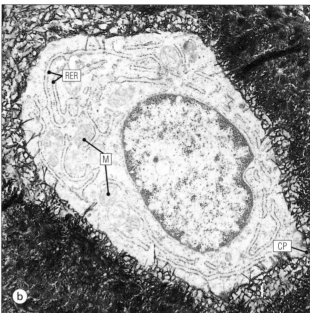

FIGURE 13.18 **Osteocytes.** (a) Micrograph of a toluidine blue-stained acrylic resin section of bone showing osteocytes trapped within mineralized bone matrix. Note their fine cytoplasmic processes, which lie in narrow canalicular channels in the mineralized bone and link one osteocyte with another. (b) Electron micrograph of a recently entrapped osteocyte. It shows some of the cytoplasmic rough endoplasmic reticulum (RER) and mitochondria (M) of the osteoblast from which it is derived. Note the origin of one of its cytoplasmic processes (CP), the rest being out of the plane of section.

osteoblasts, however, become surrounded by mineralizing bone matrix and lie within small cavities (lacunae) in the bone. When this happens, the cell is called an 'osteocyte' (Fig. 13.18).

Adjacent osteocytes can communicate with each other via long cytoplasmic processes that lie in narrow channels called 'canaliculi'. Usually, they are arranged haphazardly, but in cortical bone they assume a regular pattern (see pp. 248-249).

The function of osteocytes is not known, but each osteocyte in its lacuna maintains a narrow zone of osteoid around it and retains the prominent Golgi and a fraction of the rough endoplasmic reticulum of its parent osteoblast. This suggests that it may be able to maintain the organic matrix.

Through their interconnecting cytoplasmic processes, osteocytes receive nutrients sufficient to survive. They may also resorb formed bone matrix to release calcium (a process called 'osteocytic osteolysis'), though the evidence for this is poor.

Osteoclasts erode mineralized bone

Osteoclasts are large cells with multiple nuclei and abundant cytoplasm that are derived from precursors in the myeloid/monocyte lineage that circulate in the blood after their formation in the bone marrow. These osteoclast precursors are attracted to sites on bone surfaces destined for resorption and fuse with one another to form multinucleated cells.

Osteoclasts are found attached to the bone surface at sites of active bone resorption, often in depres-

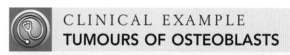

CLINICAL EXAMPLE
TUMOURS OF OSTEOBLASTS

Osteosarcoma

The most important tumour derived from bone cells is osteosarcoma, which is a malignant tumour of osteoblasts. It is most common in children and adolescents and usually involves the bones around the knee joint, either the lower end of the femur or the upper end of the tibia.

The tumour cells resemble osteoblasts in both structure and function, in that they synthesize osteoid; however, the production of osteoid is scanty, haphazard and irregular, and it does not mineralize normally.

The malignant osteoblasts are largely primitive and more closely resemble immature osteoprogenitor cells than mature osteoblasts.

Osteosarcoma spreads extensively via the bloodstream, often producing secondary (metastatic) tumours in the lungs.

Benign tumours of osteoblasts (osteoid osteomas) occur as localized swellings in bones, often painful. They may enlarge slowly, but do not spread to distant sites.

sions where they have eroded into the bone. These depressions are called 'resorption bays' or 'Howship's lacunae'.

For details of osteoclast structure and function, see Figure 13.19.

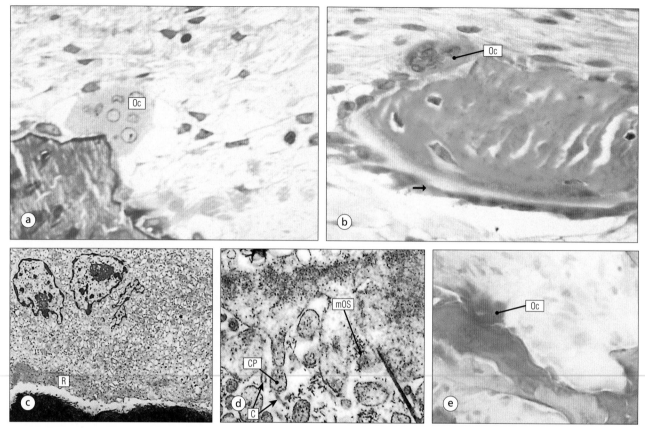

FIGURE 13.19 **Osteoclast.** (a) Micrograph of a toluidine blue-stained epoxy resin thin section showing a single osteoclast (Oc), which has alighted on an irregular spur of bone prior to reabsorption. At a later stage, the spur of bone will have been eroded and levelled as a result of osteoclast activity. (b) Micrograph of Goldner-stained acrylic resin section of bone showing active resorption of bone on one face, with a multinucleate osteoclast (Oc) lying in a Howship's lacuna. There is active osteoblast deposition of new osteoid on the other face (arrow), in a bone that is undergoing active modelling (see Fig. 13.21). (c) Electron micrograph of an osteoclast, demonstrating its richness in Golgi, lysosomes, secretory vesicles, and mitochondria. At its interface with the bone, highly complex cytoplasmic protrusions from the osteoclast's surface appear as a ruffled border (R). (d) High-power electron micrograph of the ruffled border region where numerous fine cytoplasmic processes (CP) extend from the surface of the osteoclast, some interdigitating with the collagenic fibres (C) of the osteoid. Fragments of mineralized osteoid (mOS) can be seen between the cytoplasmic processes. (e) Micrograph of a frozen section of bone demonstrating abundant acid phosphatase activity (red) in an osteoclast (Oc), which is actively eroding the bone surface.

Mineralization of Osteoid

Rigidity of bone is determined by deposition of minerals

The hardness and rigidity of bone is due to the presence of mineral salt in the osteoid matrix. This salt is a crystalline complex of calcium and phosphate hydroxides called 'hydroxyapatite' ($Ca_{10}(PO_4)_6(OH)_2$).

For mineralization to occur, the combined local concentrations of Ca^{2+} ions and PO_4^- ions must be above a threshold value. A number of factors operate to bring this about:

- A glycoprotein (osteocalcin) in osteoid binds extracellular Ca^{2+} ions, leading to a high local concentration
- The enzyme alkaline phosphatase, which is abundant in osteoblasts, increases local Ca^{2+} and PO_4^- ion concentrations
- Osteoblasts produce matrix vesicles, which can accumulate Ca^{2+} and PO_4^- ions, and are rich in the enzymes alkaline phosphatase and pyrophosphatase, both of which can cleave PO_4^- ions from larger molecules.

Matrix vesicles are round membrane-bound vesicles which are probably derived from the cell membrane. During osteoid formation they bud off from the osteoblast into the matrix and form the nidus for the initial precipitation of hydroxyapatite.

It is currently believed that osteoblast-derived matrix vesicles are the most important factor controlling the initial site of mineral deposition in osteoid, and that, once the first few crystals of hydroxyapatite have precipitated out, they grow rapidly by accretion until they join foci growing from other matrix vesicles. In this way, a wave of mineralization sweeps through new osteoid (Fig. 13.20).

Other cells that produce matrix vesicles are the ameloblasts and odontoblasts of the developing tooth (see p. 191) and chondrocytes; hence the frequent mineralization of cartilage.

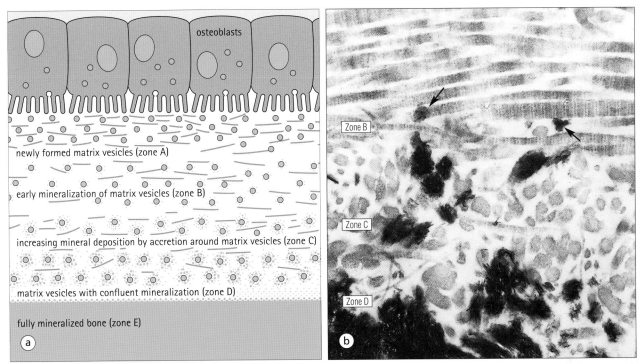

FIGURE 13.20 Mineralization of bone. (a) The events believed to occur in a newly formed osteoid. Immediately adjacent to the irregular osteoblast surface is a zone A of freshly deposited osteoid collagen and glycosaminoglycan containing newly formed matrix vesicles. Next is a zone B in which early crystals of hydroxyapatite are being deposited in slightly older matrix vesicles, and beyond it a zone C in which the foci of mineralization rapidly enlarge by accretion of mineral salts. In zone D, the individual foci of mineralization, each centred on a matrix vesicle remnant, have become almost completely confluent. In zone E, mineralization is complete and the underlying osteoid collagen is obscured. The junction between zones C and D is the so-called calcification front, but as this term is used inaccurately in an entirely different context in pathological studies of bone disease, it is best avoided unless carefully defined. (b) High-power electron micrograph showing early mineral deposition in a zone of recently formed osteoid from fetal bone. Note the early crystalline pattern of mineralization of a matrix vesicle (arrows) in zone B, enlargement of foci of mineralization in zone C, becoming confluent in zone D. Zones A and E are not shown.

If the local concentrations of Ca^{2+} and PO_4^- ions are normal, then mineralization occurs shortly after the new osteoid has been formed. However, when there is a state of high turnover, the osteoblasts produce large amounts of osteoid in a short time and mineralization lags behind, catching up only when the rate of new osteoid production falls.

During a lag phase, distinct layers of unmineralized osteoid can be seen between the layer of active osteoblasts and the previously mineralized bone. This is evident in the phases of rapid bone growth in fetal life, and also in adult life during periods of active remodelling of bone, such as following fracture or as part of some disease processes.

Bone Modelling

Following initial deposition the bone matrix and the struts forming trabecular bone are remodelled

In rapid bone growth during fetal development and childhood, large quantities of bone are produced by osteoblastic synthesis of bone matrix, which is subsequently mineralized. The subsequent pattern of remodelling is determined by local mechanical stresses, so that the bone matrix is aligned to resist local shearing and compressive stresses.

Modelling is achieved by a carefully balanced combination of:
- New bone deposition and mineralization by active osteoblasts (see Fig. 13.20)
- Selective resorption of formed bone by osteoclasts (Fig. 13.21).

Selective resorption of formed bone occurs where the osteoclast is in contact with the bone surface

Resorption of bone is believed to proceed as follows:
- Lysosomal enzymes are released from the osteoclast cytoplasm where it is in contact with the bone
- The released enzymes hydrolyze the collagenous protein and glycosaminoglycans of the adjacent bone matrix
- The disrupted bone matrix yields up its attached mineral salts
- Local acidic conditions, which possibly result from the secretion of organic acids, such as carbonic, lactic and citric acids by the osteoclasts, break up the hydroxyapatite, thereby releasing soluble Ca^{2+} and PO_4^- ions

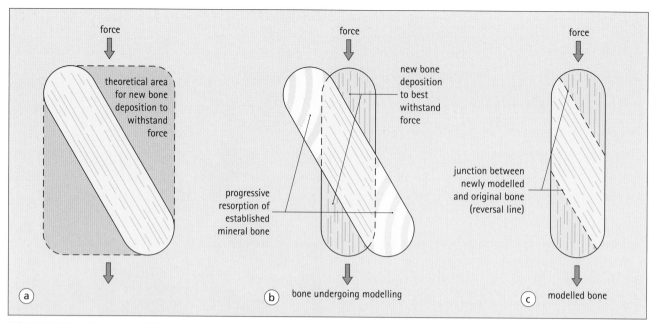

FIGURE 13.21 Bone modelling. (a) A piece of bone inappropriately orientated to best withstand the direction of the force to which it is exposed. The force could be resisted by deposition of new bone on the old in the area indicated, but this would produce a large heavy block of bone which, if repeated throughout the body as a whole, would result in such a bulky mass that movement would be impossible. A more efficient strength to weight ratio is achieved by modelling. (b) How the bone can be modelled to become more efficient. The junctions between original bone and newly modelled bone are not easily seen in histological sections of mineralized bone, but are evident when decalcified sections are examined, particularly if the section is examined in polarized light, which accentuates the different directions of the osteoid collagen fibres. The junctions between different phases of bone deposition in different directions are called reversal lines, and are particularly numerous and haphazard when bone modelling has been random and uncontrolled, as in Paget's disease. (c) Final modelled bone with reversal lines.

CLINICAL EXAMPLE
OSTEOMALACIA (FAILURE OF MINERALIZATION)

Mineralization of osteoid can take place only if there are sufficient Ca^{2+} and PO_4^- ions.

If the blood level of Ca^{2+} ions is low (e.g. due to inadequate dietary intake by vegans, or to malabsorption resulting from small intestinal disease), or if PO_4^- ion levels are low (which is uncommon, and usually due to excessive PO_4^- ion loss in the urine), then mineralization is impaired. This leads to the disease known as 'osteomalacia' (Fig. 13.22).

Patients with osteomalacia develop softening of the bone, which results in an increased tendency to fracture, either major fractures or a series of smaller microfractures producing bone pain.

Osteomalacia in the growing bones of children leads to the disease called 'rickets' and produces permanent deformity of the soft, poorly mineralized bones.

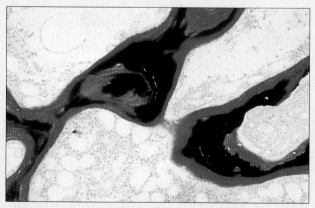

FIGURE 13.22 Osteomalacia. Micrograph of iliac crest bone embedded in acrylic resin without prior decalcification from a patient with osteomalacia. Note the broad zone of unmineralized osteoid (purple) and the central zone of mineralized bone (black) in this section stained by von Kossa's silver technique.

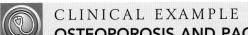

CLINICAL EXAMPLE
OSTEOPOROSIS AND PAGET'S DISEASE

Osteoporosis (Fig. 13.23) can occur as a result of disuse (e.g. prolonged bed rest, limb paralysis), and also in people who are otherwise healthy, particularly postmenopausal women. It results in an increased tendency to bone fracture, particularly compression fractures of vertebrae.

Paget's disease is of unknown cause but probably involves a combination of environmental and genetic factors, which cause uncontrolled osteoclast activity, leading to resorption of bone and osteoblastic attempts to fill in the remaining erosions (Fig. 13.24).

When the wave of osteoclastic resorption dies down or moves elsewhere, the osteoblasts continue to produce new bone in an attempt to repair the damage. Thus, paradoxically, the affected piece of bone usually ends up larger than it was originally.

The repaired bone is, however, less able to resist physical stress because the new bone deposition is haphazard and reparative, rather than organized and constructive; it is therefore more prone to fracture.

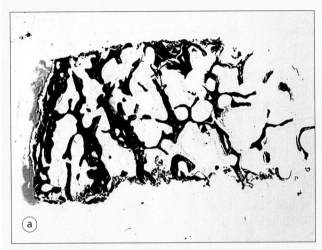

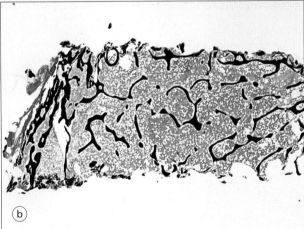

FIGURE 13.23 **Osteoporosis.** (a) Micrograph of a resin section of a bone biopsy from the iliac crest (see Fig. 1.1) showing normal cortical and trabecular bone stained with a silver method, which makes calcified bone show up as black. (b) Micrograph of bone from a patient with osteoporosis. When compared with (a), which shows bone mass of a healthy patient of the same age, it is clear that the cortical zone is narrower, and that the trabeculae are thinner and less numerous.

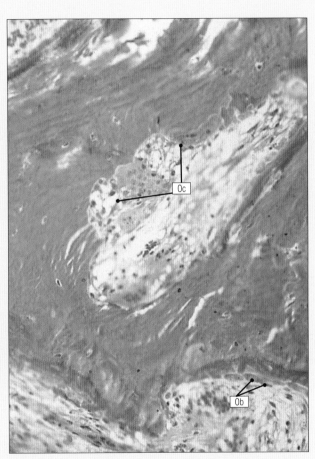

FIGURE 13.24 **Paget's disease.** Micrograph of a resin-embedded Goldner-stained section from a patient with active Paget's disease. There is uncontrolled osteoclast (Oc) resorption of a bone, and osteoblasts (Ob) are attempting to fill in sites of recent osteoclast erosion in an adjacent site.

- Some of the soluble breakdown products of demineralization and protein hydrolysis may be resorbed by the osteoclast by endocytosis.

Osteoclasts are highly mobile and resorb bone as they move along the bone surface.

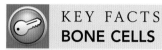

KEY FACTS
BONE CELLS

Osteoprogenitor Cells

- Are precursors of osteoblasts

Osteoblasts

- Synthesize osteoid collagen, then mineralize it by depositing calcium and phosphate hydroxides (hydroxyapatite)
- Produce matrix vesicles rich in Ca^{2+} and PO_4^- ions and the enzymes alkaline phosphatase and pyrophosphatase, essential for mineralization
- Are only large, metabolically active cells when there is a requirement for new osteoid deposition; when inactive they are insignificant spindle cells lying on the bone surface (bone lining cells)

Osteocytes

- Are inactive osteoblasts trapped within the bone they have made

Osteoclasts

- Are multinucleate cells derived from blood monocytes
- Are highly mobile cells capable of eroding mineralized bone by enzymic hydrolysis of osteoid collagen, with release of bone minerals
- Osteoclastic resorption of bone can be stimulated by parathyroid hormone in response to a low serum calcium level.

In some bone diseases, the osteoclasts are stimulated into inappropriate resorptive activity, and at the same time appear to lose their mobility so that they remain localized to one area of the bone surface. In this situation, they bore deeply into the bone at one site (tunnelling resorption) instead of sweeping bone away from a large area.

Osteoclast resorption of bone can be stimulated by parathyroid hormone (parathormone)

Parathormone is secreted by the parathyroid glands, which maintain a constant level of Ca^{2+} ions in the blood by increasing their output of parathormone in response to low serum Ca^{2+} ion concentration (see p. 273).

Parathormone increases the serum Ca^{2+} ion level by stimulating osteoclastic activity, the increased resorption of bone resulting in the release of Ca^{2+} ions into the blood. In addition, parathormone can increase blood Ca^{2+} by reducing Ca^{2+} ion loss by the kidney, and by increasing Ca^{2+} absorption by the small intestine.

The effect of parathormone activity in the bone is not usually detectable histologically, unless there is a prolonged and excessive parathormone secretion.

The elevation of blood Ca^{2+} produced by osteoclast-driven bone resorption is not matched by a rise in serum PO_4^- because parathormone also stimulates PO_4^- excretion by the kidney.

Osteoclast activity and bone resorption is inhibited by calcitonin

Calcitonin is a hormone produced by thyroid C cells (see Fig. 14.18). It antagonizes parathormone and is secreted in response to a high serum Ca^{2+} level. It has a direct effect on osteoclasts by inhibiting their activity in resorbing bone, but also has an effect on the kidney, where it increases the rate of excretion of both calcium and phosphate. The sum effect of calcitonin is to lower the levels of both calcium and phosphate ions in the blood. The ability of calcitonin to suppress the activity of osteoclasts in resorbing bone has been used in the treatment of Paget's disease; treatment with salmon calcitonin sometimes reduces the level of activity of the disease.

In the fetus, new bone formation may be intramembranous or endochondral

Bone develops in the fetus by two mechanisms:
- Condensation from sheets of mesenchymal cells which act as bone-forming membranes (intramembranous ossification)
- Transformation of previously deposited cartilage (endochondral ossification).

In intramembranous ossification, bone is formed within pre-existing membranes

Intramembranous ossification results in the formation of flat bones, such as those of the skull, and also contributes to some of the cortical bone shafts of long bones. In intramembranous ossification (Fig. 13.25), some of the primitive mesenchymal spindle cells of the mesenchymal membrane enlarge and develop abundant rough endoplasmic reticulum to become active osteoprogenitor cells and eventually osteoblasts.

The resulting osteoblasts begin to deposit bone in isolated islands, and remodelling begins instantly by combined osteoblast and osteoclast activity to form a network of trabecular bone.

Intervening residual mesenchymal tissue develops prominent blood vessels, and some mesenchymal cells eventually develop into haemopoietic bone marrow (see Chapter 7).

Further development is associated with increased bone formation on the outer and inner surfaces to form complete plates of bone (the outer and inner tables).

The external surfaces of cortical bone are continuously maintained in adult life by intramembranous ossification from the periosteum, particularly in response to changing stresses or injury.

Endochondral ossification is the method whereby the fetus forms long and short bones using preformed cartilage models

In this process, hyaline cartilage (see Fig. 4.16) is deposited in the shape of the required bone and is

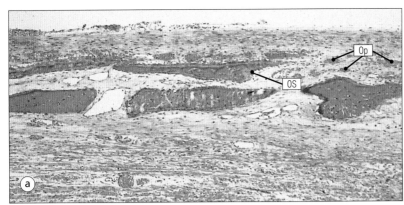 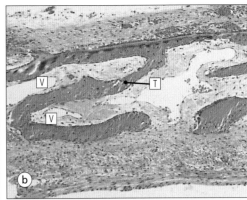

FIGURE 13.25 **Intramembranous ossification.** (a) Micrograph of an acrylic resin, Goldner-stained section from the skull of a developing fetus. Within the fibrocollagenous membrane, islands of primitive mesenchymal cells develop into clusters of osteoprogenitor cells (Op, see also Fig. 13.16), which mature into osteoblasts. The osteoblasts then lay down osteoid (OS), which becomes mineralized (blue). Although the initial bone islands are irregular in shape, remodelling by synchronized osteoblast and osteoclast activity produces flattened sheets of bone. (b) Micrograph of fetal skull showing a slightly later stage in the same process. The bone is now roughly fashioned in the shape of a plate, with almost continuous outer and inner layers bridged by trabeculae (T). The spaces between the bone are occupied by primitive mesenchymal tissue, developing fibrocollagenous tissue and a system of interconnecting vascular channels (V). Later still the bone plates thicken and haemopoietic marrow fills the spaces.

subsequently transformed into bone by osteoid deposition and mineralization.

Endochondral ossification permits elongation and thickening of the bone during fetal development and throughout childhood until bone growth ceases.

Hyaline cartilage develops from a mass of immature mesenchymal tissue and assumes the approximate shape of the bone. In the case of a long bone, this will include a shaft (diaphysis) with club-shaped expansions (the epiphyses) at either end (Fig. 13.26).

A layer of spindle-shaped mesenchymal cells, chondroblasts and some osteoprogenitor cells surrounds the hyaline cartilage model and forms a perichondrium. Later, as osteoprogenitor cells outnumber chondroblast precursors, this layer is termed the 'periosteum'.

At the midshaft of the diaphysis osteoprogenitor, cells transform into osteoblasts and lay down osteoid, which becomes mineralized to form a collar of bone around the diaphysis. Concurrently, the chondrocytes in the cartilage model multiply, so that it increases in length and breadth; chondroblasts in the perichondrium/periosteum produce new cartilage. Calcium salts are then deposited in the cartilage matrix.

Once the bony collar has been formed, the diaphysis increases in diameter by bone deposition on the outer surface of the collar and resorption of bone on the inner surface.

Capillaries grow into the diaphysis of the model by penetrating the periosteum; they carry osteoprogenitor cells, which then establish a primary ossification centre in the centre of the diaphysis.

The osteoprogenitor cells in the primary diaphyseal ossification centre transform into osteoblasts and begin to deposit osteoid, which progressively replaces the calcified cartilage of the original model.

Mineralization of the osteoid, followed by some remodelling, produces a network of trabecular bone, which progressively occupies the core of the diaphysis

and merges with the denser compact bone of the peripheral bone collar.

At about the time of birth, blood vessels and osteoprogenitor cells grow into the cartilaginous club-shaped ends of the developing bone (epiphyses) at either end of the diaphyseal shaft and form secondary (or epiphyseal) ossification centres.

Long bones continue to grow throughout childhood and adolescence

Increase in length is due to continued endochondral bone formation at each end of the long bones.

An actively proliferating plate of cartilage (the epiphyseal plate) remains across the junction between the epiphysis and diaphysis. This gives rise to the apposition of new cartilage to the ends of the diaphysis, which is converted to trabecular bone, leading to a progressive increase in length (Fig. 13.27). Activity of the epiphyseal plate normally ceases after puberty.

New bone forms on the diaphyseal side of the epiphyseal plate as follows:
- Cartilage on the epiphyseal face of the epiphyseal plate proliferates to produce columns of chondrocytes embedded in matrix
- Chondrocytes approaching the diaphyseal face of the epiphyseal plate become greatly enlarged and pale staining, and begin to produce alkaline phosphatase, which facilitates calcification of the matrix
- Osteoblasts lay down osteoid on the calcified cartilaginous matrix as the first stage in the ossification of the calcified cartilaginous trabeculae
- The deposited bone is remodelled as it is incorporated into the diaphysis.

The epiphyseal plate and the zone of ossifying cartilaginous matrix trabeculae form the metaphysis.

Increase in circumference of the diaphysis is achieved by formation of new bone on the outer surface of the

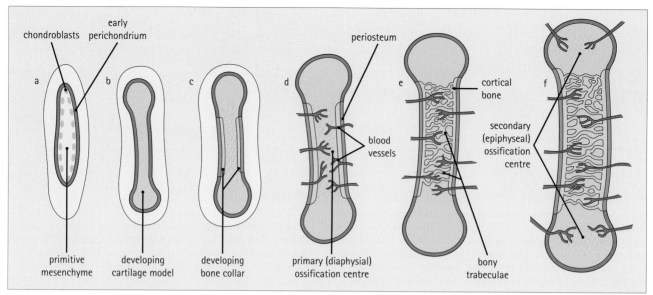

FIGURE 13.26 **Prenatal long bone development (endochondral ossification).** (a) Chondroblasts develop in primitive mesenchyme and form an early perichondrium and cartilage model. (b) The developing cartilage model assumes the shape of the bone to be formed, and a surrounding perichondrium becomes identifiable. (c) At the midshaft of the diaphysis the perichondrium becomes a periosteum through the development of osteoprogenitor cells and osteoblasts, the osteoblasts producing a collar of bone by intramembranous ossification. Calcium salts are deposited in the enlarging cartilage model. (d) Blood vessels grow through the periosteum and bone collar, carrying osteoprogenitor cells within them. These establish a primary (or diaphyseal) ossification centre in the centre of the diaphysis. (e) Bony trabeculae spread out from the primary ossification centre to occupy the entire diaphysis, linking up with the previously formed bone collar, which now forms the cortical bone of the diaphysis. At this stage, the terminal club-shaped epiphyses are still composed of cartilage. (f) At about term (the precise time varies between long bones), secondary or epiphyseal ossification centres are established in the centre of each epiphysis by the ingrowth, along with blood vessels of mesenchymal cells which become osteoprogenitor cells and osteoblasts.

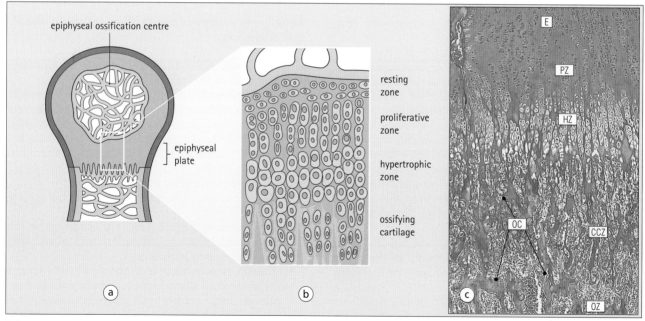

FIGURE 13.27 **Postnatal development of long bones (endochondral ossification).** (a) The initial enlargement of the secondary (epiphyseal) ossification centre within the epiphyseal cartilage, leaving an epiphyseal plate of cartilage and a surround of cartilage which will ultimately become the articular cartilage. (b) The fine detail of the epiphyseal plate between the secondary epiphyseal ossification centre on one side and the developing diaphyseal trabecular bone on the other. Chondrocytes in the epiphyseal plate proliferate in columns towards the diaphysis, becoming hypertrophied as they deposit cartilage matrix. The matrix becomes progressively mineralized before osteoblasts deposit osteoid on the calcified matrix model. (c) Low-power micrograph of decalcified H&E-stained epiphyseal region from a long bone of a fetus, for comparison with (b). Epiphyseal plate cartilage (E), the proliferative zone (PZ), the hypertrophic zone (HZ), the calcified cartilage zone (CCZ) and the beginning of the ossification zone (OZ) can be seen. At this stage, there is haemopoietic marrow in the spaces between the ossifying plates of cartilage (OC). Secondary ossification centres develop in the epiphyseal cartilage at a later stage of development.

cortical bone, which is subjected to slightly less active resorption on its inner aspect. This increases not only the diameter of the diaphysis, but also the thickness of the cortical bone, which is necessary to cope with the increased physical demands resulting from increasing body weight and physical activity.

Joints

Introduction

Bones are connected to each other by joints, which permit varying degrees of movement between the joined bones.

Joints can be divided into two main groups:
- Those that permit limited movement
- Those that permit free movement.

Some joints between bones are formed by fibrocollagenous or cartilaginous tissue.

In joints that permit only limited movement, the bones are connected by flexible fibrocollagenous or cartilaginous tissue. Such joints generally occur between bones subserving a primary supportive or protective role, for example between:
- The flat bones of the skull, which are joined by fibrous or ligamentous tissues (syndesmoses)
- The ribs and the sternum, which are joined by cartilage (synchondroses).

In old age, the support tissue forming both syndesmoses and synchondroses tends to be replaced by bone, to form a rigid immobile joint (synostosis).

A clinically important group of joints of limited movement are those between vertebrae

The bodies of the vertebrae are joined to each other by the intervertebral discs to form a long uninterrupted column (vertebral column). The discs are thick rubbery pads, which not only act as shock-absorbers but also permit some movement, so that the column is flexible within limits.

Intervertebral discs are composed essentially of fibrocollagenous tissue containing some chondrocytes and cartilage matrix (fibrocartilage, see p. 67). The two surfaces in contact with the vertebral bodies each consist of a thin layer of hyaline cartilage covering a concentrically lamellated rubbery structure of fibrocartilage (the annulus fibrosus). At the centre of the disc is a soft, semifluid core of soft gelatinous matrix (the nucleus pulposus, Fig. 13.28).

Joints that allow free movement between adjacent bones are termed synovial joints

The bone ends are held together by bands of collagenous tissue (ligaments), which may be external or internal to the joint cavity; external ligaments surround a fibrous capsule enclosing the heads of the bones, which are separated from each other by a lubricant fluid, synovial fluid.

Because the bone ends move against each other they are coated with a smooth, friction-free layer of hyaline cartilage (articular cartilage), and the synovial fluid

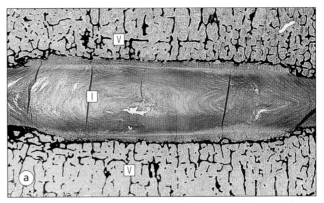
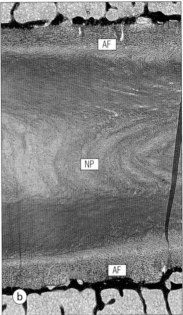

FIGURE 13.28 **Intervertebral disc.** (a) Micrograph of an acrylic resin section of an intervertebral disc (I) between two vertebrae (V) stained with H&E. (b) Micrograph of part of the same intervertebral disc at higher magnification, showing the annulus fibrosus (AF) forming a compact outer region adjacent to vertebral bone and the soft, semifluid at the centre, nucleus pulposus (NP).

CLINICAL EXAMPLE
SCIATICA

Wear and tear on the intervertebral discs may lead to degeneration of the annulus fibrosus, with outward protrusion of the nucleus pulposus. This results in:

- Impaired efficiency of the disc as a shock absorber
- Expansion of the annulus fibrosus, causing it to bulge.

If the annulus fibrosus bulges in the region of the spinal nerves as they emerge from the spinal cord, the nerves may be stretched and damaged, producing peripheral nerve symptoms.

Intervertebral disc degeneration is most common in the lumbar region of the vertebral column and causes pressure on the nerves, producing sciatica – pain traveling down the back and outer side of the leg.

provides a thin lubricant film between the opposing articular cartilages.

The internal lining of the joint capsule is a specialized secretory epithelium, the synovium, which produces synovial fluid

The synovium is composed of one to four layers of cells which merge on their deep surface with a zone of loosely arranged fibrocollagenous tissue containing adipocytes, fibroblasts, mast cells and macrophages. This deep layer merges with the denser fibrocollagenous tissue of the joint capsule.

Synovial cells vary from flat, mesothelial-like cells through to spindle-shaped, polyhedral or cuboidal cells.

Two cell types have been defined in synovial membrane: type A cells are phagocytic and contain numerous lysosomes, whereas type B cells contain abundant rough endoplasmic reticulum and are adapted for protein production. The synovial membrane has an abundant blood, lymphatic and nerve supply running in the loose fibrocollagenous tissue.

Ligaments, composed of dense collagenous tissue, stabilize joints

Structures around the joint that prevent excess movement include collagenous external ligaments and tendinous muscle attachments (Fig. 13.29). External ligaments surround articular (synovial) joints, attaching one bone to the other over the outer surface of the joint capsule.

Ligaments are composed of tightly packed collagen fibres all running in the same direction, with compressed fibrocytes in between; thus they resemble tendon, but differ from tendon in that they contain elastic fibres. Ligaments strengthen the joint; they permit normal movement but prevent overflexing or overextension. The attachment of ligament to bone is similar to that of tendons.

In some complex joints, there are internal ligaments (e.g. cruciate ligaments in the knee joints) to prevent overstretching or twisting, and fibrocartilaginous menisci (also in the knee) to stabilize and guide gliding movements.

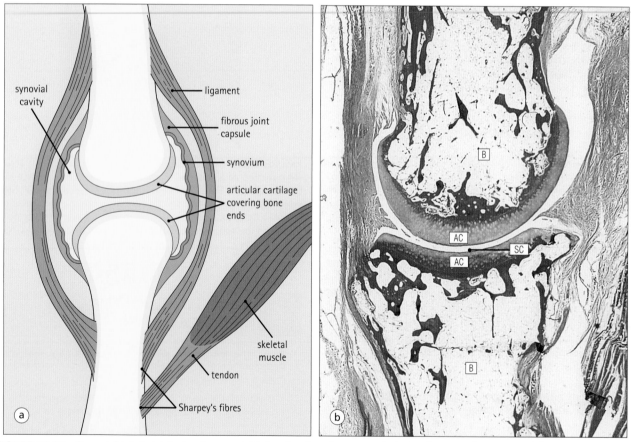

FIGURE 13.29 **Synovial joint.** (a) A simple synovial joint showing the two articulating bone ends separated from each other by synovial fluid and enclosed within a fibrocollagenous capsule. Surrounding ligaments and tendinous muscle attachments prevent excess movement. (b) Low-power micrograph of an interphalangeal joint of the finger. Note the ends of the articulating bone (B), the articular cartilages (AC) and the joint capsule enclosing the synovial cavity (SC), which contains synovial fluid. The synovial cavity is lined internally by synovium.

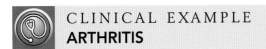

CLINICAL EXAMPLE
ARTHRITIS

Osteoarthritis

Some synovial joints, particularly the hip and finger joints, are exposed to persistent wear and tear over many years. This sometimes leads to degeneration of the articular cartilage, which loses its normal complement of hydrated glycosaminoglycans and so is unable to resist compressive forces. This leads to erosion of the cartilage and rubbing together of adjacent bone surfaces.

Eventually the surface bone becomes highly compacted and ivory like; this is called 'eburnation'.

The constant bone-to-bone trauma and excessive movement at the joint leads to a painful swollen joint with:

- Thickening of the joint capsule
- Irregular protuberances of abnormal new bone at the edges of the articular surfaces (osteophytes)
- Reduction in the synovial space.

These are the typical changes of osteoarthritis.

Rheumatoid Arthritis

Another common form of arthritis is rheumatoid arthritis, an autoimmune disease causing immune-mediated damage to the synovial membrane and articular cartilage.

The synovial membrane becomes thick and extensively infiltrated by cells of the immune system (mainly lymphocytes and plasma cells), and the damaged articular cartilage is replaced by vascular fibrocollagenous tissue (pannus).

For online review questions, please visit https://studentconsult.inkling.com.

END OF CHAPTER REVIEW

True/False Answers to the MCQs, as Well as Case Answers, can be Found in the Appendix in the Back of the Book.

1. **Which of the following features are seen in osteoblasts?**
   (a) Are derived from blood monocytes
   (b) Synthesize and secrete osteoid collagen
   (c) Produce matrix vesicles important in mineralization of bone matrix
   (d) Have abundant rough endoplasmic reticulum
   (e) Have a characteristic ruffled border on the surface closest to the bone

2. **Which of the following are true of osteoclasts?**
   (a) Are derived from osteoprogenitor cells
   (b) Erode bone
   (c) Are stimulated by parathyroid hormone
   (d) Are stimulated by calcitonin
   (e) Are rich in alkaline phosphatase

3. **Which of the following is present in skeletal muscle?**
   (a) Develops from primitive rhabdomyoblasts
   (b) Contains type 1 fast-twitch fibres
   (c) Contains satellite cells which are phagocytic
   (d) Contains stretch receptors called muscle spindles
   (e) Contains motor nerve twigs which terminate in motor endplates

4. **In bone development, which of the following features are seen?**
   (a) Chondroblasts develop in primitive mesenchyme and form an early perichondrium and cartilage model
   (b) The term diaphysis refers to the shaft region
   (c) The term epiphysis refers to the club-shaped expansion at the end of long bones
   (d) The epiphyseal plate can be divided into periosteum, bone collar and osteoprogenitor zones
   (e) Postnatal increase in length is due to endochondral bone formation near the end of long bones

CASE 13.1 A CASE OF A ROAD TRAFFIC ACCIDENT

A 23-year-old man, an amateur soccer player, sustains a compound fracture of his tibia and fibula in a road traffic accident while riding his motorbike. After the fractures have been treated surgically by insertion of pins and plates, he has great

Continued

difficulty with weight-bearing on the affected leg, his muscle mass has decreased and he enters a prolonged period of rehabilitation, which involves physiotherapy to his thigh and calf muscles.

Q. Explain the structural basis of this case. Why is physiotherapy necessary?

CASE 13.2 MUSCLE WEAKNESS IN CHILDHOOD

A 2-year-old boy is seen in a neurology clinic because he has been delayed in achieving his motor development and is clearly weak. There is a family history of similar problems, with a cousin dying following progressive muscle disease in late adolescence. A muscle biopsy shows death of many muscle fibres, evidence of muscle fibre regeneration and fibrosis. No expression of the protein dystrophin is seen.

Q. How does lack of expression of dystrophin relate to muscle disease?

CASE 13.3 A MAN WITH A LIMP

A 68-year-old man is referred by his family practitioner because of difficulty with walking, owing to pain in his right hip, gradually getting worse over about 3 years. He is now walking with a limp, favouring his left leg and supporting his right leg with the use of a walking stick. On examination, movement at the right hip is limited, mainly by pain. X-ray shows narrowing of the hip joint cavity, with flattening of the head of the femur and outgrowth of new bone (osteophyte formation) around the rim of the femoral head. A diagnosis of osteoarthritis is made.

Q. What joint structures are likely to be involved in this process and how do you think the clinical features relate to deranged function of the joint?

CASE 13.4 A WOMAN WITH BACK, BUTTOCK AND LEG PAIN

A 35-year-old woman developed sudden onset of severe pain in the lumbar region, while pruning a large rose bush. She hobbled into the house and lay down on her back on the bed, the only position in which she could tolerate the pain. She had a restless night despite taking analgesics. The next morning, the pain in her back had abated somewhat, but she had pain in the left buttock, radiating down the back of the left thigh, and by the following day, the pain also affected the back of the calf and the foot. Despite 2 days of bed rest, her symptoms persisted and she contacted her family practitioner, who visited. He found that she had some sensory loss on the sole and posterior calf, and was unable to raise her left leg when the knee was straight. She also had some weakness of ankle and toe flexion on the left. A diagnosis of prolapsed intervertebral disc was made.

Q. Describe the histological and anatomical basis for this condition.

Chapter 14

Endocrine System

Introduction

Cell communication is vital for any multicellular organism to function efficiently.

At a local level, cells communicate via cell surface molecules and gap junctions, whereas remote communication is mediated by the secretion of chemical messengers which activate cells by interacting with specific receptors. Such secretion may be one of four main types: autocrine, paracrine, endocrine or synaptic (Fig. 14.1).

Autocrine secretion occurs when a cell secretes a chemical messenger to act on its own receptors. This is particularly evident in the local control of cell growth by substances such as epidermal growth factor.

Paracrine secretion describes the secretion of chemical messengers to act on adjacent cells. This is also mainly concerned with the local control of cell growth and is also a mode of action of many of the cells of the diffuse neuroendocrine system (see p. 280).

Endocrine secretion is the secretion of chemical messengers (hormones) into the bloodstream to act on distant tissues.

Synaptic secretion refers to communication by direct structural targeting from one cell to another via synapses, and is confined to the nervous system.

The chemical messengers belong to four main molecular classes:
- Amino acid derivatives (e.g. epinephrine (adrenaline), norepinephrine (noradrenaline), thyroxine)
- Small peptides (e.g. encephalin, vasopressin, thyroid-releasing hormone)
- Proteins (e.g. nerve growth factor, epidermal growth factor, insulin, growth hormone, parathormone, thyroid-stimulating hormone)
- Steroids (e.g. cortisol, progesterone, estradiol, testosterone).

Most chemical messengers are water-soluble hydrophilic molecules that diffuse freely and usually interact with a cell surface receptor protein. However, steroids and thyroxine are hydrophobic: after carriage to a cell by special proteins in the blood, they pass through its membrane to interact with receptor proteins inside.

Endocrine Cell and Tissue Specialization

Cells whose main role is to secrete messenger substances are termed endocrine cells

Endocrine cells are found in three distinct anatomic distributions:
- Gathered together in one specialized organ to form an endocrine gland (e.g. adrenal, pituitary and pineal glands)
- Forming discrete clusters in another specialized organ (e.g. ovary, testis, pancreas)
- Dispersed singly among other cells in epithelial tissues, particularly in the gut and respiratory tract, in which case they form part of what is referred to as the diffuse neuroendocrine system.

Endocrine cells and tissues have special characteristics related to their secretory function

Certain cells termed 'neuroendocrine cells' have membrane-bound vesicles, which are granules containing the chemical messenger. Secretion is achieved by exocytosis, in which the membrane of the vesicle fuses with the cell membrane, thereby discharging its contents outside the cell. Neuroendocrine cells transiently store the messenger as specific neuroendocrine granules, which can be identified in cells using immunohistochemical staining techniques.

Endocrine tissues are usually highly vascular to facilitate rapid dissemination of secreted products into the bloodstream. In contrast to other types of secretory cell, the secretory pole of endocrine cells is adjacent to the capillary vessel wall and the nucleus is found at the opposite pole.

Autocrine and paracrine messengers act relatively slowly, having to diffuse into the bloodstream. They act on local cell receptors and are rapidly destroyed once secreted, thereby limiting their activity.

Endocrine messengers act relatively slowly, having to diffuse into the bloodstream, circulate to a target organ

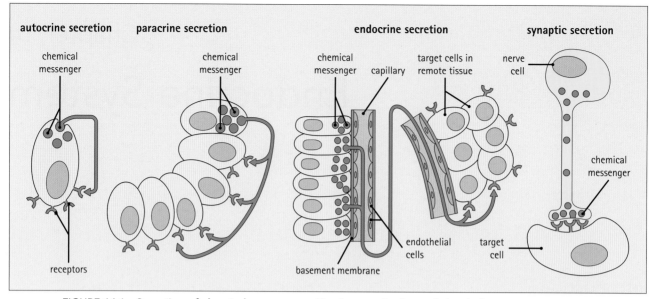

FIGURE 14.1 **Secretion of chemical messengers.** The four mechanisms of chemical messenger secretion.

and then enter a target cell. Many neuroendocrine cells secrete amines or peptides and have common metabolic features involving the uptake of amines, which then undergo decarboxylation in the process of hormone synthesis. This has led to the term 'APUD cells' (amine precursor uptake and decarboxylation).

Cells containing neuroendocrine granules and of neuroendocrine lineage have a restricted set of specific metabolic isoenzymes and structural proteins, which can be detected histochemically. γ-Enolase is an isoenzyme in the glycolytic pathway that is present in high concentration in neuroendocrine cells together with PGP 9.5 (ubiquitin-C-terminal hydrolase). In the neuroendocrine granules, chromogranin is a component of the core protein and synaptophysin is a glycoprotein in their membrane. Histochemical detection of these substances enables their use as markers of neuroendocrine differentiation.

Pituitary

The pituitary is a multifunctional endocrine gland

The pituitary gland secretes a large number of hormones to activate many peripheral endocrine cells, for example those in the adrenal glands, thyroid, testes and ovaries.

The pituitary is a bean-shaped gland approximately 12×10×9 mm in size and weighing 0.4–0.9 g in the adult. It is situated beneath the brain, to which it is linked by the pituitary stalk, and is surrounded by the bone of the base of the skull in a depression of the sphenoid bone termed the 'sella turcica' (Fig. 14.2).

Anatomically the pituitary is divided into two parts

The anterior pituitary (adenohypophysis) is an epithelial-derived tissue with three distinct components: the distal

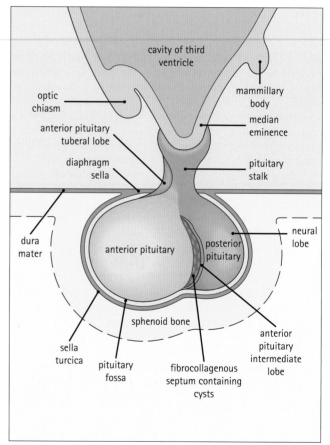

FIGURE 14.2 **Pituitary gland.** The pituitary gland and its relationship to surrounding structures.

lobe (pars distalis) forms the major portion of the gland; the intermediate lobe (pars intermedia), which is a rudimentary zone in man but prominent in other mammals; the tuberal lobe (pars tuberalis), which is a layer of cells running up the pituitary stalk.

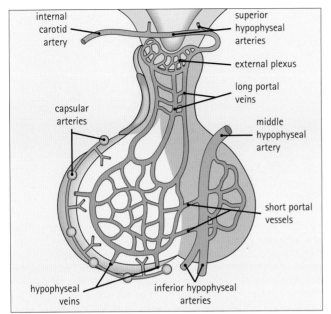

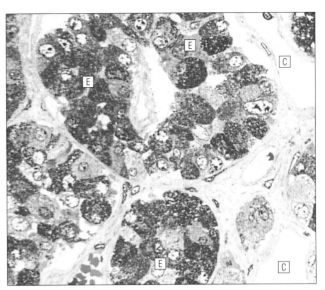

FIGURE 14.4 **Anterior pituitary cells and vessels.** Toluidine blue resin section showing pituitary endocrine cells (E) arranged in groups and surrounded by capillaries (C).

FIGURE 14.3 **Vascular supply of the pituitary.** The blood supply of the pituitary arises from three paired arteries originating from the internal carotid arteries. The superior hypophyseal arteries enter the median eminence and form the external plexus close to nerve endings from neuroendocrine cells in the hypothalamus. This gives way to a parallel capillary network which surrounds larger central muscular vessels and runs down the pituitary stalk to form the long portal vessels. Arising from the portal vessels, capillary vessels run forward into the anterior pituitary, providing a direct vascular link between the hypothalamus and the neuroendocrine cells of the anterior pituitary. Additional blood supply to the posterior pituitary is derived from the small middle and inferior hypophyseal arteries. A minor blood supply to the periphery of the anterior pituitary is derived from small blood vessels in the capsule of the gland.

The posterior pituitary (neurohypophysis) is composed of neuronal processes and glia and has three components: the neural lobe (pars nervosa, infundibular process), lying behind the anterior pituitary in the sella turcica; the pituitary stalk (infundibular stem), in which axons run from the brain above; the median eminence (infundibulum), a funnel-shaped extension of the hypothalamus.

Embryologically, the anterior pituitary is thought to be derived from an outgrowth of the foregut ectoderm called 'Rathke's pouch'. This connects with a downgrowth of the developing hypothalamus, which forms the posterior pituitary and comes to lie in the base of the skull.

The vascular supply of the pituitary integrates the functions of the endocrine and nervous systems

A special network of blood vessels (pituitary portal system, Fig. 14.3) carries hormones from the hypothalamus of the brain to stimulate or inhibit the hormone secretion of the anterior pituitary.

The major blood supply to the anterior pituitary is derived from vessels that run down the pituitary stalk.

These are easily damaged in severe head injury, resulting in death of the anterior pituitary and consequent ablation of its endocrine function.

Anterior Pituitary

The anterior pituitary secretes several hormones into the bloodstream

The anterior pituitary is served by a fine capillary network (Fig. 14.3) which, bringing blood from the hypothalamus, contains both stimulatory and inhibitory hormones (Fig. 14.4). These hormones control the neuroendocrine cells of the anterior pituitary. In turn, their secretions diffuse back into the capillary network, which subsequently drains into the pituitary veins and thence into the carotid venous sinus and systemic circulation.

The anterior pituitary contains five distinct types of endocrine cell, which vary in their distribution within the gland (Fig. 14.5). Cells were originally named by their staining characteristics, but it is more precise to name the cells according to their specific hormone product (Fig. 14.6); each cell type has the same basic ultrastructure (Fig. 14.7). These cells are:

- Somatotrophs (Fig. 14.8), which secrete growth hormone (GH)
- Lactotrophs (Fig. 14.9), which secrete prolactin (PRL)
- Corticotrophs (Fig. 14.10), which secrete adrenocorticotropic hormone (ACTH), β-lipotropin (β-LPH), α-melanocyte stimulating hormone (α-MSH), and β-endorphin
- Thyrotrophs, which secrete thyroid-stimulating hormone (TSH)
- Gonadotrophs (Fig. 14.11), which secrete the gonadotropic hormones, follicle-stimulating hormone (FSH) and luteinizing hormone (LH).

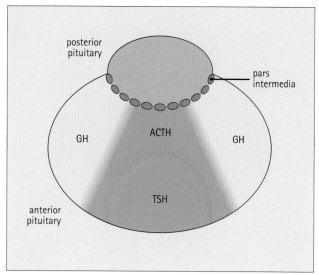

FIGURE 14.5 **Regional distribution of anterior pituitary cells.** A horizontal cross-section of the distal lobe of the pituitary. The lateral wings contain mainly somatotrophs, which secrete GH, whereas corticotrophs, which secrete ACTH, β-lipotropin, α-MSH and β-endorphin, are concentrated in the median portion of the gland just in front of the posterior pituitary. Thyrotrophs, which secrete TSH, are concentrated anteriorly. Lactotrophs secreting PRL and gonadotrophs secreting FSH and LH are uniformly scattered throughout the gland.

The intermediate lobe of the anterior pituitary is relatively small in man

The intermediate lobe of the anterior pituitary is located between the posterior pituitary and the distal lobe (see Fig. 14.2). It is poorly developed in humans compared with other mammals, consisting of a series of gland-like acini lined by a cuboidal epithelium. These cells are usually immunoreactive for corticotropic hormones, and it has been suggested that they may be producing one of the minor subunits of the pre-pro-opiomelanocortic peptides, such as β-LPH, α-MSH or β-endorphin, rather than ACTH.

The tuberal lobe is an upward extension of the anterior pituitary around the pituitary stalk

The tuberal lobe consists of a thin layer of cuboidal epithelial cells. Immunohistochemically, most of the cells are gonadotrophs.

Occasionally, nests of squamous cells can be seen, from which cysts and even tumours may develop. It has been assumed that these are embryological remnants of the ectodermal Rathke's pouch.

Posterior Pituitary

The posterior pituitary is a continuation of the hypothalamic region of the brain

The posterior pituitary extends down into the pituitary stalk and sella turcica (see Fig. 14.2) and secretes oxytocin and antidiuretic hormone (vasopressin).

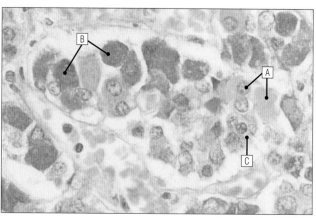

FIGURE 14.6 **Traditional methods for demonstrating cells of the anterior pituitary.** Traditionally cells of the anterior pituitary have been classified into three types: acidophils (cytoplasm staining with acidic dyes), basophils (cytoplasm staining with basic dyes and the periodic acid–Schiff (PAS) method) and chromophobes (cells with no cytoplasmic staining). In the PAS orange-G haematoxylin stain shown here, acidophils (A) stain bright yellow, basophils (B) stain darkly, and chromophobes (C) do not stain. Nuclei are stained black by the haematoxylin. It is now customary to classify cells according to their hormone content, which is demonstrable by immunohistochemical staining using antibodies to each hormone type. It is also possible to distinguish the cells of the anterior pituitary by electron microscopy. These techniques have shown that acidophils are cells secreting GH or PRL (i.e. somatotrophs and lactotrophs), and that basophils are thyrotrophs, corticotrophs and gonadotrophs. All of these cells contain abundant dense core granules. Basophils stain well with haematoxylin and PAS, which detect glycosyl groups, because TSH, LH and FSH are glycoproteins and the ACTH precursor protein is glycosylated. Chromophobes fail to stain because they contain very few granules, but may be lactotroph, somatotroph, thyrotroph, gonadotroph or corticotroph in nature. Some cells, which contain sparse dense-core granules with no recognizable immunostaining, have been termed 'null cells'.

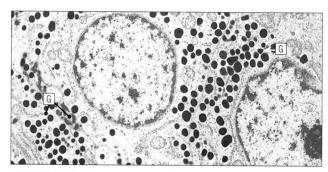

FIGURE 14.7 **Ultrastructure of anterior pituitary cells.** Electron micrograph of anterior pituitary cells showing their numerous hormone-containing dense-core granules (G).

It is composed of the axons of neuronal cells lying in the supraoptic and paraventricular nuclei of the hypothalamus, together with supporting glial cells termed 'pituicytes' (Fig. 14.13). The axons terminate in the posterior pituitary adjacent to a rich network of capillary vessels.

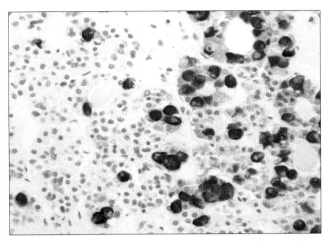

FIGURE 14.8 **Somatotrophs.** Somatotrophs make up about 50% of the anterior pituitary and are generally large, ovoid or polygonal in shape, as shown in this section stained to show GH by an immunoperoxidase method. Ultrastructurally, somatotrophs contain abundant randomly distributed electron-dense granules, which measure from 300 to 600 nm in diameter, but the majority are between 350 and 450 nm. The rough endoplasmic reticulum is arranged in parallel stacks, many positioned parallel to the cell membranes. Tumours which are derived from somatotroph cells contain spherical bundles of intermediate filaments called 'fibrous bodies'.

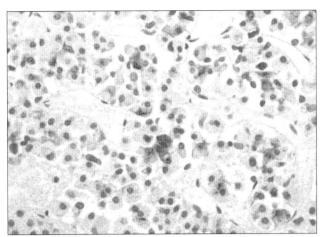

FIGURE 14.9 **Lactotrophs.** Lactotrophs make up about 25% of the anterior pituitary. Although some are rounded and polygonal, most are compressed by adjacent cells into narrow angular profiles, as shown in this section of gland stained by an immunoperoxidase method to show prolactin. They increase in size and number during pregnancy and lactation. Ultrastructurally, lactotrophs have a prominent Golgi compared with all other anterior pituitary cells and their granules measure 200–350 nm in diameter. Interestingly, exocytosis may be seen at their lateral borders (misplaced exocytosis), as well as in the usual site adjacent to capillary basement membrane. This feature can be used in diagnostic assessment, as it is limited to lactotroph-derived tumours.

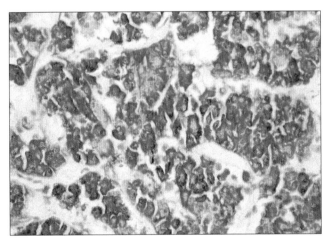

FIGURE 14.10 **Corticotrophs.** Accounting for 15–20% of the entire anterior pituitary cell population, but tending to cluster, corticotrophs are large and polygonal in shape, as shown in this micrograph stained to show ACTH by an immunoperoxidase technique. Many corticotrophs possess an unstained perinuclear vacuole called the 'enigmatic body', which is derived from secondary lysosomes. Granules in corticotrophs are large and typically measure 250–700 nm in diameter. Large perinuclear bundles of intermediate cytokeratin filaments are prominent ultrastructurally and these become even more prominent in glucocorticoid excess, when they are visible under the light microscope as pink-staining inclusions (Crooke's hyaline).

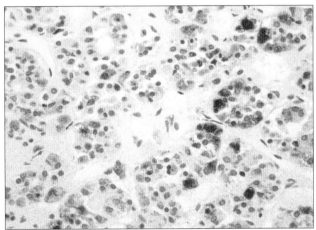

FIGURE 14.11 **Gonadotrophs.** Constituting around 10% of anterior pituitary cells, gonadotrophs are scattered as single cells or small groups throughout the gland, as seen in this section which has been stained to show the β subunit of FSH by an immunoperoxidase technique. Both FSH and LH may be evident within the same cell. Ultrastructurally, the granules are 150–400 nm in diameter. Following ablation of the ovaries or testes, gonadotrophs develop extensive cytoplasmic vacuolation. This is due to dilation of the endoplasmic reticulum by stored product and caused by the loss of feedback inhibition by gonadal steroids. Such cells, large, rounded and vacuolated on light microscopy, are called 'castration cells'.

CLINICAL EXAMPLE
TUMOURS OF THE ANTERIOR PITUITARY

The most important tumour of the anterior part of the pituitary gland is the benign **pituitary adenoma**. Although benign, this tumour causes severe symptoms for two reasons. First, it may grow large enough to push out of the small pituitary fossa and compress the optic chiasma and nerves that run over the top of the pituitary fossa; this causes severe visual disturbances and eventual blindness. The second reason is that some pituitary adenomas secrete excessive amounts of hormone, causing various endocrine syndromes. For example, the tumour illustrated in Figure 14.12 is mainly composed of somatotrophs, which secrete large amounts of growth hormone. In children this would produce gigantism; in adults the syndrome is called 'acromegaly'.

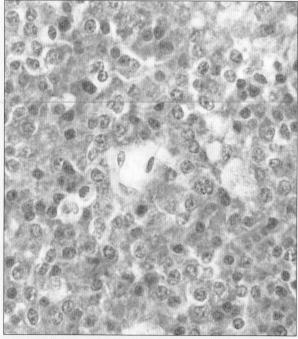

FIGURE 14.12 **Pituitary adenoma.** This photomicrograph shows a pituitary adenoma stained by an immunochemical method to demonstrate growth hormone in the cytoplasm of the somatotrophs of which this particular adenoma is composed. The patient had acromegaly.

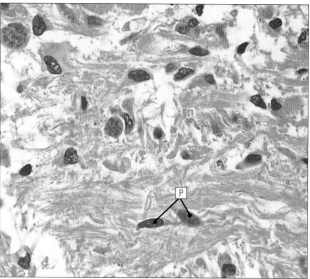

FIGURE 14.13 **Posterior pituitary.** The posterior pituitary is composed of axons which originate from cells in the hypothalamus and possess numerous neurosecretory granules containing either oxytocin or vasopressin, together with a carrier protein termed 'neurophysin', and ATP. Where axons are adjacent to capillaries, they form fusiform swellings filled with neurosecretory granules (Herring bodies). The posterior pituitary also contains specialized stellate glial cells called 'pituicytes'. In this micrograph, the axons are seen as a pale fibrillary background in which the nuclei of pituicytes (P) and small capillary vessels are present.

- A specialized system of blood vessels transports hypothalamic hormones to act locally on neuroendocrine cells in the anterior pituitary (Fig. 14.14)
- Axons project down from the hypothalamus to form the pituitary stalk, which terminates as the posterior pituitary.

KEY FACTS
PITUITARY GLAND AND HYPOTHALAMUS

- Anterior pituitary secretes prolactin, GH, ACTH, TSH, FSH, LH and others
- Posterior pituitary stores and secretes oxytocin and ADH, which are made in hypothalamic nuclei
- Hypothalamus is in direct communication with posterior pituitary via pituitary stalk, and anterior pituitary via pituitary portal vessels
- Hypothalamus produces hormones that stimulate or inhibit the release of anterior pituitary hormones.

Hypothalamus

The actions of the endocrine and nervous systems are coordinated by the hypothalamus

The hypothalamus is a region of brain composed of several clusters of neurons that secrete hormones. These hormones act as either releasing or inhibiting factors for the hormones secreted by the anterior pituitary, and are transported to the pituitary gland by two routes as follows:

Pineal Gland

The pineal gland secretes melatonin

The pineal gland is located just below the posterior end of the corpus callosum of the brain. It is a flattened conical structure 6–10 mm long and 5–6 mm wide; it is covered by leptomeninges and composed of lobules of specialized cells, which are separated by septa containing

ADVANCED CONCEPT
HYPOTHALAMIC HORMONES

At least eight hormones are known to be secreted by hypothalamic neurons. Two of these are the peptides **oxytocin** and **arginine vasopressin**, synthesized in the cell bodies of neurons in the supraoptic and paraventricular nuclei of the hypothalamus. They pass down axons into the posterior pituitary via the pituitary stalk and are released into the capillaries of the posterior pituitary.

The other hypothalamic hormones are inhibiting or releasing hormones controlling the secretion of anterior pituitary hormones. They are transported via the pituitary portal vessels (see Fig. 14.14). These are:

- Thyrotropin-releasing hormone (TRH) – mainly from dorsomedial nuclei
- Gonadotropin-releasing hormone (GnRH) – mainly from arcuate nuclei and preoptic area
- Growth hormone-releasing hormone (GHRH) – mainly from arcuate nuclei
- Corticotropin-releasing hormone (CRH) – from anterior part of paraventricular nuclei
- Growth hormone-inhibiting hormone (GIH) – also known as **somatostatin** (SS) – from paraventricular nuclei
- Prolactin release-inhibiting hormone (PIH) – also known as **dopamine** (DA) – from arcuate nuclei.

No single prolactin-releasing hormone has been found, but other hormones have this action, e.g. oxytocin, VIP and TRH.

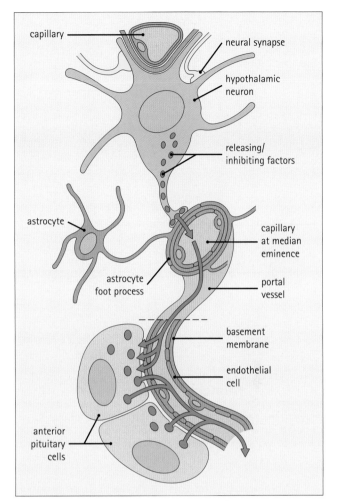

FIGURE 14.14 Hypothalamic control of anterior pituitary hormone production. Hypothalamic neurons secrete releasing/inhibiting factors in response to chemoreceptive and neural inputs. These hormones diffuse into capillaries at the median eminence and are carried to the anterior pituitary in the portal vessels. Astrocyte foot processes surrounding the capillary vessels form part of their diffusion barrier.

unmyelinated nerves and blood vessels (Fig. 14.15). The gland consists of two major cell types: pinealocytes and glial cells.

Pinealocytes are neuron-like cells that produce melatonin, which induces rhythmic changes in the secretions of the hypothalamus, pituitary and gonads, and is said to act as an endocrine transducer. They have pink-staining cytoplasm and dark-staining rounded nuclei, and are often arranged in rosettes, where several cells surround a central fibrillary area composed of cell processes directed towards a small capillary vessel.

Glial cells tend to be bipolar elongated cells that run between nests of pinealocytes. They are indistinct unless specially stained.

A common age-related change in the pineal is the accumulation of calcium particles, which are visible on a skull radiograph; thus, the gland can be used as a radiological midline landmark.

The pineal gland is innervated by sympathetic and parasympathetic nervous systems. In addition, signals from the retina arrive indirectly, as shown in Figure 14.15a.

Thyroid Gland

Introduction

The thyroid gland secretes two hormones, thyroxine and calcitonin. Thyroxine has the major role in the regulation of the basal metabolic rate, whereas calcitonin is involved in calcium homeostasis.

The thyroid gland consists of two lateral lobes and an isthmus

The lateral lobes of the thyroid are arranged on either side of the thyroid cartilage and upper trachea in the anterior portion of the neck. These lobes are joined near their lower poles by the isthmus crossing in front of the lower larynx; occasionally, a small triangular pyramidal lobe projects upwards from the midpoint of the isthmus.

Each lateral lobe is about 5 cm long, 3–4 cm wide and 2–3 cm deep. In the healthy adult, the thyroid weighs 15–20 g and is slightly heavier in males, though many factors influence its weight at any one time, for example pathological abnormalities.

The thyroid is enclosed by a thin collagenous capsule from which internal septa penetrate the parenchyma, dividing it into irregular lobules.

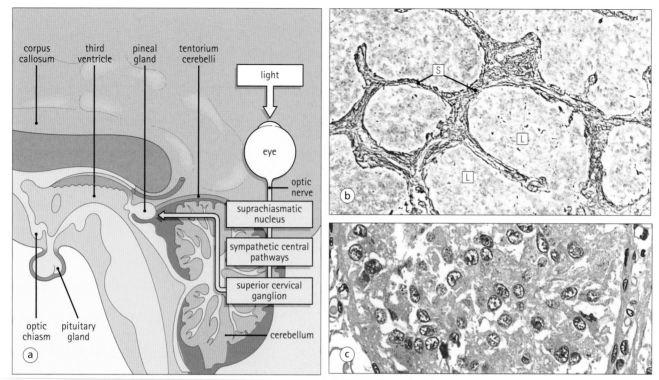

FIGURE 14.15 **Pineal gland.** (a) The location of the pineal gland. Output of pineal melatonin is modulated by light through nervous pathways which input as sympathetic innervation to the gland. (b) Low-power micrograph of a reticulin-stained section of pineal showing the septa (S) that divide it into discrete lobules (L) of pinealocytes. (c) High-power micrograph of an H&E-stained section of pineal showing a single pineal lobule surrounded by septa composed of glial processes and small vessels. In the centre of the lobule pinealocyte cell bodies are found in a background of pink-staining cell processes, some of which form a rosette structure.

Embryologically, the thyroid develops from a downgrowth of endoderm arising near the root of the tongue and called the 'thyroglossal duct', which atrophies and leaves a nodule of thyroid tissue at its correct anatomic site.

Occasionally, the thyroglossal duct fails to atrophy completely, and thyroglossal duct tissue persists in the midline of the neck, usually as a cyst or a sinus track (thyroglossal duct cyst).

The thyroid gland contains colloid, which is rich in thyroglobulin

The glandular component of the thyroid is composed of epithelium arranged as tightly packed spherical units called 'acini' (Fig. 14.16).

Each acinus is lined by a single layer of specialized thyroid epithelium, which rests on a basement membrane and encloses a lumen filled with thyroid colloid, a pink-staining (eosinophilic) homogeneous proteinaceous material rich in thyroglobulin.

Thyroglobulin is the storage form of thyroxine and is an iodinated glycoprotein (Fig. 14.17). The size of an acinus depends on whether it is in a secretory or a storage phase.

During an active secretory phase, the thyroid follicular cells show the following changes:
- The endoplasmic reticulum becomes more prominent
- Free ribosomes become more prominent

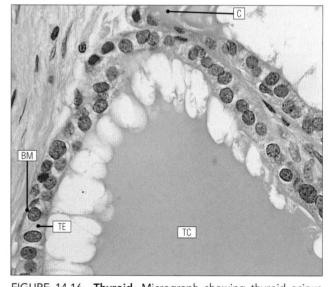

FIGURE 14.16 **Thyroid.** Micrograph showing thyroid acinus composed of specialized thyroid epithelium (TE) resting on a basement membrane (BM). These epithelial cells enclose a lumen filled with thyroid colloid (TC), and are surrounded by a fine network of capillaries (C) associated with thin fibrous septa.

- The Golgi enlarges
- The surface microvilli increase in number and length
- Intracytoplasmic droplets appear (representing colloid in endocytotic vesicles generated by

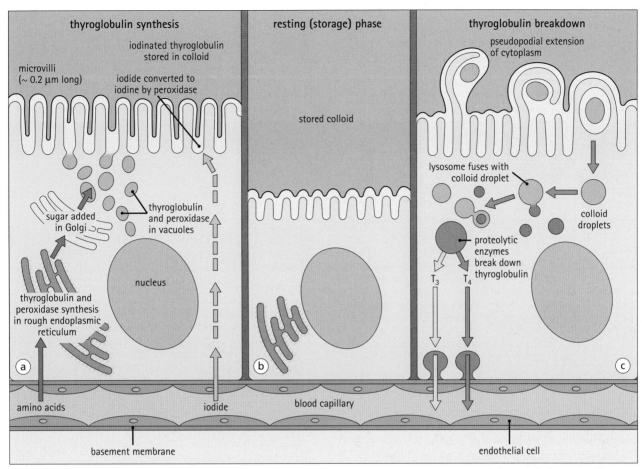

FIGURE 14.17 Thyroid colloid. (a) The formation of thyroid hormone requires the interaction of thyroglobulin and iodine. Thyroglobulin is produced by the thyroid epithelial cells, its protein component being synthesized in the rough endoplasmic reticulum and transported by the Golgi, where most of its sugar component is added by glycosylation. The thyroid epithelial cell is able to transport iodide against a concentration gradient from the capillary blood to where it is concentrated in the lumen of the follicle. However, iodide requires conversion to iodine, which is performed by the enzyme thyroid peroxidase. This enzyme is also synthesized in the epithelial cell and enters the same secretory vesicles as contain thyroglobulin. Thyroglobulin and thyroid peroxidase leave the exit face of the Golgi from small vacuoles which are transported to the luminal surface. They are released into the lumen by exocytosis. Once secreted, at the cell membrane, thyroid peroxidase becomes active and converts iodide into iodine. Iodine is then added to the tyrosine component of thyroglobulin. (b) Thyroglobulin acts as a reservoir from which thyroxine can be produced and secreted into the capillary circulation when required. (c) To release thyroxine from the stored colloid, the thyroid epithelial cell extrudes pseudopodial extensions of cytoplasm from its luminal surface; these enclose small droplets of colloid which are then incorporated into its cytoplasm. Lysosomes fuse with the small vacuoles and hydrolysis and proteolysis of the thyroglobulin occur, breaking it into smaller units, the most important of which is tetraiodothyronine (T4) or thyroxine. Another product is triiodothyronine (T3). Both are iodinated amino acids.

pseudopodial extensions of cytoplasm at the luminal surface).

The synthesis and breakdown of thyroglobulin is controlled by the hypothalamus and pituitary gland

Low blood thyroxine levels stimulate the hypothalamus to produce thyrotropin-releasing hormone (TRH), which then stimulates the anterior pituitary to produce thyroid-stimulating hormone (TSH). In turn, TSH stimulates both thyroglobulin synthesis and breakdown, with a consequent increase in thyroxine release into the capillary circulation. When thyroxine levels rise, TRH and TSH production decreases.

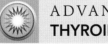

ADVANCED CONCEPT
THYROID HORMONES

The two hormones are triiodothyronine (T3) and thyroxine, which is tetraiodothyronine (T4), both of which are iodinated derivatives of tyrosine. The thyroid follicular cells produce and secrete mainly T4 (only 5–10% of the thyroid's output is T3), but T3 is functionally much more potent than T4. Most of the active T3 is produced in other tissues by the removal of one iodine molecule from T4; kidney and liver are particularly important deiodinators of T4. In the plasma, both T3 and T4 are largely bound to a protein, thyroxine-binding globulin – TBG; probably only the free non-bound hormones are physiologically active.

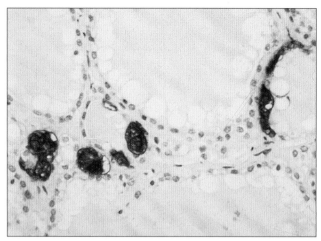

FIGURE 14.18 **Thyroid C cells.** Micrograph showing the distribution of thyroid C cells (identified using an immunoperoxidase method for calcitonin) in the adult human thyroid; they are scattered between the thyroid acinus lining cells singly, in clumps and as interstitial clusters. Cells in the acini tend to be sited on the basement membrane, apparently having no contact with the colloid-filled lumen.

The thyroid also produces the hormone calcitonin

Calcitonin inhibits calcium resorption from bones by osteoclasts, thus antagonizing the action of parathormone (see p. 256) and lowering blood calcium levels. It may increase the rate of osteoid mineralization.

Calcitonin-producing cells (C cells) are scattered between the thyroid acinus (follicle) lining cells, but are occasionally seen in small clusters in the interstitial spaces between adjacent acini. The latter location, most common in animals, such as the dog, explains the archaic name 'parafollicular cells'.

C cells are small pale-staining cells, which are difficult to see by routine light microscopy but can be identified either by electron microscopy or by immunoperoxidase techniques (Fig. 14.18). Ultrastructurally, they contain the dense-core neurosecretory granules that are characteristic of neuroendocrine cells.

Calcitonin secretion seems to be controlled directly by blood calcium levels.

Most malignant thyroid tumours are derived from the glandular epithelial cells lining the thyroid follicles, and are therefore thyroid adenocarcinomas. A rare tumour, called 'medullary carcinoma', is derived from the thyroid C cells and secretes excessive amounts of calcitonin. Both spread by lymphatics to lymph nodes in the neck, and subsequently by the bloodstream to more distant sites.

Parathyroid

The parathyroid glands secrete parathormone, which is involved in calcium homeostasis

The parathyroid glands, of which there are at least four and in some people up to eight, are small, pale tan

CLINICAL EXAMPLE
THYROTOXICOSIS

In thyrotoxicosis the thyroid epithelial cells increase in size and number and their work rate increases so that excessive thyroxine is produced (Fig. 14.19).

This is manifest clinically by weight loss and heat intolerance (due to an increased basal metabolic rate), tremor, rapid pulse and bulging of the eyes (exophthalmos) owing to an increase in the orbital support tissues.

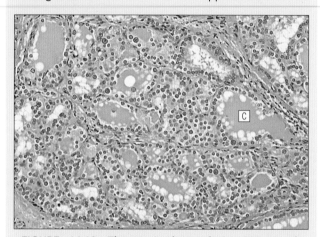

FIGURE 14.19 **Thyrotoxic hyperplasia.** Micrograph showing the characteristic features of hyperplastic thyroid. An increased number of thyroid epithelial cells is shown by the development of papillary folds of acinar epithelium; in addition, each epithelial cell is large and columnar and the edges of the colloid (C) are scalloped, indicating active removal of stored colloid for processing into thyroxine.

endocrine glands. They are usually ovoid in shape, but are occasionally flattened by moulding from adjacent organs or tissues.

Each gland is approximately 5 mm long, 3 mm wide and 1–2 mm thick, although size varies considerably with age and calcium metabolic status. In adults each gland weighs approximately 130 mg, those in women being slightly heavier than in men.

Parathyroid glands are sited in the neck in the region of the thyroid gland but their precise location is variable.

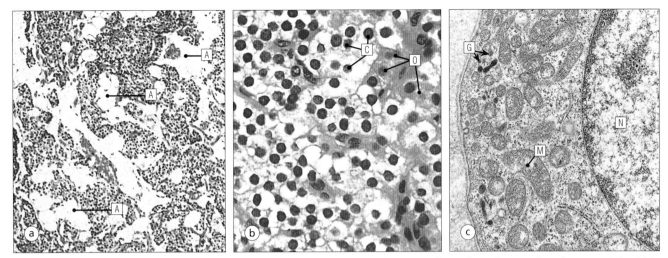

FIGURE 14.20 **Parathyroid.** (a) Low-power micrograph of an H&E-stained section of parathyroid. Note the adipocytes (A), which are seen as non-staining areas. (b) High-power micrograph of an H&E-stained section of parathyroid showing chief cells (C) and oxyphil cells (O). (c) Electron micrograph of parathyroid showing the edge of an oxyphil cell and its nucleus (N). Note the scanty peripheral neurosecretory granules (G) and numerous mitochondria (M) in this resting phase cell.

They are derived from the third and fourth branchial pouches, the glands from the third pouch being located near the lower pole of the thyroid, whereas those from the fourth lie close to the upper pole, either behind it or at the cricothyroid junction; those behind the upper pole are often sited inside the thyroid capsule and are therefore apparently intrathyroidal.

The parathyroids at the lower pole have a much more variable location. Approximately half are sited on the anterior or posterior surface of the lower pole of the lateral lobes, the other half being located in the thymic tongue just beneath the lower pole. Occasionally, parathyroid glands may be found in the mediastinum, within thymic remnants.

The parathyroid glands secrete the hormone parathormone, which is important in maintaining calcium homeostasis. It increases calcium ion concentration in the blood by mobilizing the calcium stored in mineralized bone. Parathormone achieves this by stimulating osteoclasts to erode bone from the surfaces of bone trabeculae (see p. 256). When the serum calcium level falls, an increase in parathormone secretion equalizes it by mobilizing the stored calcium in bone. Excessive secretion of parathormone leads to structural damage to bone and excess calcium in the blood (hypercalcaemia, see 'Clinical Example' box, on p. 274).

Three main histological cell types are seen in the parathyroid

The normal adult human parathyroid is surrounded by a thin fibrous capsule and is composed of three cell types:

- Adipocytes
- Chief cells, which produce parathormone
- Oxyphil cells.

Adipocytes appear in the parathyroid at puberty and gradually increase in number until about the age of 40,

from then on remaining a fairly constant proportion of the entire gland, though their number may decrease in old age. They form a background stroma in which the chief and oxyphil cells are arranged in cords and nests close to a fine network of capillary vessels.

When there is a continuous increased requirement for parathyroid hormone, for example when the serum calcium level is persistently low in renal failure, the chief cells increase in number (hyperplasia) at the expense of the adipocytes.

Parathyroid chief cells are the active endocrine component of the gland

Chief cells are about 8–10 μm in diameter and are roughly spherical in shape. Their nuclei are small, round, dark staining and central, and their cytoplasm is usually pale pinkish-purple (Fig. 14.20), although at certain stages, they become vacuolated with glycogen and lipid, when they are sometimes referred to as 'clear cells'.

Their ultrastructural appearance depends largely on whether they are in a resting, synthesizing or secreting stage of hormone response. They contain membrane-bound neuroendocrine granules of parathormone, commonly arranged towards the periphery of the cell.

In the synthesizing phase, there are stacks of rough endoplasmic reticulum and an active Golgi. In the resting phase, the neuroendocrine granules are still present but the Golgi is small and the rough endoplasmic reticulum less prominent; glycogen granules and small lipid droplets are also seen. The glycogen and lipid become less apparent during hormone synthesis but reappear when the cells are secreting the packaged hormone.

In the healthy adult with a normal calcium balance, approximately 80% of the chief cells are in the resting phase. If hypercalcaemia develops, this proportion increases to 100% (and the cells contain numerous

CLINICAL EXAMPLE
DISORDERS OF PARATHORMONE SECRETION – HYPOCALCAEMIA

Secretion of parathormone by the parathyroid glands is finely controlled by a feedback loop based on the level of calcium ions in the blood. When the level of Ca^{2+} in the blood falls below an acceptable level, a burst of parathormone secretion stimulates osteoclasts to erode just enough bone to release the appropriate amount of calcium to bring the blood level back to normal, when a feedback mechanism stops further parathormone secretion. When calcium loss is excessive and persistent (e.g. in some examples of kidney disease, when calcium ions are constantly lost in large amounts in the urine) the persistently low serum calcium levels (hypocalcaemia) act as a constant stimulus to parathormone production in an attempt to compensate. All parathyroid glands become filled with actively hormone-secreting chief cells and enlarge. This increase in cell number is called **parathyroid hyperplasia**. This massive consistent outpouring of parathormone stimulates extensive erosion of bone by osteoclasts and the architecture of the bone is destroyed, leading to severe bone disease. Parathyroid hyperplasia in response to hypocalcaemia is called **secondary hyperparathyroidism**; despite the enormous release of calcium in this way, it usually does not compensate for the vast amounts being lost in the urine by the diseased kidneys, and the serum calcium level rarely rises back to normal limits.

Hypocalcaemia can also occur when all the parathyroid glands are inadvertently removed surgically during total removal of the thyroid, usually for cancer. It may also be the result of inadequate absorption of dietary calcium.

CLINICAL EXAMPLE
TUMOURS OF THE PARATHYROID

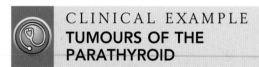

The main tumour that occurs in the parathyroid glands is the benign **parathyroid adenoma**. These tumours are almost always solitary and cause enlargement of the affected parathyroid gland. This tumour constantly secretes excess parathormone, irrespective of the serum calcium level, and constant osteoclastic erosion of the bone leads to extensive bone destruction and very high levels of calcium ions in the blood (hypercalcaemia). This is called **primary hyperparathyroidism**.

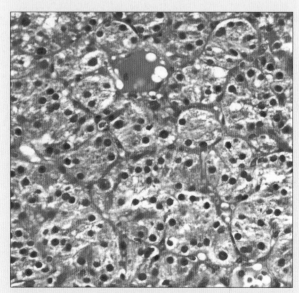

FIGURE 14.21 **Parathyroid adenoma.** Micrograph showing a benign tumour (adenoma) of the parathyroid gland. Note that the tumour is composed almost entirely of active sheets of chief cells and that the usual adipose tissue component has been replaced by tumour cells.

fine lipid droplets), but it decreases with transient or permanent hypocalcaemia. At light microscopy a synthesizing or secreting chief cell can be identified by its purplish cytoplasm and the absence of fine lipid droplets (Fig. 14.21).

> **Parathyroid oxyphil cells are larger than chief cells and have abundant eosinophilic cytoplasm**

Parathyroid oxyphil cells are greater than 10 μm in diameter and the cytoplasm is markedly eosinophilic and granular owing to the presence of many mitochondria. Their nuclei are small, spherical and dark staining.

Ultrastructurally, oxyphil cell cytoplasm is packed with large active mitochondria, with intervening cytoplasm containing only scanty free ribosomes and glycogen granules; endoplasmic reticulum and neurosecretory vacuoles are uncommon, indicating that the cells are not endocrinologically active. Transitional cell forms with features of both oxyphil and active chief cells are occasionally seen.

Oxyphil cells are rare before puberty but appear in increasing numbers in early adult life, either singly or in clumps. In the elderly, they are often numerous and sometimes form variably sized oval or rounded tumour-like nodules within a normal sized parathyroid.

Adrenals

Introduction

The adrenal glands are located on the upper poles of the kidneys and combine two distinct endocrine systems within one organ. The adrenal cortex synthesizes and secretes steroid hormones produced from cholesterol. The adrenal medulla is a neuroendocrine component, synthesizing and secreting the vasoactive amines epinephrine (adrenaline) and norepinephrine (noradrenaline).

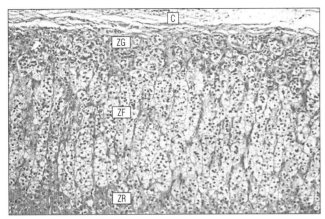

FIGURE 14.22 **Adrenal cortex (low power).** Micrograph showing the three distinct zones of the adrenal cortex, the zona glomerulosa (ZG), the zona fasciculata (ZF) and the zona reticularis (ZR), which are enclosed by a capsule (C).

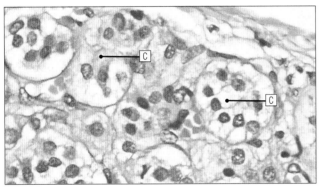

FIGURE 14.23 **Zona glomerulosa.** The zona glomerulosa is composed of small compact cells (C) arranged in clumps and separated by stroma composed largely of thin-walled capillaries. The cells contain scanty lipid droplets associated with well-developed smooth endoplasmic reticulum and comparatively little rough endoplasmic reticulum.

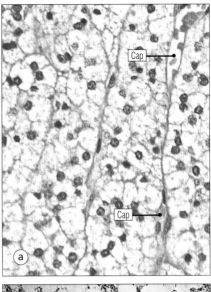

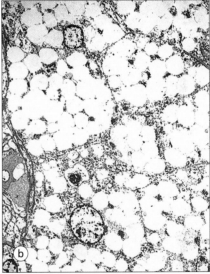

FIGURE 14.24 **Zona fasciculata.** (a) These cells are arranged in vertical columns, which are usually two to three cells wide, the columns being separated by capillaries (Cap). (b) Ultrastructurally, the cells have prominent rough endoplasmic reticulum, characteristic small round or ovoid mitochondria with tubular cristae and extensive lipid vacuoles. The surfaces of cells adjacent to capillaries may show small microvilli extending to the capillary wall.

Adrenal Cortex

The adrenal cortex secretes steroid hormones

The adrenal cortex – the outer layer of the adrenal gland in the adult – is composed of three distinct zones. These zones, the zona glomerulosa, zona fasciculata and zona reticularis, are bound externally by a thin fibrous capsule and internally by the adrenal medulla (Fig. 14.22).

The outer zona glomerulosa (Fig. 14.23) synthesizes and secretes mineralocorticoids, mainly aldosterone and deoxycorticosterone. The zona glomerulosa is the thin subcapsular zone of adrenal cortex that merges imperceptibly on its inner surface with the middle zona fasciculata. It is not always a complete layer and has a patchy distribution.

The middle zona fasciculata (Fig. 14.24) secretes glucocorticoids, mainly cortisol and corticosterone, and also small amounts of the androgenic steroid dehydroepiandrosterone (DHA). The zona fasciculata occupies most of the adrenal cortex and is composed of large rectangular cells with light-staining clear or finely vacu-

olated cytoplasm caused by intracytoplasmic accumulation of lipid droplets containing cholesterol and intermediate lipids, as well as formed glucocorticoids.

The inner zona reticularis (Fig. 14.25) produces androgenic steroids and some glucocorticoids, but normally only in small amounts. This inner zone of adrenal cortex is thinner than the zona fasciculata, but thicker than the zona glomerulosa. It is composed of cells with eosinophilic cytoplasm arranged in an anastomosing network of clumps and columns with a capillary network closely apposed to the cell membranes. A characteristic feature of this layer when stained with H&E is the presence of brown pigment (lipofuscin). To the naked eye, the layer appears pale brown, whereas the zona fasciculata is bright yellow.

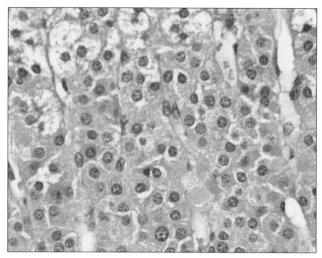

FIGURE 14.25 **Zona reticularis.**

Ultrastructurally, the cells possess prominent smooth endoplasmic reticulum and electron-dense irregular aggregations of lipofuscin, as well as lysosomes and oval or long mitochondria, with tubular cristae similar to those seen in the cells of the zona fasciculata.

The adrenal in the fetus has an extra outer cell layer

In the fetus and neonate, the adrenal cortex is proportionately much larger than in the adult and has an additional external cortical zone. This additional outer layer involutes after birth, the three layers of the adult cortex developing from the remaining cells. The cells that involute have the appearance of steroid-secreting cells, possessing a large Golgi and many lipid droplets; furthermore, they have round mitochondria with tubular cristae very similar to those of the adult zona fasciculata.

Activity of the fetal adrenal cortex is controlled partly by the fetal pituitary through the feedback of cortisol on pituitary ACTH secretion, and partly by the placenta.

Adrenal Medulla

The adrenal medulla secretes catecholamines

The adrenal medulla, the centre of the adrenal gland, is surrounded by adrenal cortex. The adrenal medulla is derived from the neural crest and is part of the neuro-endocrine system, secreting epinephrine (adrenaline), norepinephrine (noradrenaline) and associated peptides, including enkephalins. Epinephrine and norepinephrine synthesis is controlled by sympathetic and parasympathetic nerve twigs present in the gland.

Adrenal medullary cells have large, commonly pale-staining nuclei and their cytoplasm is usually finely granular, with a purplish staining reaction. They are usually polyhedral in shape, arranged in clumps, cords or columns and surrounded by a rich network of capillaries (Fig. 14.26a).

CLINICAL EXAMPLE
TUMOURS AND OTHER DISORDERS OF THE ADRENAL CORTEX

The most common disorders of the adrenal cortex are hypoadrenalism and hyperadrenalism, resulting, respectively, from a deficiency or an excess of all of the adrenal cortical steroid hormones; their clinical manifestations are, however, largely due to the hormones produced by the zona fasciculata, the glucocorticoids.

The most common cause of hypoadrenalism (Addison's syndrome) is destruction of both adrenals by disease, leaving insufficient adrenal cortex for hormone production. This usually results from autoimmune disease, but can also be due to tuberculosis.

In addition, hypoadrenalism can be induced by giving large doses of glucocorticoids therapeutically; this suppresses ACTH secretion by the pituitary, so that the adrenal cortex produces no native steroid hormone. If the therapeutic steroid is suddenly discontinued, an acute hypoadrenal crisis may develop.

Hypoadrenalism is manifest clinically by hypotension, hyponatraemia and brown skin pigmentation, and may present as a sudden collapse associated with severe shock.

The most common tumour of the adrenal cortex is the benign tumour called adrenal cortical adenoma. Most of these are non-functional but a few secrete excess glucocorticoids, producing Cushing's syndrome, or mineralocorticoids, producing Conn's syndrome. These are the most common manifestations of hyperadrenalism.

Cushing's syndrome is manifest clinically by cushingoid facies, hirsutism, acne, central obesity, striae, osteoporosis, diabetes mellitus, hypertension, hypokalaemia, muscle weakness and mental disturbance.

Conn's syndrome is associated with hypertension, hypokalaemia causing polyuria and muscle weakness, and alkalosis.

KEY FACTS
ADRENAL

- Zona glomerulosa (narrow, subcapsular zone of cortex) secretes mineralocorticoids, mainly aldosterone
- Zona fasciculata (broad, yellow mid-zone of cortex) secretes glucocorticoids, mainly cortisol and corticosterone
- Zona reticularis (narrow inner zone of cortex) secretes mainly androgenic steroids
- Adrenal medulla (central, enclosed by cortex, brown) is neuroendocrine and secretes epinephrine (adrenaline) and norepinephrine (noradrenaline).

Cells of the adrenal medulla contain neurosecretory granules

Ultrastructurally, cells of the adrenal medulla contain neuroendocrine granules. These vary in size and appearance, ranging from 150 to 350 nm in diameter.

Cells secreting epinephrine (adrenaline) have small spherical neuroendocrine granules, almost entirely

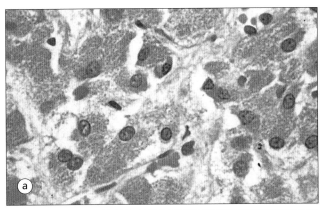

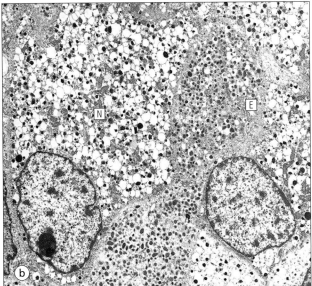

FIGURE 14.26 **Adrenal medulla.** (a) Micrograph of adrenal medullary cells showing their large nuclei and finely granular cytoplasm. (b) Electron micrograph showing large dense-core granules corresponding to norepinephrine (noradrenaline) (N) and epinephrine (adrenaline) (E).

occupied by electron-dense material with a narrow, clear halo between the central material and the thin surrounding membrane.

Cells secreting norepinephrine (noradrenaline) have larger neuroendocrine granules with a more obvious electron-lucent layer inside the membrane, the granules containing irregular and often angulated electron-dense material (Fig. 14.26b).

Adrenal medullary cells synthesize and store their respective peptide hormones, normally releasing only small amounts at a time, although during periods of acute stress or excitement larger quantities are secreted under the influence of the autonomic nervous system.

Because of their high catecholamine content, adrenal medullary cells develop an intense brown colour when exposed to air or to a strong oxidizing agent, such as potassium dichromate, owing to the formation of brown pigment when the amines are oxidized. This is the basis of their antiquated name 'chromaffin cells'.

There are two tumours of the adrenal medulla; they are uncommon but very important.

Pheochromocytoma is usually benign, in that it enlarges but does not spread to distant sites. Although benign, it produces severe symptoms and may be fatal. This is because it is derived from cells that produce epinephrine (adrenaline) and norepinephrine (noradrenaline), and the tumours produce these active chemicals in excessive amounts, leading to uncontrollable high blood pressure, which may be fatally complicated by a stroke or severe heart failure.

Neuroblastoma is a highly malignant tumour of the adrenal medulla which is derived from primitive neural crest embryonic stem cells (neuroblasts), from which the adrenal medulla develops in embryonic life. Occasionally, some of these cells persist after birth and may develop into this tumour. This is an example of a so-called 'embryonal' tumour; another type is seen in the kidney in children (nephroblastoma, see p. 308)

There is a rich vascular supply to both cortex and medulla

The adrenal glands receive a rich arterial supply, which forms an arterial plexus of capsular arteries over their surface. Two types of vessel are derived from these arteries: cortical arterioles and medullary arterioles, supplying blood to the cortex and medulla, respectively, although there is communication between the two systems at the interface between cortex and medulla. The vascular supply is shown in Figure 14.27.

Pancreas

Introduction

The neuroendocrine component of the human pancreas exists in three forms:

- Islets of Langerhans are distinct structures accounting for most of the hormone-producing cells
- Isolated nests or clumps of neuroendocrine cells form a minority population of cells gathered into small groups, which are distinct from islets
- Single cells are scattered within the exocrine (see p. 215) and ductular components of the pancreas and are demonstrable by immunocytochemical methods.

Pancreatic endocrine cells are grouped into clusters called islets of Langerhans

Islets of Langerhans are discrete, rounded clusters of cells scattered throughout the pancreatic tissue. They are embedded in its exocrine component and are most numerous in the tail region. They vary considerably in size and in the number of cells they contain. Individual cells within the islets are smaller and paler than the exocrine cells and assume spherical or polygonal shapes owing to moulding by adjacent cells. Each islet has a capillary network which is in contact with each cell (Fig. 14.28b).

Pancreatic islets develop as cellular buds from the same small ducts that ultimately supply the exocrine pancreatic components. Occasionally in humans, variably sized islets can be seen in association with a pancreatic duct in the supporting fibrous tissue.

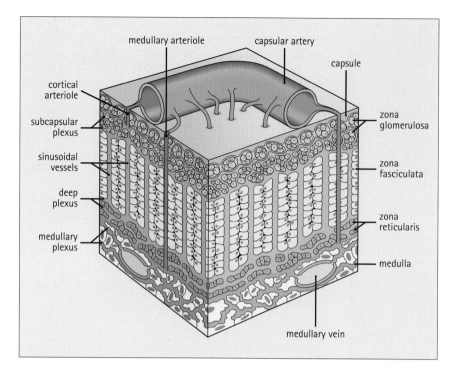

FIGURE 14.27 **Vascular anatomy of the adrenal gland.** Cortical arterioles form a subcapsular plexus. This gives rise to sinusoidal vessels running down between the columns of the zona fasciculata of the adrenal cortex before forming a further deep plexus in the zona reticularis. This deeper plexus communicates with the plexus of vessels supplying the medulla. Medullary arterioles arise directly from the capsular arteries and run straight down through the cortex into the medulla, where they form a medullary plexus. The deep medullary plexus drains by small venous vessels into the large medullary vein.

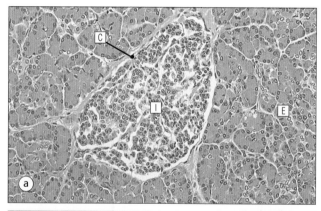

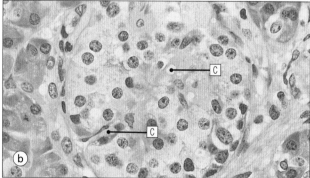

FIGURE 14.28 **Islets of Langerhans.** (a) Medium-power photomicrograph of an islet of Langerhans (I) embedded in the exocrine component (E) of the pancreas. The islets, roughly spherical, are composed of much smaller cells than the exocrine pancreas, from which they are separated by a fine fibrocollagenous capsule (C). (b) High-power micrograph showing islet cells. Note that each cell is in contact with the capillary network (C).

CLINICAL EXAMPLE
DIABETES MELLITUS

Diabetes mellitus is a disease in which there is inadequate action of the hormone insulin. It is a multi-system disease that affects carbohydrate, fat and protein metabolism.

Two main types of diabetes mellitus are identified on clinical grounds.

- Type 1 diabetes (insulin-dependent diabetes mellitus, (IDDM) or juvenile-onset diabetes). This usually develops in childhood or adolescence. It is an autoimmune disorder in which the insulin-secreting pancreatic islet cells are destroyed. The pancreas shows loss of islet cells with infiltrating lymphocytes, responsible for their destruction. This is an autoimmune process that may be caused by an abnormal immune response to certain viral infections. The destruction of insulin-secreting cells leads to insulin deficiency, which in turn leads to hyperglycaemia and other secondary metabolic complications.
- Type 2 diabetes (non-insulin-dependent diabetes mellitus (NIIDM) or maturity onset diabetes). This type of disease is more common than Type 1 diabetes. Unlike Type 1 diabetes, where there is a loss of insulin-secreting cells from the pancreatic islets, in Type 2 diabetics, disease is due to the phenomenon of peripheral insulin resistance.

In diseases that destroy the pancreas, islet cells are lost in addition to the exocrine part of the pancreas. Patients with chronic pancreatitis or patients with cystic fibrosis may develop diabetes mellitus as a result of such pancreatic pathology.

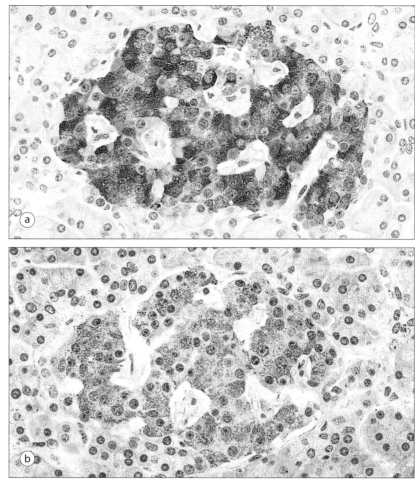

FIGURE 14.29 **Insulin-secreting cells.** (a) Immunocytochemical method for insulin. (b) Immunocytochemical method for amylin (same islet). Insulin/amylin-secreting cells occupy the central area of the pancreatic islets and are the most common cell type. These cells have well developed rough endoplasmic reticulum, a prominent Golgi, and numerous neurosecretory vesicles about 300 nm in diameter. The vesicles have a central electron-dense core in the form of a rhomboidal or polyhedral crystalline structure surrounded by an electron-lucent halo and bounded by a narrow membrane. In a few vesicles the core is missing, possibly owing to the recent discharge of insulin (the central core is thought to be composed of insulin complexed with zinc). The peptide amylin is thought to modulate the action of insulin.

Each pancreatic islet contains a number of different neuroendocrine cells

Each different cell type is mainly concerned with the secretion of a single hormone. The nomenclature of these individual cell types is confusing, and so below, each type is identified by its main hormone (with other terms being given in parentheses).

There are four main cell types and at least two minor ones. Of the total number of pancreatic endocrine cells, the proportions of the main cell types are as follows:

- Approximately 70% are insulin- and amylin-secreting cells (B or β cells) (Fig. 14.29)
- Approximately 20% are glucagon-secreting cells (A or α cells) (Fig. 14.30)
- Approximately 5–10% are somatostatin-secreting cells (D, δ or type III cells) (Fig. 14.31)
- Approximately 1–2% are pancreatic polypeptide secreting cells (PP or F cells).

The PP cells, which are comparatively scanty when a random block of the pancreas is examined, are found in greater numbers in the posterior lobe of the pancreas, in the head and neck region. They are also found as scattered cells in duct walls. Their neurosecretory vacuoles are spherical, with a central electron-dense core surrounded by a wide electron-lucent area.

The minor cell types are:
- Vasoactive-intestinal peptide (VIP)-secreting cells (D-1 or type IV cells)
- Mixed secretion cells (EC or enterochromaffin cells).

Minor cell types are present in small numbers in the islets and scattered in the exocrine and ductular components. The mixed secretion cells have been reported to produce a number of active peptides, including serotonin, motilin and substance P.

An apparent anomaly is that the gastric hormone gastrin is secreted in excess by some islet cell tumours,

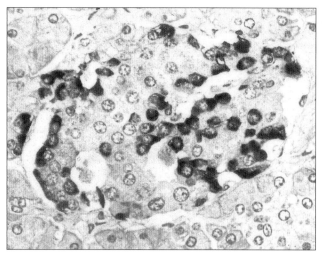

FIGURE 14.30 **Glucagon-secreting cells.** Glucagon-secreting cells are located mainly at the periphery of the pancreatic islets, as shown in this micrograph of a section stained to show glucagon by an immunoperoxidase technique. Glucagon-secreting cells possess similar ultrastructural features to those of insulin-secreting cells, except that the secretory vesicles are smaller and have a more spherical electron-dense core, which is usually eccentrically located.

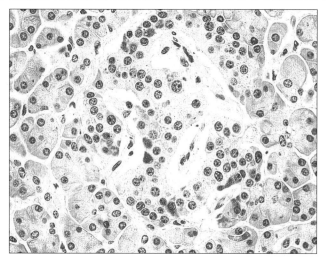

FIGURE 14.31 **Somatostatin-secreting cells.** Somatostatin-secreting cells are a minority population and, in man, are scattered apparently randomly throughout the pancreatic islets, as shown in this micrograph stained to show somatostatin by an immunoperoxidase technique. Some islets contain substantial numbers of these cells, whereas others contain none at all. Somatostatin-secreting cells contain larger neurosecretory vesicles than insulin-secreting and glucagon-secreting cells, being up to 35 nm in diameter, and their core is much less electron-dense.

but has not been satisfactorily demonstrated in the normal pancreatic islet.

The islets contain a complex network of capillaries with fenestrated endothelium

These capillaries arise from small arterioles outside the islet and, after penetrating the islet, merge with capillar-

ies supplying the exocrine component of the pancreas. Fenestrated capillary endothelium is a common feature in endocrine tissue.

Pancreatic islets are innervated by the autonomic nervous system

There are both sympathetic and parasympathetic twigs contacting the surfaces of about 10% of all the cells directly. There are well-developed gap junctions between adjacent islet cells, which may provide the mechanism whereby the neural stimulus is passed to all cells. The autonomic nervous system also innervates the blood vessels and possibly affects perfusion.

Parasympathetic stimulation increases insulin and glucagon output, whereas sympathetic stimulation inhibits insulin release.

Ovary and Testis

Although their main function is to produce female and male gametes, the testis and ovary also act as endocrine organs (see Chapters 16 and 17).

Diffuse Neuroendocrine System

Introduction

So far, only those neuroendocrine cells that are gathered together to form distinct endocrine glands have been discussed. There is, however, an extensive system of scattered neuroendocrine cells producing hormones and active peptides, many of which act on the local environment, rather than having a distant systemic impact. Almost all of these cells belong to the so-called 'APUD' or 'diffuse neuroendocrine system', and have the following common characteristics:

- Uptake and decarboxylation of amine precursor compounds, producing active amines, peptides and hormones (amine precursor uptake and decarboxylation, APUD cells)
- Possession of characteristic cytoplasmic organelles, known as dense-core granules, neurosecretory vesicles or rimmed vacuoles.

These have a common basic structure of a variably electron-dense core (usually spherical, but occasionally angulated), a clear electron-lucent halo around the dense core, a thin distinct membrane surrounding the halo, and, irrespective of the shape of the central dense core, the entire vesicle is usually spherical or oval. The vesicles vary in size (usually 100–600 nm in diameter), shape (spherical or oval), width of electron-lucent halo and electron density of the central core, depending on the nature of the amine, peptide or hormone produced. In some cases, their secretion is under neural control.

Examples of neuroendocrine cells have already been described in this chapter, for example adrenal medullary cells (see p. 276), calcitonin-secreting C cells (see p. 272) and pancreatic islet cells (see p. 279). Further examples occur in other chapters, for example renin-producing juxtaglomerular cells (see p. 306).

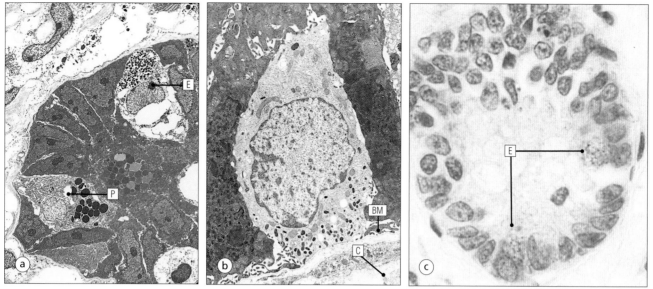

FIGURE 14.32 **Enteroendocrine cell.** (a) Low-power electron micrograph showing enteroendocrine cells (E) in the base of a small bowel gland. This contrasts with a Paneth cell (P) (see also Fig. 11.40). (b) High-power electron micrograph showing neuroendocrine vesicles facing the basement membrane (BM) of the gland, and an adjacent capillary vessel (C). (c) Micrograph showing enteroendocrine cells (E) demonstrated by an immunoperoxidase method to detect synaptophysin, a glycoprotein specific to the neuroendocrine vesicle membrane.

The important cells of the diffuse neuroendocrine system are gut-associated endocrine cells and respiratory-associated endocrine cells.

Gut-associated endocrine cells are seen throughout the intestinal tract

Throughout the alimentary tract, the lining epithelium contains scattered endocrine cells termed 'gut-associated endocrine cells' or 'enteroendocrine cells'. Enteroendocrine cells are mainly concentrated in the stomach and small intestine (see Figs 11.32, 11.41). They are also present in the lower oesophagus and large intestine, and in the ducts of organs draining into the gut (i.e. the bile and pancreatic ducts).

In general, enteroendocrine cells are small, with a spherical nucleus and pale-staining cytoplasm, and lie in contact with the basement membrane on which the mucosal epithelial cells sit (Fig. 14.32); many are not in contact with the lumen. Neurosecretory vesicles are concentrated mainly in the basal portion of these cells.

Enteroendocrine cells are difficult to identify by routine H&E staining but can be highlighted by certain silver stains, which is why they were formerly termed 'argentaffin' or 'argyrophil cells'. Another old synonym, 'enterochromaffin cells', is based on their reaction with potassium dichromate to produce a brown pigment. Immunocytochemical methods have demonstrated many more enteroendocrine cells than are visible by silver methods; they also indicate the cells' main secretion. These methods, therefore, have effectively replaced silver staining methods for demonstrating such cells.

The ultrastructural features of enteroendocrine cells, particularly the size, shape and number of neurosecretory vesicles, vary according to the amine or peptide hormone produced, and more than 20 such products have been identified. Most of these hormones cannot be accurately matched with an ultrastructurally characteristic cell type, and it is likely that some or all of the cells can produce more than one active secretion.

Tumours of the gut-associated endocrine cells occur but are rare; for historical reasons they are given the uninformative and unsatisfactory name of **carcinoid tumours**. They are most often seen in the small intestine and are malignant, but grow for a long time before spreading to different sites.

Respiratory-associated endocrine cells are seen throughout the respiratory tract

Pulmonary neuroendocrine cells in humans exist in two forms: scattered and aggregated.

Individual neuroendocrine cells are scattered throughout the trachea, the intrapulmonary airways, and occasionally in the alveolar wall. These cells are pale when stained by H&E and are difficult to distinguish without the aid of special methods such as immunocytochemical techniques. Most of the cell sits on the epithelial basement membrane in a manner similar to that of enteroendocrine cells (see Fig. 14.32a), but a cytoplasmic process extends towards the lumen between adjacent epithelial cells.

Small aggregates of neuroendocrine cells form small mounds protruding into the airway lumen or alveoli. These aggregates, which are particularly prominent where airways branch, receive unmyelinated axons from peribronchial and peribronchiolar nerves and have been called 'neuroepithelial bodies' (see Fig. 10.13b).

The cytoplasm of both individual and clumped pulmonary neuroendocrine cells contains numerous neurosecretory vesicles. Serotonin, bombesin, calcitonin and Leu-enkephalin have all been demonstrated within these cells.

In humans, respiratory-associated neuroendocrine cells are most numerous and prominent at birth, decreasing rapidly thereafter, whereas in some other animals, particularly rodents, they remain in significant numbers throughout life.

A malignant tumour of neuroendocrine cells in the bronchial mucosa (called a small cell undifferentiated carcinoma) is one of the most common and important types of 'lung cancer'. It is highly malignant, and spreads rapidly and widely (see p. 174).

Paraganglia

The paraganglia are specialized neuroendocrine glands associated with the autonomic nervous system

Paraganglia consist of prominent neuroendocrine cells containing neurosecretory vesicles. Those that have been adequately investigated have been shown to contain active amine or peptide hormones and are therefore regarded as part of the neuroendocrine system.

In many cases, their precise function and the nature of their secretions is not clear, but it is known that some of the larger paraganglia in the thorax and neck (e.g. aortic body and carotid body), act as chemoreceptors.

Paraganglia vary in size from clumps of a few cells associated with nerves, visible only with microscopy, to structures up to 3 mm in diameter, which are anatomically distinct. The largest are the intercarotid paraganglia (carotid bodies) and the aortic sympathetic paraganglia (organ of Zuckerkandl).

Paraganglia are composed of chief cells, sustentacular cells and blood vessels

Chief cells are neuroendocrine cells containing neurosecretory vesicles arranged into roughly round clumps or nests (zellballen). Each clump is surrounded by an intimate network of capillaries with fenestrated endothelium and a basement membrane. The neuroendocrine cells are of two types.

Most are termed 'light cells' and have pale vacuolated cytoplasm containing moderate numbers of spherical electron-dense neurosecretory vesicles about 100–150 nm in diameter.

A small proportion are termed 'dark cells' and have darker staining cytoplasm containing large numbers of pleomorphic, often angulated, neurosecretory vesicles 50–250 nm in diameter.

Between the neuroendocrine cells and the capillaries are occasional flattened support cells, the sustentacular cells (Fig. 14.33).

Sustentacular cells, which account for 35–45% of paraganglion cells, have elongated spindle-shaped nuclei and pale-staining cytoplasm with ill-defined cell borders. Concentrated at the periphery of the clumps of neuroendocrine cells, they send cytoplasmic processes into

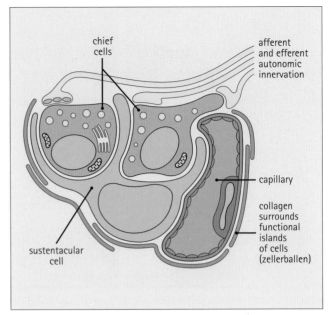

FIGURE 14.33 **Paraganglion.** A paraganglion, showing that it is composed of chief cells arranged into clumps surrounded by sustentacular cells and capillaries.

the clumps and also around nerve axons, thus behaving in a similar manner to Schwann cells (see Chapter 6), which they closely resemble both histologically and ultrastructurally.

Paraganglia are richly innervated by both the sympathetic and parasympathetic nervous systems.

 KEY FACTS
CAROTID BODY FUNCTION

The human carotid body contains a mixture of peptides, particularly methionine enkephalin and leucine enkephalin, with smaller amounts of neurotensin and bombesin. In addition, some of the neurosecretory vacuoles contain active amines, including epinephrine (adrenaline), norepinephrine (noradrenaline), serotonin and dopamine.

The carotid body acts as a peripheral chemoreceptor, responding to significant alterations in arterial blood gas tensions and blood pH. Acute hypoxia is countered by an increase in the respiratory rate; this is thought to be mediated by the release of some of the above transmitters, which in turn stimulate afferent nerve terminals.

Chronic hypoxia (such as that seen physiologically in people living at high altitude and pathologically in patients with chronic lung disease or cyanotic congenital heart disease) leads to persistent enlargement of the carotid bodies, up to two or three times the normal size, due to hyperplasia of both sustentacular and chief cells.

With old age, the carotid bodies may show progressive lymphocytic infiltration and fibrosis.

The carotid and aortic bodies are important paraganglia

A single oval carotid body lies in the fibrocollagenous support tissue between the bifurcation of each common carotid artery into internal and external branches. Each carotid body measures about 3×2×2 mm and weighs 5–15 mg.

Carotid bodies are most prominent in children and teenagers, becoming progressively less obvious with increasing age, except in people with chronic hypoxia due to lung disease, or those living in low oxygen tension at high altitudes; in these people, the carotid bodies increase in size as a result of hyperplasia (an increase in cell numbers) and may reach 40 mg in weight.

The carotid body has the general structure of all paraganglia (see Fig. 14.33) and in humans the main peptides identified in it are enkephalins. In other species, such as the cat, other active peptides are also found, including VIP, substance P and catecholamines.

Similar in structure to the carotid bodies, but smaller, are the aortic pulmonary paraganglia (aortic bodies), located on the concave surface of the arch of the aorta, close to where the right pulmonary artery passes beneath.

The carotid and aortic bodies act as chemoreceptors, monitoring the arterial oxygen tension and pH of the blood, the precise mechanism of which is not known.

Numerous aortic sympathetic paraganglia lie around the abdominal aorta

Aortic sympathetic paraganglia are mainly situated around the abdominal aorta from above the level of origin of the renal arteries to the iliac bifurcation and beyond. On the anterior surface of the aorta they are particularly numerous around the coeliac axis and around the origin of the inferior mesenteric artery. Although prominent in infants, they are much less obvious in adults and are rarely discernible with the naked eye.

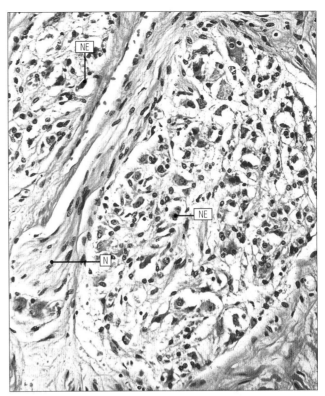

FIGURE 14.34 **Aortic sympathetic paraganglion.** Low-power micrograph showing a small aortic sympathetic-type paraganglion. Note the afferent nerve fibres (N) and the nests of neuroendocrine cells (NE).

Collectively, they are known as 'the organs of Zuckerkandl', particularly the cluster around the origin of the inferior mesenteric artery.

Histologically, aortic sympathetic paraganglia have the same general structure of paraganglia, but the neuroendocrine cells have larger neurosecretory granules than those in the carotid body and more closely resemble those of the adrenal medulla (Fig. 14.34).

 PRACTICAL HISTOLOGY

FIGURE 14.35 **Thyroid.** Micrograph showing normal human thyroid composed of variable-sized follicles (F) filled with pink-staining thyroid colloid. In this illustration the thyroid follicles are in a storage phase, so the lining epithelium (E) is cuboidal or flat and the stored colloid fills the follicle. There is a complex intimate capillary network between adjacent follicles. The details of the thyroid epithelial cell in an active phase are illustrated in Figure 14.17, and the calcitonin-secreting component of the thyroid in Figure 14.18.

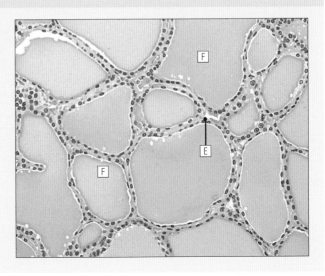

PRACTICAL HISTOLOGY

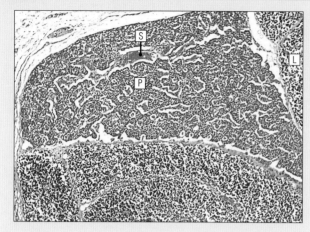

FIGURE 14.36 **Parathyroid gland.** Micrograph showing a child's parathyroid gland (P) closely associated with lymphoid tissue (L). The gland is almost entirely composed of endocrine cells separated by fibrocollagenous septa (S) rich in blood vessels. With increasing age, progressively more adipose tissue develops in the parathyroid gland (see p. 272). The details of the cell types present in the parathyroid are illustrated in Figure 14.20.

 PRACTICAL HISTOLOGY

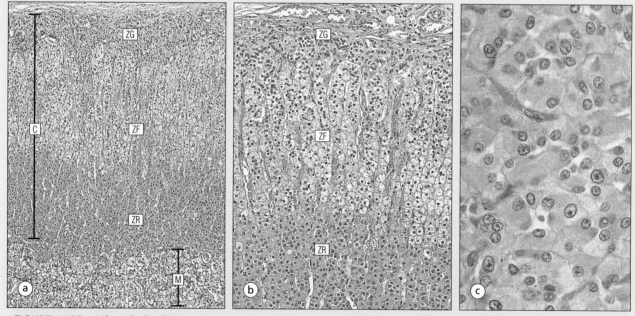

FIGURE 14.37 **Adrenal gland.** (a) Low-power micrograph showing adrenal cortex (C) and medulla (M). Three distinct zones can be seen in the cortex, the zona glomerulosa (ZG), zona fasciculata (ZF) and zona reticularis (ZR). (b) Micrograph showing the adrenal cortex at higher magnification. Note the zona glomerulosa (ZG), zona fasciculata (ZF) and zona reticularis (ZR). The zona fasciculata is the middle zone and is composed of pale-staining cells rich in lipid droplets. The histological details of the cells in these zones are shown in greater detail in Figures 14.23–14.25. (c) Medium-power micrograph of adrenal medulla, which is composed of irregularly shaped cells with granular cytoplasm. These cells contain abundant neuroendocrine vesicles and secrete epinephrine (adrenaline) and norepinephrine (noradrenaline) (see Fig. 14.26). There is an intimate capillary supply.

For online review questions, please visit
https://studentconsult.inkling.com.

END OF CHAPTER REVIEW

True/False Answers to the MCQS, as Well as Case Answers, Can be Found in the Appendix in the Back of the Book.

1. Which of the following features are seen in the epithelial cells of the thyroid acinus?
   (a) Synthesize and secrete calcitonin
   (b) Can convert iodide into iodine
   (c) Can break down thyroglobulin with the release of active thyroid hormones
   (d) Are controlled by TSH from the hypothalamus
   (e) May proliferate and produce a hyperthyroid state

2. Which of the following features are true of the parathyroid glands?
   (a) Are always four in number
   (b) Secrete parathormone in response to a high serum calcium
   (c) Contain chief cells, which are the main hormone secretors
   (d) Contain a variable amount of adipose tissue
   (e) May develop benign tumours which lead to bone destruction

3. Match the components of the adrenal with the relevant major secretion product.
   (a) Zona reticularis
   (b) Medulla
   (c) Zona fasciculata
   (d) Zona glomerulosa
      i. Cortisone
      ii. Aldosterone
      iii. Androgens
      iv. (nor)epinephrine ((nor)adrenaline)

4. Which of the following features are seen in the pituitary gland?
   (a) Is divided into two parts, anterior (neurohypophysis) and posterior (adenohypophysis)
   (b) Is supplied by blood vessels which run from the hypothalamus
   (c) Secretes ADH from the adenohypophysis
   (d) Has most of the GH-secreting cells in the lateral wings of the adenohypophysis
   (e) Is located in the sella turcica

CASE 14.1 A WOMAN WITH MULTIPLE SYMPTOMS

A 37-year-old woman was referred to hospital by her family practitioner for investigation and treatment. For about 6 months, she had noticed that she had become increasingly clumsy in the home, dropping many things and becoming very irritable and 'stressed'. At times of great 'stress' she noticed that her hands trembled and her palms were often hot and sweaty. She slept badly and described 'palpitations', where she felt her heart was racing. A major problem was her constant restlessness, being unable to complete a task before moving on to another, and this caused her great distress, as she felt she was losing her grip at work and antagonizing her workmates. On direct questioning, she admitted to diarrhoea and irregular periods over the preceding few months and considerable loss of weight. Blood tests showed features of thyrotoxicosis and further investigations were arranged to look at the likely cause.

> **Q. Describe the functional and histological background to this case. Concentrate on describing the normal control of thyroid hormone production and speculate where this may become deranged, leading to oversecretion.**

CASE 14.2 A MAN WHO BECAME OBESE AND HYPERTENSIVE

A 56-year-old man is referred to hospital for investigation. At a recent Well Man clinic, he had been found to be hypertensive and the community doctor noted that he was obese, with abdominal striae. A possible diagnosis of Cushing's disease, caused by the effects of excessive corticosteroid, was considered.
   Investigations show an elevated cortisol level and further tests are considered to investigate the cause.

> **Q. Describe the structural and functional background to this case. Concentrate on describing the normal regulation of cortisol production and speculate where this could go wrong to produce disease.**

Chapter 15

Urinary System

Introduction

The main function of the urinary system is the production, storage and voiding of urine.

Urine is an aqueous solution of excess anions and cations and many of the breakdown products of the body's metabolic processes, particularly those that would be toxic if allowed to accumulate.

The most important toxic metabolites are the nitrogen-containing products of protein breakdown, such as urea and creatinine. The composition and concentration of urine can be varied to maintain internal homeostasis.

Urine production and the control of its composition are the responsibility of the kidneys, whereas storage and voiding are performed by the bladder.

The pelvicalyceal systems and ureters transfer urine from the kidneys to the bladder, and the urethra is the channel through which stored urine is voided from the bladder.

The pelvicalyceal systems, ureters, bladder and urethra have a relatively uncomplicated structure (see p. 311). The kidney, however, performs a wide range of biochemical and physiological tasks during the production of urine, and its structure is accordingly complex.

Outline of the Urinary System

The general arrangement of the urinary system is illustrated in Figure 15.1.

The kidneys are solid, bean-shaped organs, located high on the posterior abdominal wall beneath the peritoneum

The concave aspect of each kidney faces toward the midline, where the major channels of arterial supply (the aorta) and venous drainage (the inferior vena cava) run. This concave area is called the 'hilum'. It is the site of entry of the renal arterial supply, and of the emergence of the renal venous drainage and urinary transport systems.

The pelvicalyceal system and ureters are hollow muscular tubes lined by a specialized epithelium

The epithelium is resistant to damage by the variable osmolarity of urine and by the concentration of toxic solutes within it. The walls of the tubes are composed of smooth muscle capable of pushing the fluid towards the bladder by alternate coordinated contraction and relaxation; this process is called 'peristalsis'.

The bladder acts as both a reservoir and a pump

The bladder has basically the same structure as the pelvicalyceal system and ureters but its arrangement of muscle fibres is more sophisticated to allow it to act as both a capacious reservoir for urine and as a pump to force out the urine through the urethra under voluntary control.

Kidney Structure

The kidney is divided into cortex and medulla

Each kidney has two distinct zones: an outer cortex and an inner medulla (Fig. 15.2).

The cortex forms an outer shell and also forms columns (the so-called 'columns of Bertin') that lie between the individual units of the medulla.

The medulla is composed of a series of conical structures (medullary pyramids), the base of each cone being continuous with the inner limit of the cortex and the pointed peak of the pyramid protruding into part of the urine collecting system (the calyceal system) towards the hilum of the kidney. This pointed tip of the medullary pyramid is known as the 'papilla'.

Each human kidney contains 10–18 medullary pyramids, thus 10–18 papillae protrude into the collecting calyces.

Each medullary pyramid, with its associated shell of cortex, comprises a functional and structural lobe of the kidney. This lobar architecture is clearly visible in the fetal kidney (see Fig. 15.1) but becomes less obvious as the kidney increases in size with increasing age.

Kidney Function

The kidney is essential for fluid, electrolyte and acid–base balance, and also has an endocrine function

Urine is produced in the kidney by the selective removal of substances from the blood plasma. Subsequent controlled reabsorption of water, ions, salts, sugars and other carbohydrates, and small molecular weight proteins, allows the kidney to produce urine, the composition of which is appropriate to the body's internal environment and requirements at the time.

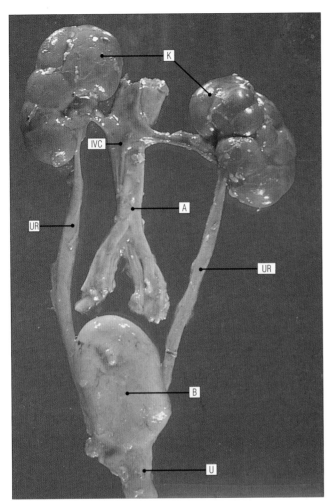

FIGURE 15.1 **Urinary system.** A dissected urinary system from a term male stillbirth demonstrating the interrelationship between the aorta (A), inferior vena cava (IVC), kidneys (K), ureters (UR), bladder (B) and urethra (U). In the adult, the bladder is more spherical.

For example, if the plasma volume is expanded and diluted by a substantial ingestion of water, the kidney will then excrete the excess water by producing large quantities of dilute urine. Conversely, if fluid ingestion is restricted, the kidney will produce a small amount of highly concentrated urine.

Whatever the quantity and concentration of the urine, it will contain the required amount of waste products and ions to maintain internal biochemical homeostasis.

An inability to produce concentrated or dilute urine is an important feature of kidney failure, as it is evidence of inadequate excretion of nitrogenous waste products and other substances, for example potassium ions (see p. 309).

It is important to realize that the kidneys (and the lungs) differ from most other organs in one important respect. In most organs, the vascular supply is the servant of the parenchymal tissues, providing them with oxygen and other raw materials required for the tissue's metabolic processes, and carrying synthesized cell products and waste materials away from the organ. In the kidney, however, the parenchymatous components of the organ are the servants of the blood supply, as the function of

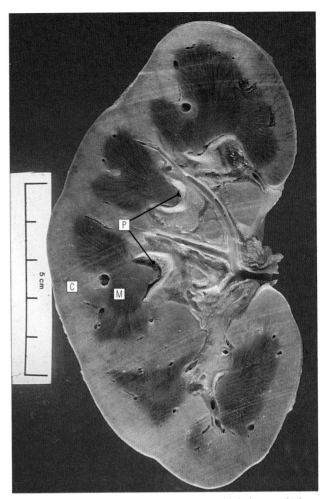

FIGURE 15.2 **Adult human kidney.** An adult human kidney cut longitudinally to show the arrangement of the cortex (C), medulla (M) and papillae (P).

the kidney, in broad terms, is the filtration and cleansing of the blood.

Thus, the parenchymal unit of the kidney, the nephron, which is composed of the glomerulus and cortical and medullary tubular systems, can be regarded as an appendage of the renal blood vascular system, attached to it for servicing purposes. It is not surprising, therefore, that the blood vascular system of the kidney is both substantial and structurally unusual, reflecting its central role. The two kidneys receive 25% of the total cardiac output. Consequently, many of the important and common diseases of the kidney result from abnormality in the blood vascular component (see p. 309).

The kidney also produces the hormones erythropoietin and renin.

Kidney Vasculature

Arteries supplying the kidney branch within the renal substance to supply distinct regions

In most cases, the arterial supply to each kidney comes from a single renal artery, which is a substantial, direct lateral branch of the abdominal aorta. A common variant

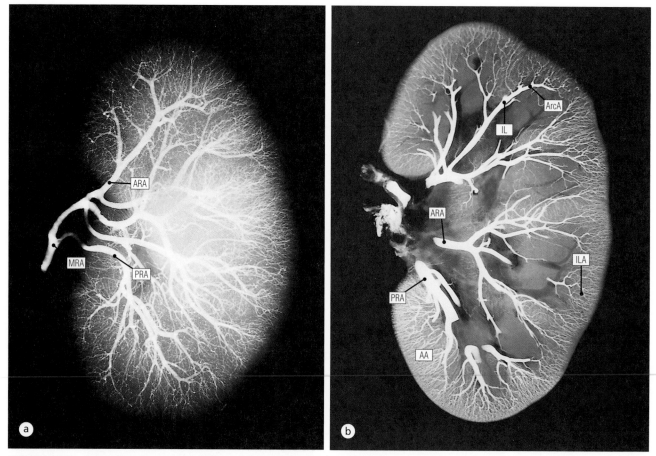

FIGURE 15.3 **Arterial system of the kidney.** (a) Arteriogram of a whole postmortem human kidney showing the division of the main renal artery (MRA) into two branches, a comparatively minor posterior branch (PRA) and a more substantial anterior branch (ARA). The posterior branch supplies the lower pole, whereas the larger anterior branch divides, in this case, into four segmental arteries, which together supply the mid-zone and upper pole of the kidney. (b) In this section, the posterior (PRA) and anterior (ARA) branches of the renal artery can be seen, although some segments are missing owing to the tortuosity of the arteries at the hilum. Note the interlobar arteries (IL), the arcuate arteries (ArcA) and the fine network of interlobular arteries (ILA). The faint haziness (AA) in some areas of the cortex indicates filling of the afferent arterioles.

is the presence of a separate artery arising directly from the aorta and supplying one or other pole.

The renal artery runs towards the concave hilum of the kidney and divides into two main branches, one anterior, one posterior (Fig. 15.3), each of which divides into a number of interlobar arteries that run between the medullary pyramids, one branch to each developmental lobe.

At about the midpoint of the thickness of the kidney parenchyma, where the cortex abuts on the broad base of the medullary pyramid (the corticomedullary junction), the interlobar artery divides into several arcuate arteries, which make a right angle turn and run laterally along the corticomedullary junction.

The arcuate arteries then give rise to a series of side branches (interlobular arteries), which again make a right angle turn and run vertically upwards into the cortex.

Interlobular arteries give rise laterally to a series of arterioles, called 'afferent arterioles', usually directly, but sometimes via a short intralobular artery. These arteries terminate at the periphery of the kidney, just beneath

the capsule, supplying a stellate subcapsular arteriolar and capillary plexus.

Thus far, the arterial supply has been anatomically unremarkable. From the afferent arterioles onward, however, the renal vascular system becomes unique.

Renal Microcirculation

The renal microcirculation contains two capillary systems

In almost every other organ, the capillary network lies between the terminal part of the arterial/arteriolar system and the proximal part of the venular/venous system, and is the major site of oxygen/carbon dioxide exchange. The renal vascular system, in contrast, has a highly specialized preliminary capillary network, the glomerular tuft, which receives blood from an afferent arteriole and which is the site of filtration of waste products from plasma, together with a second capillary system arising from the efferent arteriole, which varies in

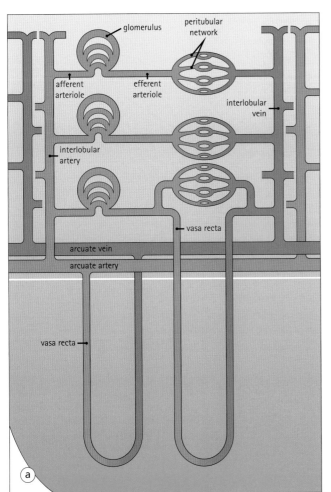

FIGURE 15.4 **Renal microcirculation.** (a) The principles of renal microcirculation. The afferent arteriole, which is a branch of the interlobular artery, enters the glomerular capillary tuft at the vascular hilum. The emerging vessel, the efferent arteriole, normally divides into a complex system of capillaries, the peritubular capillary network, which surrounds the cortical tubules. The venous tributaries arising from the peritubular capillary network drain into small veins opening into the interlobular vein, which runs vertically alongside the interlobular artery and drains into the arcuate vein, running alongside the arcuate artery at the corticomedullary junction. Close to the corticomedullary junction, some of the efferent arterioles give rise to vertically running vessels, the vasa recta, which pass down into the medulla alongside the medullary duct and tubular systems. Some vasa recta arise as direct branches of the arcuate artery and drain directly into the arcuate vein. (b) A carmine–gelatin injection specimen, showing a vertically running interlobular artery (ILA) in the renal cortex, with glomerular capillary tufts (G) arising from lateral branches of the artery and the afferent arterioles (AA). Some peritubular capillary networks (PCN) can also be seen. (c) A carmine–gelatin injection specimen showing the interlobular artery (ILA), the afferent (AA) and efferent arterioles (EA), the glomerular tuft (G) and the peritubular capillary network (PCN). (d) A carmine–gelatin injection specimen of the corticomedullary junction. Note the arcuate artery (ArcA), an interlobular artery (ILA), glomeruli (G) and a number of peritubular capillary networks (PCN) in the cortex. The medulla contains parallel bundles of straight blood vessels, the vasa recta (VR), some of which arise as direct vertical branches of the arcuate artery and others from the efferent arterioles of some glomeruli close to the corticomedullary junction.

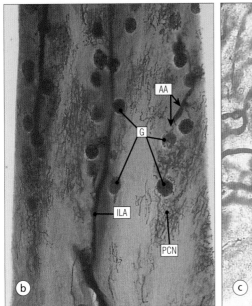

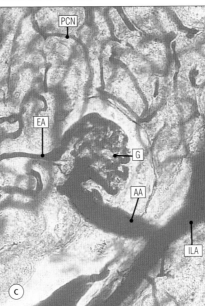

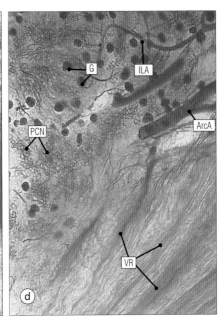

structure and function according to its location within the kidney (Fig. 15.4).

In most cases, after leaving the glomerulus, the efferent arteriole divides into a complex capillary system, which runs in the interstitial spaces between the components of the system of cortical tubules. Each capillary is in intimate contact with these tubules, and is thus ideally placed to take up any substances reabsorbed from the glomerular filtrate by tubular epithelial cells (see p. 298).

However, the capillary system originating from efferent arterioles leaving glomeruli situated deep in the cortex, close to the corticomedullary junction (juxtamedullary glomeruli), is different (see Fig. 15.4). These efferent arterioles divide into a series of long, thin-walled vessels, the vasa recta, which run straight down into the medulla alongside the medullary components of the tubular systems. These vessels play an important role in the ionic and fluid exchanges occurring in the medulla (see p. 301). Some vasa recta arise as direct, vertically running side branches of the arcuate artery.

The first capillary system, the glomerular tuft, does not transfer its contained oxygen to the tissues, nor does it take up a significant amount of carbon dioxide. The major exchange of dissolved gases takes place in the second capillary system. Oxygen is supplied to the cortical and medullary parts of the renal parenchyma, which have the highest demand because of their high metabolic activity.

The venous drainage of the kidney mirrors the arterial supply

In general, the renal venous drainage mirrors the arterial supply, except that there is no venous equivalent of the glomerular capillary tuft. The subcapsular arteriolar and capillary plexuses drain into a subcapsular venular and venous plexus of stellate veins that forms the origin of the interlobular veins. As they proceed towards the corticomedullary junction, the interlobular veins receive venous tributaries from the peritubular capillary network and, as the juxtamedullary zone is approached, from some of the venous tributaries from the medulla, which are the venous equivalent of the arterial vasa recta.

Many of the medullary venous vessels drain directly into the arcuate veins, which run laterally with the equivalent artery at the corticomedullary junction. These in turn drain into large interlobular veins lying between adjacent medullary pyramids, and then into the major vein tributaries at the renal hilum. The major renal vein opens end-to-side into the inferior vena cava.

Nephron

The functional unit of the kidney parenchyma that serves the blood supply is called the nephron

The nephron has two main components:
- The glomerulus, which is associated with the first capillary system
- The cortical and medullary tubular systems, which are associated with the second capillary system.

The glomerulus is the site of initial blood filtration and the tubular systems are the site where the concentration and chemical content of blood returned to the general systemic circulation, and hence the concentration and content of the urine to be voided from the body, are controlled.

Figure 15.5 shows the structure of a nephron and its relationship to its microcirculation. The simplified overview of the various homeostatic functions of the tubular

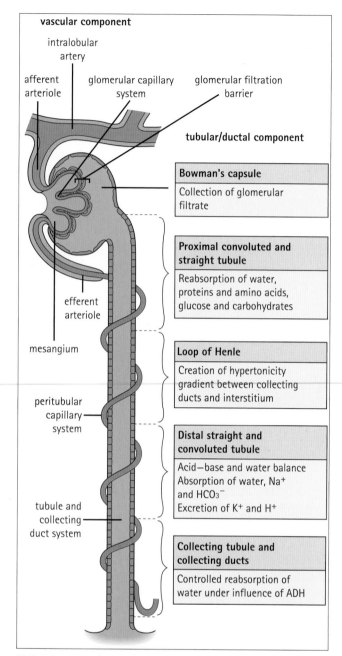

FIGURE 15.5 **The nephron.** A simple diagram to show different parts of the nephron and associated blood vessels.

component of the nephron will be dealt with in greater detail later in the chapter.

Within the renal cortex, the nephrons are organized into a distinct repeated lobular pattern

The glomeruli, and proximal and distal tubules, are aligned mainly on either side of the interlobular arteries that supply them with blood (see Fig. 15.4).

At the midpoint between adjacent interlobular arteries is a vertically running arrangement of tubules and ducts known as the 'medullary ray' (see Fig. 15.36c), at the centre of which is a main collecting duct that collects all of the largely unconcentrated urine from the

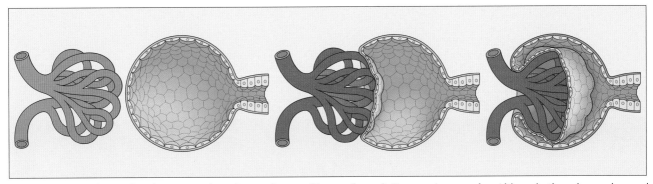

FIGURE 15.6 **Relationship between the glomerular capillary tuft and Bowman's capsule.** Although the glomerulus and Bowman's capsule do not in fact develop in this way, the relationships between the two are best conceived by imagining the intrusion of the glomerular tuft into the spherical, distended and closed end of the tubular system. This is particularly helpful in conceptualizing the glomerular tuft with its outer coating of epithelial cells, which is continuous with the cells lining Bowman's capsule.

nephrons on either side. The other tubular components of the medullary ray are the straight collecting tubules carrying urine from the end of the distal tubule to the main cortical collecting duct. The duct systems of the medullary ray run vertically downward into the medulla.

The subunit of the cortex, comprising a centrally placed medullary ray and the nephrons on either side of it, is called the 'renal lobule' and each interlobular artery runs upward in the cortex between adjacent lobules. This lobular arrangement and the medullary ray system can be seen in Figure 15.36.

Glomerulus

The first functional component of the nephron encountered by the microcirculation is the **glomerulus**, which is the site of initial filtration of the blood arriving by the afferent arterioles.

The afferent arteriole enters the glomerulus at the vascular pole

The afferent arteriole, which enters the glomerulus immediately, splits up into about five main branches. Each branch then subdivides into its own capillary network (see Fig. 15.4), the short main branch and its capillaries being supported by its own strip or stalk of mesangium (see p. 297).

The division of the glomerular capillary network into about five independent segments gives the glomerular tuft an implicit lobulation, which is rarely apparent by routine light microscopy in health, but which becomes evident in some forms of primary glomerular disease, particularly when the mesangial component of each segment is enlarged (see Fig. 15.15). The independence of each glomerular segment is also demonstrated by disease affecting only one segment (e.g. segmental glomerulonephritis).

The glomerular capillaries converge to form a single efferent arteriole, which leaves the glomerulus at the same vascular pole as the afferent arteriole enters.

The glomerulus is a complex structure in which capillaries are in intimate contact with a specialized epithelium

In simple terms, the structure of the glomerulus is best conceived as a globular capillary network intruding into a hollow sphere of epithelial cells called 'Bowman's capsule', which represents the bulbous, distended closed end of a long hollow tubular system (Fig. 15.6). This means that the glomerular capillary system, which is lined internally by endothelial cells, acquires an outer layer of epithelial cells that is continuous at the vascular pole with the cells lining Bowman's capsule.

The epithelial cells of Bowman's capsule are flat and simple, except near the opening of the tubular system, where they become more cuboidal and acquire some of the cytoplasmic organelles of the proximal convoluted tubule epithelial cells (see pp. 298-299).

In contrast, the epithelial cells coating the glomerular capillary tuft are larger and have a highly specialized and unusual structure, which has led to their being named 'podocytes' (see p. 295).

The epithelium-lined space between the coated glomerular capillary network and the parietal shell of Bowman's capsule is called the 'urinary space', and is continuous with the lumen of the long tubular system of the nephron.

As well as the outer epithelial (podocyte) coating, the glomerular capillary network has other unusual features, including the possession of an unusually thick basement membrane (the glomerular basement membrane) and the presence of a supporting strip or stalk, analogous to the mesentery of the small bowel, called the 'mesangium' (Fig. 15.7 and see p. 296).

Blood enters the glomerular capillary network from the afferent arteriole. Ultrafiltration of the blood then occurs in the glomerular capillary network and the filtrate passes into the urinary space before passing down the tubular system. The partly filtered blood leaves the glomerulus via the efferent arteriole and flows onward to provide an oxygenated blood supply to the tubular systems.

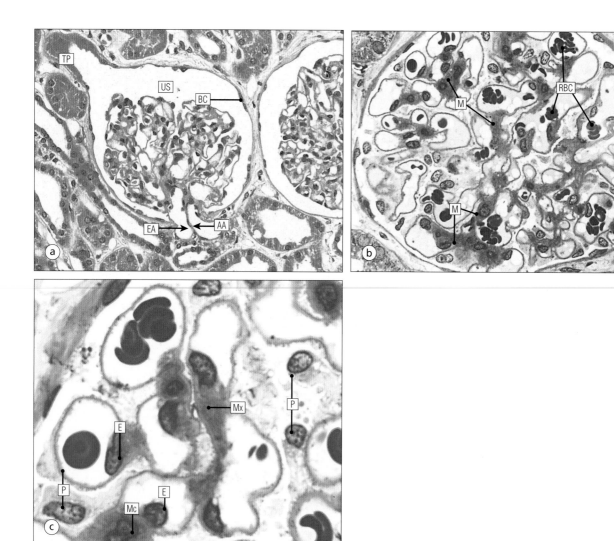

FIGURE 15.7 **Normal human glomerulus.** (a) An H&E paraffin section of normal human kidney, which has been inflation fixed to distend the blood vessels. Note the afferent arteriole (AA) and efferent arteriole (EA) at the vascular pole. Opposite the vascular pole is the tubular pole (TP), where the urinary space (US) empties into the first part of the tubular system. Although fine details of the glomerular structure are not apparent in this micrograph, the suggestion of glomerular lobulation is evident. The flattened epithelial lining of Bowman's capsule (BC) is easily seen. (b) A thin epoxy-resin section of a normal human glomerulus stained with toluidine blue. This technique permits much greater resolution of the structure of the glomerulus. The dilated capillary loops contain red blood cells (RBC) and are supported by the darkly stained mesangium (M). (c) High-power micrograph of a thin epoxy-resin section of a segment of the glomerular tuft stained with toluidine blue. At this magnification, details of the glomerular capillary wall, endothelial and epithelial cells and mesangium become apparent. The capillary loops are supported by darkly stained mesangial stalks, comprising acellular matrix (Mx) and nucleated mesangial cells (Mc). The capillary basement membrane is lined internally by endothelial cytoplasm and endothelial cell nuclei (E) are apparent. External to the glomerular basement membrane are the epithelial podocytes (P).

Glomerular Filtration Barrier

The barrier between circulating blood and the urinary space is the glomerular filtration barrier (Fig. 15.8). It is composed of:

- The capillary endothelial inner layer
- The unusually thick glomerular capillary basement membrane
- The podocyte (the outer epithelial) layer.

An additional component of the functional barrier is a high polyanionic charge on some of the above structural components.

Glomerular capillary endothelial cells are attenuated and fenestrated

The endothelial cells in the renal glomeruli are adapted for their specialized filtration role. The cytoplasm forms a thin sheet broken by numerous small circular pores or fenestrations, each about 70 nm in diameter. Their nuclei are usually located near the mesangium. Normal glomerular capillary endothelium is shown ultrastructurally in Figure 15.8. A diagrammatic representation, illustrating the structure of the endothelium and its relationships with other glomerular components, is shown in Figure 15.14b.

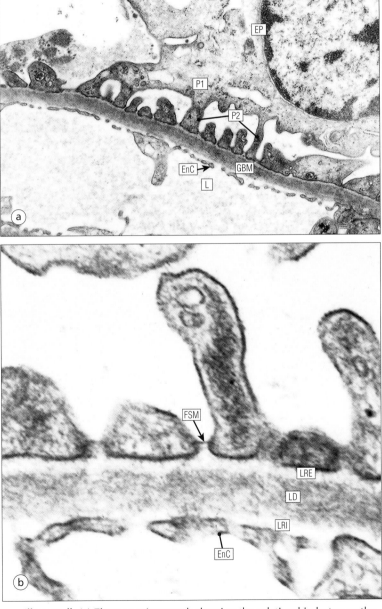

FIGURE 15.8 **Glomerular capillary wall.** (a) Electron micrograph showing the relationship between the glomerular basement membrane (GBM), capillary lumen (L), endothelial cytoplasm (EnC) and the epithelial podocyte (EP), with its primary (P1) and secondary (P2) foot process system. (b) High-power electron micrograph of the glomerular filtration barrier, comprising fenestrated endothelial cytoplasm (EnC), glomerular basement membrane and podocyte foot processes. Note the filtration slit membrane (FSM, see p. 295). In this high-magnification electron micrograph, the three layers of the basement membrane can be seen, although they are indistinct in adult humans (as here). The layers are lamina densa (LD) and, on either side of it, lamina rara interna (LRI) and lamina rara externa (LRE).

GLOMERULAR ENDOTHELIAL ABNORMALITIES

In some primary glomerular diseases, there is a great increase in the size and number of endothelial cells, and the glomerular capillary lumina become blocked (Fig. 15.9). This produces the acute nephritic syndrome, which is characterized by:

- An increase in blood pressure owing to the increased peripheral resistance following blockage of the vast glomerular capillary network
- A rise in the blood levels of nitrogenous waste products (azotaemia) owing to the failure of filtration by the abnormal glomeruli
- Haematuria (loss of red blood cells in the urine), the mechanism of which is not known
- Oedema (fluid accumulation in support tissues).

Primary structural abnormalities of the glomerulus, such as that illustrated here, are known by the name 'glomerulonephritis'. The micrograph shows an example of acute endocapillary glomerulonephritis.

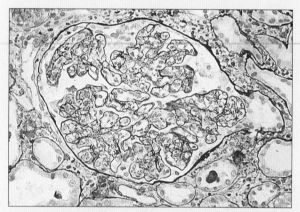

FIGURE 15.9 **Acute nephritic syndrome.** This paraffin section of kidney from a child with acute nephritic syndrome has been stained by the Jones methenamine silver technique to highlight the basement membranes and mesangium of the glomerular capillary loops (brown-black). The capillary lumina are obliterated by proliferation of cells within the basement membrane, which are therefore largely endothelial cells. If this occurs in all of the glomeruli, as is usually the case, blood flow through the glomerular capillary network is reduced.

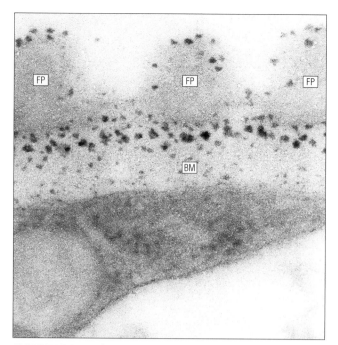

FIGURE 15.10 **Glomerular basement membrane–polyanionic sites (polyethylenimine method).** Electron micrograph of the glomerular filtration barrier identifying the sites of high polyanionic charge both in the basement membrane (BM) and on the surfaces of the podocyte foot processes (FP). Loss of this surface anionic charge leads to leakage of excess protein.

- Electron-lucent lamina rara externa on the epithelial podocyte, or urinary space, side.

This layered structure is clearly seen in rodents and children but becomes less apparent in most adults (see Fig. 15.8b).

The lamina densa is partly composed of type IV collagen (see p. 56), and the fibril network acts as a physical barrier to the passage of large molecules from the blood into the urinary space.

The lamina rara layers, and the surfaces of some podocyte secondary foot processes, contain fixed negatively charged (polyanionic) sites composed of glycosaminoglycan (see p. 55). In the basement membrane, this is heparan sulfate, and on the foot process surfaces it is a sialic acid-rich substance named 'podocalyxin'. When demonstrated ultrastructurally using a cationic substance, such as ruthenium red or polyethylenimine (Fig. 15.10), such sites appear to be organized to form fairly regular lattice with a spacing of approximately 60 nm.

It is thought that the polyanionic sites act as a charge barrier, preventing the passage of cationic molecules.

The combination of layers in the glomerular basement membrane produces both a physical and an electrical barrier to the passage of large molecules (i.e. over 70 kDa) and highly cationic molecules of many sizes. Nevertheless, certain large molecules, including some proteins, may pass through into the urinary space and require reabsorption in the tubular system.

The full thickness of the glomerular basement membrane does not completely surround the circumference of the capillary wall, but instead occupies about

The glomerular basement membrane is divided into three distinct zones

Glomerular basement membrane is much thicker than normal capillary basement membranes elsewhere. It measures approximately 310–350 nm in healthy young adults, being slightly thicker in males. Both the inner endothelial and outer epithelial cell populations contribute to its production. It has three layers:

- A central electron-dense lamina densa
- Electron-lucent lamina rara interna on the endothelial or capillary lumen side

three-quarters of it, being partly deficient at the site of the attachment of the capillary to the mesangium. The lamina rara interna continues as an ill-defined layer between the endothelial cytoplasm and the cytoplasmic and matrix components of the mesangium (see Fig. 15.14b).

The podocyte layer lies on the outer surface of the glomerular capillaries

The podocyte layer is composed of specialized epithelium which is continuous at the vascular hilum with the flat, relatively inert epithelium lining Bowman's capsule. It is highly specialized in structure, and presumably in function as well, though much of its functional detail is not known.

The podocyte is so named because the main body of the cell hovers above the external surface of the glomerular capillary and sends down cytoplasmic extensions (foot processes) that make contact with the basement membrane (see Figs 15.8 and 15.11).

Between adjacent foot processes on the glomerular basement membrane is a fairly consistent gap of 30–60 nm, the filtration slit. A thin membrane, the filtration slit membrane, bridges the gap between adjacent foot processes. This filtration slit membrane contains a cell adhesion molecule called 'nephrin', which connects with actin filaments within the adjacent foot processes.

The functional aspects of this complex cytoplasmic arrangement are not understood, but it obviously plays an important role in preventing certain molecules from passing into the urinary space. Loss of the podocyte foot process pattern in some renal diseases is associated with such excessive protein loss (mainly albumin) that the patient develops the nephrotic syndrome (see below).

CLINICAL EXAMPLE
BASEMENT MEMBRANE ABNORMALITIES IN GLOMERULAR DISEASE

Abnormalities in the structure of the glomerular basement membrane are responsible for some important kidney diseases which are characterized by an excessive loss of protein in urine (proteinuria). Sometimes so much is lost in the urine that the capacity of the liver to synthesize fresh protein (particularly albumin) is outstripped. The patient then develops a low blood albumin (hypoalbuminaemia), and oedema due to the low oncotic pressure of the blood.

The combination of proteinuria, hypoalbuminaemia and oedema is called the nephrotic syndrome.

There are many causes of the nephrotic syndrome, but all appear to be related to a structural or functional abnormality of the glomerular basement membrane.

Diseases in which the abnormality is structural include diabetes mellitus and membranous nephropathy.

In nephrotic syndrome associated with diabetes mellitus the glomerular basement is thickened three- to fivefold and the demarcation into three laminae is lost (Fig. 15.12a).

In membranous nephropathy, the basement membrane is damaged by the deposition of antigen–antibody complexes (Fig. 15.12b).

Although in these examples the basement membrane is physically thickened, it is functionally leaky and many large molecules pass into the urinary space, including large molecular weight proteins.

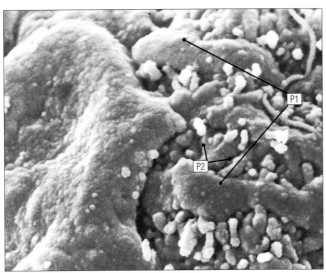

FIGURE 15.11 **Epithelial podocyte.** Scanning electron micrograph of the epithelial podocyte and its foot processes in a healthy human adult. Arising from the main cell body of each epithelial cell are a number of broad cytoplasmic processes, the primary processes (P1), which extend along and wrap around the capillary, giving rise at regular intervals to a series of smaller processes, the secondary processes (P2), which rest on the glomerular basement membrane. There is interdigitation of secondary processes so that adjacent foot processes may be derived from different podocytes. The foot process pattern in the adult human is not so neatly arranged as it is in the neonate or the rodent.

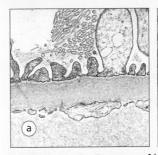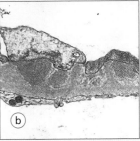

FIGURE 15.12 **Patterns of basement membrane thickening in disease.** (a) Electron micrograph of a uniformly thickened basement membrane from a patient with diabetes mellitus who presented with the nephrotic syndrome. Photographed at the same magnification as Figure 15.8a. (b) Electron micrograph of a basement membrane thickened by deposition of antigen–antibody complexes on the epithelial side. It was taken from a patient with membranous nephropathy who presented with the nephrotic syndrome. Photographed at same magnification as Figure 15.8a.

CLINICAL EXAMPLE
PODOCYTE ABNORMALITIES IN GLOMERULAR DISEASE

In children, the most common cause of the nephrotic syndrome is the so-called 'minimal change nephropathy'. By light microscopy, the glomerulus appears normal but electron microscopy reveals loss of the foot process pattern, with the outer surface of the glomerular capillaries being covered by an almost continuous sheet of podocyte cytoplasm, probably representing primary process remnants (Fig. 15.13). The abnormality is usually only temporary; structure and function return to normal in time. The podocyte abnormalities are associated with loss of the polyanionic charge (see p. 294), which possibly explains the protein leak.

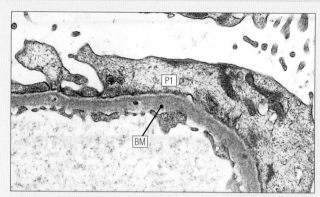

FIGURE 15.13 **Foot process fusion.** Compare the foot process arrangement in this electron micrograph with that seen normally (Fig. 15.9). In this kidney from a child with the nephrotic syndrome due to minimal change nephropathy, the complex secondary foot process arrangement is lost and the primary foot processes (P1) lie directly on the basement membrane (BM). Minimal change nephropathy is the commonest cause of the nephrotic syndrome in childhood and resolves spontaneously with no long-term renal impairment.

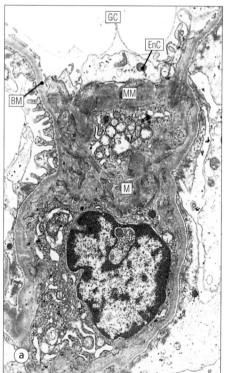

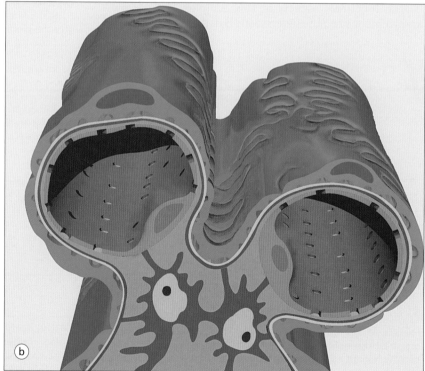

FIGURE 15.14 **Mesangium.** (a) Electron micrograph of mesangium (M) and its relationship with the glomerular capillary (GC). The capillary wall is deficient in basement membrane (BM) at the site of attachment to the mesangium, the wall being composed of endothelial cell cytoplasm (EnC) lying directly on mesangial matrix (MM). The basement membrane continues over the surface of the mesangium to the next capillary loop. (b) The podocytes with their foot processes (green) are separated from the fenestrated endothelium (red) by the glomerular basement membrane. Note the supporting role of the mesangium (matrix beige, cytoplasm brown). The lamina densa (purple) and lamina rara externa (blue) of the basement membrane are not continuous around the capillary, but are reflected over the mesangial surface to the next capillary. The lamina rara interna (beige) appears to blend with the mesangial matrix where the capillary is attached to the mesangium.

Mesangium

The mesangial support to the glomerular capillary network has two components, mesangial cells and extracellular mesangial matrix. The role of the mesangium as a support for the glomerular capillary system can be seen in Figure 15.7, and Figure 15.14 illustrates the details of the structure of the mesangium and its relationship to the glomerular capillary and the glomerular basement membrane.

Mesangial cells are irregular in shape and have a number of cytoplasmic processes

The mesangial cell processes run in an apparently haphazard fashion through the extracellular mesangial matrix. The mesangial cell nucleus is round or oval and is larger than the endothelial cell nucleus (see Fig. 15.7). There is a dense rim of nuclear chromatin inside the nuclear membrane and numerous small chromatin clumps are scattered throughout the nucleoplasm.

The mesangial cell cytoplasm contains myosin-like filaments and bears angiotensin II receptors. In experimental animals, contraction of mesangial cell filaments has been shown to be stimulated by angiotensin II.

Mesangial matrix is an acellular material produced by the mesangial cell

The mesangial matrix largely encloses the mesangial cells but is permeated by mesangial cell cytoplasmic processes. Ultrastructurally, it is of variable electron density, the more electron-lucent parts closely resembling the lamina rara interna of the glomerular basement membrane, with which it is in continuity where the glomerular capillary and mesangium meet.

The mesangium may have roles in phagocytosis, maintaining basement membrane and glomerular blood flow

The precise mechanisms of action of the mesangium in humans are not known. It has four postulated functions:

- Support of the glomerular capillary loop system
- Possible control of blood flow through the glomerular loop by the myosin–angiotensin mechanism described above
- Possible phagocytic function
- Possible maintenance of the glomerular basement membrane.

CLINICAL EXAMPLE
MESANGIAL ABNORMALITIES

Abnormalities of the mesangium are an important component of many glomerular diseases.

In some forms of immunological damage to the glomerulus, there is a proliferation of mesangial cells, which leads to compression of the glomerular capillaries (mesangial glomerulonephritis); this is often associated with the deposition of immune complexes within the mesangium (Fig. 15.15).

In diabetes mellitus, the mesangial cells of one or more of the glomerular segments produce excessive amounts of acellular matrix to form spherical nodules known as 'Kimmelstiel–Wilson nodules' (Fig. 15.16).

In permanently damaged glomeruli, whatever the cause, excessive formation of mesangial matrix in all segments eventually converts the glomerular tuft into an acellular spherical mass (hyalinization, see end-stage kidney, Fig. 15.30).

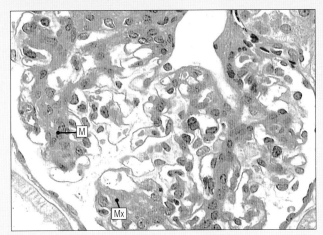

FIGURE 15.15 **Mesangial glomerulonephritis.** A paraffin section of kidney showing proliferation of the mesangial cells (M) and excessive production of mesangial matrix (Mx) expanding the lobules of the glomerular tuft and beginning to compress the glomerular capillary lumina. This pattern of disease is called 'mesangial glomerulonephritis'.

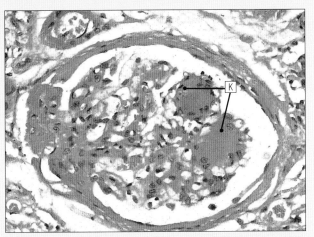

FIGURE 15.16 **Kimmelstiel–Wilson nodule.** An H&E-stained paraffin section of kidney from a patient with diabetes mellitus showing a localized nodule of mesangial matrix (Kimmelstiel–Wilson nodule, K) in two of the glomerular lobules.

KEY FACTS
THE GLOMERULUS

- The glomerulus is the site of ultrafiltration of blood
- Filtration occurs across the highly specialized glomerular capillary wall, with filtrate entering the urinary space enclosed by Bowman's capsule
- The filtration barrier comprises glomerular capillary endothelium, glomerular basement membrane (GBM) and epithelial podocyte attached to outer surface of GBM
- Further physicochemical barrier is the high polyanionic charge on the outer surface of GBM and podocyte surface, preventing passage of cationic molecules
- Initial glomerular filtrate passes down tubular and collecting duct systems, where controlled reabsorption and further excretion of small molecules (including water) occurs
- Filtered blood leaving the glomerulus via efferent arteriole enters a second capillary system around the tubules.

Intravenously injected particulate matter (e.g. colloidal carbon, ferritin, etc.) in experimental animals, and circulating immune complexes in man, appear in the mesangium in some disease states. The incompleteness of the basement membrane over the area of attachment to the mesangium would facilitate phagocytic function.

Note the close resemblance and continuity of mesangial matrix and lamina rara interna. The importance of the mesangium in human glomerular disease suggests that it is a vital functional component of the glomerulus and that its significance has been underestimated.

Tubular and Collecting System

Introduction

The glomerular filtrate leaves the urinary space at the tubular pole of the glomerulus and enters a tubule, which modifies its composition. The names of the different parts of this tubule and the course of the glomerular filtrate after leaving the glomerulus on its way to being excreted are illustrated in Figure 15.17.

The convoluted parts of both proximal and distal tubules are found close to the glomeruli, which are usually clustered around the ascending interlobular arteries from which their afferent arterioles are derived.

In contrast, the straight parts of the tubular system and the cortical parts of the collecting duct system are concentrated together in the segments of cortex virtually devoid of glomeruli; these segments are inaccurately called 'medullary rays'.

Such zoning divides the cortex into lobules. Each lobule is the segment of cortex between adjacent interlobular arteries and has a medullary ray at its centre.

The proximal tubule is vital for reabsorption of glomerular filtrate

In the proximal tubule, there is extensive reabsorption of various components of the glomerular filtrate (Fig. 15.18).

The cells that line the proximal tubule are continuous with the cells lining Bowman's capsule and there is an abrupt transition of cell form at the tubular pole of the glomerulus.

The proximal tubule lining cells are adapted for fluid and ion exchange

Proximal tubule cells are cuboidal or columnar and have a centrally placed nucleus and a well-developed luminal brush border. The brush border is composed of numerous closely packed microvilli about 1 mm in length. At the base of the microvilli brush border are pinocytotic vesicles that lie close to lysosomes. Each cell rests on a basement membrane, which is continuous with the basement membrane of Bowman's capsule.

The basal membrane of each tubule cell shows extensive basal interdigitation and some lateral interdigitation, which makes the lateral borders irregular and difficult to define except apically, where the intercellular space is sealed off from the tubule lumen by a tight junction (Fig. 15.19).

Although the lateral intercellular space of proximal tubule cells is narrow and difficult to define throughout its length from apex to base, it is often easy to see places where the space is distended into roughly spherical saccules.

In the lower half of each proximal tubule cell, numerous elongated mitochondria are closely associated with the basal interdigitations from adjacent cells and are arranged in parallel with the interdigitating basal cytoplasmic membranes.

The membrane and cytoplasmic specializations are most developed in the convoluted part of the proximal tubule. In the straight descending portion, as the thin loop of Henle is approached, the microvilli become smaller and less numerous, the degree of basal and lateral interdigitation less marked, and mitochondria and lysosomes fewer. The cells also become more cuboidal.

The loop of Henle is divided into thick and thin parts

Traditionally, the loop of Henle is regarded as having thick descending and ascending components, and a thin-walled section in between. It is better, however, to regard the thin-walled part as a distinct functional and structural entity for the following two reasons.

First, the thick descending and ascending components are ultrastructurally closely identifiable with the proximal and distal convoluted tubules.

Second, the transitions between thick and thin tubules are abrupt, whereas the thick ascending and descending parts merge gradually with the proximal and distal convoluted tubules.

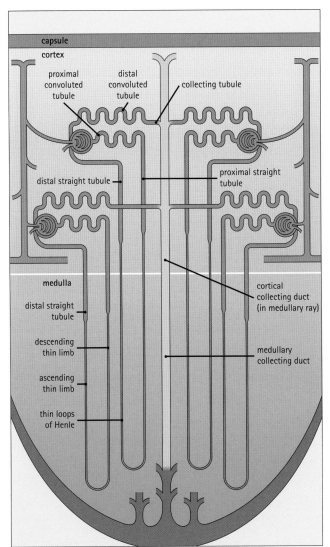

FIGURE 15.17 **Tubular and collecting system of the nephron.** The first part of the tubular system is the proximal tubule, which is a continuation of Bowman's capsule and initially pursues a convoluted course (the proximal convoluted tubule), remaining close to the glomerulus from which it arises. The proximal tubule then straightens and descends toward the medulla (proximal straight tubule, or the thick descending limb of the loop of Henle), merging with a thin-walled part of the tubular system (thin limb of the loop of Henle). This runs down in the cortex, and then in the medulla, toward the papillary tip (descending thin limb). It then loops back on itself (ascending thin limb) and re-enters the cortex. The wall then becomes thicker, forming the straight segment of the distal tubule (the thick ascending limb of the loop of Henle or the distal straight tubule). In the cortex, close to the glomeruli, the distal tubule becomes convoluted (distal convoluted tubule), and empties into a collecting tubule, which in turn empties into a collecting duct lying within the medullary ray. The collecting ducts descend into the medulla where a number converge to produce large-diameter ducts in the papillae (papillary ducts or ducts of Bellini). These ducts open into the calyces at the tips of the papillae, the concentration of the openings producing a sieve-like surface appearance to the papillary tip (the area cribrosa). The lengths of the various components of the tubular system vary, mainly according to the location of the glomerulus from which each is derived. The main variation in length occurs in the thin ascending and descending limbs of the loop of Henle. The proximal convoluted tubule is longer than the distal convoluted tubule.

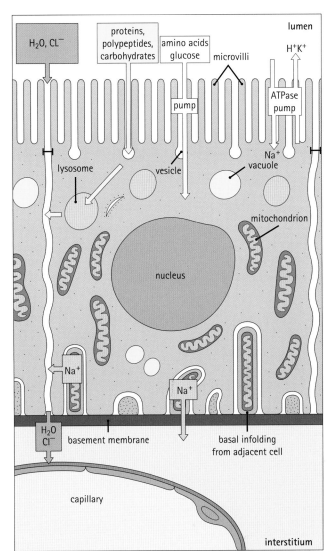

FIGURE 15.18 **Functional aspects of proximal convoluted tubule cells.** In the proximal tubule there is extensive reabsorption of components of the glomerular filtrate. The apical microvilli of the proximal tubule cells provide an immense surface area for absorption and the mitochondria, which are particularly numerous and prominent in the convoluted portion, provide the energy for the active transport of various components against gradients. In the brush border, membrane ion pumps (ATPases) bring Na^+ ions into the cell from the glomerular filtrate passing through the tubular lumen. Other ions, e.g. H^+, K^+ may be exchanged and pass into the lumen from the cell. Once in the cell, further membrane pumps in the basolateral membranes push Na^+ into the intercellular space, where their presence creates a high osmotic force. This force pulls water and Cl^- ions from the lumen, past the tight junctions and into the intercellular space (paracellular route). From here, water and Cl^- ions pass through the basement membrane into the interstitium, where hydrostatic pressure forces them into the adjacent peritubular capillaries. Proteins, polypeptides and some carbohydrates are also reabsorbed into the cell by endocytosis, and are broken down by lysosomal enzymes (see p. 24) into amino acids and small molecular sugars, which then pass into the intercellular space and thence into the interstitium and capillaries. Glucose and certain amino acids in the tubular lumen are transported into the cell by specific transport systems at the microvillar surface.

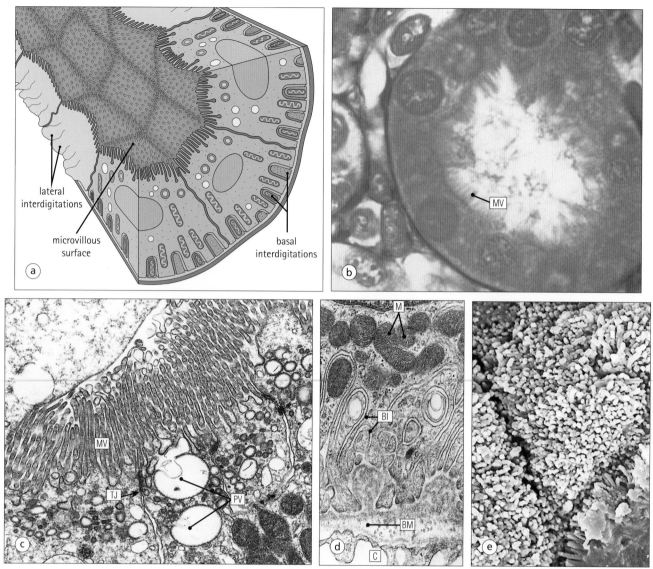

FIGURE 15.19 **Proximal convoluted tubule.** (a) The microvillous surface, the complex basal interdigitations and the lateral inter-digitations of proximal convoluted tubule cells. (b) High-power micrograph showing the microvillus brush border (MV) lining the lumen of the azan-stained proximal tubule. (c) High-power electron micrograph of the microvillus brush border (MV) and the system of pinocytotic vesicles (PV). Note the tight junction (TJ) joining adjacent cells near the base of the brush border. (d) Electron micrograph showing the system of basal interdigitations (BI) at the site of attachment of the proximal convoluted tubule cell to its basement membrane (BM). Note the abundant large mitochondria (M) and the proximity of an interstitial capillary (C). (e) Scanning electron micrograph of the lumen of a proximal convoluted tubule showing the complex system of microvilli.

The thin limbs of the loop of Henle are lined by a flat epithelium and vary in length

The thin limbs of the loop of Henle vary in length. Those associated with juxtamedullary glomeruli are long and extend deep into the medulla towards the papillary tip, whereas those associated with mid-cortical or subcapsular glomeruli extend only partway into the medulla. Thus thin Henle loops may be found in the cortex and medulla, and in the human kidney a few loops of Henle are located entirely within the cortex.

The thin limbs, both ascending and descending, have flat lining epithelium showing very little cytoplasmic specialization (Fig. 15.20). At its simplest, the thin loop resembles a dilated capillary by light microscopy and can be difficult to distinguish in routine paraffin sections.

In other areas, however, the epithelium, although flat, is rather more prominent, and ultrastructurally has short microvilli and some of the basal and lateral inter-digitations seen to a greater degree in proximal tubules. In some rodents, this taller, more specialized epithelial pattern is consistently found in the descending thin limb of short-looped nephrons from more superficial glomeruli, but such consistent placement is not apparent in man.

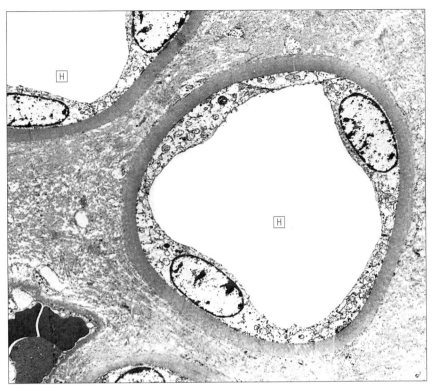

FIGURE 15.20 **Loop of Henle.** This electron micrograph shows the structural simplicity of the thin loops of Henle (H) in the medulla.

The thin limb of the loop of Henle maintains an osmotic gradient in the renal parenchyma

The thin limb of the loop of Henle creates a gradient of hypertonicity. The gradient is from the corticomedullary junction to the tip of the renal papilla, and is effected by the variable passage of sodium and chloride ions between the lumen of the Henle loop and the interstitium. This gradient allows concentration of the urine in the collecting duct system as it passes through the medulla. The widely accepted explanation of this mechanism is called the 'countercurrent multiplier hypothesis' (see Fig. 15.21).

The distal tubule starts after the loop of Henle

The ascending thin limb of the loop of Henle opens into the short straight part of the distal tubule, which passes into the cortex running in a medullary ray and then becomes convoluted before opening into the collecting tubule. At about the junction between the straight and convoluted parts, the distal tubule runs close to the glomerular hilum to form a specialized segment called the 'macula densa' (see p. 306).

The cells lining the distal tubule are adapted for fluid and ion exchange

The distal tubule is lined by cuboidal epithelial cells with extensive basal and lateral interdigitations. These are similar to those seen in the proximal tubule, but the microvilli on the luminal surface are less well formed and comparatively scanty (Fig. 15.22). Mitochondria are numerous and mainly situated close to the lateral and basal interdigitations. There are none of the luminal invaginations and vesicles seen close to the microvillus border in the proximal convoluted tubule.

The structure of the distal tubule is virtually identical in the convoluted and straight segments (ascending thick limb of loop of Henle), but the macula densa shows a local variation in structure.

The distal tubule is crucial to the control of acid–base balance, and is also important in urine concentration

As can be deduced from its rich mitochondrial content, the distal tubule cell has the ability to pump ions against concentration gradients.

In the distal tubule:
- Sodium ions are reabsorbed from the dilute urine in the lumen and potassium ions are excreted
- Bicarbonate ions are reabsorbed and hydrogen ions are excreted, thus rendering the urine acidic.

These functions are dependent on the presence of the hormone aldosterone, a mineralocorticoid secreted by the adrenal cortex (see p. 275).

Antidiuretic hormone controls the permeability of the distal tubular epithelium to water

Antidiuretic hormone (ADH) secreted by the posterior pituitary acts on the last part of the distal convoluted

ADVANCED CONCEPT

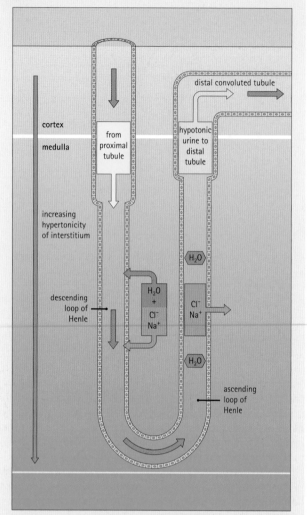

FIGURE 15.21 **Countercurrent multiplier hypothesis.** The descending thin limb of the loop of Henle is freely permeable to water and Na^+ and Cl^- ions, whereas the ascending thin limb, which is impermeable to water, actively pumps Cl^- ions out of the lumen into the interstitium, whereupon Na^+ ions follow to maintain ionic neutrality. Thus the ascending limb discharges Na^+ and Cl^- ions into the interstitium but retains water within its lumen. Some of the Na^+ and Cl^- ions diffuse back into the tubular lumen at the descending thin limb but are pushed out again when they reach the ascending limb. This produces the multiplier effect and leads to hypertonicity of the interstitial tissue in relation to the fluid in the tubular lumen, particularly near the papillary tip. The fluid emerging from the end of the ascending limb of the loop of Henle into the distal tubule system is hypotonic.

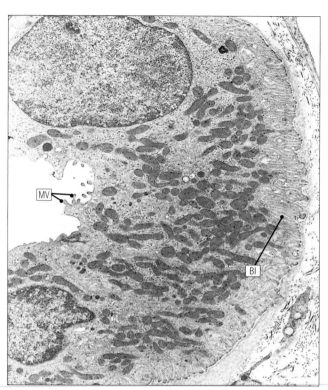

FIGURE 15.22 **Distal tubule.** Electron micrograph showing the features of a distal convoluted tubule cell. Note that it exhibits similar basal interdigitations (BI) to those of the proximal convoluted tubule cell, but that the luminal microvilli (MV) are scanty and poorly formed.

duct lumen into the hypertonic interstitium, and thence into the blood system (vasa recta). This movement of water is dependent on the countercurrent exchanger system (see Fig. 15.26).

CLINICAL EXAMPLE
DIABETES INSIPIDUS

In the permanent absence of ADH, as occurs in diabetes insipidus, vast quantities of dilute urine are formed because of the failure of water reabsorption at the distal convoluted tubule and collecting ducts.

Fatal body water depletion is only prevented by drinking large quantities of water, which is stimulated by a constant feeling of thirst.

Abnormalities of Tubular Function

The renal tubular and duct system is almost entirely dependent for its oxygen supply on the integrity of the glomerular capillary network and the arterial vessels supplying the glomeruli, as they receive oxygen from the peritubular capillary networks, which are branches

tubule. Its effect is to increase the permeability of the tubule, thus permitting the absorption of water to produce a more concentrated urine.

ADH also acts on the collecting ducts in a similar manner, permitting the absorption of water from the of the efferent arterioles leaving the glomeruli (see Fig. 15.4).

Thus, the tubular epithelial cells can become significantly hypoxic if there is arterial or glomerular disease that reduces the blood flow into the efferent arterioles. For example, obliteration of the glomerular capillary lumina by proliferation of the lining endothelial cells (see Fig. 15.9) leads to impaired oxygenation of the tubular epithelial cells. The clinical and biochemical picture is, however, usually dominated by features resulting from retention of nitrogenous waste products and the increase in peripheral vascular resistance (acute nephritic syndrome, see p. 294).

If such damage to the glomeruli persists, then the tubular epithelial cells become so starved for oxygen that their enzyme systems and various pumping mechanisms are unable to function, and biochemical abnormalities develop as a result of the loss of the sensitive homeostatic mechanisms.

The most important biochemical abnormalities resulting from impaired tubular function are due to failure of excretion of H^+ and K^+ ions. The blood therefore contains a high concentration of H^+ ions (acidosis) and K^+ ions (hyperkalaemia). These, along with the retention of nitrogenous waste material due to failure of glomerular function, are features of renal failure (see p. 309).

The collecting tubules and ducts start after the distal tubule

The convoluted segment of the distal tubule opens into the collecting system of tubules and ducts. This transition is not abrupt, as there is a variable segment (sometimes called the 'connecting segment'), where the epithelial lining contains both distal tubule and collecting tubule cell types in an apparently random fashion.

The collecting tubules are lined by two cell types

The collecting tubule (Fig. 15.23) is lined by two types of cell: clear cells (the majority) and intercalated dark cells.

The clear cells are cuboidal or rather flat in the proximal part of the collecting system; they have light, poorly-staining cytoplasm, which contains few cytoplasmic organelles (mainly randomly arranged small round mitochondria). Basal membrane infoldings are present in the proximal part of the collecting system but become less apparent further along, but microvilli are short and sparse.

The intercalated or dark cells are richer in cytoplasmic organelles, possessing numerous mitochondria. Their luminal surface has a well-developed microvillus system, with vesicles in the cytoplasm at the base of the microvilli. Normally, there are no basal infoldings.

The collecting tubules in the cortex pass towards the medullary rays and open into collecting ducts

The collecting ducts run vertically within the rays into the medulla. All of the medullary collecting ducts merge near the papilla to form large straight papillary ducts that

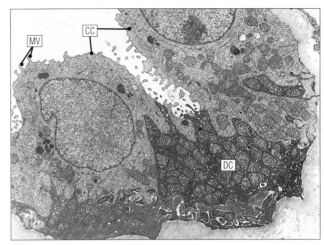

FIGURE 15.23 **Collecting tubule.** Electron micrograph of collecting tubule which connects the end of the distal convoluted tubule and the collecting duct in the medullary ray of the cortex. Note the intercalated dark cell (DC), which is rich in mitochondria, and the sparse, short microvilli (MV) of the clear cells (CC).

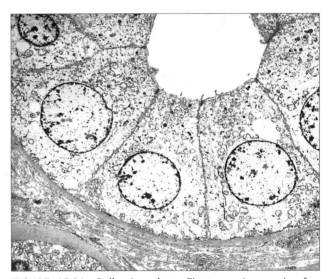

FIGURE 15.24 **Collecting duct.** Electron micrograph of a large collecting duct in the medulla. Note the lining of regular cuboidal or columnar clear cells and the sparse organelles.

run to the tip of papilla, where they open out into the pelvicalyceal system.

The collecting ducts are lined initially by epithelium that is identical in type to that of the collecting tubules. As they pass down the medullary rays and into the medulla, however, the number of intercalated dark cells decreases and the clear cells become progressively taller and more prominent, so that, as the papilla is approached, the ducts are lined by regular straight-sided columnar clear cells (Fig. 15.24).

In humans, the basement membrane of the collecting duct system becomes progressively thicker as it nears the papillary tip. This feature becomes exaggerated with age.

CLINICAL EXAMPLE
ACUTE TUBULAR NECROSIS

Failure of tubular function due to poor oxygenation can also occur in the absence of any significant disease of arteries or glomeruli. The most common cause is a central failure of blood circulation owing to poor cardiac output, which in turn is usually due either to low blood volume (hypovolaemia), for example following massive blood loss through haemorrhage, or to low blood pressure (hypotension), for example following a myocardial infarction.

Poor perfusion through the peritubular capillary network leads to inadequate oxygen supplies for the tubular epithelial cells, and this leads to failure of enzyme systems and pump mechanisms, with consequent biochemical abnormalities, particularly acidosis and hyperkalaemia. Because the glomeruli are not being perfused with arterial blood at an adequate pressure, little filtration takes place, so the production of urine falls or may even cease. The syndrome of acute renal failure comprises:

- Oliguria or anuria (partial or total cessation of urine production)
- Hyperkalaemia (elevated K^+ level in the blood)
- Acidosis (elevated H^+ level in the blood).

When the tubular failure is due to a central cause such as hypovolaemia or hypotension, the tubular epithelial cells degenerate (Fig. 15.25). Their histological appearance is due to accumulation of water within the cytosol.

If hypovolaemia or hypotension are treated promptly, tubular epithelial cells can recover normal structure and function; otherwise, the tubular epithelial cells die (acute tubular necrosis). If adequate oxygenation is re-established the tubules can become repopulated with epithelial cells.

In renal grafting, the tubular epithelial cells of the donor kidney die after the kidney is removed. When the kidney is transplanted (usually many hours after its removal) and its arterial supply is re-established, the tubules are eventually repopulated with functioning epithelial cells and normal homeostatic control is established.

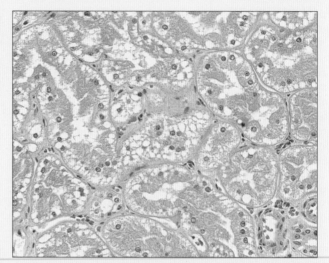

FIGURE 15.25 **Acute tubular damage.** Micrograph of an H&E-stained paraffin section from a patient with early acute renal failure caused by hypovolaemic shock. The proximal convoluted tubule epithelium shows early degenerative changes resulting from inadequate oxygenation following a prolonged fall in blood pressure. The individual cells are swollen with water as a result of failure of the Na^+/K^+ ATPase pump, leading to inadequate excretion of water into the interstitium. Note that the microvilli are largely lost and many cells have lost their nuclei. Compare with Figure 15.19.

KEY FACTS
TUBULAR AND COLLECTING DUCT SYSTEM FUNCTIONS

- Proximal convoluted tubule – reabsorption of water, glucose and amino acid by Na^+/K^+/ATPase pump, whereas larger molecules are reabsorbed by endocytosis
- Thin loop of Henle – creates gradient of hypertonicity to allow concentration of urine in collecting duct system
- Distal tubule – Na^+ and HCO_3^- ions reabsorbed from urine in exchange for K^+ and H^+, which are excreted, dependent on aldosterone
- Collecting tubules and ducts – control final concentration of urine by regulated reabsorption of water from urine under influence of hypertonicity gradient and antidiuretic hormone.

The collecting tubules and ducts play an important role in the final concentration of urine

The collecting tubules and ducts are not solely conduits for the transfer of urine into the pelvicalyceal system but are instrumental in concentrating urine to a degree appropriate to the level of blood hydration. This is achieved by interplay between the collecting tubules and ducts, the interstitium and the vasa recta, to produce a countercurrent exchanger system (Fig. 15.26). Controlled water transport is made possible by the variable permeability of the collecting duct under the influence of ADH (see p. 302). The amount of ADH released depends on the body's requirement for water excretion or retention.

In the presence of high levels of ADH, water is lost from the collecting duct lumen into the interstitium, from where it passes into the blood circulation via the ascending vasa recta. This results in the production of a small amount of highly concentrated urine. When low levels of ADH are present, water remains within the collecting duct lumen and is lost in the form of copious dilute urine.

The vascular networks of the vasa recta also play a role in the concentration of urine in the medulla

On the descending (arterial) side of the looped vessels, the walls are permeable to water and salts; water passes out into the interstitium and sodium and chloride ions pass in. Thus, blood in the vasa recta is more or less in equilibrium with the hypertonic medullary interstitium.

On the ascending (venous) side of the vascular loop, sodium and chloride ions pass from the vessel lumen to the interstitium and water is reabsorbed into the venous blood from the interstitium.

Renal Interstitium

The renal interstitium contains vessels and specialized interstitial cells

 ADVANCED CONCEPT

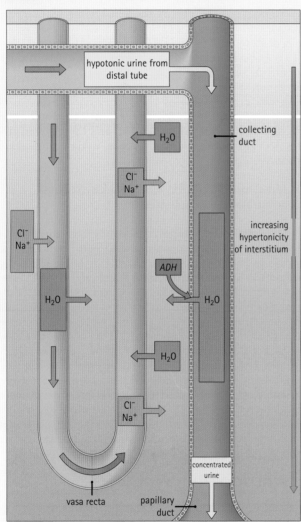

FIGURE 15.26 **Countercurrent exchanger system.** Dilute urine in the collecting tubule and duct system is progressively concentrated by the osmotic transfer of water from the lumen into the hypertonic medullary interstitial tissue, whence it is reabsorbed into the vasa recta. The hypertonicity is due to the high concentration of Na^+ and Cl^- ions in the medulla, resulting from the countercurrent multiplier activity of the loops of Henle. Thus, an increasingly concentrated urine is produced.

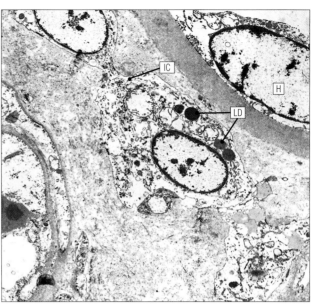

FIGURE 15.27 **Medullary interstitial cell and matrix.** Electron micrograph showing a typical human medullary interstitial cell (IC) located in the loose matrix near to the loop of Henle (H). The characteristic cytoplasmic feature is the presence of electron-dense spherical lipid droplets (LD); there is abundant rough endoplasmic reticulum and a few mitochondria.

In the cortex of the human kidney, the interstitial space is small and largely occupied by small blood vessels and lymphatics. In the medulla, the interstitium becomes a significant component, both in bulk and in function. The interstitium increases in both size and importance as the tip of the papilla is neared (see Figs 15.35, 15.41).

Ultrastructurally, the medullary interstitium is largely composed of loose electron-lucent acellular material, partly protein and partly glycosaminoglycans, in which collagen fibres, lipid droplets and basal lamina-like material are scattered. Variable numbers of interstitial cells are also present (Fig. 15.27).

In humans, the most frequently seen interstitial cell is irregular in outline with narrow, stellate cytoplasmic processes extending in all directions into the interstitial matrix. In rodents, these cell processes can often be seen to contact thin loops of Henle and adjacent medullary capillaries, sometimes seeming to act as a bridge between the two, but this is rarely apparent in man.

The cytoplasm of interstitial cells in man contains mitochondria, lysosomes, lipid droplets and a small amount of rough endoplasmic reticulum.

Another type of interstitial cell, which is often spindle shaped and contains abundant rough endoplasmic reticulum, resembles a fibroblast.

The importance of the medullary interstitium in salt and water homeostasis has already been described in relation to the functions of the loops of Henle, vasa recta and collecting ducts. The function of the interstitial cells is, however, not known. Although the renal medulla is known to be an important site of prostaglandin synthesis, it is currently believed that the epithelial cells of the collecting ducts, and not the interstitial cells, are responsible.

Juxtaglomerular Apparatus

The juxtaglomerular apparatus is involved in maintaining blood pressure and volume by the production of the hormone renin. It is a specialized adaptation of vascular and tubular tissues that allows blood flow to affect renin output. The juxtaglomerular apparatus comprises:
- Renin-producing cells located in the walls of the afferent and efferent arterioles at the vascular hilum of the glomerulus
- Lacis cells
- The macula densa area of distal tubule (Fig. 15.28).

Renin-secreting cells contain neuroendocrine granules

In man, renin-producing cells are concentrated mainly in the walls of the afferent arteriole, although small numbers are present in the efferent arteriole.

Renin-producing cells have the ultrastructural features of highly specialized myoepithelial cells, with some contractile filaments. They also contain neuroendocrine granules of many shapes and sizes, although two distinct types can be recognized.

Type I granules are irregular in shape and contain rhomboidal crystalline bodies (protogranules), which are believed to be the precursors of the other types of granules.

Type II granules are larger, spherical, uniformly electron dense, and have an ill-defined membrane; they are thought to represent the mature renin-secreting granules.

The lacis cells resemble mesangial cells

Lacis cells have a network (lacis) of thin interwoven processes, which are separated by an acellular matrix of basement membrane-like material. Lacis cells occupy the triangular region bordered by the macula densa at the base and the afferent and efferent arterioles at the sides; the apex is formed by the base of the glomerular mesangium.

Because of their apparent continuity with the glomerular mesangium at the vascular pole of the glomerulus, these cells have also been called 'extraglomerular mesangial cells'. Their function is not definitively known but they have numerous processes containing gap junctions and are thought to provide electrical coupling among themselves and to the mesangium and glomerular arterioles.

The macula densa is a specialized adaptation of distal tubular epithelium

The macula densa is a specialized zone of the distal tubule where it is in close contact with the vascular hilum of the glomerulus.

In this region, the epithelial cells of the distal tubule are taller and more tightly packed than elsewhere in the tubule and the nuclei lie closer to the luminal surface; the Golgi is located between the nucleus and the basement membrane.

The precise function of this specialized zone of distal tubule is not known but it may act as a sensor, regulating juxtaglomerular function by monitoring sodium and chloride levels in the distal tubule lumen.

Renin converts angiotensinogen to active angiotensin which then causes the adrenals to secrete aldosterone

Renin produced in the juxtaglomerular apparatus catalyses the conversion of inactive angiotensinogen. Angiotensinogen is an α2-globulin produced in the liver, converted by renin to the decapeptide angiotensin I. Angiotensin I is then converted to angiotensin II, which stimulates the secretion of aldosterone by the zona glomerulosa of the adrenal cortex (see p. 275).

Aldosterone is a mineralocorticoid hormone that regulates body sodium and potassium ion levels through its effect on the sodium pump mechanism at cell membranes.

In the distal tubule of the kidney, aldosterone promotes the reabsorption of sodium ions and water from the glomerular filtrate (Fig. 15.29), and thereby contributes to the maintenance of plasma volume and blood pressure.

Renin synthesis may be modulated by sodium concentration or blood pressure

Macula densa cells monitor the sodium concentration in the distal tubule lumen contents and signal renin release by the juxtaglomerular cells in the arteriole walls via production of prostaglandins (PGI2 and PGE2) and nitric oxide. Renal renin release is inversely related to renal perfusion pressure such that a drop in perfusion pressure stimulates renin secretion, whereas an increase in perfusion pressure inhibits it. This is the so-called 'renal baroreceptor mechanism'. The precise signal-effector coupling between renal arterial pressure and renin secretion has not yet been characterized precisely. It is now widely accepted that blood pressure changes are detected within the afferent arteriole itself and pressure-dependent regulation of renin release is not absolutely dependent on macula densa function.

Erythropoietin Synthesis

The kidney secretes erythropoietin (EPO) in adults but the site and mechanism are unknown

Erythropoietin (EPO) acts as a major regulator of erythropoiesis by promoting the survival, proliferation, and differentiation of erythroid progenitor cells and regulating the number of erythrocytes in peripheral blood.

Despite the application of modern techniques, the precise site of erythropoietin formation within the

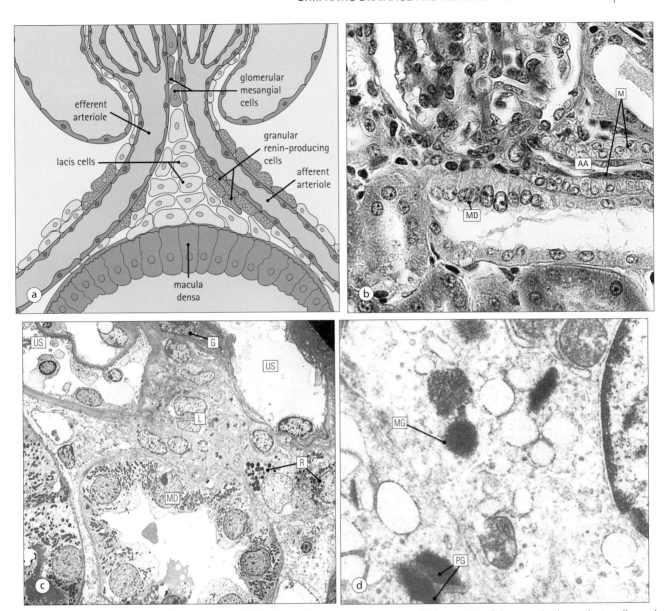

FIGURE 15.28 **Juxtaglomerular apparatus.** (a) The juxtaglomerular apparatus, which consists of the macula densa, lacis cells, and the afferent and efferent arterioles. Within the walls of the arterioles are granular renin-secreting cells. (b) Masson's trichrome stain showing the macula densa (MD) and afferent arteriole (AA) with prominent muscle cells (M) containing renin granules. The efferent vessel and lacis cells are not visible in this section. (c) Electron micrograph of human juxtaglomerular apparatus. Note the macula densa (MD), renin-producing cells (R), lacis cells (L), glomerular mesangial cells (G), and urinary space (US). (d) High-power electron micrograph of the renin-secreting granular cells in the afferent arteriole wall. Note the protogranules (PG) (type I) and mature granules (MG) (type II).

kidney remains unknown. Recently investigators identified EPO-producing kidney cells as peritubular interstitial cells expressing neuronal markers showing a unique stellar or arborizing configuration with long multidirectional projections. When the number of interstitial cells exhibiting EPO mRNA was calculated in relation to anaemia, the numbers increased in parallel with both total EPO mRNA and serum EPO levels. Thus, EPO production appears to correlate with increased numbers of peritubular interstitial cells producing EPO mRNA. In the fetus, the liver is the primary site of EPO production, especially in the hepatocytes surrounding central veins.

Lymphatic Drainage and Nerve Supply of the Kidney

The importance of the lymphatic drainage and nerve supply of the kidney in normal function is probably minimal, as both are destroyed during renal transplantation with no obvious serious side-effects.

Lymphatics in the kidney run with blood vessels

The lymphatic drainage of the cortex of the kidney is mainly by a series of lymphatics that run in parallel with

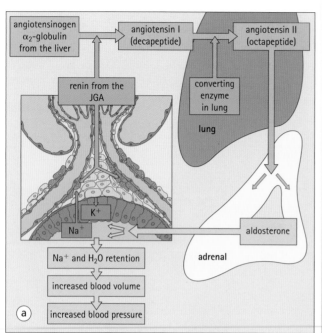

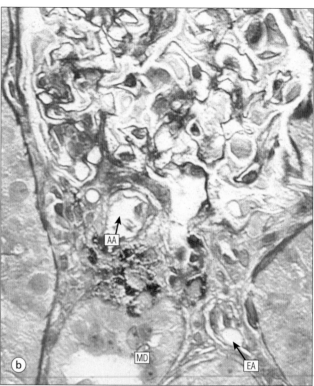

FIGURE 15.29 **Renin–angiotensin–aldosterone system.** (a) Renin secreted by the juxtaglomerular apparatus (JGA) catalyses the production of angiotensin I from its inactive precursor, angiotensinogen. Angiotensin I is then converted in the lung into the active octapeptide angiotensin II, which stimulates the release of aldosterone from the adrenal cortex. Aldosterone mediates the absorption of sodium and water from the glomerular filtrate at the distal tubule. The feedback control of renin secretion is not known. (b) Immunocytochemical method for renin (brown) showing its location at the vascular hilum in relation to the afferent (AA) and efferent (EA) arterioles. Note the macula densa (MD).

the cortical blood vessels. The main channels follow the interlobular, arcuate and interlobar blood vessels and emerge at the kidney hilum. A minor lymphatic system runs in the renal capsule and receives small tributaries from the outer cortex. There is some communication between these two systems within the cortex.

The kidney is supplied by autonomic innervation

The nerve supply to the kidney arises mainly from the coeliac plexus. Both adrenergic and cholinergic fibres have been demonstrated. In general, these nerves have been seen to follow the course of blood vessels throughout the cortex and the outer medulla.

Lower Urinary Tract

The lower urinary tract is a series of conduits and reservoirs for urine

The lower urinary tract is a functional rather than a geographical entity, as it extends from an intrarenal component high in the abdominal cavity to the tip of the urethra. It comprises:

- The calyceal collecting system, into which the large collecting ducts of Bellini in the medullary papillae discharge the urine

- The renal pelvis, which is the reservoir at the hilum of the kidney into which the various calyces pass the urine
- The ureter, which is a long muscular tube that conducts urine down to the bladder
- The bladder, which acts as a major reservoir, holding the urine until it can be voided
- The urethra, through which the urine stored in the bladder is voided to the exterior.

CLINICAL EXAMPLE
IMPORTANT TUMOURS OF THE KIDNEY

The most common tumour arising from the kidney parenchyma (renal cell carcinoma) is malignant and is derived from the glandular cells lining the tubules, and is therefore an adenocarcinoma. It occurs in the middle-aged and elderly and can spread extensively to other sites of the body via the bloodstream.

The other important type occurs only in young children and the cell of origin is a multipotential stem cell called the 'nephroblast', which, during embryonic life, differentiates to produce all the specific cells of the kidney. Rarely, some of these persist after birth and can give rise to rapidly growing malignant tumours called **nephroblastomas**.

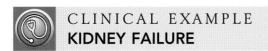

CLINICAL EXAMPLE
KIDNEY FAILURE

Because the blood circulatory system in the kidney is its most important component, it is not surprising that many renal diseases are the result of abnormalities in this system. Common vascular diseases, such as systemic hypertension, diabetes mellitus and atherosclerosis, frequently damage the kidney, leading to impaired excretory and homeostatic functions.

Chronic renal failure

Decreased blood flow through the glomerular capillary system because of thickening of the arterial and arteriolar walls, and the consequent reduction in the lumina of these vessels, produces chronic ischaemia of the tubular system and reduces glomerular filtration. If prolonged, this leads to disuse shrinkage of the components of the glomerulus (glomerular hyalinization) and atrophy of the tubules (Fig. 15.30). When these changes affect most of the glomeruli and their associated tubular systems, all of the functions of the kidney are impaired and the patient develops symptoms of chronic renal failure.

Failure of the kidney's excretory function leads to retention in the blood of toxic metabolic waste materials, particularly urea and creatinine, from the endogenous breakdown of body protein. This is called uraemia; the accumulation of urea and creatinine can be measured chemically. Eventually, without treatment this intoxication leads to coma, fitting and death. Failure of homeostatic functions carried out by the renal tubules leads to a loss of control of the body's water and electrolyte concentration; hydrogen and potassium ions accumulate in the blood, producing acidosis and hyperkalaemia.

The kidneys are unable to produce a urine with a concentration or dilution commensurate with the body's needs. Instead a urine of constant specific gravity is produced, irrespective of the degree of haemoconcentration or haemodilution.

These biochemical disorders are the result of inexorable destruction of all of the activities of all nephrons. Chronic renal failure is irreversible.

Acute renal failure

In acute renal failure, there is a sudden transient cessation of all nephron activity, which is usually due to damage to all tubules, or all glomeruli, or both. Depending on the cause, some recovery is usually possible if the patient can be sustained by haemodialysis through the period of intense metabolic upset, while the nephrons are inactive.

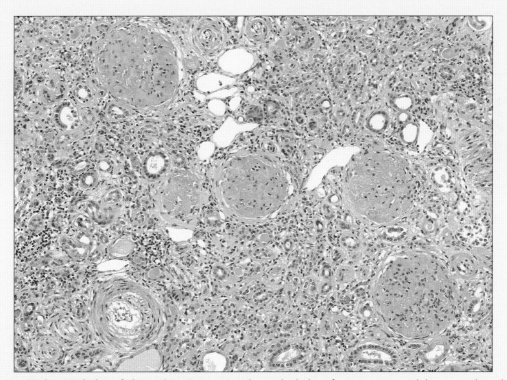

FIGURE 15.30 **End-stage kidney failure.** This H&E section shows the kidney from a patient with long-standing chronic renal failure due to progressive disease of the renal arterial supply. Little remains of the normal structure of the nephron. The glomeruli have been converted into acellular spheres containing no capillary network and the tubules have atrophied, the epithelial cells being flattened or cuboidal.

At various points, there are sphincters capable of closing off parts of the lower urinary tract so that it can act as a reservoir. The most important of these muscular sphincters are located at the junction between the bladder and urethra and are under voluntary control.

These excretory passages are essentially hollow tubes with muscular walls. With the exception of part of the urethra, they are lined by a specialized epithelium that is capable of withstanding contact with a fluid of variable concentration containing a number of toxic substances. This specialized lining is a form of stratified epithelium, known as 'transitional epithelium' or, in this site, the 'urothelium' (Fig. 15.31).

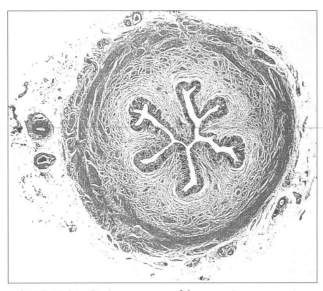

FIGURE 15.31 Basic structure of lower urinary tract. Low-power micrograph of a transverse section of human ureter showing the basic structure of the lower urinary tract. The walls are muscular and there is an internal lining of specialized urothelium.

The lower urinary tract is lined by specialized transitional epithelium termed urothelium

The urothelium is a multilayered epithelium that varies in thickness at various sites in the lower urinary tract. In the small calyces, it is only two to three cell layers thick, but in the empty bladder, it may contain up to five or six layers; presumably this reflects the different degrees of distension to which the two components are usually subjected. As these epithelial cells have the ability to stretch, shift on each other and flatten, a distended bladder may appear to be lined by only a two- to three-cell layer of stretched, flat cells.

In the non-distended state, urothelium has a rather compact, cuboidal basal layer, polygonal-celled middle layers, and a surface layer composed of tall, rather columnar cells, which are often binucleate, with a convex luminal surface bulging into the lumen.

By light microscopy, the luminal surface of urothelium often appears fuzzy in the undistended bladder owing to the relaxation of the complex and convoluted cell surface membrane (Fig. 15.32).

Urothelial cells have specialized plaques in the apical cell membrane

Ultrastructurally, the surface layer of urothelium is highly specialized. The luminal aspect of each cell is convoluted, with deep clefts running down into the cytoplasm, which also contains fusiform vesicles lined by cell membrane, identical to that seen on the luminal surface (Fig. 15.33).

It is not yet clear whether all these vesicles communicate with the lumen (i.e. represent clefts that have been sectioned obliquely) or whether they represent reserve segments of surface membrane that can be incorporated into the surface layer when the lumen is distended with urine and a greater surface area is required.

In conditions of distension, the tall cells of the surface layer become flattened and lose their convex apical bulge, whereas ultrastructurally the deep clefts and

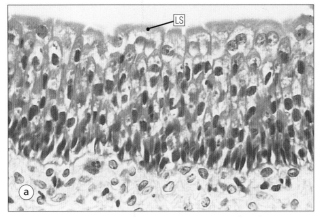

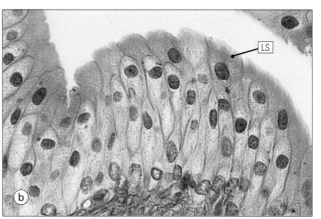

FIGURE 15.32 Urothelium. (a) High-power micrograph showing the characteristic appearance of the H&E-stained urothelium in the undistended state. When the lumen is distended with urine, the cells flatten and form a thinner layer. Note the five to six layers, the occasional binucleate surface cell, and the indistinct luminal surface (LS). (b) Masson's trichrome stain showing the lateral cell borders of urothelium and its stratified nature. Note the indistinct luminal membrane (LS).

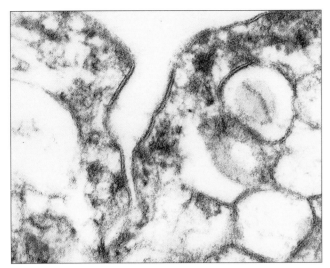

FIGURE 15.33 **Urothelial cell surface.** Electron micrograph of a non-distended human bladder postmortem, showing something of the unique structure of the surface of the urothelial cell. The luminal surface shows areas of a three-layered cell membrane (asymmetric membrane), most clearly seen in the invagination forming membrane plaques. The membrane has a central lucent lamina between a thick electron-dense outer lamina and a thinner dense inner lamina. Immediately beneath the surface the cytoplasm contains numerous round or oval vesicles (multilaminate vesicles) lined by identical trilaminar membrane. These vesicles become incorporated into the luminal surface by fusing with the frequent invaginations as the bladder fills and the surface urothelium stretches.

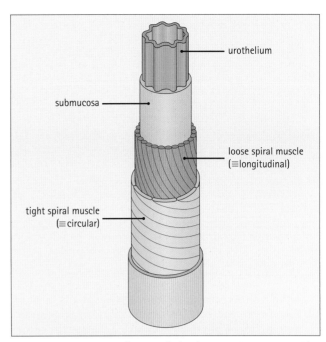

FIGURE 15.34 **Musculature of the lower urinary tract.** The arrangement of the muscle layers in the ureter is shown, emphasizing that the muscles are not truly circular and longitudinal, but rather are tight spirals and loose spirals.

multilaminate vesicles largely disappear. Throughout most of the lower urinary tract the urothelium stands on a thin, indistinct basement membrane supported by a variable layer of dense subepithelial support tissue which is mainly collagen (the lamina propria).

The lamina propria and muscle layers are external to the urothelium

The urothelium is supported by a vascular lamina propria. Beneath the lamina propria are the layers of smooth muscle which, in the pelvicalyceal system and ureters, are responsible for the peristaltic contractions forcing urine down into the bladder in one direction only.

The ureter has a spiral arrangement of smooth muscle in its wall

In the simple tubular ureter, there appear to be two distinct layers of muscle: an inner longitudinal layer and an outer circular layer (see Fig. 15.31). However, three-dimensional studies suggest that both muscle layers are in fact helical arrangements, with a loosely spiralled internal helix and a more tightly spiralled outer helix (Fig. 15.34), which appear to be respectively longitudinal and circular when the ureter is sectioned transversely.

In the architecturally more complex pelvicalyceal system, and in the virtually spherical bladder, the arrangement of the muscle layers is less clearly defined.

The urinary bladder has three layers of smooth muscle

The bladder is considered to have three muscle layers:

- An inner layer continuous with the inner longitudinal layer of the ureter
- A middle layer continuous with the outer circular layer of the ureter
- An additional outer layer in which the fibres run in approximately the same direction as the innermost layer (i.e. approximately longitudinal).

Because the bladder is roughly spherical instead of cylindrical, and the bladder musculature is, in any case, a distorted continuation of the helical arrangement seen in the ureter, the terms longitudinal and circular have little meaning.

The arrangement of muscle often appears rather haphazard in histological sections, except at the narrow bladder neck, where the layers again become more distinct (Fig. 15.35).

A functional 'valve' prevents urine reflux during micturition

In the normal ureter, which is a narrow-bore tube, urine is forced downward by peristalsis to prevent reflux back toward the kidney. In the larger spherical bladder, however, this cannot be achieved, as the lumen of the fully distended reservoir is too large for a segment of it to be closed off by muscle contraction; thus, when the bladder musculature contracts during micturition, urine could reflux back up the open ureters and damage the kidney.

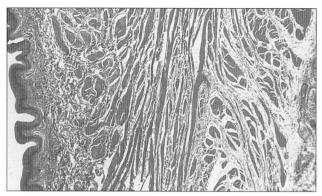

FIGURE 15.35 Bladder wall. Beneath the urothelium is a fibrocollagenous submucosal region. The bulk of the wall is composed of smooth muscle, which is loosely organized into three layers. This arrangement is most clearly seen at the bladder neck, as in this micrograph.

Although there are no anatomic valves at the junction of the ureters and bladder, potentially damaging reflux is prevented by a physiological valve, which results from the oblique path by which the ureters enter the posterolateral bladder wall musculature.

As the bladder distends and enlarges, the ureteric openings close, partly due to compression of the ureter lumen by extrinsic pressure from the musculature of the bladder wall and partly by acute angulation at the site of opening produced by bladder distension.

CLINICAL EXAMPLE
TUMOURS OF THE BLADDER

The most common tumour of the bladder is derived from the epithelium that lines the organ internally, the urothelium, which is a specialized type of transitional cell epithelium. The tumours range in behaviour from virtually benign to aggressively malignant, but all are called transitional cell carcinomas. This tumour can affect any part of the lower urinary tract which is lined by urothelium, so can also occur in the ureters and in the pelvicalyceal epithelium within the kidney.

At the junction between the bladder and the urethra is a muscular sphincter, the internal sphincter, which when closed permits the bladder to act as a reservoir of urine. When this sphincter relaxes, micturition occurs.

The bladder is supplied by autonomic innervation

The bladder nerve supply is from the autonomic nervous system, and both sympathetic and parasympathetic nerves are found.

Sensory fibres from the bladder transmit signals as to the degree of bladder distension to the sacral spinal cord.

Parasympathetic fibres ending in the muscles and adventitia of the bladder act as the effector nerves for micturition.

Sympathetic nerves innervate the blood vessels to the bladder.

The urethra conducts urine from the bladder to be voided

The urethra is the final conduit through which urine passes to the exterior. The anatomy of the urethra differs in the male and female.

The human female urethra is short, being approximately 5 cm long. It runs from the bladder and opens to the exterior in the midline of the genital vestibule just between the clitoris and the superior border of the vaginal introitus.

The urethra is lined mainly by stratified squamous epithelium and its lamina propria contains many vascular channels as well as a few small mucus-secreting glands.

Although the urethral muscular wall is a continuation of the involuntary smooth muscle of the bladder, there is a sphincter, the external sphincter. This is composed of striated muscle and is under voluntary control; it is found around the midportion of the urethra where it passes through the striated muscles of the pelvic floor.

The male urethra is 20–25 cm long and is more complex than the female urethra, as it serves two purposes. Not only is it the final conduit of the urinary system, but it is also the terminal conduit of the male reproductive system (see Fig. 16.1). It can be divided into three segments: the prostatic urethra, the membranous urethra and the penile urethra.

The prostatic urethra begins at the bladder neck and runs through the prostate gland, from which many periurethral glands open into it through short ducts. It also receives the openings of the ejaculatory ducts.

The membranous urethra is the short segment (i.e. approximately 1 cm long), which runs through the pelvic floor muscles. This is the site of voluntary control of micturition, as it is here that the external sphincter, of striated muscle, surrounds the urethra.

The penile urethra is the distal part of the urethra and runs through the corpus spongiosum of the penis, opening to the exterior at the external meatus of the glans penis; small mucous glands, analogous to those in the female, open into the penile urethra.

The male urethra is lined proximally by transitional epithelium similar to that in the remainder of the lower urinary tract, but this becomes progressively less urothelial in character in the membranous and penile segments, where it changes to a rather non-specialized, pseudostratified columnar epithelium. This finally changes to a stratified squamous epithelium at the distal penile urethra close to the external urinary meatus, where the epithelium merges with the stratified squamous epithelium of the glans penis.

PRACTICAL HISTOLOGY

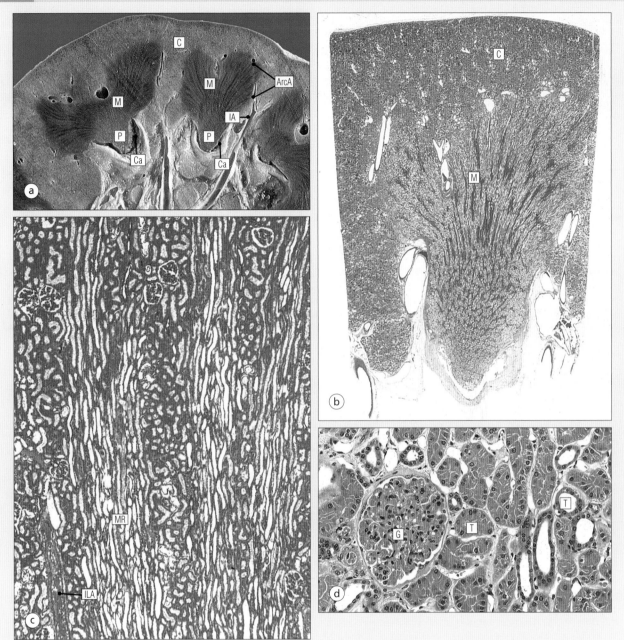

FIGURE 15.36 **Anatomy of adult kidney.** (a) Sectioned adult kidney, which has been fixed in formalin and the near-natural colour restored in alcohol. Note the cortex (C), the medullary pyramid (M) culminating in the papillary tip (P), which protrudes into the lumen of a calyx (Ca). Interlobar arteries (IA) and arcuate arteries (ArcA) can also be seen. Little detail of cortical structure is visible with the naked eye, but the vertical linearity of the components of the medulla is highlighted by clusters of prominent blood vessels (vasa recta). (b) In this H&E-stained paraffin section the distinction between cortex (C) and medulla (M) is easily seen. This section also shows the vertical linearity of the components of the medulla, both tubules and vessels. At this low magnification, glomeruli can be seen as small dots in the cortex. Note that some areas of the cortex are free of glomeruli but contain vertically running duct systems; these areas are known as 'medullary rays' and represent the sites where cortical tubules drain into the collecting ducts. (c) In this micrograph of cortex at a higher magnification than in (b) it can be seen that the medullary ray (MR) area is devoid of glomeruli and that the interlobular arteries (ILA) run in the glomeruli-rich area. (d) Renal cortex – glomerulus (G) and cortical tubules (T).

PRACTICAL HISTOLOGY

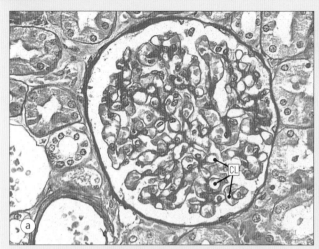

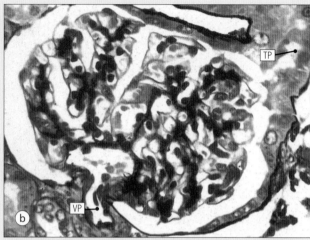

FIGURE 15.37 **Glomerulus.** (a) The details of the structure of the glomerular tuft are not easily seen in routine paraffin sections without the assistance of special stains to delineate capillary basement membranes. In this high-power micrograph occasional capillary lumina (CL) can be seen, but it is difficult to distinguish clearly between endothelial, mesangial and epithelial podocyte cells. (b) A glomerulus stained by the Jones methenamine silver method to show the mesangium and capillary basement membranes. Clear delineation of the capillary basement membrane permits the recognition of endothelial cells (inside the membrane) and epithelial podocytes (outside the membrane). Note that this fortuitous section shows both the vascular (VP) and tubular (TP) poles.

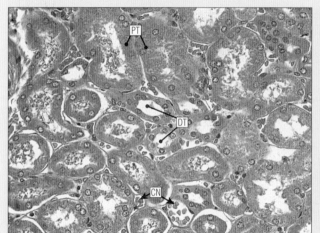

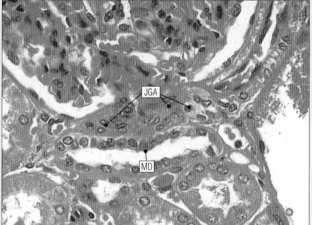

FIGURE 15.38 **Cortical tubules.** In this high-power micrograph of cortical tubules the proximal tubules (PT) are most numerous and prominent, having tall epithelium and small lumina. Distal tubules (DT) are smaller and have a cuboidal epithelium and proportionately larger lumina. Note the intimate capillary network (CN). Collecting ducts on their way to the medullary ray and thick and thin loops of Henle are also visible.

FIGURE 15.39 **Juxtaglomerular apparatus.** Any glomerulus sectioned through the vascular hilum may show part of the juxtaglomerular apparatus (JGA), though the detailed structure is rarely apparent. The most easily seen component in a paraffin section is the macula densa (MD), and the afferent and efferent arterioles are sometimes visible. Without the assistance of special stains, the juxtaglomerular and lacis cells cannot be specifically identified.

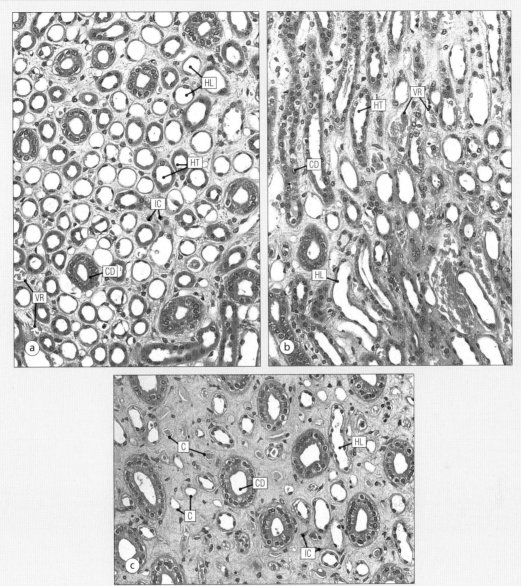

FIGURE 15.40 **Medulla.** In the medulla, all the various tubules, ducts and vessels run in the same direction: towards the papillary tip. The appearance on histological examination depends on whether the section has been cut longitudinally to the axis of the tubules (in which case the tubules and ducts are cut in longitudinal section) or transversely. In most randomly selected tissue blocks, the section is usually oblique to the longitudinal plane of the medulla to a greater or lesser extent. (a) In this micrograph of outer medulla, just below the corticomedullary junction, the tubules and ducts are seen in transverse section. The outer medulla contains a mixture of thick descending and ascending portions of loops of Henle (HT), which are histologically very similar to proximal and distal convoluted tubule, thin loops of Henle (HL), small collecting ducts (CD) and vasa recta (VR). In this region, there is a small amount of interstitium in which a few interstitial cells (IC) can be seen. (b) Micrograph of the same area of outer medulla shown sectioned almost longitudinally. (c) In this micrograph of the lower medulla note the difference in the content of tubules and ducts from that of the outer medulla shown in (a) and (b). There are now no thick portions of loops of Henle but thin Henle loops (HL) are numerous, as are thin-walled capillaries (C). The collecting ducts (CD) are larger and lined by distinct, clear-celled cuboidal epithelium. The pale-staining interstitium now forms a substantial part of the tissue, and scattered small stellate and spindle-shaped interstitial cells (IC) are numerous. In this micrograph, the loops of Henle, vessels and collecting ducts are in transverse section.

PRACTICAL HISTOLOGY—cont'd

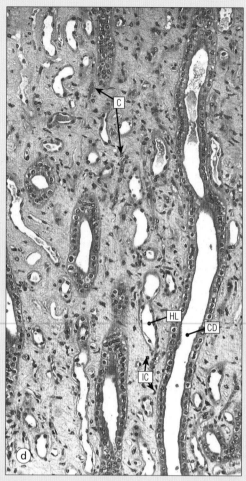

FIGURE 15.40, cont'd (d) Micrograph of same area of lower medulla shown in (c) sectioned longitudinally. Note the prominent straight collecting ducts running down towards the papilla; the nearer the tip of the papilla, the larger the ducts become.

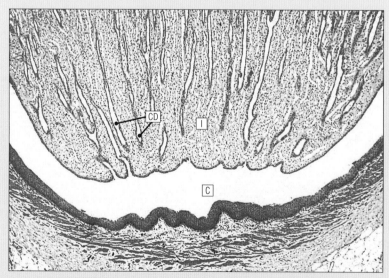

FIGURE 15.41 **Papilla.** The large collecting ducts (CD) are few in number as a result of fusion; they open into the calyx (C) at the papillary tip. At the papilla, the distal medulla consists almost entirely of large collecting ducts embedded in bulky interstitium (I), with very few thin Henle loops and a number of vasa recta vessels. Interstitial cells are numerous.

For online review questions, please visit
https://studentconsult.inkling.com.

❓ END OF CHAPTER REVIEW

True/False Answers to the MCQS, as Well as Case Answers, Can be Found in the Appendix in the Back of the Book.

1. **The glomerular filtration barrier comprises which of the following?**
   (a) Endothelial cells
   (b) Podocyte cytoplasm
   (c) Attenuated Bowman's capsule epithelium
   (d) Capillary basement membrane
   (e) Polyanionic charge barrier

2. **Which of the following features are seen in the proximal convoluted tubule epithelium?**
   (a) Shows extensive microvilli on luminal surface
   (b) Shows extensive basal interdigitation
   (c) Reabsorbs water from glomerular filtrate
   (d) Excretes glucose into the glomerular filtrate
   (e) Is partly controlled by the level of antidiuretic hormone (ADH) secreted by the posterior pituitary

3. **Which of the following features are seen in the juxtaglomerular apparatus?**
   (a) Is located in the glomerular mesangium
   (b) Contains highly specialized myoepithelial cells which also contain neuroendocrine granules
   (c) Secretes angiotensin
   (d) Secretes renin
   (e) Is important in maintaining plasma volume and blood pressure

4. **Which of the following features are present in the lower urinary tract?**
   (a) The renal pelvis, ureter and bladder are lined by transitional epithelium
   (b) The ureter has two muscle layers
   (c) The bladder has two muscle layers
   (d) The male urethra is lined by a pseudostratified columnar epithelium throughout its length
   (e) The female urethra is lined mainly by a stratified squamous epithelium

CASE 15.1   A CHILD WITH BLOOD IN THE URINE

A 6-year-old boy is admitted because his mother noted that he had been passing reduced amounts of concentrated dark brown urine. He had also been unwell, lethargic and tearful, and she noticed that his face had become puffy. She had taken a sample of the child's urine to the family practitioner, who applied a simple test, which showed that the dark brown colour was due to the presence of blood (haematuria), and the urine also contained abundant protein. On admission, the test was repeated and severe haematuria confirmed. The paediatrician also noted the facial puffiness, particularly around the eyes, and found that the child had high blood pressure. Laboratory tests showed that he had a raised blood urea. A clinical diagnosis was made that the child was developing renal failure and the possibility that this was caused by glomerular disease was considered. It was felt that the child had developed the nephritic syndrome. Further investigations were planned to investigate the underlying cause.

> **Q. Describe the structural and functional background to this case. Concentrate on describing the normal structure of the glomerulus and what normally prevents blood and protein from entering the urine. Speculate how the glomerular structure can become abnormal in disease to cause leakage of red cells in the urine and reduced glomerular filtration leading to uraemia. Why do you think there is associated hypertension?**

CASE 15.2   A MIDDLE-AGED MAN WITH SEVERE PROTEINURIA

A 46-year-old man who had had diabetes mellitus since his teens, developed proteinuria (excessive protein loss in the urine) as noted by his family practitioner, and an appointment was made for him to see his diabetic physician. In hospital, the presence of severe proteinuria was confirmed but it was also noted that he had puffy swelling (oedema) of his hands, feet, fingers and toes. Laboratory tests also showed that he had a low serum albumin. He was admitted and transferred to the care of a renal physician for further investigation of his nephritic syndrome.

> **Q. Describe the structural and functional background to this case. Concentrate on describing how the renal glomerulus normally prevents protein loss into the urine. Speculate what structural or functional changes may have developed to cause disease.**

Continued

CASE 15.3 A YOUNG MAN WITH MULTIPLE INJURIES

A 23-year-old man was involved in a road traffic accident and was trapped in the car for some hours. An intravenous infusion was set up by paramedics, but his blood pressure remained low and he lost consciousness while he was being extricated from the wreckage by fire officers with metal-cutting equipment. It was obvious that he had sustained compound fractures of the tibia and fibula in both legs, and it was suspected that he had internal bleeding from either a fractured pelvis or a ruptured internal organ. Despite intravenous plasma expanders and blood transfusion, he remained hypotensive and hypovolaemic in the ambulance. In the Emergency Room it was considered that his persistent hypotension was due to intra-abdominal bleeding, and emergency laparotomy showed a ruptured spleen. This was removed and good haemostasis was obtained at the site; and with the aid of blood transfusion his hypotensive and hypovolaemic state improved sufficiently that the orthopaedic surgeons operated on the compound fractures of tibia and fibula in the same operation. After the operation, he remained hypotensive for a further 24 h despite blood transfusion. It was noted that he was not passing urine, and blood samples were sent for analysis. This showed that he had a raised hydrogen ion concentration in his blood (acidosis) and that his serum potassium level was raised (hyperkalaemia). It was thought that he had acute renal failure.

Q. Describe the structural and functional background to this case. Concentrate on describing how which part of the kidney regulates hydrogen ion and potassium levels and speculate what might have happened to cause disease.

Chapter 16

Male Reproductive System

Introduction

The male reproductive system is responsible for:

- Production, nourishment and temporary storage of the haploid male gametes (spermatozoa)
- Intromission of a suspension of spermatozoa (semen) into the female genital system
- Production of male sex hormones (androgens).

Whereas the first two functions are important only during the years of sexual maturity, hormone production is required throughout life, even in-utero.

The male genital system (Fig. 16.1) comprises:

- Testes, which produce spermatozoa, and synthesize and secrete androgens
- Epididymis, vas deferens, ejaculatory duct and part of the male urethra, which form the ductal system responsible for the carriage of spermatozoa to the exterior
- Seminal vesicles, the prostate gland and the bulbo-urethral glands (of Cowper), which are secretory glands providing fluid and nutrients to support and nourish the spermatozoa, and forming the bulk of the semen
- Penis, which is an organ capable of becoming erect for insertion into the female vagina during sexual intercourse.

The testes, epididymis and vas deferens are located in the scrotal sac (Fig. 16.2), which is a skin-covered pouch enclosing a mesothelium-lined cavity continuous with the peritoneal cavity at the inguinal canal.

Testes

Anatomy and Development

The testes are paired organs located outside the body cavity in the scrotum

The location of the testes in the scrotum means that they are maintained at a temperature approximately 2–3°C below body temperature; this is essential for normal spermatogenesis.

Embryologically, the testes develop high on the posterior abdominal wall and migrate to the scrotum, usually arriving there in the 7th month of intrauterine life.

Sometimes a testis fails to migrate from the posterior abdominal wall and does not arrive in the scrotum. It may stay on the posterior abdominal wall at its site of original development, or it may become stuck on its way down to the scrotum, the common site being within the inguinal canal. This is called 'undescended testis' or 'mal descent of the testis'. Because the testis does not arrive in the cooler environment of the scrotal sac, the germ cells in the seminiferous tubules degenerate and die, without ever producing spermatozoa. This is called **cryptorchidism**, and the testis remains small and non-functional throughout life, although the testosterone-producing Leydig cells (see p. 325) remain undamaged and functional. Undescended testes have a high risk of developing malignant tumours.

CLINICAL EXAMPLE
SCROTAL SWELLINGS

Common causes of scrotal swelling are hydrocele, haematocele and inguinal hernia.

A hydrocele results when excessive fluid forms or accumulates within the scrotal cavity.

After trauma, bleeding into the scrotal cavity may produce a haematocele.

An inguinal hernia occurs when loops of intestine pass into the sac through the inguinal canal.

Less common, but more important, are tumours of the testis, which present as a solid scrotal mass. Almost all testicular tumours arise from germ cells, and there are two main types. Seminoma affects older males; tumour cells resemble spermatocytes (see Fig. 16.6). Teratoma affects younger males; tumour cells resemble structures seen in the developing embryo.

Each mature adult testis is a solid ovoid organ approximately 4–5 cm long, 3 cm deep and 2.5 cm wide, and usually weighs 11–17 g. The right testis is commonly slightly larger and heavier than the left.

Each testis has an epididymis (see p. 328) attached to its posterior surface and is suspended in the scrotal sac by the spermatic cord containing the vas deferens (see p. 328), the arterial supply and the venous and lymphatic drainage.

The testis is completely enclosed by the tunica albuginea, which is thickened posteriorly to form the mediastinum of the testis, projecting some way into the body of the testis (Fig. 16.3). Blood and lymphatic vessels, and the channels carrying spermatozoa, pass through this area (rete testis, see p. 326). Fibrous septa from the mediastinum divide the body of the testis into 250–350 lobules, each lobule containing one to four seminiferous tubules.

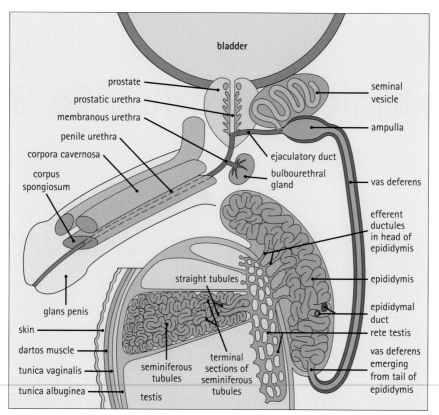

FIGURE 16.1 **The male genital system.** Spermatogenesis occurs in the seminiferous tubules; the resulting spermatozoa pass into the rete testis at the hilum (mediastinum) of the testis. From the rete testis, spermatozoa are transported by about a dozen efferent ductules into the head of the epididymis, where the ductules fuse to form the single, highly coiled epididymal duct. Within this duct they acquire their motility. The spermatozoa then pass into a long straight tube, the vas deferens, which transports them from the scrotal sac into the short ejaculatory duct, receiving abundant secretions from the seminal vesicles. The ejaculatory ducts from the right and left sides run through the tissue of the prostate gland and open into the prostatic urethra. Prostatic secretions and the secretions of the bulbourethral glands accompany or precede the semen along the penile urethra.

Seminiferous Tubules

A seminiferous tubule is a coiled, non-branching closed loop, both ends of which open into the rete testis

The rete testis is a system of channels located at the posterior hilum of the testis, close to the mediastinum.

Each seminiferous tubule is approximately 150 μm in diameter and 80 cm long. It has been calculated that the combined total length of all the seminiferous tubules in each testis is 300–900 m.

In a sexually mature adult, each seminiferous tubule has a central lumen lined by an actively replicating epithelium, the seminiferous or germinal epithelium, mixed with a population of supporting (sustentacular) cells, the Sertoli cells.

The lining cells sit on a well-defined basement membrane lying inside a collagenous layer containing fibroblasts and other spindle-shaped cells. These are contractile myoid cells containing intermediate filaments and desmin, like smooth muscle cells. In some animals, these myoid cells form a continuous peritubular layer and contract rhythmically, possibly propelling the non-motile spermatozoa towards the rete testis (spermatozoa only acquire their motility after they have passed through the epididymis). In human testis, the myoid cells form a less distinct layer and are not usually circumferential.

The outer wall of the tubule, comprising basal lamina, collagen layer and myoid cell layer, is sometimes called the 'tunica propria'.

Blood vessels and clusters of hormone-producing interstitial (Leydig) cells are found between adjacent seminiferous tubules (Fig. 16.4).

Germinal epithelium and spermatogenesis The germinal epithelium lining the seminiferous tubules produces the haploid male gametes (spermatozoa) by a series of steps called, in sequence, 'spermatocytogenesis, meiosis and spermiogenesis' (Fig. 16.5).

In spermatocytogenesis, the stem cells (spermatogonia) undergo mitosis

This mitotic division (see Fig. 2.26) produces not only more spermatogonia but also cells that differentiate into primary spermatocytes (Fig. 16.6).

In man, spermatogonia can be divided into three groups according to their nuclear appearances: type A-dark (Ad) cells, type A-pale (Ap) cells, and type B cells. It is thought that type Ad spermatogonia are the stem cells of the system, their mitotic division producing more type Ad cells and some type Ap cells, which further replicate by

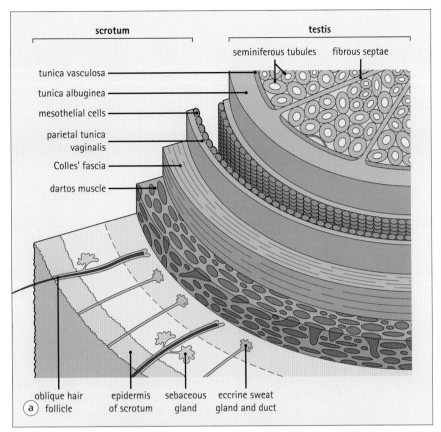

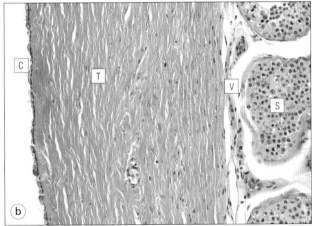

FIGURE 16.2 **Scrotum and tunica vaginalis.** (a) The scrotum is covered externally by skin with oblique hair follicles (producing curly hair) and numerous eccrine sweat glands. In the deeper layers of the skin, smooth muscle fibres, arranged in a rather haphazard manner, form the poorly-defined dartos muscle, contraction of which produces wrinkling of the scrotal skin. Beneath the dartos muscle lies fibrocollagenous fascia (Colles' fascia), the deepest layer being compacted to form the dense parietal layer of tunica vaginalis, which is lined internally by flattened mesothelial cells similar to those lining the peritoneal cavity, with which it is continuous. This smooth mesothelial-coated parietal tunica vaginalis forms the inner layer of the scrotal sac and is separated from the external surface of the testis by a potential space containing a watery fluid. This fluid acts as a lubricant, allowing the testis to move smoothly within the scrotal sac without friction. The testis is covered externally by a thick collagenous capsule, the visceral layer of the tunica vaginalis (the tunica albuginea), the outer surface being coated with flattened mesothelial cells. Beneath the tunica albuginea lies a narrow variable layer of loosely arranged collagen containing superficial blood vessels; internal to this are the seminiferous tubules. (b) Micrograph of the tunica albuginea of the testis. Note the scrotal cavity (C), the collagenous tunica albuginea (T) covered externally by small mesothelial cells, the narrow vascular layer (V), which is sometimes called the 'tunica vasculosa', and the seminiferous tubules (S).

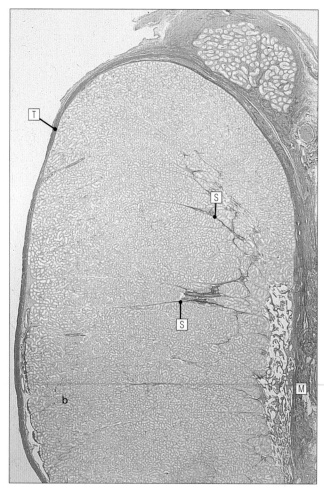

FIGURE 16.3 **Testis.** Low-power micrograph of a sagittal section through a testis stained by the van Gieson method, which colours collagen red. Note the tunica albuginea (T), which is thickened posteriorly to form the mediastinum testis (M). From the mediastinum, fibrous septa (S) enter the testis, separating it into lobules.

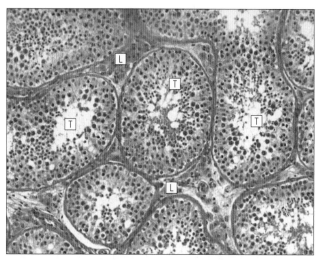

FIGURE 16.4 **Seminiferous tubules and interstitium.** Micrograph showing seminiferous tubules (T) cut in transverse, longitudinal and oblique section, lined by germinal epithelium and enclosed by tunica propria. In the interstices are blood vessels and clumps of Leydig (interstitial) cells (L).

mitosis to form clusters of daughter cells linked to each other by cytoplasmic bridges. These type Ap spermatogonia mature into type B cells, which divide mitotically to produce further type B cells; these cells then mature in a cluster to produce primary spermatocytes.

Primary spermatocytes replicate their DNA shortly after their formation (i.e. they are 4n). Primary spermatocyte formation marks the end of spermatocytogenesis.

Meiotic division occurs at the spermatocyte stages

Primary spermatocytes pass through a long prophase lasting about 22 days, during which changing patterns of nuclear chromatin enable preleptotene, leptotene, zygotene, pachytene and diplotene stages to be identified (see Fig. 16.5). Meiosis is described on page 33.

The first meiotic division occurs after the late pachytene/diplotene stages, with the formation of diploid secondary spermatocytes which rapidly (i.e. within a few hours) undergo the second meiotic division to produce haploid spermatids.

Spermiogenesis is the process by which haploid spermatids are transformed into spermatozoa

Spermiogenesis can be divided into four phases, all of which occur while the spermatids are embedded in small hollows in the free luminal surface of the Sertoli cells (see p. 327). These four phases are:
- The Golgi phase
- The cap phase
- The acrosome phase
- The maturation phase.

The details of these phases are shown diagrammatically in Figure 16.7.

Mature spermatozoon. The mature spermatozoon comprises a head and a tail region, the latter being composed of a neck, a middle piece, a principal piece and an end-piece (Fig. 16.8).

The head of a mature spermatozoon is composed of the nucleus covered by the acrosomal cap

The spermatozoon head is flattened and pointed, and the chromatin of the nucleus is condensed and broken only by occasional clear nuclear vacuoles.

The acrosomal cap covers the anterior two-thirds to three-quarters of the nucleus; it is a glycoprotein containing numerous enzymes, including a protease, acid phosphatase, neuraminidase and hyaluronidase, and can be regarded as a specialized giant lysosome.

The acrosomal enzymes are released when the spermatozoon contacts the ovum; they facilitate penetration of the corona radiata and zona pellucida of the ovum (see Chapter 17) by the spermatozoal nuclear head.

The tail region of a mature spermatozoon is composed of the neck region, and middle, principal and end-pieces

Running throughout the tail is the axoneme, which is responsible for spermatozoon motility; it is essentially a

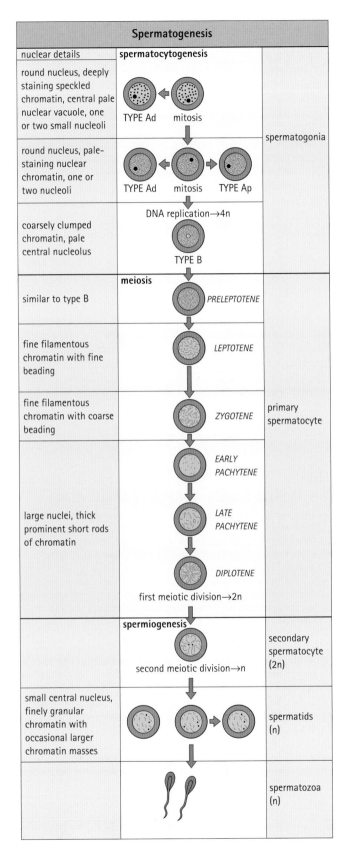

Spermatogenesis		
nuclear details	**spermatocytogenesis**	
round nucleus, deeply staining speckled chromatin, central pale nuclear vacuole, one or two small nucleoli	TYPE Ad ← mitosis	spermatogonia
round nucleus, pale-staining nuclear chromatin, one or two nucleoli	TYPE Ad ← mitosis → TYPE Ap	
coarsely clumped chromatin, pale central nucleolus	DNA replication→4n TYPE B	
	meiosis	
similar to type B	PRELEPTOTENE	
fine filamentous chromatin with fine beading	LEPTOTENE	
fine filamentous chromatin with coarse beading	ZYGOTENE	primary spermatocyte
large nuclei, thick prominent short rods of chromatin	EARLY PACHYTENE	
	LATE PACHYTENE	
	DIPLOTENE first meiotic division→2n	
	spermiogenesis second meiotic division→n	secondary spermatocyte (2n)
small central nucleus, finely granular chromatin with occasional larger chromatin masses		spermatids (n)
		spermatozoa (n)

FIGURE 16.5 **Spermatocytogenesis and meiosis.** Spermatocytogenesis begins with the development of spermatogonia, of which three types are recognized: the type A-dark (Ad) cell, the type A-pale (Ap) cell, and the type B cell. It is thought that the Ad cells are the precursor cells, which divide to produce new Ad cells and some Ap cells, the latter giving rise to type B cells, which subsequently pass through a meiotic phase to produce spermatocytes. The B cells pass through several stages of maturation before the first meiotic division, and in these early stages are known as 'primary spermatocytes'. The preleptotene cell is similar to the type B cell, but is not in contact with the basement membrane of the seminiferous tubule. The cell then undergoes its first meiotic division to produce a secondary spermatocyte, which is smaller than its parent primary spermatocyte and has fine granular chromatin. This immediately undergoes a second meiotic division to produce the haploid spermatids from which the spermatozoa will develop. The spermatids are located toward the lumen of the seminiferous tubule and have spherical central nuclei with finely granular chromatin and occasional larger chromatin masses. Their nuclear diameter is about half that of the primary spermatocytes from which they are derived.

long, specialized cilium, with nine outer doublet tubules around a central tubule pair (see Fig. 3.17)

The proximal part of the tail is the neck. This is a short narrow segment containing the pair of centrioles and a connecting piece that form the nine fibrous rings surrounding the axoneme.

The axoneme runs through the centre of the middle piece and is surrounded by the nine coarse longitudinal fibres from the connecting piece in the neck and an outer zone of tightly packed, elongated mitochondria. The lower limit of the middle piece is marked by a sudden narrowing, sometimes associated with an annular thickening of the cell membrane, the annulus.

The principal piece is the longest part of the tail and comprises the axoneme surrounded by the nine coarse longitudinal fibres, which are in turn enclosed by numerous external sheath fibres orientated circumferentially. As one of the anterior and one of the posterior longitudinal fibres are fused with the circumferential fibres, the remaining seven fibres are distributed asymmetrically, four in one lateral compartment and three in the other.

At the junction between the principal piece and the short end-piece, the longitudinal and circumferential fibres cease. Thus the end-piece is composed of axoneme only.

Sertoli Cells

The Sertoli cell sits on a basement membrane with its irregular apex extending into the lumen of the seminiferous tubule

Sertoli cells are tall, columnar cells (Fig. 16.9) and are the main cell type until puberty, after which they comprise only about 10% of the cells lining the seminiferous tubules. In elderly men, however, a decrease in the number of germinal epithelial cells is common, so Sertoli

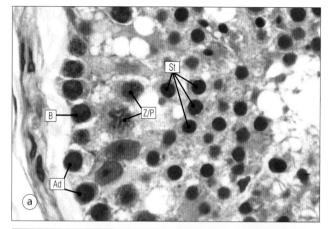

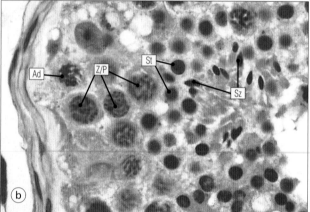

FIGURE 16.6 **Spermatocytogenesis and spermiogenesis in seminiferous tubules.** Spermatogenesis occurs in waves along the length of the seminiferous tubules, and thus adjacent areas of the same tubule show spermatocytogenesis and spermiogenesis at various stages. (a) Micrograph showing spermatogonia of various types, including Ad and B types, and zygotene/pachytene (Z/P) stages of primary spermatocytes. Some spermatids (St) are also present. (b) Micrograph showing a later stage in which there is spermiogenesis as well as spermatocytogenesis. (Ad) spermatogonia, and zygotene/pachytene (Z/P) stages of primary spermatocytes, and spermatids (St) are shown, as well as developing spermatozoa (Sz) embedded in Sertoli cell cytoplasm. Sertoli cells are poorly defined in light microscopic sections of human testis.

which roughly divide the seminiferous tubule lining into basal and adluminal compartments.

Other forms of intercellular junctions (see Chapter 3) between Sertoli cells, including gap junctions and (occasionally) desmosomes, have been described, and intercellular junction-like structures have been seen between Sertoli cells and developing germinal epithelial cells.

Sertoli cell cytoplasm is eosinophilic and finely granular; it may contain lipid vacuoles. Ultrastructurally, it has abundant endoplasmic reticulum, often arranged as flat-stacked cisternae (annulate lamellae) with associated ribosomes. The lipid vacuoles are usually found close to the larger cisternae.

Endoplasmic reticulum is also prominent in the cytoplasmic processes interdigitating between the developing germ cells, and clusters of free ribosomes are numerous at the base of the cell. Microfibrils and microtubules are common in areas of cytoplasm close to the developing spermatids.

Spermatogonia and preleptotene spermatocytes occupy the basal compartment, whereas remaining primary spermatocytes, secondary spermatocytes and spermatids are located in the adluminal compartment. These compartments are clearly distinguishable in some animal species, including primates, but not in man.

ADVANCED CONCEPT
SERTOLI CELLS

In the mature testis, Sertoli cells secrete androgen-binding protein (ABP), which binds testosterone and hydroxytestosterone produced outside the seminiferous tubule; high concentrations of these hormones are required within the germinal epithelium and tubule lumen for normal germ cell maturation.

ABP secretion is dependent on follicle-stimulating hormone (FSH) secretion by the pituitary and FSH receptors are present on Sertoli cells. FSH promotes spermatogenesis, probably by inducing Sertoli cells to produce varying amounts of ABP.

Sertoli cells also secrete the hormone inhibin, which inhibits the secretion of FSH by the pituitary gland and therefore plays an important feedback role in controlling the rate of spermatogenesis.

cells again become a significant component of the tubule cell population.

Sertoli cells are not affected by any of the factors that injure the sensitive germinal epithelium. For example, they do not degenerate when exposed to normal body temperature and can therefore survive in the undescended testis.

The cell nucleus is irregular with deep folds, but tends towards an oval shape, with the long axis at right-angles to the basement membrane. The nucleus has a vesicular chromatin pattern and a prominent nucleolus.

The Sertoli cell outline is irregular, with many ramifying cytoplasmic extensions that make contact with those from neighbouring Sertoli cells to form a meshwork of cytoplasm. This encloses the developing cells of the germinal epithelium and forms tight junctions (see Fig. 3.6),

Sertoli cells have supportive, phagocytic and secretory functions

Sertoli cells were originally thought to be supporting or sustentacular cells, but are now known to be polyfunctional.

Supportive functions probably include the provision of nutrients to developing germinal cells via their intimate cytoplasmic processes, and the transport of waste materials from spermiogenesis to the blood and lymph vascular systems surrounding the seminiferous tubules.

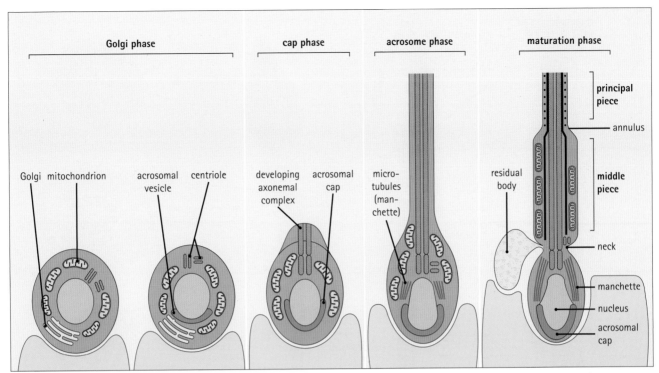

FIGURE 16.7 Spermiogenesis. In the Golgi phase, PAS-positive granules (pre-acrosomal granules) appear in the Golgi apparatus and fuse to form a membrane-bound acrosomal vesicle close to the nuclear membrane. This vesicle enlarges and its location marks what will be the anterior pole of the spermatozoon. The two centrioles migrate to the opposite (posterior) pole of the spermatid, the distal centriole becoming aligned at right-angles to the cell membrane. It then begins the formation of the axoneme complex of the sperm tail. In the cap phase, the acrosomal vesicle changes shape to enclose the anterior half of the nucleus and become the acrosomal cap. The nuclear membrane beneath the acrosomal cap thickens and loses its pores and the nuclear chromatin becomes more condensed. In the acrosome phase, the increasingly dense nucleus flattens and elongates; an anterior pole, capped by the acrosomal cap, and a posterior pole closely related to the developing axonemal complex can be identified. With the changed shape of the nucleus, the cytoplasm between the acrosomal cap and the anterior cell membrane migrates to the posterior part of the cell. The entire cell orients itself so that the anterior pole is embedded in the luminal surface of the Sertoli cell, pointing down toward the base of the seminiferous tubule; the cytoplasm-rich posterior pole of the spermatid protrudes into the tubule lumen. At the same time, a sheath of microtubules, called the 'manchette', extends from the posterior part of the acrosomal cap toward the developing tail. The centrioles (see Fig. 2.22), have migrated posteriorly from the neck of the developing spermatozoon, which is the connecting piece between the head (containing the nucleus and acrosomal cap) and the developing tail. One centriole continues to synthesize the axonemal complex of the sperm tail, producing a regular tubular complex comprising two central microtubules surrounded by a ring of nine peripheral doublets. In the neck region, nine coarse fibres are produced which extend down into the tail around the microtubules of the axonemal complex. Prominent mitochondria aggregate in and below the neck to surround the nine coarse fibres; this forms the segment known as the 'middle piece'. The mitochondria finish abruptly at a ring (annulus) demarcating the middle piece from the main parts of the tail (the principal piece and end-piece). The maturation phase is characterized by the pinching-off of surplus cytoplasm, particularly from the neck and middle piece regions, and its phagocytosis by Sertoli cells. The immature spermatozoa then become disconnected from the Sertoli cell surface and lie free in the seminiferous tubule lumen, marking the end of spermiogenesis. The immature male gametes are later modified in the ductular systems leading to the penis. The duration of spermatocytogenesis from spermatogonium type Ad to released immature spermatozoon is about 70 days.

It has long been assumed that Sertoli cells phagocytose any residual cytoplasm (residual bodies) shed by maturing spermatids during spermiogenesis. They may also phagocytose any effete cellular material derived from degenerate germinal cells that fail to complete spermatogenesis.

Secretory functions vary with sexual maturity. In the male embryo at about the 8th or 9th week of fetal development, Sertoli cells secrete müllerian inhibitory substance (MIS), which is thought to suppress further development of the müllerian duct system. In the pre-pubertal testis they may secrete a substance preventing meiotic division of the germinal epithelial cells.

The testicular interstitium contains hormone-secreting Leydig (interstitial) cells

The interstitial tissue lying between the seminiferous tubules is a loose network of fibrocollagenous tissue composed of:

- Fibroblasts
- Collagen, in which occasional macrophages and mast cells are present
- Blood and lymphatic vessels
- Clumps of interstitial or Leydig cells.

Leydig cells synthesize testosterone and, although they are most common in the tubular interstitium, they

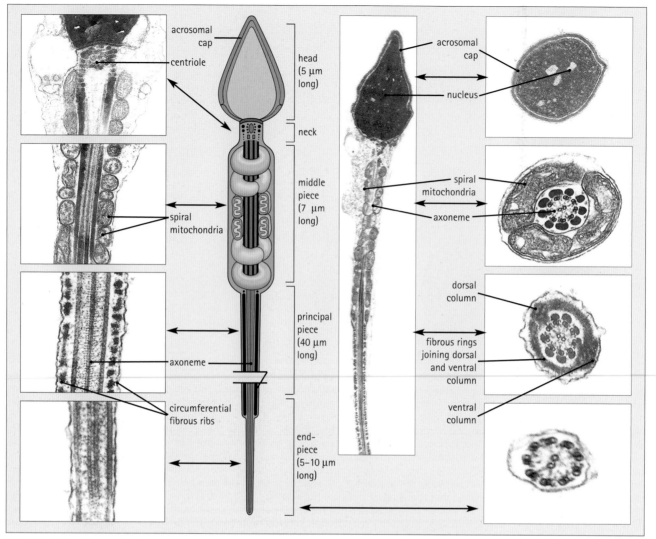

FIGURE 16.8 **Mature human spermatozoon.** A mature spermatozoon accompanied by electron micrographs confirming its structure.

can occasionally be found in the mediastinum of the testis, the epididymis, or even in the spermatic cord. They are often closely related to nerves, like their female equivalent the hilus cells of the ovary (see Chapter 17).

Leydig cells have round vesicular nuclei with prominent nuclear membranes and one or two nucleoli. Some of the cells are small and spindle shaped and are thought to be immature forms, but most are round or polygonal.

Leydig cells have granular eosinophilic cytoplasm containing lipases, oxidative enzymes, esterases and a number of steroid dehydrogenases.

A characteristic feature of Leydig cells is Reinke's crystalloid, which is an intracytoplasmic, eosinophilic, elongated, rectangular or rhomboid mass, approximately 3 μm thick and up to 20 μm long (Fig. 16.10).

Reinke's crystalloids are not seen before puberty. They increase in number during the years of sexual maturity, becoming most common in old age.

Yellow-brown lipofuscin pigment is present in most Leydig cells.

The rete testis is a complex arrangement of interconnecting channels located at the mediastinum of the testis

Spermatozoa formed in the seminiferous tubule loops pass to the terminal portions, which are lined entirely by Sertoli cells (see Fig. 16.9), and thence via the short straight tubules into the rete testis (Fig. 16.11) embedded in a fibrous stroma continuous with the tunica albuginea.

Both straight tubules and rete testis are lined by a simple epithelium of cuboidal or low columnar cells bearing microvilli on their luminal surface. Most of the rete testis epithelial cells bear a single long central flagellum.

Channels of the rete testis fuse to form about a dozen efferent ductules

These emerge from the upper end of the mediastinum of the testis, penetrating the tunica albuginea (see

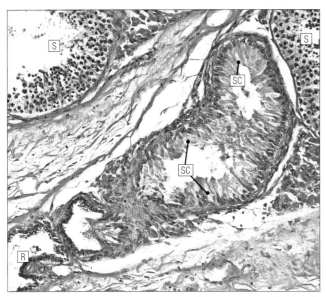

FIGURE 16.9 **Sertoli cells.** Sertoli cells (SC) are rarely clearly identifiable in the lining of seminiferous tubules (S) in which active spermatogenesis is occurring, but form the entire lining of the tubule for a short distance at its distal end shortly before it drains into the rete testis system (R) at the mediastinum testis. This micrograph is taken from such an area.

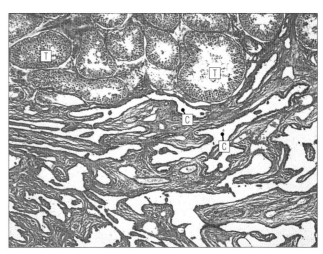

FIGURE 16.11 **Rete testis.** The rete testis is a network of interconnecting channels (C) into which the seminiferous tubules (T) empty. Spermatozoa are transferred from the rete testis to the epididymis via the efferent ductules.

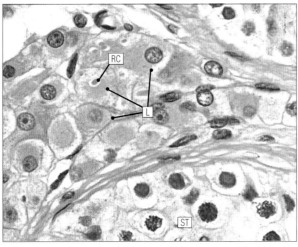

FIGURE 16.10 **Leydig (interstitial) cells.** Micrograph showing a cluster of Leydig cells (L) situated in the interstitium between seminiferous tubules (ST). They have abundant eosinophilic cytoplasm, and some of the cells contain Reinke's crystalloids (RC).

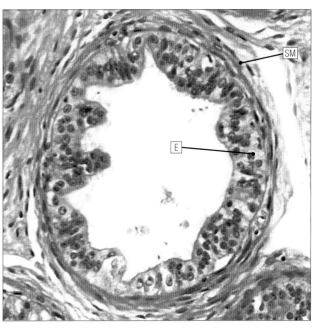

FIGURE 16.12 **Efferent ductules.** Note the mixed columnar and cuboidal epithelium (E), the typical fringed internal lumen, and the circumferential ring of smooth muscle (SM) fibres.

Fig. 16.1) and entering the head of the epididymis. Here, they gradually merge to become a single tube, the epididymal duct.

The efferent ductules are lined by a mixed epithelium of tall ciliated columnar cells and non-ciliated cuboidal or low columnar cells with microvilli on their luminal surface (Fig. 16.12). The cilia beat toward the epididymis and propel the spermatozoa onward, whereas the non-ciliated cells absorb some of the testicular fluid, which is the transport medium for the immature and still immotile spermatozoa.

The efferent ductules are highly convoluted and have a narrow sheath of circumferential smooth muscle cells interspersed with elastic fibres; peristaltic contractions of this muscle enhance the progression of the spermatozoa.

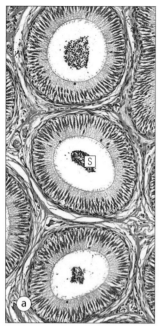
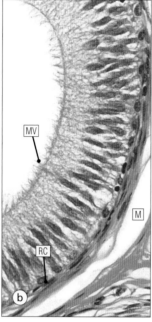

FIGURE 16.13 **Epididymal duct.** (a) Micrograph of epididymal duct lined by tall columnar epithelium with basal nuclei; the lumina contain clumps of spermatozoa (S). (b) High-power micrograph showing a single duct. Note the unusually tall microvilli (MV), the scattered small round cells at the base of the columnar epithelium (RC) and the narrow band of circular muscle fibres (M).

Epididymis

The epididymal duct (ductus epididymis) is formed by the fusion of the efferent ductules

The epididymal duct is a single highly convoluted tube about 5 m long. It is embedded in a loose vascular supporting stroma of fibroblasts, collagen and glycosaminoglycan matrix, and is surrounded by a dense fibrocollagenous capsule, to form the comma-shaped body called the 'epididymis'.

The epididymis can be divided into head, body and tail regions, with the efferent ductules entering the head and the distal end of the epididymal duct emerging at the tail to become the vas deferens.

The human epididymis is usually 5 cm long and 1 cm wide, and, as the entire 5 m of epididymal duct is contained within it, it is clear that the duct is enormously convoluted.

The epididymal duct is lined by a tall columnar epithelium bearing numerous very long, atypical microvilli

These giant microvilli (Fig. 16.13) are largely immotile and are inaccurately named stereocilia; they neither contain the internal microtubular structures of cilia (see Fig. 3.17) nor function like cilia. They are about 80 μm long in the epididymal head and 40 μm long in the tail. The cells also possess coated vesicles and lysosomes, rough endoplasmic reticulum and a prominent Golgi.

They have the following absorptive/phagocytic and secretory functions:

- Absorption of testicular fluid commenced by the efferent ductules
- Phagocytosis and digestion of degenerate spermatozoa and residual bodies
- Secretion of glycoproteins, sialic acid and a substance called 'glycerylphosphorylcholine', which is believed to play a role in the maturation of the spermatozoa, though the precise mechanism is unknown. The glycoproteins bind to the surface membranes of the spermatozoa, but their function is also unknown.

In addition to the tall columnar cells, there is a population of small round cells with a high nucleus/cytoplasm ratio that lie on the epithelial basement membrane and are thought to be the precursors of the tall cells.

The entire epididymal duct is surrounded by a narrow sheath of circular muscle similar to that in the efferent ductules, but in the tail there is also a longitudinal layer internal to the circular layer, and an outer longitudinal layer.

All of the muscle layers thicken within the epididymal tail, becoming significant layers where the duct emerges to become the vas deferens.

Vas Deferens

The ductus (vas) deferens is a straight tube running vertically upward behind the epididymis within the spermatic cord

The spermatic cord also contains arteries, veins, lymphatics and nerves. The veins form a complex anastomotic plexus called the 'pampiniform plexus'. Externally, the spermatic cord contains longitudinal fibres of voluntary striated muscle, the cremaster muscle.

The vas deferens has a thick, muscular wall composed of a middle circular and outer and inner longitudinal layers. Internal to the inner layer is a fibroelastic lamina propria covered with a tall columnar epithelium almost identical to that of the epididymis, but thrown up into longitudinal folds by the lamina propria; this produces a small stellate lumen (Fig. 16.14). Peristalsis of the thick muscular wall propels spermatozoa forward during emission.

Each vas deferens enters the pelvic cavity via the inguinal canal and then passes downward and medially to the base of the bladder. Near its distal end, close to the base of the bladder, each vas deferens has a dilatation (the ampulla) where the muscle layer becomes thinner; the mucosal layer in the ampulla appears thicker because the folds, some of which are branched, are taller.

At the distal end of the ampulla, the vas deferens is joined by a short duct from the seminal vesicles.

Seminal Vesicles

Each seminal vesicle is a highly convoluted, unbranched tubular diverticulum of the vas deferens.

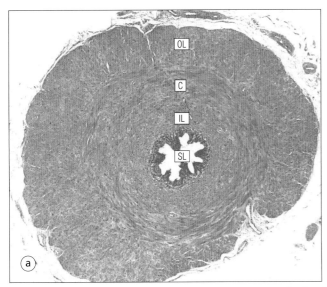

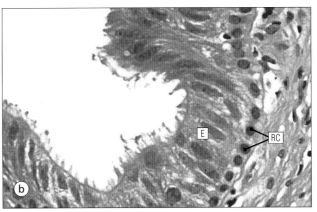

FIGURE 16.14 **Vas deferens.** (a) Low-power micrograph showing the three muscle layers (a central circular (C) layer between outer (OL) and inner longitudinal (IL) layers) and the stellate lumen (SL). (b) High-power micrograph showing the tall ciliated columnar epithelium (E), the basal layer of small regular round cells (RC), and the pattern of folds.

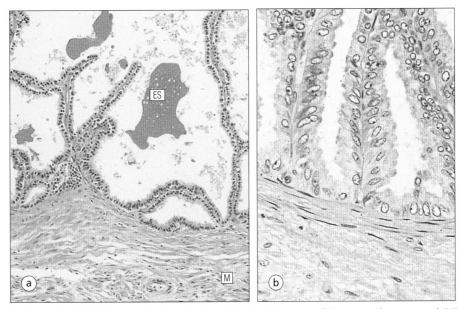

FIGURE 16.15 **Seminal vesicle.** (a) Micrograph of seminal vesicle showing part of the muscular surround (M) and the pattern of tall mucosal folds. The lumen contains blobs of eosinophilic secretion (ES). (b) Micrograph showing the tall columnar secretory epithelium at high magnification.

The seminal vesicle is 15 cm long but is coiled on itself to form a body about 5–6 cm long. This tube is surrounded by an inner circular and an outer longitudinal smooth muscle layer, with an external layer of fibrocollagenous tissue containing many elastic fibres.

Seminal vesicle mucosa is composed of a fibroelastic lamina propria thrown up into tall, narrow complicated folds (Fig. 16.15) covered by non-ciliated, tall columnar epithelial cells and a population of non-specialized basal round cells similar to those seen in the proximal ducts and ductules. The tall cells have the characteristics of secretory cells, with large secretory vacuoles near their luminal surface and abundant rough endoplasmic reticulum; they may also contain small, yellow-brown lipofuscin granules.

The complexity of the mucosal folding produces a vast surface area for secretion and 70–80% of the human ejaculate is a thick, creamy-yellow secretion of the seminal vesicles. This secretion contains abundant fructose and other sugars, prostaglandins, proteins, amino acids, citric acid and ascorbic acid. Fructose is the major nutrient of spermatozoa.

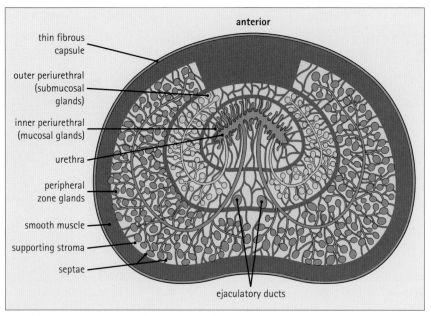

FIGURE 16.16 **Prostate.** The prostate is surrounded by a thin fibrous capsule internal to which is a substantial layer of smooth muscle giving rise to septa (mainly muscular but with a fine fibrocollagenous component) that penetrate the organ to provide an intimate stroma supporting and demarcating the glandular elements. Division into central and peripheral zones is indistinct. The inner periurethral (mucosal) glands are small and open directly into the urethra around its entire surface; the outer periurethral glands are more numerous and open into the urethra through short ducts that enter the posterolateral urethral sinuses on their posterior surface on either side of the central ridge, the urethral crest. These two groups of glands comprise the central zone. The glands of the peripheral zone empty their secretions into the urethra by way of long ducts opening alongside the urethral crest.

Contraction of the seminal vesicle smooth muscle propels accumulated secretion into the ejaculatory duct

The ejaculatory duct is formed by the merging of the short duct from the seminal vesicle with the vas deferens distal to the ampulla.

Each ejaculatory duct is only 1 cm long and is lined by an epithelium of tall columnar and small round cells identical to that of the ampulla; there is no smooth muscle in its wall. The right and left ejaculatory ducts run through the prostate gland and open into the prostatic urethra at the prostatic utricle.

Prostate

Introduction

The prostate is composed of secreting glands that open into the urethra, which runs through its body. These prostatic glands and ducts are embedded in a supporting stroma of fibroblasts, collagen and smooth muscle.

The entire prostate gland is surrounded by a fibrocollagenous capsule from which septa extend partway into its body, dividing it into ill-defined lobes.

The prostate gland progressively enlarges from about 45 years of age and may become very large in elderly men.

The prostatic glands are arranged in three concentric groups

A small group of mucosal glands open directly into the urethra; a larger group of submucosal glands open into the urethra via short ducts; a substantial outer group of so-called main prostatic glands open into the urethra via long ducts (Fig. 16.16).

The ducts of the submucosal and main prostatic glands open posteriorly into the urethral sinuses on either side of a longitudinal ridge called the 'urethral crest'.

The epithelium lining of the prostate glands is thrown up into complex folds accompanied by a narrow supporting lamina propria. There are two types of epithelial cell:
- Tall columnar or cuboidal cells with pale foamy cytoplasm and basal pale-staining nuclei
- Scanty flat basal cells with small dark-staining nuclei in contact with the basement membrane (Fig. 16.17c).

Ultrastructurally, the tall columnar cells have a prominent Golgi located between the basal nucleus and the luminal surface; lysosomes, secretory granules and rough endoplasmic reticulum are numerous.

The secretory products of these cells include acid phosphatase (produced in large quantities by the lysosomes), citric acid, fibrinolysin, amylase and other proteins. The gland lumina usually contain some stored secretions; in older men, small spherical corpora

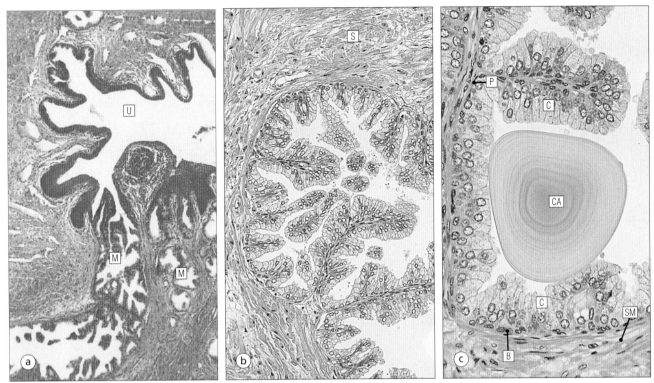

FIGURE 16.17 **Prostatic glands.** (a) Micrograph of prostatic mucosal glands (M) opening directly into the urethra (U). (b) Micrograph showing the general architecture of a typical prostatic gland with its papillary pattern of ingrowths. Note the smooth muscular and fibrocollagenous stroma (S). (c) Micrograph showing the cytological detail of prostatic gland lining epithelium. It is composed of tall, pale-staining columnar cells (C) and occasional small basal cells (B) with darker-staining nuclei. Note the delicate supporting stroma of the papillary ingrowth (P) and the narrow periglandular layer of smooth muscle fibres (SM). The lumen contains an uncalcified, concentrically laminated corpus amylacea (CA).

amylacea, which are mainly condensed glycoprotein and often calcified, are found.

The ducts of the prostate gland may also be lined by tall columnar epithelium, but as they near the urethra, this becomes progressively more cuboidal, and even transitional, like that of the urethra itself.

Bulbourethral Glands

Seminal fluid enters the prostatic urethra from the right and left ejaculatory ducts, passing through the short membranous urethra and the penile urethra, before entering the vagina during sexual intercourse. Opening into the membranous urethra are the long narrow ducts from the paired small bulbourethral glands.

The bulbourethral glands are lined by tall mucus-secreting epithelium

The bulbourethral glands are about 5 mm in diameter and the epithelium produces a watery, slightly mucoid fluid containing abundant sugars (mainly galactose) and some sialic acid. This fluid precedes the thicker semen along the penile urethra during emission and may have a lubricating function.

ADVANCED CONCEPT
PROSTATIC EPITHELIUM

The prostatic epithelium depends on adequate testosterone levels to maintain its structural and functional integrity; any inadequacy is manifest by a change of epithelium from tall secretory to cuboidal, with loss of, or reduced, secretory activity. This change is seen increasingly from the middle years onwards, and in extreme cases, the epithelium may be converted to a stratified squamous pattern, often with keratin formation.

Penis

The penis is composed of erectile tissue and contains part of the male urethra.

The erectile tissue is arranged into two dorsal cylinders (corpora cavernosa) and a smaller central ventral cylinder (corpus spongiosum) through which the penile urethra runs. The cylinders are each surrounded by a dense fibrocollagenous sheath, the tunica albuginea, which also holds them together (Fig. 16.18).

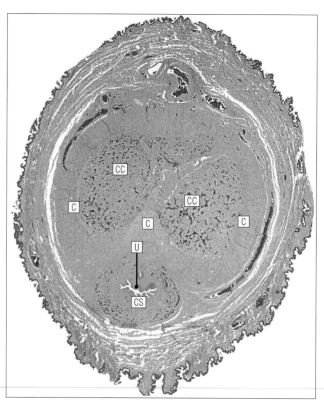

FIGURE 16.18 **Penis.** Transverse section of penis showing the arrangement of the vascular erectile tissue into two dorsal corpora cavernosa (CC) and a single ventral corpus spongiosum (CS) through which the penile urethra (U) runs. Small mucous glands in the corpus spongiosum are particularly concentrated around the penile urethra, into which they open. The corpora are enclosed within, and divided by, a broad fibrocollagenous capsule (C). The erectile core is surrounded by a sheath of skin to which it is connected by a very loose subcutis containing a number of blood vessels, including the small paired dorsal arteries and the midline superficial and deep dorsal veins.

 CLINICAL EXAMPLE
BENIGN PROSTATIC HYPERPLASIA

The commonest disorder of the prostate is benign prostatic hyperplasia and occurs in elderly men. This is characterized by considerable enlargement of the prostatic glands in the mucous and submucosal gland groups owing to an increase in the number and size of the glands and ducts, and an increase in the bulk of the supporting fibromuscular stroma. Many glands are overdistended with secretion (Fig. 16.19).

The increase in bulk of the prostatic tissue leads to compression of the urethra and micturition difficulties, including retention of urine.

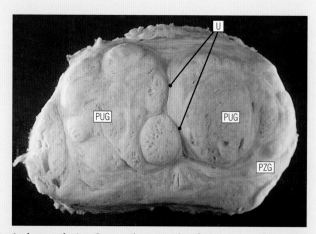

FIGURE 16.19 **Benign prostatic hyperplasia.** Gross photograph of the cut surface of a prostate removed at autopsy showing the typical appearance of benign prostatic hyperplasia. There is nodular overgrowth of the periurethral glands (PUG), which is causing compression and distortion of the urethra (U). Note that the peripheral zone glands (PZG) are not involved.

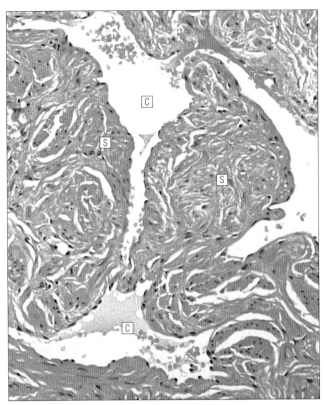

FIGURE 16.20 **Corpus spongiosum.** Micrograph of corpus spongiosum showing large, irregular interconnecting vascular channels (C) lined by flat endothelium and separated by a fibrocollagenous stroma (S) containing some smooth muscle bundles.

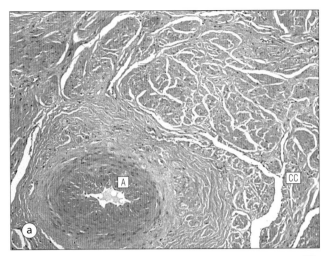

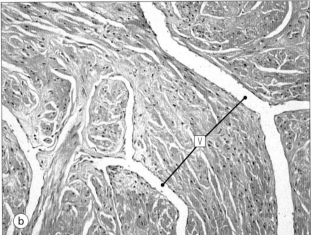

FIGURE 16.21 **Corpora cavernosa.** (a) Micrograph of part of the corpora cavernosa (CC) with the central deep artery (A). (b) Micrograph showing the system of interconnecting vascular channels (V) of the corpora cavernosa in the non-erectile state.

The erectile tissues are essentially interconnecting vascular spaces which are empty when the penis is flaccid (Figs 16.20, 16.21) but which fill with blood during erection to form an enlarged, rigid organ.

The blood supply to the penis is provided by the dorsal and the deep arteries. From the deep arteries arise arteries supplying the tunica albuginea, and the helicine arteries, which supply the erectile tissue.

The helicine arteries are so named because they are spiral in the flaccid penis but during erection they straighten and dilate, filling the corpora with blood.

This filling effect is partly due to closure of the arteriovenous shunts existing between the helicine arteries and deep veins, which constitute the normal route of helicine artery blood flow in the flaccid state.

Parasympathetic nerve discharges cause the closure, leading to diversion of the helicine artery blood into the cavernous spaces, while increased pressure in the corpora compresses the thin-walled veins, preventing emptying.

After ejaculation the parasympathetic stimulation ceases, the arteriovenous shunts open and blood passes from the corpora into the veins.

During erection the two corpora cavernosa become more turgid than the corpus spongiosum. The pressure exerted by the corpus spongiosum on the urethra running through it is not sufficient to prevent passage of the semen, which is forcibly ejected by contraction of the smooth muscle, but is usually sufficient to prevent successful, pain-free micturition.

The erectile component of the penis is surrounded by skin, which has a very loose subcutis, permitting it to move considerably during intercourse.

At the distal end of the penis the corpus spongiosum terminates on the glans penis, which is covered with non-keratinizing squamous epithelium containing sebaceous glands.

The penile urethra opens to the exterior at the meatus at the centre of the glans penis

For most of its length the penile urethra is lined by non-secreting columnar epithelium into which small mucous glands embedded in the corpus spongiosum drain. Within the glans penis, however, the urethra dilates (navicular fossa) and becomes lined by non-keratinizing stratified squamous epithelium identical to that covering the glans.

The end of the penis is normally covered by an overlap of penile skin (the prepuce), which is rich in elastic fibres

CLINICAL EXAMPLE
CARCINOMA OF THE PROSTATE

Cancer in the prostate gland almost always originates in the main glands arranged around the periphery and is often advanced before symptoms arise due to blockage of the urethra (Fig. 16.22).

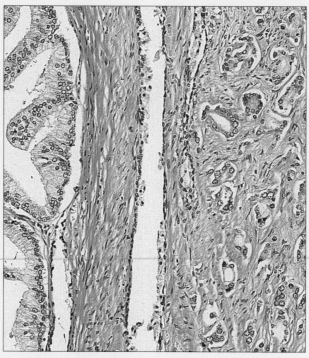

FIGURE 16.22 **Adenocarcinoma of the prostate.** Micrograph showing cancerous transformation of the prostatic glands. Those on the left have a normal arrangement with regular tall columnar epithelium. The cancerous prostatic glands on the right have lost their tall columnar pattern as well as their regular architecture.

permitting it to retract over the glans penis during intercourse.

Endocrine Control

The male sex hormone testosterone is essential for the male reproductive system to function successfully

In the embryo, testosterone and other androgens produced by the immature testes are responsible for the development of the penis and accessory sex glands, such as the prostate and epididymis.

With the onset of puberty, male secondary sexual characteristics develop under the influence of testosterone (Fig. 16.23). This hormone also induces maturation and division of spermatogonia in the seminiferous tubules, leading eventually to full spermatogenesis with the production of mature spermatozoa.

In addition, testosterone is responsible for the maturation of the characteristic epithelia of the male genital ducts and the accessory glands that discharge secretions into them.

In the adult male, continued production of spermatozoa, and maintenance of the normal structure and function of the ducts and accessory glands, is dependent on continued testosterone production.

Failing testosterone production in old age leads to partial or complete cessation of spermatogenesis and alteration of the specialized secretory, absorptive and microvillus epithelium of the ducts and accessory glands to a more simplified cuboidal or squamous epithelium, which is unable to perform its previous functions.

Thus, testosterone is the hub of the structure and function of the male genital system. It is produced by Leydig (interstitial) cells from cholesterol under the influence of luteinizing hormone secreted by the gonadotroph cells of the pituitary (see p. 265).

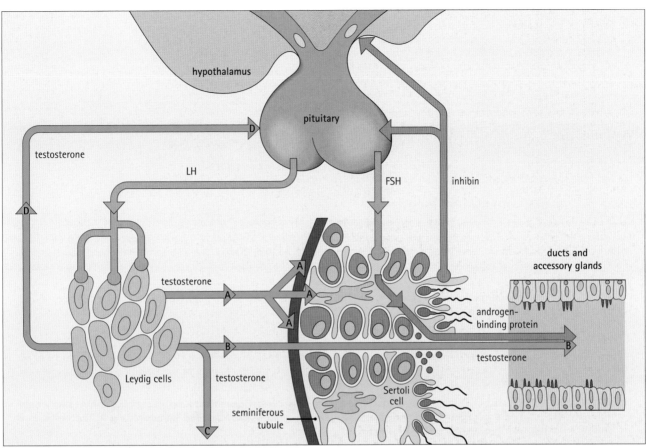

FIGURE 16.23 **Hormonal control of the male reproductive system.** Testosterone stimulates spermatogenesis in seminiferous tubules (A), maintains the structure and function of the ducts and accessory glands (B), stimulates and maintains secondary sexual characteristics (C), and provides a feedback mechanism (D) controlling pituitary output of luteinizing hormone (LH). Secretion of testosterone by Leydig cells is stimulated by LH. Sertoli cells secrete androgen-binding protein under the influence of follicle-stimulating hormone (FSH) from the pituitary, and also produce inhibin, which is responsible for feedback control.

 For online review questions, please visit https://studentconsult.inkling.com.

(?) END OF CHAPTER REVIEW

True/False Answers to the MCQs, as Well as Case Answers, can be Found in the Appendix in the Back of the Book.

1. **Which of the following features are seen in the germinal epithelium of the testes?**
   (a) Lines the seminiferous tubules and rete testes
   (b) Produces haploid male gametes
   (c) Is dependent on testosterone for its functional integrity
   (d) Is supported by Sertoli cells
   (e) Is an example of a renewing stem cell population

2. **Which of the following features are true for the spermatozoon?**
   (a) Contains the haploid nucleus in the head region
   (b) Has an acrosomal cap which contains several enzymes believed to help with penetration of the ovum
   (c) Contains an axoneme which is based on actin filaments
   (d) Is rich in mitochondria in the middle piece
   (e) Is formed by maturation of spermatids and takes place adjacent to the luminal surface of Leydig cells

Continued

3. **Which of the following features are seen in the prostate gland?**
   (a) Discharges its secreted products into the seminal vesicles
   (b) Has three zones of glands termed mucosal, submucosal and main prostatic glands
   (c) Has both glandular and fibromuscular components
   (d) Has glandular elements lined by transitional epithelium
   (e) Is sensitive to endocrine stimulation, especially from testosterone

4. **Which of the following are seen in the penis?**
   (a) There are two dorsal corpora spongiosa and one ventral corpus cavernosum
   (b) Blood is supplied to the erectile tissue by the helicine arteries
   (c) The urethra runs through the corpus spongiosum
   (d) The urethra is lined by squamous epithelium in its distal portion in the glans penis
   (e) There are small mucous glands which secrete into the urethra

CASE 16.1 A MAN WITH URINARY PROBLEMS

A 63-year-old man presented with a 1-year history of problems with micturition. After a period when his only problem was increasing nocturia (having to get up to pass urine in the night), he then found that he needed to go more frequently day and night, had a poor stream, and often dribbled when he thought he had finished. He also sometimes had to wait a long time before the stream started. The urological surgeon performed a rectal examination and found that the prostate gland was enlarged.

Q. Describe the histological and structural background to this case. What might happen to the bladder if the prostate gland is enlarged?

CASE 16.2 A COUPLE WITH SUBFERTILITY

A young married couple are being investigated for subfertility. In a semen analysis, the male partner is found to have no spermatozoa, and both testes are smaller than normal and rather firm. It transpires that, as a young boy, he had surgery for bilateral undescended testes.

Q. Describe the structural and functional background to this case. Concentrate on describing what one would normally expect in the postpubertal testis and speculate on what you might find histologically in the testis in a patient who has no spermatozoa in his ejaculate.

Chapter 17

Female Reproductive System

Introduction

The female reproductive system:
- Produces haploid female gametes (ova)
- Receives haploid male gametes (spermatozoa) prior to fertilization
- Provides a suitable environment for fertilization of ova by spermatozoa
- Provides a suitable physical and hormonal environment for implantation of the embryo
- Accommodates and nourishes the embryo and fetus during pregnancy
- Expels the mature fetus at the end of pregnancy.

The structure of the human female reproductive system changes considerably from childhood into reproductive maturity, and later the menopause, under the control of tropic hormones.

Furthermore, the various components undergo structural and functional modification at different stages in the monthly cycle.

The system (Figs 17.1, 17.2) comprises the ovaries, uterine tubes, uterus and vagina (collectively referred to as the **internal genitalia**), together with the mons pubis, vulva (labia majora and labia minora) and clitoris (referred to as the **external genitalia**).

Unlike many other mammals, the human female ovulates at regular intervals (approximately every 28 days) throughout the year.

As tissues from other animals do not accurately reflect the changes seen in the human, only human tissues are described and shown in this chapter.

Mons Pubis, Labia Majora and Labia Minora

The mons pubis, labia majora and labia minora all consist of modified skin (see Chapter 18) as given below.

The mons pubis (mons veneris) is skin superimposed on a substantial pad of subcutaneous fat

The mons pubis is the area overlying the symphysis pubis. It is characterized by the presence of unusually oblique hair follicles, which produce the coarse, curly pubic hair common to most races. Underneath the skin is a pad of fat.

The labia majora are posterolateral extensions of the mons pubis on either side of the vaginal introitus

The labia majora are similarly richly endowed with subcutaneous fat and oblique hair follicles (see Fig. 17.1c). There are smooth muscle fibres in the subcutaneous fat.

The accumulation of subcutaneous fat and the development of the oblique hair follicles and pubic hair is hormone dependent and begins with the onset of sexual maturity, usually between the ages of 10 and 13 years.

This area is also rich in apocrine glands and prominent sebaceous glands, both of which mature and become active at the onset of sexual maturity, but eccrine sweat glands, which are present from birth, show no change.

The labia minora are thin flaps of skin devoid of adipose tissue but with abundant blood vessels and elastic fibres

Although hair follicles are absent, there are many sebaceous glands that open directly on to the epidermal surface (see Fig. 17.1d).

The epidermis of both the labia majora and minora becomes pigmented by melanin with the onset of puberty. The outer, lateral aspect of the labia minora is usually more pigmented than the inner medial aspect, and the epidermis has a well-developed rete ridge system.

On the inner aspect, the melanin pigmentation becomes progressively reduced as the vaginal introitus is approached and the keratinized, stratified, squamous epithelium becomes thinner, with flattening of the rete ridges and thinning of the keratin layer.

This keratinized epithelium extends into the vaginal vestibule as far as the hymen, which is a thin fibrous membrane that is rarely completely intact and usually appears as an irregular 'frill' in the lining of the lower vagina, the hymeneal tegmentum. On its exterior (vulval) surface the hymen is covered with the keratinized stratified squamous epithelium, whereas the inner (vaginal) surface is covered with non-keratinized stratified squamous epithelium, rich in glycogen, which is similar to that lining the vagina (Fig. 17.3).

The hymen can be regarded as the junction between the internal and external genitalia.

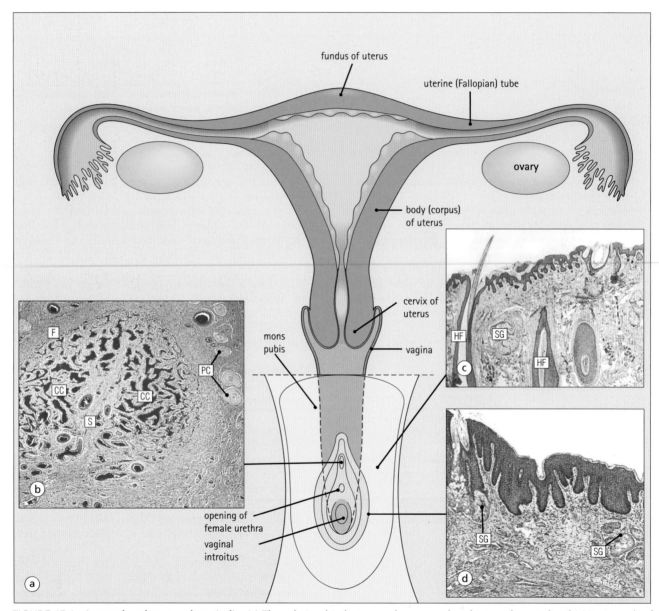

FIGURE 17.1 **Internal and external genitalia.** (a) The relationship between the external and internal genitalia. (b) Micrograph of clitoris; note the two corpora cavernosa (CC), arranged side by side and engorged with blood, the incomplete central septum (S) and the fibrocollagenous sheath (F), outside which are prominent nerve endings (mainly Pacinian touch corpuscles (PC), see also Chapter 18). (c) Micrograph of labia majora. The skin contains many hair follicles (HF), sebaceous glands (SG) and eccrine sweat glands and ducts. (d) Micrograph of labia minora. The skin is devoid of hair follicles but is rich in sebaceous glands (SG), which open directly on to the surface. Note that the dermis is highly vascular.

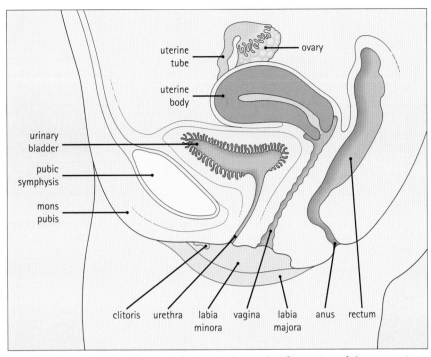

FIGURE 17.2 **Lateral view of female genitalia.** Note the angle of insertion of the uterus into the vagina.

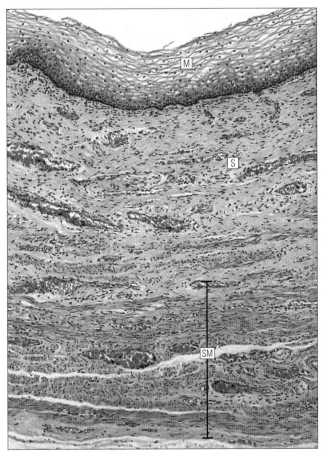

FIGURE 17.3 **Vagina.** Micrograph of vaginal wall showing glycogen-rich stratified squamous epithelial mucosa (M), a highly vascular submucosa (S) and irregular smooth muscle (SM).

Clitoris

The clitoris is located below the mons pubis and is the female equivalent of the penis

The clitoris is composed of two corpora cavernosa of erectile vascular tissue which lie side by side surrounded by a fibrocollagenous sheath; an incomplete central septum partly separates the two corpora (see Fig. 17.1b).

The clitoris is covered by thin epidermis that is devoid of hair follicles, sebaceous glands, eccrine and apocrine glands, but is richly equipped with sensory nerves and a variety of receptors.

Over the superior surface of the clitoris, the skin forms an incomplete hood (the clitoral prepuce), and, on the inferior surface, a thin midline frenulum. At the base of the clitoris, the corpora cavernosa diverge to lie along the pubic rami, where they contain fibres of the ischio-cavernosus muscle.

The clitoris, which is small before puberty, enlarges to a greater or lesser extent with the onset of sexual maturity. During sexual arousal, it becomes engorged in a manner similar to that of the penis.

The urethral meatus opens to the exterior in the midline below the clitoris

On either side of the meatus are the openings of the paraurethral glands (of Skene). These glands are located around the urethra, mainly posteriorly and laterally, and are lined by pseudostratified columnar epithelium.

Vagina

The vagina is a fibromuscular tube extending from the vestibule to the uterus

In the mature female, the vagina is 7–9 cm long, but is capable of both marked distension and elongation (see Fig. 17.1). It forms an angle of more than 90° with the normal anteverted uterus (see Fig. 17.2).

At its inner end, the vagina forms a cuff around the protruding cervix of the uterus, forming anterior, posterior and lateral pouches known as the 'fornices'.

The vagina has four layers (see Fig. 17.3) as follows:
- Stratified squamous epithelial mucosa
- Lamina propria (subepithelial region), which is rich in elastic fibres and thin-walled blood vessels, mainly veins and venules
- A fibromuscular layer containing ill-defined bundles of circularly arranged smooth muscle and a more prominent outer layer of longitudinally arranged smooth muscle
- Adventitia, which is composed of fibrocollagenous tissue containing numerous thick elastic fibres, large blood vessels, nerves and clumps of ganglion cells. At the lower end the fibromuscular layer also contains some skeletal muscle, which is found

mainly around the vaginal introitus in the hymeneal region.

The rich meshwork of elastic fibres in the vaginal wall is responsible for its elasticity and permits the great temporary distension required during parturition. The extensive submucosal plexus of thin-walled blood vessels is thought to permit the diffusion of watery fluid across the epithelium and to contribute to vaginal fluid.

Although structurally a tube, at rest, the vagina is collapsed so that the anterior wall is in contact with the posterior wall, and for much of its length there are shallow longitudinal grooves in the midline of both these walls. In addition, the vaginal mucosa is rugose, being thrown up into a series of closely packed transverse mucosal folds or ridges.

The structure of the vagina varies with age and hormonal activity

Changes occur in the non-keratinizing, stratified squamous epithelium which lines the vagina.

Before puberty the epithelium is thin, a state to which it reverts after the menopause, but during the reproductive years the epithelium responds to the activity of oestrogens and thickens. The basal cells and the distinct parabasal layer show increased mitotic activity, and the more superficial cells increase not only in number but also in size as a result of the accumulation of stored glycogen and some lipid within the cytoplasm.

Glycogen content is maximal at the time of ovulation, and some glycogen-rich surface squames are shed into the vaginal cavity after ovulation, during the secretory phase of the menstrual cycle.

Breakdown of the glycogen by commensal lactobacilli in the vaginal cavity produces lactic acid, resulting in an acid pH. This restricts the vaginal bacterial flora to acid-loving commensals and deters invasion by bacterial pathogens and fungi, such as *Candida albicans*, which is the cause of vaginal 'thrush'.

Bartholin's (vulvovaginal) glands are located around the lower vagina

The Bartholin's glands are composed of acini lined by tall columnar mucus-secreting cells with pale cytoplasm and small basal nuclei.

These glands open into the vagina posterolaterally at the level of the hymeneal remnants through a duct lined by a transitional epithelium with a surface mucin-secreting layer.

Uterus

The uterus is a muscular organ and receives the right and left uterine (fallopian) tubes. It is lined by columnar epithelium and at its lower end, it opens into the vagina.

The uterus can be divided into three parts: the fundus, the body and the cervix (Fig. 17.4). Whereas the fundus and body have the same histological structure (see p. 344), that of the cervix is different.

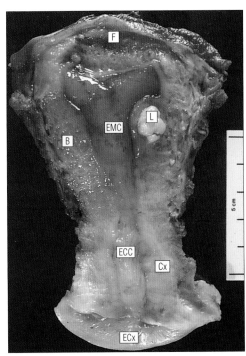

FIGURE 17.4 **Uterus.** Section through the uterus of a 35-year-old woman showing the fundus (F), body (B) and cervix (Cx). Note the endometrial cavity (EMC), endocervical canal (ECC) and ectocervix (ECx). The smooth muscle of the body contains a small tumour, a leiomyoma (L) (see also Fig. 17.11).

Cervix

The cervix is the lower part of the uterus, part of which protrudes into the vagina

The junction between the cervix and the uterine body is the internal os, and at this point the nature of the lining epithelium and the uterine wall changes (Fig. 17.5).

The cervical lumen opens into the vaginal cavity at the external os, where again there is an important change in the nature of the lining epithelium. This zone is the site of many important pathological changes (see Figs 17.8, 17.9).

The cervix is cylindrical and symmetrical, being about 3 cm long and 2–2.5 cm in diameter, but becomes more barrel-shaped after pregnancy and parturition. After childbirth, the external os becomes a transverse slit dividing the distal end of the cervix into anterior and posterior lips, whereas the external os of the nulliparous cervix is circular.

The cervical stroma is important in childbirth

The cervical stroma is composed of smooth muscle fibres embedded in collagen, the proportions of the two components varying with age and parity. Normally, the cervix is firm and rubbery and the cervical lumen is a narrow channel, but the cervix can be dilated under some circumstances, a fact which is used in investigative gynaecological practice to obtain samples of the uterine lining epithelium for histological examination. A measure of the capacity of the cervix for dilatation is the fact that a

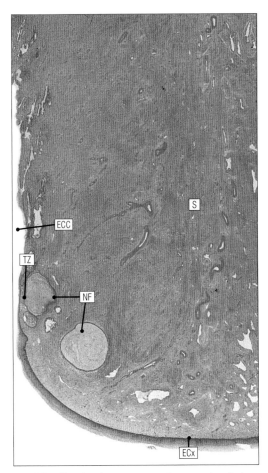

FIGURE 17.5 **Cervix.** Low-power micrograph of the cervix. The stroma (S) is composed of smooth muscle fibres embedded in collagen, the proportions of muscle and fibrous tissue varying according to age and parity; blood and lymphatic vessels are prominent and numerous. The ectocervix (ECx) is covered with stratified squamous epithelium, and the endocervical canal (ECC) is lined by tall columnar epithelium. The junction between the squamous and columnar epithelium is located in the region of the external os. In this example there is a transformation zone (TZ) (see p. 343) of squamous epithelium, which has extended into the endocervical canal; note the Nabothian follicles (NF) (see Fig. 17.8c).

cervical lumen, which is normally a narrow canal incapable of taking a pencil, becomes, at childbirth, capable of allowing the passage of a baby. Furthermore, after delivery, the cervix reverts to normal in a very short time.

This capacity depends on radical alterations in the nature of the cervical stroma, attended by a change in texture ('cervical softening').

The Epithelial Content of the Cervix

The external surface of the part of the cervix that protrudes into the vagina is the ectocervix and the lining of the lumen is the endocervix.

The ectocervix is covered by epithelium continuous with that of the vagina at the vaginal fornices

Like vaginal squamous epithelium, the ectocervical epithelium is non-keratinizing, stratified, squamous and rich

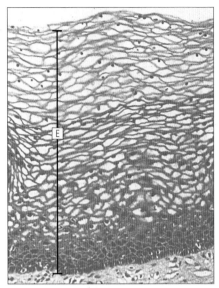

FIGURE 17.6 **Ectocervix.** Stratified squamous epithelium (E) covers the ectocervix. Like those of the vagina, the cells are rich in glycogen during the period of sexual maturity.

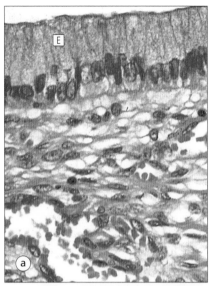

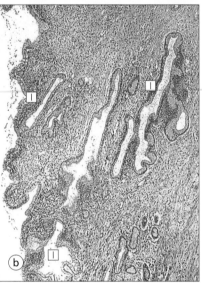

FIGURE 17.7 **Endocervix.** (a) The endocervical canal is lined by a single layer of tall columnar mucus-secreting epithelium (E). (b) Numerous deep invaginations (I) of the mucus-secreting epithelium extend into the cervical stroma and greatly increase the surface for mucus production.

ADVANCED CONCEPT
THE CERVIX IN CHILDBIRTH

The normally firm and rubbery uterine cervix with a narrow lumen of less than 1 cm in diameter dilates to approximately 10 cm during labour. This is achieved by softening and increased elasticity in the cervical stroma. The changes in the cervix in late pregnancy are complex.

In the glycosaminoglycan matrix, hyaluronic acid concentration between collagen fibres increases, drawing in water molecules, which increase the bulk and softness of the matrix and separate the collagen fibres of the cervical stroma. Dermatan sulfate concentration decreases, leading to weakening of the dermatan sulfate bridges holding adjacent collagen and elastin fibres together. This further contributes to the separation of collagen fibres.

There are also changes in collagen and elastin fibres. Type I and type II collagen fibres become separated from each other, lose their strong parallel alignment and become shorter. The separation of collagen fibres, their rearrangement from a compact parallel pattern to a more haphazard arrangement, and the shortening of individual fibres all lead to a reduction in tensile strength and a decreased resistance to the pressure exerted by the presenting part of the fetus being expelled from the uterine body. Similar changes probably occur in elastin fibres.

The endocervical canal runs between the uterine and vaginal cavities

The canal is lined by a single layer of tall columnar mucus-secreting epithelium, the endocervical epithelium (Fig. 17.7a).

Longitudinal or transverse histological sections of the cervix have given the impression that there are glandular structures (endocervical mucous glands) extending into the underlying stroma. Three-dimensional studies, however, indicate that the structures are in fact deep, slit-like invaginations of the surface epithelium, with blind-ended tubules arising from the clefts (Fig. 17.7b). Thus, there is a large surface area for the production of cervical mucus, which fills the endocervical canal. Before puberty and after the menopause, the amount of cervical mucus is greatly reduced.

in glycogen in the sexually mature period (Fig. 17.6). It undergoes cyclical changes during the menstrual cycle under the influence of oestrogens and progesterone.

Before menarche and after menopause, the epithelium is much thinner, with fewer layers and smaller cells containing less glycogen.

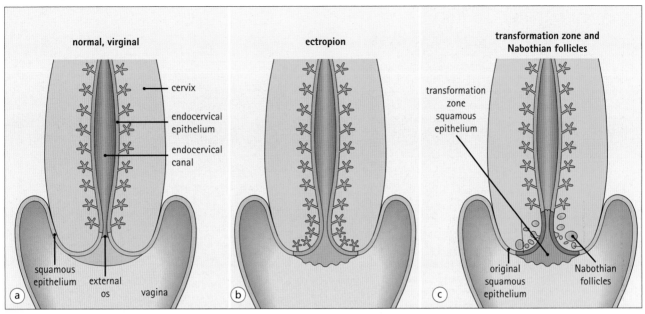

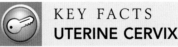

FIGURE 17.8 Squamous/columnar junction of the cervix. The mobility of the squamous/columnar junction, the development of ectropion and the formation of the transformation zone. (a) The squamous/columnar junction is originally situated in the region of the external os. (b) At puberty, the endocervical epithelium extends distally into the acid environment of the vagina and forms an ectropion. (c) A transformation zone forms as squamous epithelium regrows over the ectropion. The openings of the crypts may be obliterated in the process, resulting in the formation of mucus-filled Nabothian follicles (see Fig. 17.5).

As well as contributing to vaginal lubrication during sexual intercourse, the mucin in the endocervical canal acts as a protective barrier, preventing bacterial ascent into the endometrial cavity.

Movement of endocervical mucus into the vaginal canal is facilitated by a few ciliated columnar epithelial cells scattered among the mucus-secreting endocervical cells, particularly at the upper end of the canal, close to the junction with the endometrium.

Both the mucin-secreting and ciliated cells have fine microvilli, which are only visible ultrastructurally.

The columnar epithelium of the endocervical canal and the squamous epithelium of the ectocervix meet at the squamocolumnar junction of the cervix

This is the most likely area of the cervical epithelium to be affected by disease.

The original squamous columnar junction is usually located in the region of the external os, but its precise location at birth is influenced by maternal hormone exposure in utero.

At about puberty, hormonal influences lead to extension of the columnar epithelium on to the ectocervix, forming an ectropion or cervical erosion (Fig. 17.8), which is augmented by a first pregnancy, particularly when this occurs shortly after menarche.

Before puberty, the pH of the vagina and cervix is alkaline, but afterwards, bacterial breakdown of the glycogen in the vaginal and cervical squamous epithelium renders an acidic environment, with a pH of about 3.

Exposure of the sensitive columnar epithelium of the ectropion to the postpubertal acidic environment of the vagina induces squamous metaplasia and a transformation zone between the endocervical columnar epithelium and the ectocervical squamous epithelium.

Thus, the squamous columnar junction is of variable size but its site always approximates to the external os. In older women, it may retreat into the endocervical canal.

The transformation zone is composed of new squamous epithelium in an area previously occupied by columnar epithelium.

One almost invariable consequence of squamous metaplasia near the external os is that the openings of some of the deep crypts of previously everted endocervical mucous glands become obliterated so that mucin produced deep in the crypts cannot be excreted into the endocervical lumen or vagina. Instead, it accumulates within the blocked clefts and produces spherical cystic masses of inspissated mucus lined by flattened endocervical mucus-secreting epithelium; these are called **Nabothian follicles**. Other consequences of this constant change of epithelium include the development of abnormal epithelium, which may progress to cancer.

KEY FACTS
UTERINE CERVIX

- Lower part of uterus, protruding into vagina
- Canal is lined by tall columnar mucin-secreting epithelium
- Surface protruding into vagina is covered by stratified squamous epithelium
- Squamo-columnar junction is an important site of disease (transformation zone)
- Has a stroma of smooth muscle fibres embedded in collagen; proportions of each vary according to age and parity

CLINICAL EXAMPLE
CARCINOMA OF THE CERVIX

The transformation zone of the cervical epithelium is the most common site of origin of carcinoma of the cervix. Current research suggests that the vast majority of cervical cancers are caused by infection with 'high-risk' cancer inducing human papillomaviruses (HPV). The development of cervical cancer is usually preceded by histological abnormality of the squamous epithelial cells in this transformation zone. The abnormal cells:

- Lose their regular stratified pattern
- Have a high nucleus-to-cytoplasm ratio
- Show variation in shape and size and increased mitotic activity.

These cytological features are characteristic of malignant tumour cells and are usually associated with evidence of invasive behaviour. However, in the cervix the cytological changes of malignancy may be present for years before the abnormal epithelium begins to invade the underlying stroma; they are referred to as carcinoma-in-situ or cervical intraepithelial neoplasia (CIN) (Fig. 17.9a).

Eventually, the abnormal epithelial cells breach the basement membrane and invade the cervical stroma (Fig. 17.9b), gaining access to blood and lymphatic vessels, which are their route for spread to other sites, such as the lymph nodes around the iliac arteries. This is invasive carcinoma. Early diagnosis of CIN can be obtained by cervical cytology (cervical smear); cells are scraped from the epithelial surface in the region of the cervical os and examined microscopically for abnormal cells. Abnormal areas can then be treated, usually by surgical removal, thus preventing the future development of invasive cancer.

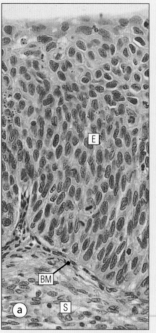
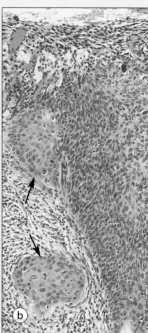

FIGURE 17.9 **Carcinoma of the cervix.** (a) The cervical epithelial cells (E) have lost their regular stratified pattern, have high nucleus to cytoplasm ratios and show increased mitotic activity (compare with Fig. 17.6). As the basement membrane (BM) between the epithelium and underlying stroma (S) is intact, this is carcinoma-in-situ or cervical intraepithelial neoplasia. (b) Some of the abnormal epithelial cells have breached the basement membrane and invaded the cervical stroma (arrows); this is invasive carcinoma.

Uterine Body

The body and fundus of the uterus have thick walls composed of smooth muscle (myometrium)

The myometrial smooth muscle is arranged into three ill-defined layers.

Myometrium is hormone sensitive and undergoes both hypertrophy (an increase in cell size) and hyperplasia (an increase in cell numbers) during pregnancy (Fig. 17.10), progressively returning to its normal size (involution) in the weeks after delivery.

Within the myometrium are prominent blood vessels, both arterial and venous, which undergo marked dilation and thickening of their walls during pregnancy.

With cessation of hormonal stimulation after the menopause, the myometrial cells atrophy and the uterus shrinks. The fibrocollagenous tissue between the muscle bundles, which is comparatively insignificant when the myometrial smooth muscle is prominent during sexual maturity, then becomes obvious.

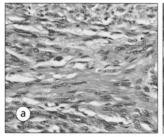
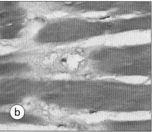

FIGURE 17.10 **Myometrium.** (a) Normal myometrium from a non-pregnant 35-year-old woman. The muscle cells are small and tightly packed. (b) Myometrium from a 28-year-old woman in the 8th month of pregnancy, photographed at the same magnification as (a). Note the enormous increase in size of the individual muscle fibres, due almost entirely to an increase in cytoplasm. This is an example of physiological hypertrophy and is a common response of muscle cells to an increased workload, in this case the need to increase the propulsive power of the uterus to expel the fetus at childbirth.

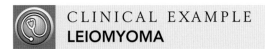
The myometrium is the site of one of the most common benign tumours, the leiomyoma or fibroid (Fig. 17.11, see also Fig. 17.4), which is derived from smooth muscle of the uterine wall.

Like normal uterine smooth muscle, leiomyomas are hormone dependent and progressively enlarge until the menopause, after which time they regress.

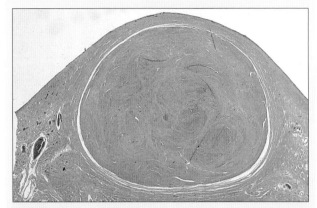

FIGURE 17.11 **Leiomyoma.** Micrograph of a typical small leiomyoma.

The body of the uterus is lined by the endometrium, which is composed of glands and supporting stroma

Before puberty, the endometrium is simple and composed of low cuboidal epithelium supported by a scanty spindle-celled stroma. Downgrowths of epithelium into the stroma produce a small number of rudimentary tubular glands.

Between menarche (the first menstrual period) and menopause, the endometrium can be differentiated into two layers, a deep basal layer at the junction with the myometrium, and a superficial functional layer lining the lumen. It is the functional layer that is hormone responsive and undergoes the monthly cycle of proliferation, secretion, necrosis and shedding. The endometrium is sensitive to the fluctuating levels of oestrogen and progesterone secreted by the ovary, and the changes are known as the **menstrual cycle**. The relationships between the histological changes in the endometrium and the ovarian and pituitary hormone secretions are discussed below and illustrated in Figure 17.24, p. 355.

If fertilization and successful implantation of an ovum occur, the endometrium remains unshed and forms the decidua (see p. 360).

The basal layer, which is not shed at menstruation, provides a cellular reserve from which a new functional layer develops after menstrual shedding. The endometrium does not respond evenly to ovarian hormonal stimulation: functional endometrium in the lower segment close to the junction with the cervix, and patches around the entrances of the uterine tubes, may show little proliferative or secretory activity, and often

resembles the basal layer. As menopause approaches, more and more of the endometrium may fail to respond fully to the hormonal stimulus.

At menopause, when hormonal stimulation ceases, the endometrium reverts to the simple prepubertal pattern, although the tubular downgrowths may undergo cystic distension and the stroma may become compact (atrophic cystic endometrium).

Uterine Tubes

The uterine (fallopian) tubes convey ova from the ovary to the lumen of the body of the uterus (endometrial cavity)

They are also the site of fertilization of the ovum by spermatozoa. After fertilization, the tube transmits the fertilized ovum to the endometrial cavity where implantation can take place.

Each uterine tube is 10–12 cm long and extends from a dilated open end close to the ovary to a narrow portion which passes through the myometrial wall of the uterus before opening into the uterine cavity. There are four recognizable tubal segments (Fig. 17.12), each differing histologically, particularly in their proportions of muscle and epithelium and the degree of convolution of their epithelium.

The infundibulum is surrounded by a fringe of epithelial-coated **fimbriae**, some of which may become adherent to the nearby ovary. Medial to the infundibulum is a thin-walled zone called the 'ampulla', where ovum fertilization usually takes place.

The ampulla leads into a narrower, thick-walled segment called the 'isthmus'. In turn, the isthmus is continuous with the short intramural segment, which opens into the uterus.

The uterine tube is essentially a muscular tube lined by specialized epithelium, which is variably folded and plicate, differing in appearance at different sites.

The smooth muscle wall of the uterine tube is composed of two layers

The inner layer of smooth muscle in the uterine tube appears to be circular in histology sections and the outer layer appears to be longitudinal. In reality, these layers are almost certainly arranged as a tight spiral (circular) and a loose spiral (longitudinal), as seen in the ureter (see Fig. 15.34). Close to the uterus, a third muscular layer is also present.

Internal to the muscle layers, a delicate vascular lamina propria supports the tubal epithelial lining.

There are two types of epithelial cell lining the uterine tube: ciliated cells and secretory cells

The ciliated cells are particularly numerous near the ovarian end of the tube where they form the majority population (about 60–80%), but close to the uterus they are the minority population (about 25%) and secretory cells predominate (see Fig. 17.12).

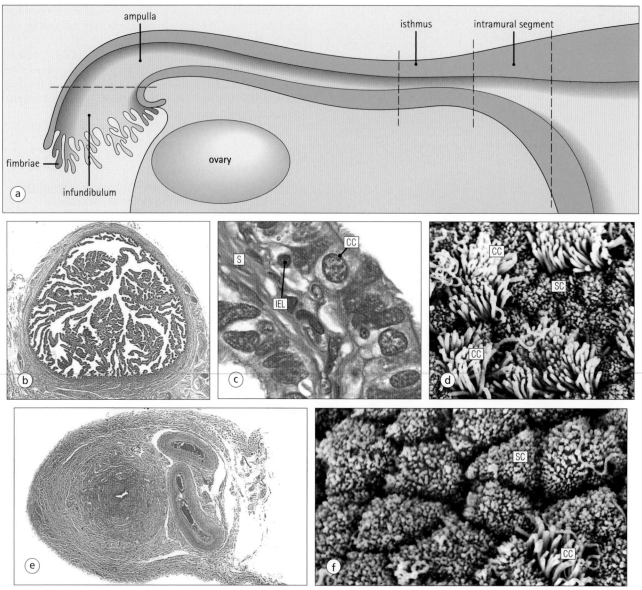

FIGURE 17.12 **Uterine (fallopian) tube.** (a) The uterine tube, ovary and uterus. (b) Low-power micrograph of the ampulla, showing its thin muscular wall and large lumen with markedly papillary mucosa. (c) High-power micrograph of tubal epithelium at the ampulla, showing a high proportion of ciliated cells (CC), thin delicate stroma (S) and an occasional intraepithelial lymphocyte (IEL). (d) Scanning electron micrograph of tubal mucosa at the ampulla, showing numerous ciliated cells (CC) and relatively scanty secretory cells (SC). (e) Low-power micrograph of the isthmus, showing its thick muscular wall and small lumen with simpler, non-papillary mucosa. (f) Scanning electron micrograph of tubal mucosa at the isthmus, showing few ciliated cells (CC) and many secretory cells (SC) with abundant microvilli.

Two other cell types have been described in the tubal epithelium: the peg cell and the reserve basal cell. The peg cell is currently considered to be an effete secretory cell and the reserve basal cells have been shown to be intraepithelial cells of the lymphoid series.

The ciliated tubal epithelial cell is a columnar cell, the height of which varies during the menstrual cycle

The ciliated tubal epithelial cell is at its tallest and most ciliated at about the time of ovulation, after which it progressively shortens and loses some cilia until menstruation. The decrease in height and ciliation is presumably a progesterone effect, as similar changes occur and

persist throughout the duration of a pregnancy. With the resumption of oestrogen secretion after menstruation or delivery, the cells again lengthen and become more ciliated.

The ciliated cells may be responsible for movement of the ovum through the infundibulum and ampulla, though tubal peristalsis probably plays a greater role. They may also have a role in propelling the spermatozoa in the opposite direction.

The secretory cells are columnar cells with surface microvilli

The secretory cells produce a watery tubal fluid (see Fig. 17.12), which is rich in potassium and chloride ions

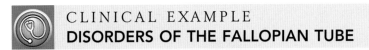

CLINICAL EXAMPLE
DISORDERS OF THE FALLOPIAN TUBE

An important disorder of the uterine tube is tubal ectopic pregnancy.

Tubal Ectopic Pregnancy

Occasionally, the fertilized ovum is held up in the tubal lumen and implants in the wall of the uterine tube, producing a tubal ectopic pregnancy.

Partial development of the embryo and placenta proceeds for a time, but the thin-walled uterine tube is an unsatisfactory site for implantation and the embryo cannot survive. The vascular placental tissues penetrate into the thin tubal wall (Fig. 17.13a) and often perforate through, producing brisk bleeding into the lumen of the tube and into the peritoneal cavity. This produces lower abdominal pain and, if the blood loss is severe, shock.

Acute and Chronic Salpingitis

Bacterial infection of the tube (e.g. by *Gonococcus*) produces acute inflammation in the papillary folds and muscular wall and pus formation in the lumen (Fig. 17.13b).

Such infections may persist, with abscess formation and chronic inflammation, or may heal with scarring, leaving a blocked or distorted lumen, which may obstruct the passage of the fertilized ovum and predispose to tubal ectopic pregnancy or infertility.

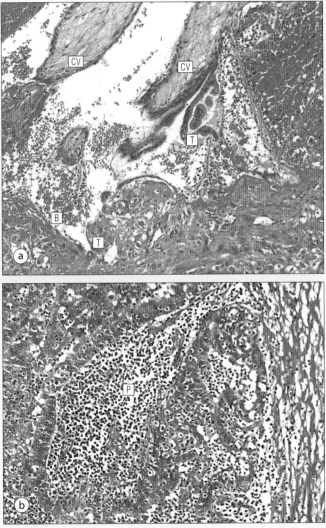

FIGURE 17.13 **Disorders of the fallopian tube.** (a) Micrograph of a tubal ectopic pregnancy; chorionic villi (CV) are developing in the lumen of the tube, and trophoblast (T) is eroding into the tubal wall, producing bleeding (B). (b) In this section from an infected tube, the papillary folds and muscular wall are infiltrated by neutrophils and there is pus (P) in the lumen.

and also contains normal serum proteins, including immunoglobulins.

The tubal fluid is assumed to have a nutritive function for spermatozoa and fertilized or unfertilized ova.

Ovary

Introduction

The paired ovaries are small, flattened ovoid organs lying in the right and left lateral pelvic cavities. They have two major functions:
- They are the source of mature ova
- They are endocrine organs, producing the steroid hormones that prepare the endometrium for conception and maintain pregnancy should fertilization occur.

The surface of the ovary is covered by a single layer of epithelium

This surface layer is usually cuboidal or low columnar in type (see Fig. 17.16), but commonly flattens with increasing age and when the ovary is enlarged.

The epithelium is continuous with the pelvic peritoneum at the hilum of the ovary (though the cells differ structurally from the peritoneal mesothelial cells). It is called the 'germinal epithelium', which is, however, a misnomer because the epithelial cells are not the source of the female gametes.

The surface epithelial cells have prominent surface microvilli and occasional cilia; mitochondria are abundant and small pinocytotic vesicles are associated with the base of some microvilli.

The ovarian surface is usually irregularly fissured, and the fissures are also lined by the surface epithelium. The necks of the fissures may seal over, leaving islands of surface epithelium within the ovarian cortex. Fluid secretion by the cells then converts these islands into cysts (germinal inclusion cysts), which are common.

The surface epithelial cells show little alteration during the menstrual cycle but usually lengthen during pregnancy.

A substantial basement membrane (the tunica alba-ginea) separates the surface cells from the underlying ovarian tissue in the mature ovary.

The ovary can be divided into three components: hilum, medulla and outer cortex

The ovarian **hilum** is the route whereby blood vessels, lymphatics and nerves enter and leave the ovary, and is continuous with the medulla, the central core of the ovary (Fig. 17.14).

In addition to the vessels and lymphatics, the medulla and hilum also contain vestigial remnants of the embryonic Wolffian duct and clusters of hilus or hilar cells.

The Wolffian duct remnants persist as irregular tubules lined by flat or cuboidal epithelium (rete ovarii).

The hilus cells are histologically identical to the interstitial (Leydig) cells of the testis (see Fig. 16.10) and are

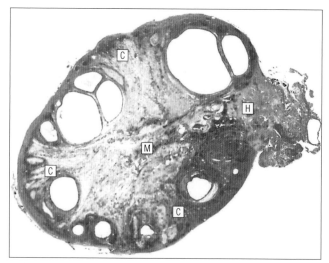

FIGURE 17.14 **Ovary.** Micrograph of ovary showing the hilum (H), medulla (M) and cortex (C). Gamete formation and maturation occur in the cortex and are responsible for the cystic spaces seen here.

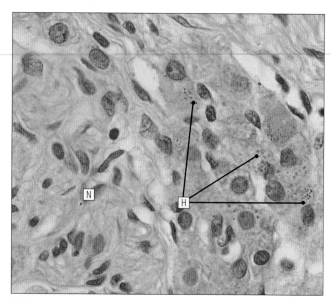

FIGURE 17.15 **Ovary – hilus cells.** A clump of hilus cells (H) is shown adjacent to a nerve (N) in the ovarian hilum, a characteristic location. These cells have ill-defined borders, foamy eosinophilic cytoplasm and granules of brown lipofuscin pigment.

round or oval, with eosinophilic granular or foamy cytoplasm containing brown lipofuscin-like pigment. They are densely packed (Fig. 17.15).

Occasional hilus cells contain Reinke's crystalloids (see p. 326) and some contain round eosinophilic hyaline bodies as well. The small clumps of hilus cells are often found close to nerves and blood vessels.

The ovarian **medulla** often contains clusters of stromal cells identical to those occupying the bulk of the cortex.

The ovarian **cortex** has two components:
- A supporting stroma
- Gamete-producing structures and their derivatives.

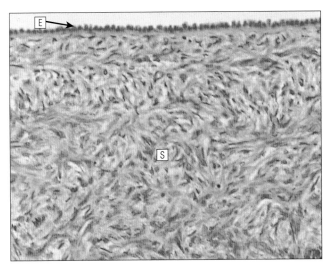

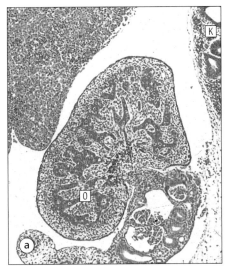

FIGURE 17.16 **Ovarian cortical stroma and surface epithelium.** Note the whorled pattern of the spindle-shaped ovarian stromal cells (S) and the single layer of cuboidal surface epithelial cells (E).

The proportions and appearances of these two components in any individual ovary will depend on both age and hormonal stimulation.

The cortical stroma is composed of closely packed, spindle-shaped fibroblast-like cells

The stromal cells are arranged haphazardly or in a variable whorled pattern (Fig. 17.16). The cytoplasm of these cells is rich in ribosomes and microfilaments; mitochondria are also numerous and tend to collect around the nucleus. Micropinocytotic vesicles are found in association with the cell surface, and there are small numbers of lipid droplets.

Reticulin and collagen fibres between the stromal cells are particularly prominent in the outer part of the cortex. Progressive collagenization of this area begins early in reproductive life and becomes more marked with time, so that by menopause it is almost universal.

The cellularity of the ovarian stroma, and the amount of lipid the cells contain, is dependent on hormonal stimulation. An increase in lipid accumulation in the stromal cells is called **luteinization of stromal cells** and is particularly prominent during pregnancy.

The ovarian stroma has three main functions:
- It provides structural support for the developing ova
- It gives rise to the theca interna and theca externa around the developing follicle (see Fig. 17.19b)
- It secretes steroid hormones.

Although it is probable that all stromal cells have the potential to produce steroid hormones under appropriate circumstances, three types of steroid-secreting stromal cells are recognized:
- The cells that surround the follicle (i.e. theca layers, see Figs 17.19b, 17.21b)
- The scattered lipid-rich luteinized stromal cells
- A population of stromal cells, called enzymically active stromal cells (EASC), which exhibit marked oxidative and other enzyme activity.

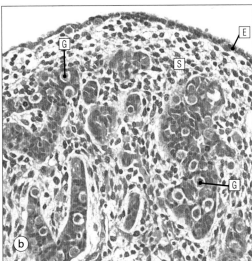

FIGURE 17.17 **Ovary in embryo.** (a) The developing ovary (O) in a 9-week-old embryo is shown close to the developing kidney (K). (b) At this stage of development, the columns of primordial germ cells (G) are embedded in a mesenchymal stroma (S) covered by a layer of cuboidal surface cells (E).

EASC are particularly numerous in postmenopausal women. They are disseminated in clusters in the cortex and medulla, and have been shown to secrete testosterone and other androgenic steroids.

Gamete Production and Maturation in the Ovary

The number of gametes in an ovary, and their appearance, varies with age. Embryologically, they are derived from primordial germ cells, which develop in the yolk sac and migrate to the developing ovary (Fig. 17.17).

Mitotic divisions of primordial germ cells produce small oogonia

Oogonia multiply by further mitotic divisions within the developing fetal ovary.

During the second trimester of pregnancy, the mitotic divisions cease, and the large numbers of oogonia increase in size and are called **primary oocytes**. At this

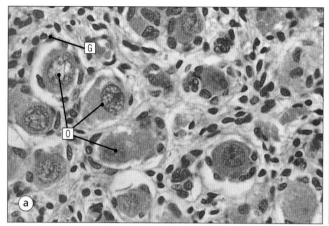
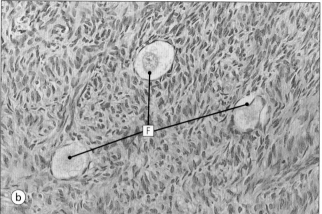

FIGURE 17.18 **Primordial follicles.** (a) Ovarian cortex from a 32-week-old fetus; it is packed with primordial follicles, each comprising a large primary oocyte (O) with a single surrounding layer of flat granulosa cells (G). Most primordial follicles undergo continuing atresia throughout infancy, childhood and the years of sexual maturity. (b) Ovarian cortex from a 25-year-old woman showing persistence of some primordial follicles (F).

stage, they number several million in each ovary, but many degenerate, so that by birth, each ovary contains about 1 million oocytes.

The oocytes continue to degenerate throughout life and at the onset of puberty oocyte numbers are reduced to a quarter of a million or so.

The primary oocytes that survive degeneration in the second trimester enter the prophase of the first meiotic division

Primary oocytes remain in this phase for many years and acquire a single layer of flat surrounding cells (granulosa cells); these structures are called **primordial follicles** (Fig. 17.18a). At birth, the ovarian cortex is packed with large numbers of primordial follicles embedded in the cellular cortical stroma, and some of these persist in the ovarian cortex throughout the period of sexual maturity (Fig. 17.18b).

Some primordial follicles develop further at puberty to produce primary follicles

At puberty, the cyclical secretion of follicle-stimulating hormone (FSH) from the pituitary stimulates the further development of a small number (probably 30–40) of the primordial follicles.

The first step is enlargement of the oocyte, which is associated with an increase in size of the surrounding granulosa cells, so that they become cuboidal or columnar; at this stage the structure is called a **unilaminar primary follicle**.

Continuing FSH secretion then induces the granulosa cells to divide to produce a multilayered surround to the enlarging oocyte, and a distinct glycoprotein layer of eosinophilic (PAS-positive) material forms between the oocyte and these cells (Fig. 17.19a). This layer is called the **zona pellucida** and is traversed by microvilli protruding outwards from the oocyte and by thin cytoplasmic processes from the inner layer of the granulosa cells. The follicle is now known as a **multilaminar primary follicle**.

Meanwhile, ovarian stromal cells come to lie in roughly concentric layers around the enlarging follicle to form a capsule-like arrangement. At about this stage, most follicles then degenerate by a process called **atresia** (see p. 353).

A small number of follicles, however, continue to develop, although atretic degeneration still occurs at all subsequent stages; thus only a few follicles reach full maturity.

Continuing maturation leads to the formation of secondary follicles

With continuing follicle maturation, the granulosa cell layers increase in thickness and the outer capsule of ovarian stromal cells begins to differentiate into two layers.

The inner layer of stromal cells (the **theca interna**) increases in size as the cells develop prominent smooth endoplasmic reticulum and mitochondria with tubular cristae (features characteristic of cells producing steroid hormones) and begin to secrete oestrogens; this layer also acquires a prominent capillary network.

The outer layer of stromal cells (the **theca externa**) remains small and compact and has no known secretory function. The follicle is now known as a **secondary follicle** (Fig. 17.19b).

The fully mature follicle is called the tertiary (Graafian) follicle and is ready for ovulation

A small fluid-filled split appears in the layers of granulosa cells surrounding the oocyte. It enlarges to form a fluid-filled cavity (the **antrum**) that progressively increases in size; the fluid is slightly viscous and is rich in hyaluronic acid.

The oocyte lies to one side of the by now large follicle, and is separated from the follicle fluid by a coat of granulosa cells called the 'cumulus oophorus'. The follicle is now known as a **tertiary** or **Graafian follicle** and is ripe for ovulation (Fig. 17.20).

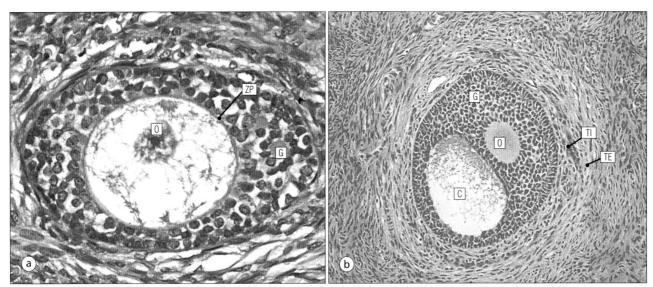

FIGURE 17.19 **Follicle maturation.** (a) Micrograph of a multilaminar primary follicle. The granulosa cells (G) have divided to produce a layer 3–5 cells thick, and the pink-staining zona pellucida (ZP) becomes apparent between the oocyte (O) and the granulosa cells. (b) Further maturation to a secondary follicle occurs by continuing proliferation of the granulosa cells (G), the appearance of a fluid-filled cavity (C) within them, and condensation of stromal cells around the follicle to form an inner layer of plump cells (theca interna, TI) and an outer layer of smaller spindle-shaped cells (theca externa, TE). O, oocyte.

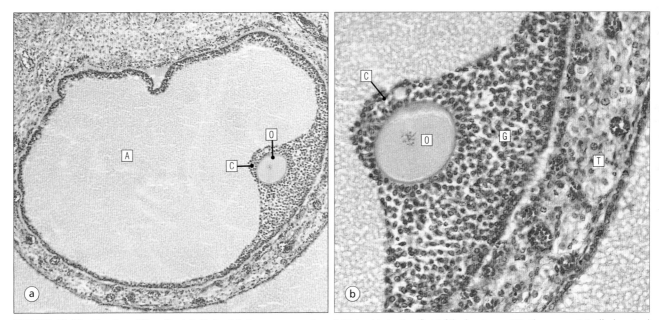

FIGURE 17.20 **Tertiary (Graafian) follicle.** (a) A mature tertiary follicle. Note the fluid-filled antrum (A), the eccentrically located oocyte (O) and the cumulus oophorus (C) of granulosa cells around the oocyte. (b) Micrograph of the oocyte (O), cumulus oophorus (C) and granulosa cell layer (G) at higher magnification. The theca layer (T) is highly vascular.

The first stage of meiosis is then completed to produce a haploid gamete and a small polar body, which can sometimes be seen attached to the oocyte (now called a **secondary oocyte**). Follicle maturation takes approximately 15 days, by which time the mature follicle is ready for ovulation.

The theca interna secretes increasing amounts of oestrogen to stimulate proliferation of the endometrium (see Fig. 17.24) in preparation for possible implantation of a fertilized ovum.

Ovulation is stimulated by luteinizing hormone from the anterior pituitary

At ovulation, the Graafian follicle is usually so large that it distorts the surface of the ovary; it appears to the naked eye as a small cystic mass bulging from the ovarian surface, covered only by a thin layer of germinal epithelium and membrane, and an attenuated zone of cortical stromal cells.

The stimulus to ovulation is probably a surge of luteinizing hormone (LH) from the pituitary, which induces completion of the first stage of meiosis, and probably leads to disruption of the structure of the follicle as well.

Before leaving the ovary, the oocyte may break free from its attachment in the follicle wall and float freely in the follicle fluid, surrounded by an irregular ring of granulosa cells, which remain attached to it (the **corona radiata**).

The area of follicle wall in intimate contact with the germinal epithelial covering of the ovarian surface breaks down and the follicular fluid containing the oocyte is disgorged into the peritoneal cavity.

The oocyte with its surrounding corona radiata is then drawn into the infundibular opening of the uterine tube, possibly by the waving action of the fimbriae at the infundibular margin.

With rupture of the follicle, there is bleeding from the decompressed lining (particularly from the highly vascular theca interna), filling the follicle antrum with blood clot. Small quantities of blood may pass into the peritoneal cavity.

The disgorgement of blood and follicular fluid on to the pain-sensitive peritoneal surface is thought to be responsible for the transient midcycle (days 14–16) lower abdominal pain experienced by some women.

The ruptured follicle becomes a corpus luteum after ovulation

After ovulation the remains of the follicle change under the influence of continuing LH secretion by the pituitary gland. The clot-filled lumen of the follicle (corpus haemorrhagicum) undergoes progressive organization and fibrosis over the following weeks.

The main changes occur in the granulosa and theca interna cells. In these cells, LH induces changes (luteinization) that convert the follicle remnants into an endocrine structure known as the corpus luteum.

Thus, the granulosa cells enlarge, acquire a substantial network of smooth endoplasmic reticulum, become distended with lipid (granulosa lutein cells) and secrete progesterone (Fig. 17.21).

Some of the theca interna cells, already well equipped with smooth endoplasmic reticulum, also accumulate lipid and persist as theca lutein or paralutein cells, continuing to secrete oestrogens as they did before ovulation. However, many theca interna and externa cells involute, becoming small, compact and spindle-shaped.

The formed corpus luteum therefore has a central area of fibrosing blood clot surrounded by a broad zone of yellow, lipid-rich granulosa lutein cells, with scantier collections of smaller theca lutein cells scattered around the periphery.

Fibrous septa partly separate the granulosa lutein masses, and clusters of theca lutein cells are particularly prominent in the regions of these septa (Fig. 17.21b).

At its maximum size (usually on about day 20 of the menstrual cycle), a corpus luteum is commonly an ovoid structure up to 2 cm long and 1.5 cm wide; it then begins to involute, unless the cycle has been interrupted by fertilization of the oocyte in the uterine tube (see p. 357).

The corpus luteum changes into a corpus albicans

Normally, involution of the corpus luteum begins by a decrease in the size of the granulosa and theca lutein

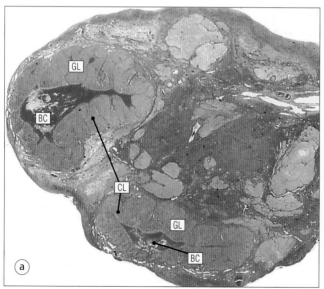
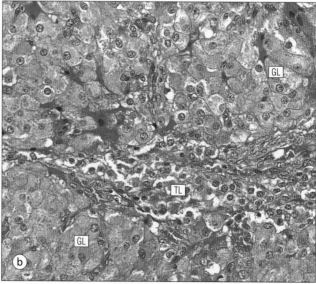

FIGURE 17.21 **Corpus luteum.** (a) Micrograph of an ovary containing two corpora lutea (CL), two follicles having ripened to maturity in the same ovary in the same menstrual cycle, providing the potential for non-identical twins. Each corpus luteum shows central blood clot (BC) surrounded by a thick layer of lipid-rich granulosa lutein cells (GL); (b) Micrograph of the large pale-staining granulosa lutein (GL) cells and the small compact theca lutein (TL) cells, which are mainly concentrated along fibrous septa at the periphery of the corpus luteum.

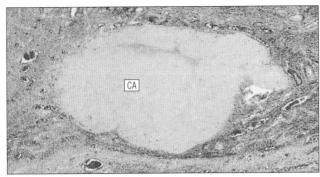

FIGURE 17.22 **Corpus albicans.** The corpus luteum involutes to form a shrunken mass of collagenous tissue, the corpus albicans (CA), which maintains approximately the shape of the original corpus luteum. Incomplete involution of a corpus luteum may produce a luteal cyst, which is a cyst lined by attenuated granulosa and theca lutein cells.

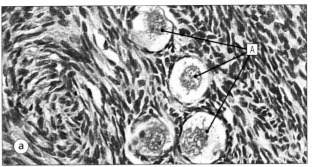

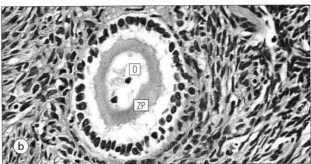

FIGURE 17.23 **Follicle atresia.** (a) Micrograph showing a cluster of four primordial follicles, of which three are undergoing atresia (A); they will leave no scar. (b) Micrograph showing a primary follicle undergoing atresia which is mainly manifest by a degenerate oocyte (O) and a collapsing zona pellucida (ZP).

cells, with the appearance of vacuoles in their previously uniformly eosinophilic cytoplasm. Progression of this change leads to reduced secretion of progesterone and oestrogen by the two cell types.

At the same time, the spindle-shaped cells of the theca externa and the spindle-shaped fibroblasts forming the fibrous septa rapidly produce collagen, which replaces the involuting lutein cells.

By about the 26th day of the cycle the hormone-secreting cells are completely eliminated and the progesterone and oestrogen levels fall dramatically, with a significant impact on the endometrium (see Fig. 17.24g).

The end-result of corpus luteum involution is a small ovoid mass of relatively acellular (hyaline) collagenous tissue with the general physical configuration of the corpus luteum. This structure is a corpus albicans (Fig. 17.22) and remains in the ovary, decreasing in size with the passing years but never disappearing.

Most female gametes do not grow to maturity, but undergo atresia

Of the vast number of oogonia formed in utero by mitotic division of primitive germ cells, only about 500–600 reach full maturity and ovulation during a woman's reproductive life. Some fail to develop, and others undergo a process called **atresia**.

Atresia can occur at any stage but is most marked during intrauterine life, when primary oocyte numbers are enormously reduced. As atresia continues throughout infancy, childhood and the reproductive years, degenerating primary and secondary oocytes can be seen on histological examination of any ovary.

Atresia can supervene at any stage of follicle development. When the follicles are small (primary and secondary stages), the components of the follicle undergo cellular degeneration and complete resorption, leaving no scar (Fig. 17.23a). However, larger follicles (tertiary stage) with a substantial cellular component undergo gradual disintegration and replacement by hyaline fibrous tissue. The oocyte disintegrates and the granulosa cells

separate and degenerate, whereas the zona pellucida collapses and wrinkles but remains identifiable.

Often a glassy membrane develops between the degenerating granulosa cells and the outer thecal layers; this may proliferate transiently, perhaps providing the source of the fibrocollagenous fibrous tissue that ultimately replaces the atretic follicle.

When a large follicle has undergone atresia, a substantial collagenous scar may form, a **corpus fibrosum**, which resembles a small corpus albicans in shape.

Menstrual Cycle

Introduction

During the reproductive years, the histological appearance of the superficial functional zone of the endometrial lining varies from day to day on a regular cyclical basis, the **menstrual cycle**.

A complete cycle normally takes about 28 days, but there is considerable variation between women and also some variation in individual women at different times. For example, the first few cycles after menarche and after a pregnancy tend to be irregular, and increasing irregularity of the cycle is common prior to menopause.

At the end of every cycle the superficial functional endometrium undergoes necrosis and is shed via the cervix and vagina with bleeding (**menstruation**), leaving only the basal endometrium to act as a reservoir for the development of a new functional layer during the next cycle.

Menstruation lasts for about 4 days and the day it starts is taken as the first day of the menstrual cycle.

The cyclical changes in the functional endometrium are governed by the changing pattern of hormone secretion by the ovaries, which in turn is influenced by the cyclical secretion of hormones (FSH and LH) by the pituitary gland. The secretion of the gonadotropic hormones is in turn controlled by the secretion of gonadotropin-releasing hormones by the hypothalamus. Thus the histological appearance of endometrial curettings can be used to stage (within a few days on either side) the endometrial cycle.

The sequence of changes in the menstrual cycle is repeated throughout the period of sexual maturity, from menarche to menopause, and is interrupted only by pregnancy or hormone therapy, for example oestrogen and progesterone given as a contraceptive.

The proliferative (oestrin or follicular) phase of the menstrual cycle lasts from day 4 to about day 15 or 16

During menstruation, the entire superficial functional zone of endometrium is shed (days 1–4), leaving the compact basal endometrium behind.

At the same time, a new cycle of ovarian follicle maturation begins, the resulting increasing oestrogen secretion by the developing follicle stimulating mitotic activity in the basal endometrial glands and stroma (Fig. 17.24a,b). Continued proliferation of these cells over 10–12 days re-establishes a substantial functional endometrial layer comprising straight tubular endometrial glands embedded in stroma.

As the levels of oestrogen continue to rise in the latter stages of this phase, the glands usually become slightly tortuous and their lumina may distend, and continued mitotic proliferation of endometrial gland columnar cells may produce some heaping up of cells, and therefore a pseudostratified appearance.

Ovulation occurs at about days 14–16

Ovulation is accompanied by the development of subnuclear vacuolation in the endometrial glands (Fig. 17.24c), which coincides with peak levels of LH secretion by the pituitary gland. Eventually all of the glands show this change.

The secretory (luteal) phase lasts from about day 16 to day 25

The onset of the next (secretory or luteal) phase in the menstrual cycle is marked by the appearance of supranuclear secretory vacuoles at the apical poles of the endometrial gland cells. Secretory material is shed into the gland lumen by the apocrine method (see Fig. 3.24) and the luminal surfaces of the gland cells become irregular and ill-defined. The glands themselves become tortuous (Fig. 17.24d) and their lumina distend with secretion (Fig. 17.24e).

This phase of gland secretion occurs in response to progesterone secreted by the corpus luteum.

The premenstrual phase lasts from about day 25 to menstruation at day 28

At about day 22, the secretory activity of the endometrial glands declines and they begin to show involutional changes; the luminal secretion diminishes and that which remains becomes inspissated. The glands become irregular and begin to collapse and there are significant changes in the stroma, including prominent spiral arterioles (Figs 17.24f,g) and swelling of the stromal cells, particularly around the arterioles.

These changes are precipitated by the sudden fall in progesterone and oestrogen secretion due to involution of the corpus luteum.

FIGURE 17.24 **Menstrual cycle.** The interrelationships between pituitary hormones and ovary, and ovarian hormones and the endometrium in the menstrual cycle. The cycle starts on the first day of menstruation, when the functional endometrium from the previous cycle is shed, with bleeding (days 1–4). Release of pituitary follicle-stimulating hormone (FSH) stimulates the maturation of an ovarian follicle, some of the cells of which secrete oestrogen, which initiates and maintains the proliferation of new functional endometrium. (a) A new layer of functional endometrium (F) in the early proliferative stage arising from the compact basal endometrium (B). (b) High-power detail of one of the proliferating endometrial glands. Nuclei are prominent and some cells are in mitosis (arrow). The proliferative stage lasts from day 4 to day 14, at which time a surge of pituitary luteinizing hormone initiates ovulation (days 15–16) and luteinization of the wall of the ovarian follicle. The luteinized cells of the follicle begin to secrete progesterone, which initiates early secretory changes in the endometrium. (c) The earliest changes of secretory activity in the endometrial glands. They develop subnuclear vacuoles (V) and the previously straight tubular glands begin to become convoluted. Continuing secretion of progesterone by the corpus luteum produces further convolution of the endometrial glands, increase in bulk of the stroma and increasing secretory activity of the gland epithelium. (d) A low-power photomicrograph of the endometrium at about day 22 of the cycle. The glands (G) are markedly convoluted and distended by secretion. (e) High-power detail of a late secretory endometrium with secretory vacuoles (V) now in a supranuclear position and secretion (S) in the lumen of the convoluted gland. At about day 25 of the cycle, the secretion of LH and FSH by the pituitary ceases, causing involution of the corpus luteum in the ovary with consequent abrupt reduction in progesterone and oestrogen secretion. This reduction in hormones leads to ischaemic necrosis of the late secretory endometrium, initiating menstruation. Just before undergoing necrosis, the endometrium is very bulky, with early decidual change in the stroma and prominent spiral arterioles. (f) Part of the premenstrual endometrium at low magnification. Note the highly convoluted glands and the very bulky decidualized endometrial stroma (DC), particularly near the surface. (g) A high-power photomicrograph showing the thick-walled and contorted spiral arterioles (SA).

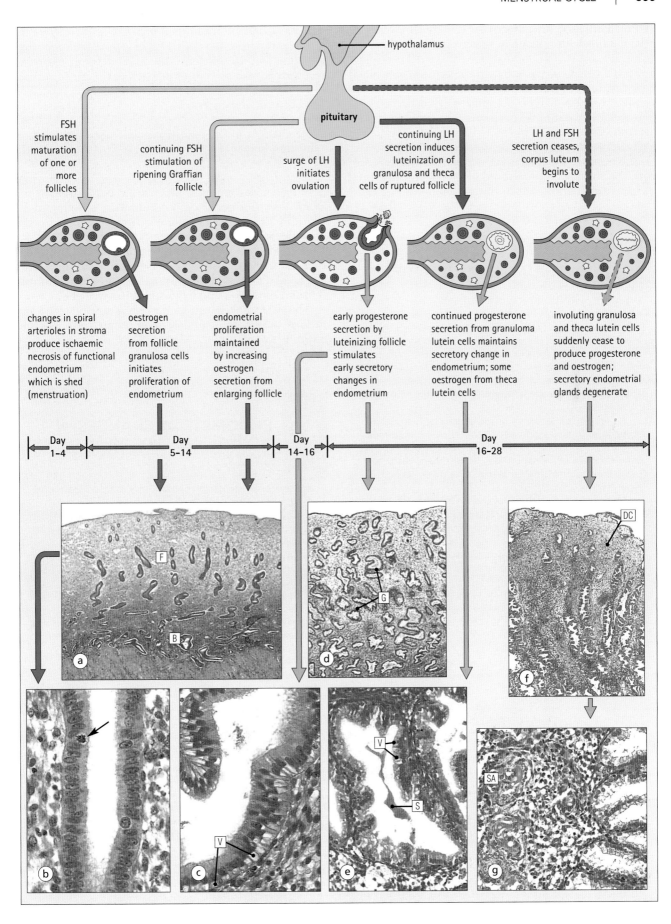

hypothalamus

pituitary

FSH stimulates maturation of one or more follicles

continuing FSH stimulation of ripening Graffian follicle

surge of LH initiates ovulation

continuing LH secretion induces luteinization of granulosa and theca cells of ruptured follicle

LH and FSH secretion ceases, corpus luteum begins to involute

changes in spiral arterioles in stroma produce ischaemic necrosis of functional endometrium which is shed (menstruation)

oestrogen secretion from follicle granulosa cells initiates proliferation of endometrium

endometrial proliferation maintained by increasing oestrogen secretion from enlarging follicle

early progesterone secretion by luteinizing follicle stimulates early secretory changes in endometrium

continued progesterone secretion from granuloma lutein cells maintains secretory change in endometrium; some oestrogen from theca lutein cells

involuting granulosa and theca lutein cells suddenly cease to produce progesterone and oestrogen; secretory endometrial glands degenerate

Day 1–4 | Day 5–14 | Day 14–16 | Day 16–28

At menstruation, the superficial functional layer of the endometrium undergoes necrosis and is shed

Increased coiling of the spiral arterioles decreases blood flow and further constriction of the arterioles leads to significant ischaemia of the functional endometrium. Subsequent dilatation of deeper vessels, combined with necrosis of the walls of the more superficial vessels, then leads to haemorrhage into the stroma.

The necrotic endometrial glands and stroma, together with the stromal accumulations of blood, are then shed as menstrual debris, usually piecemeal, with the most superficial endometrium shed first; the deeper layers are lost over the next 4–5 days until only basal endometrium remains. During this time, the endometrium begins to regenerate, with re-epithelialization of the naked surface of remaining basal endometrium. This healing process is not hormone-dependent.

The changes in the menstrual cycle are suspended during pregnancy

The cyclical changes in the ovary and endometrium described above are seen either when fertilization of the ovum does not occur or if fertilization is followed by death of the zygote or failure of implantation into the endometrium.

In the event of successful fertilization and implantation, the cyclical changes are suspended until some time after childbirth, and almost all of the tissues of the female genital tract undergo structural changes.

The structural changes in the cervix, myometrium and uterine tube have been described on pp. 342, 344 and 346.

CLINICAL EXAMPLE
MENSTRUAL IRREGULARITIES

Irregularity and abnormality of menstruation is a common and important complaint in women of reproductive age. There is a normal tendency for menstrual periods to be irregular in interval, duration and intensity at three times in a woman's life: for the first few cycles after puberty, for the first one or two cycles after pregnancy and for a variable number of cycles before the menopause. The following clinical features imply some form of pathology.

Amenorrhoea (absence of menstruation) is complete absence of menstruation after puberty, which is termed 'primary amenorrhoea' and the cause is usually an endocrine abnormality. Amenorrhoea, where there has previously been normal menstruation, is termed 'secondary amenorrhoea'.

Menorrhagia describes excessive bleeding at menstruation, in both intensity and duration of blood loss. There is often an underlying endometrial or myometrial abnormality.

Dysmenorrhoea is excessively painful menstruation often caused by an endometrial or myometrial disorder.

Intermenstrual bleeding is usually caused by an abnormality in the cervix, vagina or vulva.

Postmenopausal bleeding is a most important symptom, as it is the way in which most malignant tumours of the uterus present.

KEY FACTS
ENDOMETRIAL CHANGES IN NORMAL (28-DAY) MENSTRUAL CYCLE

- Days 1–4: menstrual phase – necrotic endometrium from previous cycle shed
- Days 4–14: proliferative phase – new straight tubular endometrial glands and stroma grow from residual basal endometrium. Much mitotic activity
- Days 14–16: ovulatory phase – earliest sign of secretory activity in endometrial glands in subnuclear vacuolation
- Days 16–25: secretory phase – endometrial glands become tortuous and lumina fill with secretion
- Days 25–28: premenstrual phase – spiral arterioles prominent in stroma; ischaemia leads to degeneration, then necrosis, of secretory endometrium.

CLINICAL EXAMPLE
ENDOMETRIAL DISORDERS

There are many abnormalities that can occur in endometrium, most resulting from inappropriate ovarian hormone stimulation and causing abnormal patterns of menstruation.

Because the endometrium is largely shed once a month, many abnormalities are transient, but persisting endometrial abnormalities are important.

Benign cystic hyperplasia (Fig. 17.25a) of the endometrium is the result of unopposed oestrogen secretion and may occur in the presence of an oestrogen-secreting ovarian tumour.

Atypical endometrial hyperplasia is marked by hyperplastic endometrial glands, which show disorganization of architectural arrangement, whereas the epithelial cells show atypical dysplastic features similar to those seen in malignant tumours of endometrial glands. This condition (Fig. 17.25b) is considered capable of conversion into an invasive endometrial tumour.

The typical malignant tumour of the endometrium, the endometrial adenocarcinoma (Fig. 17.25c), occurs mainly in postmenopausal women and presents as postmenopausal bleeding.

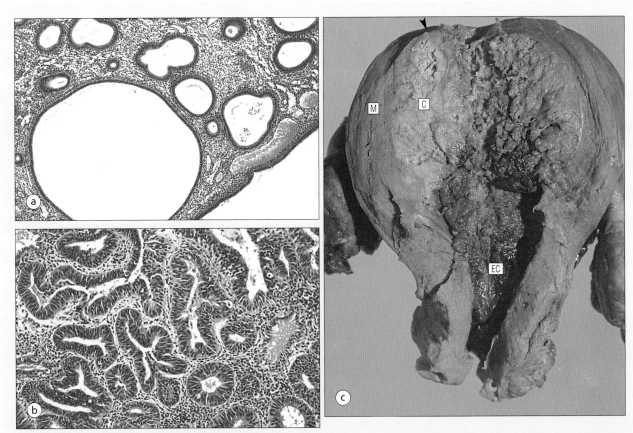

FIGURE 17.25 **Important endometrial growth disorders.** (a) Simple cystic hyperplasia of the endometrial glands. Note the cystically dilated glands. (b) Atypical complex hyperplasia. Note the crowded irregular glands composed of tall epithelial cells, in which some dysplastic features will be present. (c) Invasive endometrial adenocarcinoma (C) fills the endometrial cavity and is invading into the myometrium (M) and part of the way down the endocervical cavity (EC). Note that near the fundus (arrowhead) the malignant tumour has almost infiltrated through the myometrium to the serosal surface of the uterus.

Pregnancy

Fertilization of the ovum usually occurs in the uterine tube (oviduct)

When the ovum is disgorged from the ovary at ovulation, it enters the open infundibular end of the uterine tube and passes into the dilated ampullary portion, which is the most common site for its fertilization (Fig. 17.26).

The second meiotic division of the ovum is only completed once the ovum has been successfully penetrated by a spermatozoon. The nuclear material of the penetrating haploid spermatozoon then joins with that of the haploid ovum, forming a diploid zygote, which immediately begins a series of mitotic divisions to produce a solid ball of cells, the **morula**.

The morula migrates down the uterine tube and enters the endometrial cavity about 4–5 days after fertilization

In the endometrial cavity, further cell divisions of the morula rapidly produce a cystic mass called the **blastocyst**, comprising a fluid-filled cavity (the **blastocoele**)

surrounded by a cellular wall (the **trophoblast**). A solid collection of cells, internal to the trophoblast at one pole of the blastocyst, is called the **inner cell mass** and gives rise to the embryo.

After a day or so floating free in the endometrial cavity, the blastocyst must implant in the secretory endometrium if the pregnancy is to continue.

Attempts at implantation begin about 6 days after fertilization

Implantation is usually 7–8 days after ovulation, and on days 21–22 of the menstrual cycle. If unsuccessful, the blastocyst degenerates and is expelled with the degenerate endometrium and blood with the onset of menstruation at 28 days.

Sometimes implantation occurs but cannot be maintained; menstruation eventually supervenes, often after some delay, and the menstrual loss may be greater than usual.

When implantation is successful, the blastocyst gains access to the endometrial stroma, probably directly across the endometrial surface, and by about 11 days after fertilization (i.e. day 27 of the cycle) is completely embedded in endometrial stroma.

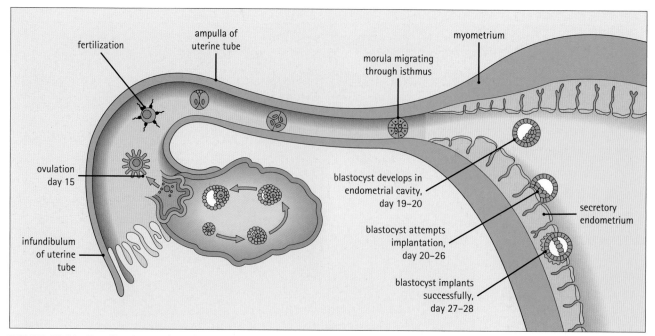

FIGURE 17.26 Fertilization and implantation. The main features of fertilization and implantation. The timing is from the onset of the last menstrual period, and is approximate, there being great individual variation between women and from cycle to cycle.

After implantation, the pregnancy is initially maintained by progesterone secreted by the persisting corpus luteum

From about the time of ovulation, the corpus luteum secretes progesterone. If fertilization and implantation occur it does not regress, but increases in size up to 3–4 cm in diameter (the **corpus luteum of pregnancy**). This persists throughout the first trimester of pregnancy and is a constant source of progesterone, which is necessary to sustain the pregnancy; thereafter the placenta takes over this function and the corpus luteum of pregnancy involutes.

At the time of implantation, the endometrium is in its late secretory phase (see Fig. 17.24e), being characterized by bulky tortuous secretory glands and a stroma which may be demonstrating early decidual change (see Fig. 17.24f).

Implantation stimulates the development of true decidual change under the influence of the continuing progesterone secretion from the **corpus luteum of pregnancy**.

Because of the progesterone secretion, the endometrial glands develop exaggerated secretory appearances which, taken in conjunction with the stromal decidual change, produce the appearance known as **pregnancy pattern endometrium**.

Further development of the trophoblast and some of the decidual endometrial stroma produce the placenta

The placenta is responsible for continued nourishment of the developing embryo and also for continued

secretion of hormones necessary for maintaining the pregnancy.

Further development of the embryo from the inner cell mass is beyond the scope of this book.

Trophoblast

Introduction

On implantation, the single layer of trophoblast, which forms the outer wall of the blastocyst, becomes a double layer.

The outer layer is characterized by the loss of its lateral cell margins so that it forms a thin syncytial layer, the **syncytiotrophoblast**. The inner layer begins as a continuous monolayer of cuboidal cells with pale-staining cytoplasm, the **cytotrophoblast**.

The syncytiotrophoblast has numerous surface microvilli and the ability to erode or invade adjacent tissue

This ability of the syncytiotrophoblast ensures successful erosion of the endometrial tissues and vessels at implantation. The blastocyst initially attaches to the surface epithelium of the endometrium by adhesion. Individual trophoblast cells then intrude between the epithelial cells so that the blastocyst can insinuate itself through the epithelium and into the endometrial stroma, where erosion of an endometrial capillary ensures it an adequate blood supply (Fig. 17.27a).

The breach in the endometrial surface is covered by a small blood clot and the surface is quickly re-epithelialized.

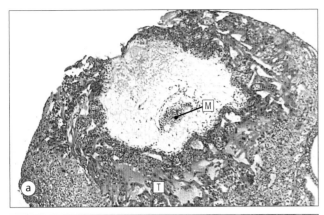

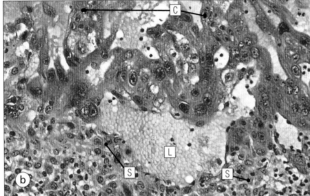

FIGURE 17.27 **Implantation site.** (a) Low-power micrograph showing an early human implantation site. The blastocyst has infiltrated the superficial endometrium and the trophoblast (T) is beginning to infiltrate the endometrial stroma. Part of the inner cell mass (M) can be seen. (b) High-power micrograph from the area of trophoblast infiltration. Cords of syncytiotrophoblast (S) have eroded blood vessels and produced lakes of maternal blood (L). Islands of cytotrophoblast (C) are extending into the syncytial masses.

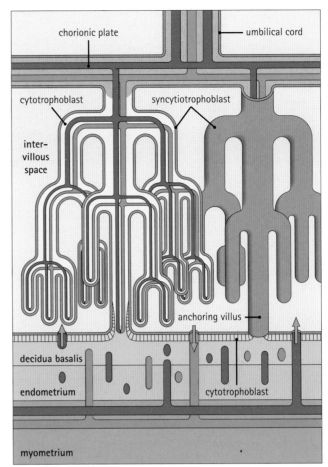

FIGURE 17.28 **Placental structure.** The basic structure of the placenta and the relationship between the fetal and maternal blood.

The presence of the blastocyst within the endometrial stroma induces early decidualization of the stromal cells, which rapidly involves all of the endometrium and leads to marked thickening.

Once the blastocyst is embedded in the endometrial stroma, the trophoblast rapidly proliferates and the outer syncytial layer extends as irregular protrusions into the surrounding stroma, eroding the walls of small blood vessels as it goes.

Lakes of maternal blood form between the protrusions (Fig. 17.27b), and the surface microvilli of the syncytiotrophoblast probably assist in transferring oxygen and nutrients from the maternal blood to the developing blastocyst.

The cytotrophoblast grows into the syncytial protrusions as finger-like extensions

The solid masses of cytotrophoblast covered by syncytium form the **primary** or **stem chorionic villi**.

With the development of a loose mesenchymal core, the origin of which is uncertain, the villi are known as **secondary villi**, and soon acquire a system of capillaries that become part of the blood circulatory system of the embryo.

Fully vascularized villi are referred to as **tertiary villi** (see Fig. 17.29).

As the villi mature, the mesenchymal core contains interlacing vascular channels, fibroblasts, some smooth muscle cells and large pleomorphic cells with vacuolated cytoplasm (**Hofbauer cells**). These cells have some of the ultrastructural and immunocytochemical features of macrophages, and are believed to be motile macrophages with a particular facility for protein ingestion and pinocytosis.

The early chorionic villi subdivide in an arborizing pattern to form a complex system that provides an immense surface area for exchange between the maternal and fetal circulations.

After the complex branching of the villi, the terminal villi contain small, thin-walled capillaries, all of which connect with larger vessels in the larger 'twigs', 'branches' and 'trunks' of the tree-like proliferation; these vessels ultimately combine to form the two arteries and single vein that run in the umbilicus to the blood circulation of the embryo (Fig. 17.28).

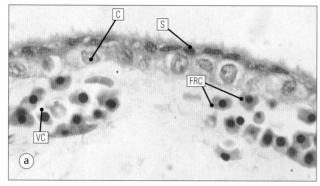

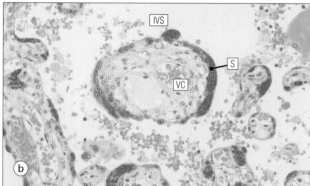

FIGURE 17.29 **Chorionic villi.** (a) Micrograph showing part of an early chorionic villus, which is covered by a layer of cuboidal cytotrophoblast (C) and an outer layer of syncytiotrophoblast (S). Note the villus capillaries (VC) filled with nucleated fetal red cells (FRC). (b) Micrograph of chorionic villi close to end of pregnancy; note the prominent heaped-up syncytiotrophoblast (S), maternal blood in the intervillous space (IVS), and fetal blood in the villous capillaries (VC).

The appearances of the chorionic villi change with time

In early pregnancy, the villi contain central capillaries embedded in bulky mesenchyme, but later, the capillaries proliferate and come to lie close to the trophoblast surface.

As the capillaries become more numerous and dilated, the mesenchyme is reduced in bulk and its cellular component is reduced; in particular, Hofbauer cells become scarce.

Initially, the cytotrophoblast cells predominate and the syncytiotrophoblast is a thin layer (Fig. 17.29a). Division of the cytotrophoblast probably maintains the syncytial cell mass throughout gestation. As the pregnancy progresses, the syncytiotrophoblast becomes the predominant layer and the cytotrophoblast appears to partly regress, becoming a discontinuous layer, then collections of scattered cells beneath the syncytiotrophoblast.

At term, the villi show increasing hyalinization of the mesenchymal stroma, and fibrin is deposited in the blood-filled intervillous spaces, often coating the outer surface of the villi.

The arrangement of complex chorionic villi of fetal origin intruding into a constantly blood-filled intervillous

space of maternal origin provides an efficient means of transferring oxygen, nutrients, maternal antibodies and hormones from the mother to the fetus, and waste metabolites from the fetus to the mother (see Fig. 17.28).

ADVANCED CONCEPT
ENDOCRINE FUNCTIONS OF THE PLACENTA

In addition to being a site of exchange, the placenta also acts as an endocrine organ.

- The syncytiotrophoblast secretes human chorionic gonadotropin (hCG) (Fig. 17.30), which is responsible for maintaining the corpus luteum of pregnancy (see p. 358) after cessation of the LH stimulus from the pituitary gland
- The syncytiotrophoblast secretes human chorionic somatomammotropin (hCS), which is believed to stimulate lactogenesis
- The placenta secretes progesterone and oestrogens; oestrogen precursors produced by the adrenal cortex and liver of the fetus are converted into active oestrogens in the placenta.

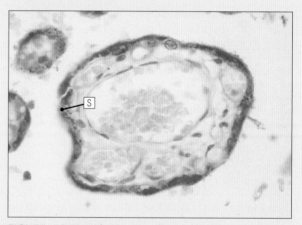

FIGURE 17.30 **Chorionic villi and hCG.** Micrograph showing a chorionic villus from a term placenta demonstrating localization of human chorionic gonadotropin (hCG), stained brown, to the syncytiotrophoblast (S).

Decidua

After implantation, the endometrial stroma undergoes decidualization

The normally small compact cells of the endometrial stroma undergo remarkable enlargement; this process is known as **decidualization**.

Decidualization begins in the stromal cells around the implanted blastocyst, but soon spreads to involve the rest of the pregnancy endometrium. As the stromal cells enlarge, they dominate the endometrium and the glandular component becomes insignificant. The thickened

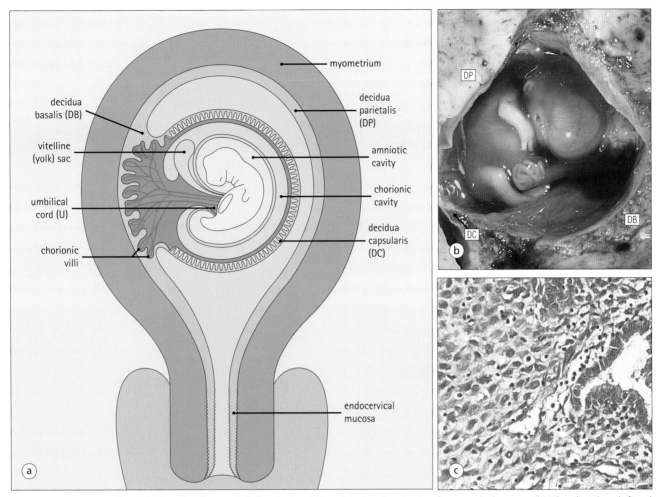

FIGURE 17.31 **Decidua.** (a) The decidua and their relationships with the developing fetus and placenta. (b) The decidua defined in (a). Note the decidua parietalis (DP), decidua capsularis (DC) and decidua basalis (DB). (c) Micrograph of decidual cells. They are large polygonal cells with pale-staining nuclei and granular eosinophilic cytoplasm.

superficial endometrial layers become the decidua, as follows (Fig. 17.31):

- The endometrium immediately beneath the implantation site, into which the major trophoblast growth occurs, becomes the **decidua basalis**
- The thin rim of endometrial stroma overlying the blastocyst becomes the **decidua capsularis**
- The endometrium lining the rest of the uterine cavity is called the **decidua parietalis**.

Of the decidua, the decidua basalis is the most important, as the vessels in this part of the modified endometrium supply maternal arterial blood to the lacunae between the fetal chorionic villi and receive venous blood from the lacunae. The villous trophoblast (from the fetus) and the decidua basalis (from the mother),

and the intervillous spaces between them, comprise the placenta.

Decidual stromal cells have prominent, pale-staining, round or ovoid nuclei, often with finely granular chromatin and one or two nucleoli; their cytoplasm is bulky, and usually eosinophilic, and granular or slightly foamy, although some cells may have a basophilic tinge (see Fig. 17.31c).

Ultrastructurally, the decidualized stromal cells contain prominent, often long mitochondria, together with variable amounts of rough endoplasmic reticulum.

The eosinophilia or basophilia of the cytoplasm in individual cells depends on the relative proportions of mitochondria (eosinophilic) and rough endoplasmic reticulum (basophilic).

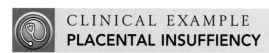

CLINICAL EXAMPLE
PLACENTAL INSUFFIENCY

The placenta is essential for growth of the fetus and any abnormality can lead to problems in growth and development. If this happens early in pregnancy, there may be a reduction in growth of the fetus, termed 'intrauterine growth restriction' (IUGR). This problem develops in about 5% of all pregnancies. It can be suspected if the size of the uterus is smaller than that which would be expected for the stage of pregnancy.

Several conditions are recognized as being associated with placental insufficiency and IUGR:

- Poor maternal nutrition
- Maternal diabetes
- Alcohol abuse
- Heavy smoking
- Twin or triplet pregnancies
- Pre-eclampsia or eclampsia, both of which are conditions associated with elevated maternal blood pressure
- Infection with cytomegalovirus, toxoplasmosis, rubella or syphilis, known collectively as TORCH infections
- Structural defects of the placental membranes or the umbilical cord
- Abnormal implantation of the placenta in the uterus

One of the functions of regular examinations in pregnancy is to check that the growth of the fetus and placenta are both satisfactory.

Babies born after IUGR and placental insufficiency are recognized to be physically small with risks for neurological problems.

**For online review questions, please visit
https://studentconsult.inkling.com.**

END OF CHAPTER REVIEW

True/False Answers to the MCQs, as Well as Case Answers, Can be Found in the Appendix in the Back of the Book.

1. **Which of the following is true of the transformation zone of the cervix?**
   (a) Is the site where endometrium changes to endocervix at the internal os
   (b) Is the result of vaginal acid acting on the lower endocervical epithelium
   (c) Is an important site for the development of cervical cancer
   (d) Results in Nabothian follicles
   (e) Develops shortly after birth

2. **The sexually mature endometrium has which of the following characteristics?**
   (a) Is the site of implantation of the fertilized ovary
   (b) Is shed every month at the time of ovulation
   (c) Is regenerated every month from its basal portion
   (d) Undergoes atrophy after the menopause
   (e) Fails to respond to oestrogens and progesterone after the menopause

3. **Which of the following features are seen in the corpus luteum of the ovary?**
   (a) Develops from a ruptured tertiary Graafian follicle
   (b) Secretes progesterone but not oestrogens
   (c) Undergoes involution at the end of each menstrual cycle
   (d) Converts into a corpus fibrosum after involution
   (e) Persists as a progesterone-secreting source in the first 3 months of pregnancy

4. **Which of the following features are present in the ovary?**
   (a) The cortex consists of a spindle-cell stroma which surrounds the gamete-producing structures
   (b) Most primordial follicles undergo atresia
   (c) A primary follicle is composed of an oocyte surrounded by granulosa cells and Sertoli cells
   (d) A tertiary follicle is also called a Graafian follicle
   (e) The thecal cells that surround the secondary follicle are derived from stromal cells

CASE 17.1 A WOMAN WHO CANNOT BECOME PREGNANT

A 26-year-old woman is seen because she has not been able to become pregnant despite trying with her partner for 2 years. She has normal regular periods, and endocrinological investigations suggest that ovulation is taking place normally. Investigations have excluded a likely male factor.

Q. Describe the structural and functional features that allow successful fertilization and implantation. Speculate where abnormalities may develop that might explain infertility.

Chapter 18

Skin and Breast

Introduction

The skin is an extensive organ covering the exterior of the body. It varies in structure from site to site according to specific functions, which include:
- Protection from external damaging agents
- Thermoregulation
- Sensation (touch, heat, pressure, pain)
- Secretion of protective lipids, milk, etc.

The breast is a highly modified area of skin with specialized sweat glands to produce nutritious secretions under hormonal influences.

The skin is composed of two main layers: the epidermis and dermis, and a variable third layer, the subcutis.

The **epidermis** is the surface epithelial layer in contact with the external environment. Downgrowths of this layer produce sweat glands, hair follicles and other epidermal appendages.

The **dermis** is a middle supporting layer containing the epidermal appendages, blood vessels, nerves and nerve endings, which are embedded in an elastocollagenous stroma produced by fibroblasts.

The **subcutis** is the deepest layer and varies in size and content, but is usually composed mainly of adipose tissue (Fig. 18.1).

Epidermis

The epidermis is the protective skin layer in contact with the external environment

A stratified epithelium (see p. 38), the surface of the epidermis bears closely packed flat plates of protein (**keratin**), which form a tough, water-repellent layer (**stratum corneum**).

Keratin is produced by the main cell type in epidermis, the keratinocyte. Note that, contrary to traditional teaching, the stratum corneum is not cellular but is composed entirely of intracytoplasmic keratin remnants bound to the skin surface after the death of the keratinocytes that produced them (see Fig. 3.28). Each keratin plate conforms roughly to the shape of the keratinocyte shortly before its death.

Although normally thin, the stratum corneum is very thick in skin exposed to constant trauma, such as that on the soles and palms.

Epidermis is traditionally regarded as a stratified squamous epithelium, but in fact only the most superficial two or three living cell layers of the epidermis approach a squamous or flat configuration, most keratinocytes being cuboidal or polyhedral.

The surface plates of keratin, and the flat dying keratinocytes that precede them, are known as squames, and result from the maturation of the other layers of keratinocytes comprising the epidermis. These layers are the basal layer, the prickle cell layer and the granular layer (Fig. 18.2).

ADVANCED CONCEPT
NOMENCLATURE OF THE EPIDERMAL LAYERS

In this book, we use the English nomenclature for the layers of the epidermis, rather than their Latin equivalents:

- Basal layer ≡ stratum basale or stratum germinativum
- Prickle cell layer ≡ stratum spinosum
- Granular layer ≡ stratum granulosum
- Keratin layer ≡ stratum corneum.

In addition, a further layer, the stratum lucidum, is described in the skin of the sole. This refers to a narrow, pale-staining layer of compact keratin sometimes seen between the granular layer and the more intensely staining bulk of the thick keratin layer. It has no structural or functional significance and may be an artifact of staining (see Fig. 18.20).

Keratinocytes are separated from the underlying support tissues of the dermis by a basement membrane

The junction between the dermis and epidermis is an important area, tethering the two layers together (Fig. 18.3) and structured to minimize the risk of dermoepidermal separation by shearing forces as follows:
- Tethering fibres connect the dermis and epidermis to the intervening basement membrane
- The basal cell membrane of individual basal cells, and the underlying basement membrane, are convoluted (see Fig. 18.6)
- There is a system of **rete ridges** (i.e. downgrowths of epidermis into dermis), which varies markedly from site to site. In protected areas, where the skin is not normally subjected to shearing stress (e.g. the trunk), rete ridges are barely evident and the dermoepidermal junction appears flat, but in areas

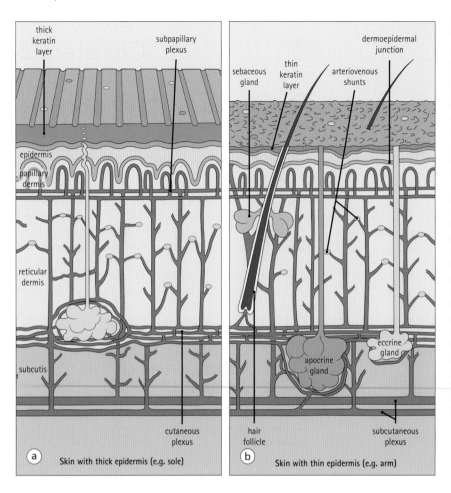

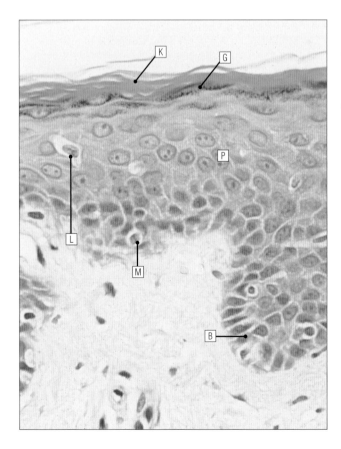

FIGURE 18.1 **Architecture of the skin.** The most superficial layer of the skin is the epidermis. (a,b) This varies in thickness from site to site and is covered by acellular keratin, which is mainly thin but is thick in special sites, e.g. the sole. Beneath the epidermis is the dermis, which has two components: a more superficial loose papillary dermis and a denser reticular dermis, which comprises the bulk of the layer. The dermis is mainly composed of collagen, with some elastic fibres. The deepest layer of the skin, the subcutis, has a variable structure; when prominent it is composed largely of adipose tissue intersected by fibrocollagenous septa. The subcutis contains the main subcutaneous network of arteries and veins from which vessels extend upwards and form a network (the cutaneous plexus) at the dermosubcutaneous junction. From here, smaller vessels penetrate the dermis, giving branches to the skin appendages and culminating in a superficial network of small venules and arterioles (the subpapillary plexus). Capillary loops from this plexus extend upward into the dermal papillae to lie close to the dermoepidermal junction. Blood vessels do not penetrate the epidermis.

FIGURE 18.2 **Epidermis layers.** The basal layer (B) sits on the basement membrane and is covered by the prickle cell layer (P), and then the granular layer (G), which contains dark-staining keratohyaline granules. The surface layer is dense acellular keratin (K). Two non-keratinocyte cells of the epidermis, a melanocyte (M) and a Langerhans' cell (L) (see pp. 368-369), are also evident.

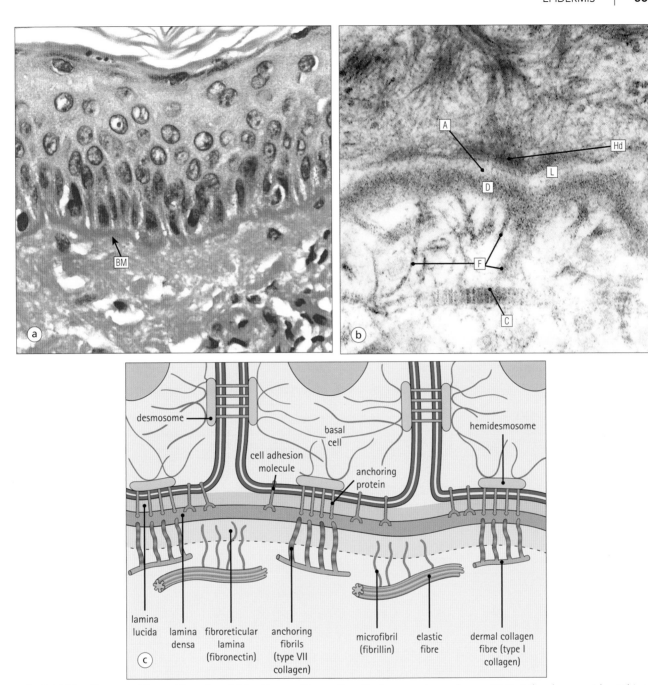

FIGURE 18.3 Dermoepidermal junction. (a) In this paraffin section, the basement membrane (BM) at the dermoepidermal junction is demonstrated by the PAS stain. (b) In this electron micrograph of dermoepidermal junction, the basement membrane can be seen to consist of three main layers: a superficial electron-lucent lamina lucida (L), an electron-dense lamina densa (D) and an ill-defined fibroreticular lamina. The basal cells are tethered to the lamina densa by hemidesmosomes (Hd), from which anchoring proteins (A) cross the lamina lucida. On the dermal aspect, fine anchoring fibrils (F) of type VII collagen attach the lower surface of the lamina densa to collagen fibres (C) in the papillary dermis, and fibrillin microfibrils attach it to elastic fibres. In addition, the zone immediately beneath the lamina densa contains abundant fibronectin (see p. 59). (c) The dermoepidermal junction showing the components of the basement membrane and its attachments to basal cells and dermal fibres.

constantly exposed to shearing stress (e.g. tips of fingers, palms and soles) the rete ridge system is highly developed (see Figs 18.1a, 18.5, 18.12). The basement membrane at the dermoepidermal junction can be seen to consist of three main layers, specifically:

- An electron-lucent lamina lucida on the epidermal side

- An electron-dense lamina densa in the middle
- An ill-defined fibroreticular lamina, which contains abundant fibronectin, on the dermal side.

The basal cells are tethered to the lamina densa by hemidesmosomes from which anchoring proteins cross the lamina lucida. On the dermal aspect, fine anchoring fibrils of type VII collagen attach the lower surface of the lamina densa to collagen fibres in the papillary dermis, whereas fibrillin microfibrils attach it to upper dermal elastic fibres. In addition, the zone immediately beneath the lamina densa contains abundant fibronectin (see p. 59 and Fig. 18.3c).

The basal layer is the deepest cell layer of the epidermis and is responsible for the constant production of keratinocytes

The basal layer cells are cuboidal or low columnar in shape and are attached to the basement membrane, which separates it from the underlying dermis, by hemidesmosomes, and to adjacent basal cells by true desmosomes.

Basal cells have round or oval nuclei (Fig. 18.4) with prominent nucleoli, and their cytoplasm is rich in ribosomes and mitochondria; tonofilaments are present in small numbers. In pigmented skin the cytoplasm also contains melanin granules and lysosomes.

It is in the basal layer that cells in mitosis are seen, as well as scattered non-keratinocyte cells, melanocytes and Merkel cells (see p. 376).

The keratinocytes above the basal cells form the prickle cell layers

The cells are polyhedral with central round nuclei and pinkish-staining cytoplasm.

Prickle cells are in contact with each other by a system of intercellular bridges, formed from small cytoplasmic projections from the cell surface terminating in desmosomal junctions (Fig. 18.6; see also Fig. 3.11). The prickle cells form a layer of variable thickness, sometimes called the 'stratum spinosum'.

The cytoplasm of the prickle cells contains many tonofilaments (see Fig. 3.28), which are particularly concentrated in the cytoplasmic projections leading into the desmosomes and are more numerous in the cell layers closest to the granular layer.

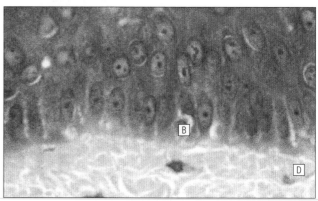

FIGURE 18.4 **Basal cells (acrylic).** The basal cells (B) are smaller than the other keratinocytes and may show a regular, regimented arrangement (palisading). They have rounded or oval nuclei, and rest on the basement membrane marking the junction between epidermis and dermis (D).

CLINICAL EXAMPLE
BASAL BLISTERS

The dermoepidermal junction is a site where fluid can accumulate in sufficient quantity to lift the epidermis away from the dermis, thereby forming a basal blister. This can result from:

- Excessive shearing force
- Structural abnormality.

Excessive shearing forces are the most common cause and are usually due to constant shearing friction, such as occurs with tight-fitting shoes.

Structural abnormalities may be primary or secondary, and the most important primary cause is the rare inherited skin disease epidermolysis bullosa, in which the dermoepidermal junction is intrinsically weak and unable to resist even minimal shearing trauma. There are a number of different types of epidermolysis bullosa, depending on the site of separation, which can be ascertained by electron microscopy.

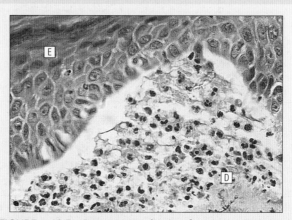

FIGURE 18.5 **Dermatitis herpetiformis.** Micrograph showing a secondary cause of basal blistering, dermatitis herpetiformis, in which patients develop an intensely itchy blistering eruption. In dermatitis herpetiformis the immunoglobulin IgA becomes deposited in the tips of the dermal papillae close to the basement membrane. This activates the complement cascade via the alternative pathway, and neutrophil polymorphs are attracted to the site by the release of chemotaxins. As a result, the dermis (D) is damaged just below the dermoepidermal junction and the epidermis (E) separates, leaving a basal blister containing fluid and some remnants of neutrophil polymorphs. Note the numerous neutrophils in the small early blister shown here.

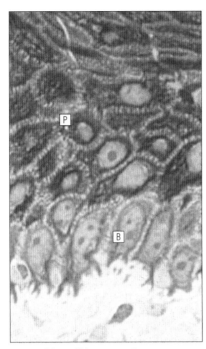

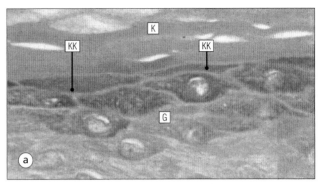

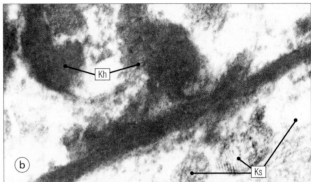

FIGURE 18.6 **Prickle cell layer.** A thin epoxy resin section of skin stained with toluidine blue showing the basal layer (B) and the prickle cell layer (P) above it. Prickle cell cytoplasm stains more intensely than the basal cell cytoplasm because of its high content of tonofilaments. The characteristic intercellular bridges to which the prickle cells owe their name are easily seen and are the site of desmosomal attachments between adjacent prickle cells.

The cells of the upper prickle cell layer are flatter than the polyhedral cells of the deeper layers. The narrow interstices between the prickle cells are partly occupied by the cytoplasmic projections of melanocytes and Langerhans' cells.

The granular cell layer produces the surface keratin and non-wettable substances

The granular keratinocytes contain small or oval haematoxyphilic round bodies (**keratohyaline granules**) composed of proteinaceous material containing abundant sulfur-rich amino acids (e.g. cysteine). They also contain abundant tonofibrils and small round lamellated **keratinosomes** or **Odland bodies**.

In the upper layer, the cytoplasm of granular keratinocytes is largely composed of masses of keratohyaline material and tightly packed tonofibrils, with little cytosol and few cytoplasmic organelles, and at this level, the cells are flat. Death of the nucleus and cytoplasm leaves the keratohyaline and tonofibrils, which combine to form the keratin (see Fig. 3.28) of the acellular surface layer, the stratum corneum (Fig. 18.7).

Keratinosomes produce a complex hydrophobic glycophospholipid, which is released when the superficial granular keratinocytes die, and probably acts as a glue, cementing together the flakes of keratin. This substance also renders the skin surface relatively non-wettable, although prolonged exposure will wash it away, permitting the keratin to absorb water, swell and soften. This

FIGURE 18.7 **Granular cell layer.** (a) Micrograph (acrylic) showing the granular layer (G) of the epidermis with acellular keratin (K) above it. The cytoplasm becomes progressively darker staining near the surface, owing to its increasing content of keratohyaline granules. The most superficial cells have lost their nuclei and are flat plates of keratohyaline and keratin (KK). (b) Electron micrograph showing part of the cytoplasm of a cell in the granular layer; it is packed with irregular masses of electron-dense keratohyaline (Kh) and round or oval keratinosomes (Ks), some of which show lamellation.

feature is obvious in the skin of the hands after prolonged immersion in water, particularly when the water is hot and contains some form of lipid-dissolving detergent.

 CLINICAL EXAMPLE
TUMOURS OF THE EPIDERMAL CELLS

Tumours of the epidermal cells in skin are very common, and most are associated with prolonged exposure of the skin to ultraviolet light. They are therefore most common in sun-exposed areas of skin such as the face and the backs of the hands, and particularly in the elderly or those who have had excessive sun exposure at an early age through their lifestyle.

The commonest tumour is derived from the basal cells of the epidermis and is therefore called basal cell carcinoma. These tumours are malignant and, unless treated by complete excision when they are first noticed, may continue to grow slowly and destroy skin and deep tissues locally; they never metastasize to distant sites. Slightly less common are tumours derived from the keratinocytes from the stratum spinosum (prickle cell layer). These are called squamous cell carcinomas and, like basal cell carcinomas, are locally invasive and destructive, but these tumours also spread to distant sites via lymphatics.

Surface keratin is constantly lost due to normal wear and tear from surface friction, washing and scrubbing

Surface keratin needs to be constantly replenished from the granular layer, which in turn is constantly repopulated by cells from the prickle layer. The prickle cells are produced by proliferation of cells in the basal layer.

Turnover, from basal cell to desquamated keratin, varies from site to site, being faster (i.e. 25–30 days) in traumatized areas (e.g. soles); slow turnovers range from 40 to 50 days. The turnover period is considerably shortened in some skin diseases, particularly psoriasis.

Non-keratinizing Epidermal Cells

In addition to keratinocytes, the epidermis also contains melanocytes, Langerhans' cells and Merkel cells.

Melanocytes produce the protective pigment melanin

Melanin is largely responsible for skin colour and minimizes tissue damage by ultraviolet radiation.

Melanocytes are derived from neuroectoderm and are located in the basal layer of keratinocytes in contact with the basement membrane. They are pale staining, with large ovoid nuclei and abundant cytoplasm, from which numerous long cytoplasmic processes extend into the spaces between the keratinocytes.

Melanocyte cytoplasm contains characteristic membrane-bound ovoid granules (**premelanosomes** and **melanosomes**), which have a striated electron-dense core and produce melanin (Fig. 18.8c). In the production of melanin, tyrosine is converted into an intermediate pigment, which polymerizes into melanin.

Melanin binds to proteins to form the active melanoprotein complex, which appears ultrastructurally as spherical masses of homogeneous electron-dense material, and often obscures the premelanosomes.

Melanoprotein complexes pass along the cytoplasmic processes of the melanocyte and are transferred into the cytoplasm of basal and prickle cell layer keratinocytes, the highest concentration being in the basal layers.

Melanocyte numbers remain more or less constant but their degree of activity is genetically variable, accounting for racial and individual variation in skin colour.

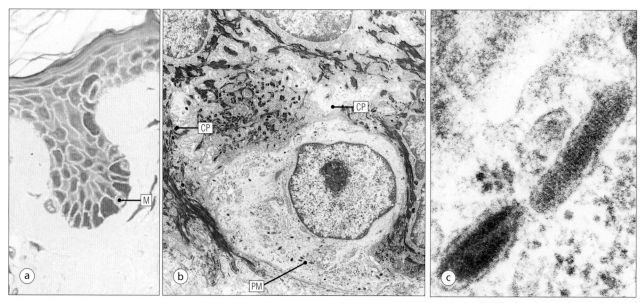

FIGURE 18.8 **Melanocyte.** (a) Micrograph showing a melanocyte (M), with its pale-staining cytoplasm. In this section of black skin, it can be clearly seen against the pigment-laden basal cells. (b) Ultrastructurally, melanocytes contain premelanosomes (PM) and melanosomes, and their cytoplasmic processes (CP) extend between keratinocytes of the basal and lower prickle cell layers. (c) High-magnification electron micrograph showing the characteristic boat shape of premelanosomes; both coarse longitudinal and fine transverse striations can be seen.

Langerhans' cells are antigen recognition cells

Langerhans' cells are located in all layers of the epidermis but are most easily seen in the prickle cell layer. They recognize antigen and are an important component of the immune system (see pp. 128-129).

Like melanocytes, Langerhans' cells have an ovoid, pale-staining nucleus surrounded by pale-staining cytoplasm from which cytoplasmic (dendritic) processes extend between the keratinocytes.

Langerhans' cell cytoplasm contains scattered characteristic Birbeck granules, which are rod-like structures with periodic cross-striations and are most numerous near the Golgi. Sometimes one end of the rod is distended to form a spherical saccule, giving the appearance of a tennis racket (Fig. 18.9d).

Although present in small numbers in healthy skin, Langerhans' cells are increased both in number, and in the extent and complexity of their dendritic processes, in many chronic inflammatory skin disorders, particularly those with an allergic or immune aetiology, such as chronic atopic dermatitis.

Merkel cells are sensory receptors in the epidermis

Merkel cells are scanty and difficult to demonstrate in normal skin. They are found in the basal layer and resemble melanocytes by routine light microscopy, but electron microscopy reveals rounded membrane-bound cytoplasmic neuroendocrine-type granules.

Merkel cells form synaptic junctions with peripheral nerve endings at the base of the cell and also scanty desmosomal attachments to adjacent keratinocytes (Fig. 18.10). They occur either as scattered solitary cells or as aggregates, when they are associated with a so-called hair disc, located immediately beneath the basement membrane. Such aggregates are thought to be touch receptors and are sometimes called 'tactile corpuscles'.

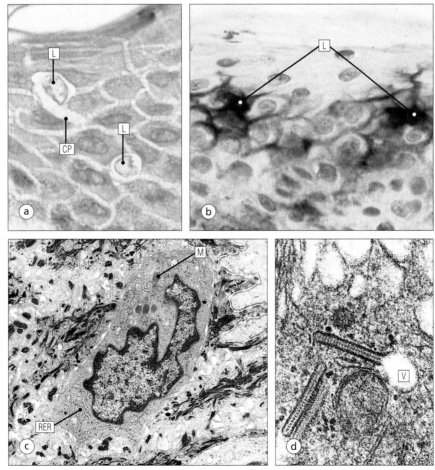

FIGURE 18.9 **Langerhans' cells.** (a) In paraffin or resin sections stained with H&E, Langerhans' cells (L) are irregular, pale-staining cells in the prickle cell layer, with pale-staining oval or reniform nuclei, which are often cleft. Their numerous cytoplasmic processes (CP) pass between the keratinocytes. (b) Langerhans' cells (L) carry CD1 marker and can be clearly visualized by immunoperoxidase techniques. (c) Ultrastructurally, Langerhans' cells have an irregular cleft nucleus and are devoid of tonofilaments. They have prominent mitochondria (M), lysosomes and rough endoplasmic reticulum (RER). Birbeck granules are not seen at this magnification. (d) High-magnification electron micrograph showing characteristic Birbeck granules, one with a distended vesicle (V) at one end.

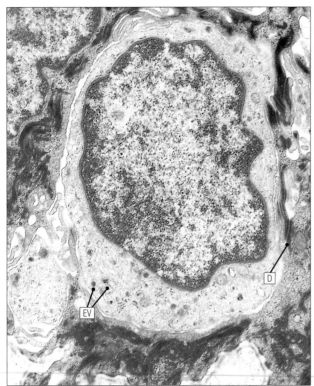

FIGURE 18.10 **Merkel cells.** Merkel cells can be distinguished from melanocytes by their ultrastructural features (compare with Figure 18.8b,c). They have a convoluted nucleus, which occupies much of the cell, and no cytoplasmic processes insinuating between keratinocytes, but may have short protrusions, which contact adjacent keratinocytes at occasional desmosomes (D). Round neuroendocrine vesicles (EV) are present in the cytoplasm, particularly at the base of the cell, close to the basal nerve terminal, which communicates with the underlying nerve disc (not shown here). The cytoplasm also contains a prominent Golgi, smooth endoplasmic reticulum and scattered ribosomes.

Skin Appendages

The skin appendages are the pilosebaceous apparatus, isolated sebaceous glands, eccrine sweat glands and ducts and apocrine sweat glands and ducts.

The pilosebaceous apparatus produces hair and sebum, which is a non-wettable secretion that protects the hair and augments the non-wettable characteristics of the keratin.

The components of a pilosebaceous apparatus are hair follicle, hair shaft, sebaceous glands and erector pili.

Pilosebaceous Apparatus

Hair is derived from the epithelium of the follicle

The **hair follicle** is a tubular epithelial structure opening on to the epidermal surface. At its lower end, a bulbous expansion (the **hair bulb**) with a concave lower surface contains a specialized area of dermis called the **hair papilla**. This is richly supplied with myelinated and nonmyelinated nerve endings and abundant small blood vessels.

CLINICAL EXAMPLE
DERMATITIS (INFLAMMATION OF SKIN)

The skin is exposed to many damaging agents, such as chemicals and ultraviolet irradiation, which produce a wide variety of common rashes. A common type of dermatitis, seborrhoeic dermatitis, is shown in Figure 18.11.

In addition, the skin reacts to internal abnormalities, and produces rashes in response to disorders, such as viral infections (e.g. measles) and drug allergies (e.g. penicillin rash).

The cause of most skin diseases is not known.

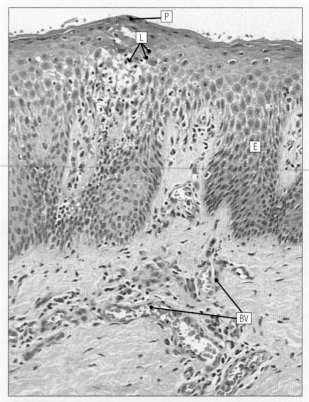

FIGURE 18.11 **Seborrhoeic dermatitis.** The epidermis (E) is thickened, and is disrupted by an infiltration of lymphocytes (L) associated with an accumulation of water (clear areas) between keratinocytes. Note that the surface keratin layers still contain remnants of keratinocyte nuclei. This is termed 'parakeratosis' (P) and is a manifestation of disordered keratinocyte maturation in areas of epidermal damage. Blood vessels (BV) in the upper dermis are dilated and surrounded by lymphocytes and macrophages. In seborrhoeic dermatitis, the damaging agent is thought to be a fungus.

In the hair bulb, numerous small, actively proliferating germinative cells produce the hair shaft and the internal root sheath, which lie within the external root sheath.

Germinative hair bulb cells have dark basophilic cytoplasm with a scattering of melanocytes.

The internal root sheath of the hair follicle is composed of three layers:

- Henle's layer, which is a single cell layer
- A thicker layer characterized by the presence of large eosinophilic trichohyalin granules
- The cuticle, which consists of overlapping keratin plates.

The cuticle is continuous with the cuticle of the hair shaft (see below) in the lower regions of the hair follicle.

The internal root sheath undergoes keratinization to produce the hair shaft. It extends up from the hair bulb to about the level of the insertion of the sebaceous glands, where it disintegrates, leaving a potential space around the hair shaft into which the sebaceous gland products are secreted.

The external root sheath of the follicle is modified epidermis

Near the opening of the follicle on to the skin surface, it consists of all three epidermal layers (basal, prickle cell and granular). In the deeper parts of the hair follicle, below the point of insertion of the sebaceous glands, it is composed of highly modified prickle cells, with large, pale-staining cells rich in glycogen.

Outside the external root sheath is a thick basement membrane, which is strongly eosinophilic and is known as the glassy membrane (Fig. 18.12).

Each hair shaft is composed of two or three layers of highly organized keratin

Each hair can be divided into an inner medulla, an outer cortex and a superficial cuticle.

The **medulla** is a variable component and is not present in the finer vellus and lanugo hairs. When present, it is composed of layers of tightly packed polyhedral cells. The **cortex** is composed of tightly packed keratin, which is produced without the incorporation of keratohyaline granules; it is 'hard' keratin and differs in composition from the soft keratin of the epidermal surface. The **cuticle** consists of a single layer of flat keratinous scales, which overlap in a highly organized manner.

Hair shafts contain variable amounts of melanin depending on melanocyte activity in the germinative cells of the hair bulb.

The erector pili muscle positions the hair follicle and hair shaft

A further component of the pilosebaceous apparatus is a narrow band of smooth muscle, the **erector pili**, which originates in the fibrocollagenous sheath surrounding the hair follicle and runs obliquely upward into the upper dermis. Its contraction makes the hair follicle and shaft more vertical, so that the hair appears to stand on end.

Sebaceous glands develop as lateral outgrowths of the external root sheath

Sebaceous glands secrete a mixture of lipids called sebum. They are largely inactive until puberty, after which they enlarge and become secretory.

Sebaceous glands are composed of lobules of large polyhedral pale-staining cells containing abundant lipid droplets and small dark-staining central nuclei. There is a single layer of cuboidal or flattened precursor cells between the basement membrane of each lobule and the central mass of cells. The sebaceous gland lobules are connected to the hair follicle, usually about two-thirds to three-quarters of the way up from the hair bulb, by short ducts lined by stratified squamous epithelium, showing all the layers seen in the normal epidermis.

Sebum is a lipid mixture which includes triglycerides and various complex waxes

Sebum is produced by large-scale death of sebaceous cells, resulting in the release of their lipid content into the ducts (Fig. 18.13), and thus into the space between the formed hair shaft and the external root sheath, following degeneration of the internal root sheath. This pattern of secretion is called 'holocrine secretion' (see Fig. 3.24).

The number, size and activity of sebaceous glands varies from site to site within the skin

Sebaceous glands are particularly abundant on the face, scalp, ears, nostrils and vulva, and around the anus, but are absent from the soles and palms.

In certain areas of the body, the sebaceous glands do not empty into hair follicles, but open directly on to the epidermal surface. This occurs in:

- The labia minora (see p. 339)
- Areolar skin around the nipple, where they are known as Montgomery's tubercles (see p. 378)
- The eyelids, where they are known as Meibomian glands (see p. 401)
- The lips and buccal mucosa (Fordyce spots).

Eccrine Sweat Glands and Ducts

Eccrine glands produce sweat and are controlled by the autonomic nervous system

Sweat is a hypotonic watery solution with a neutral or slightly acid pH that contains various ions, particularly sodium, potassium and chloride ions.

Eccrine sweat glands and ducts are found everywhere in the skin

Eccrine glands are particularly numerous on the forehead, scalp, axillae, palms and soles. They arise as downgrowths of the epidermis at about the 16th week of intrauterine life.

The secretory gland component, which is situated deep in the dermis or in the upper subcutis near the dermosubcutaneous junction, communicates with the exterior by a duct. Proximal to the gland the duct is coiled, but thereafter it proceeds in a single direction up to the dermoepidermal junction. Within the epidermis, it again becomes coiled, but this is only seen to any extent where the epidermis is thick, for example in the soles of the feet (see Fig. 18.20).

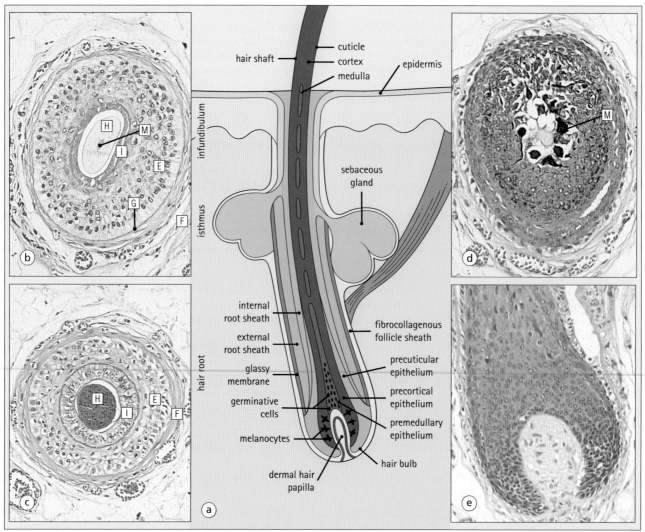

FIGURE 18.12 **Pilosebaceous apparatus.** (a) The general architecture of the pilosebaceous apparatus. The hair bulb is a collection of compact epithelial cells surrounding a vascularized fibrocollagenous dermal papilla, and produces the various components of the hair shaft (i.e. medulla, cortex and cuticle). In dark-haired people, abundant active melanocytes in the basal layer of the hair bulb supply melanin to the precortex cells; the medulla and cuticle are not pigmented. The outer cells of the hair bulb epithelium produce the internal root sheath, the middle layer of which contains numerous red-staining trichohyalin granules. The external root sheath is derived from the epidermis by downgrowth and is bound externally by a distinct homogeneous membrane: the glassy membrane. This separates it from the fibrocollagenous follicle sheath, which surrounds the entire follicle and also encloses the sebaceous glands as a thin, variably distinct layer. Attached to the fibrocollagenous follicle sheath at, or just below, the level of the sebaceous glands is the erector pili muscle, which extends obliquely upward from this lower attachment to its upper attachment in the papillary dermis. The lower parts of the hair shaft consist of partly keratinized cells in which the nuclei of the progenitor epithelium can still be seen, but higher up the hair is composed of anuclear hard compact keratin, which does not stain with eosin. (b) Transverse section through a hair follicle just below the sebaceous glands. The hair shaft (H) is anuclear and composed of non-staining hard keratin; a central medullary remnant (M) can be seen. The outer fibrocollagenous root sheath (F) and glassy membrane (G) around the external root sheath (E) are well formed, but the internal root sheath (I) is acellular and degenerate. (c) Transverse section through a hair follicle just above the hair bulb. The hair shaft (H) contains nuclear remnants and is strongly eosinophilic. The cellular internal root sheath (I) is well formed and contains eosinophilic trichohyalin granules. Note the external root sheath (E) and the outer fibrocollagenous root sheath (F). (d) Transverse section through a hair bulb showing melanocytes (M) supplying melanin to the precortex epithelium. (e) Longitudinal section through a hair bulb. There are no active melanocytes in this example.

Eccrine sweat glands are composed of two layers of cells: an inner layer of secretory cells and an outer flat layer of contractile myoepithelial cells which is bounded by a distinct, sometimes thick membrane. The dermal ducts consists of two layers of dark-staining cuboidal cells surrounding a distinct lumen, the surface of which is often strongly eosinophilic (Fig. 18.14).

Apocrine Glands

Apocrine glands produce a viscid, slightly milky secretion

External stimuli, such as fear, sexual excitement, etc. cause secretion from apocrine glands, the function of

FIGURE 18.13 **Sebaceous gland.** (a) Micrograph showing a sebaceous gland (G) opening through a narrow duct (D) into the hair follicle (HF). The sebum is formed by necrosis (N) of the lipid-packed cells of the gland. (b) A sebaceous gland at higher magnification showing the single layer of cuboidal or flat precursor cells (P) and the large sebaceous cells (S) distended with lipid droplets.

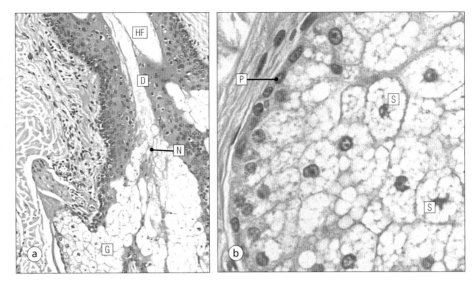

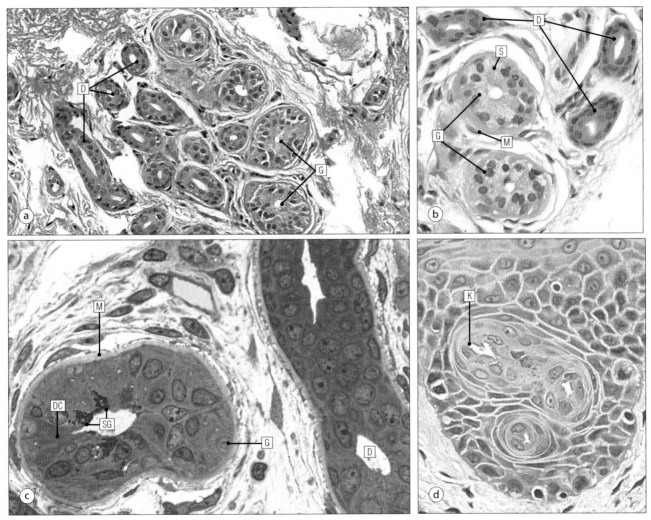

FIGURE 18.14 **Eccrine gland and duct.** (a) Micrograph showing eccrine glands (G) and ducts (D) in the deep dermis at low magnification. (b) High-power micrograph showing that the glands (G) are composed of pale-staining secretory cells (S) with an outer layer of indistinct myoepithelial cells (M). The ducts (D) have a more distinct double layer of dark-staining cells. (c) Thin epoxy resin section stained with toluidine blue showing that the gland (G) is composed of large, pale-staining glycogen-rich cells, some of which contain dark secretory granules (SG) and a smaller number of narrow darker-staining cells (DC) that secrete sialomucins. Eccrine glands are surrounded by a thick amorphous membrane (M) and their ducts (D) are lined internally by a homogeneous cuticle, which is composed of microvilli covered by an amorphous glycocalyx. (d) Micrograph showing intraepidermal portion of eccrine duct, which is spiral and is sometimes called the 'acrosyringium'. There is a single layer of cells lining the lumen, and two or three layers of outer cells. The lining cells develop small keratohyaline granules (K) and become keratinized where they emerge through the granular layer of the epidermis. The spiral course continues through the keratin layer and is most clearly seen in skin with a thick epidermis.

which is not known in humans; similar glands in mammals act as scent organs and produce scent for the delineation of territory and sexual attraction.

Apocrine glands develop as downgrowths of the epidermis and are scanty in humans but well developed in many other mammals. They are small and insignificant in childhood but become more prominent and probably functionally active after puberty.

In the human, apocrine glands are concentrated mainly in the perineal region, around the anus and genitalia, and in the axillae. Modified apocrine glands are found in the eyelids (**Moll's glands**), in the areolar skin around the nipple, and in the external auditory canal, where they form the **ceruminous glands** responsible for the production of ear wax.

Apocrine glands are composed of:
- A secretory glandular unit situated, like the eccrine gland, in the lower dermis or at the dermo-subcutaneous junction
- A more or less straight duct, which opens into a pilosebaceous unit near the surface, usually above the entrance of the sebaceous duct.

The secretory unit of an apocrine gland is composed of an inner layer of cuboidal epithelial cells and an outer layer of discontinuous flat cells, surrounded by basement membrane. It has a large lumen (Fig. 18.15). The duct resembles the eccrine duct (see Fig. 18.14), having a double layer of cuboidal epithelium.

Dermis

Dermis is the supporting tissue on which epidermis sits

In the dermis are located the epidermal appendages, blood supply, nerve supply and lymphatic drainage (Fig. 18.16). It is composed of:

- Fibroblasts, fibrocytes and their extracellular products (see p. 63)
- Collagen and elastic fibres
- Glycosaminoglycan-containing matrix
- Blood vessels and nerves
- Small numbers of macrophages, lymphocytes and mast cells.

Two distinct zones of dermis can usually be identified: an upper narrow papillary dermis, which is close to the dermoepidermal junction, and a thicker reticular dermis, between the papillary dermis and the subcutaneous adipose tissue.

Papillary dermis is paler than reticular dermis and contains less collagen and elastin, but more matrix. The thin collagen and elastin fibres are more randomly arranged, with a high proportion perpendicular to the skin surface. It contains small blood vessels of capillary size, fine nerve twigs and nerve endings (Fig. 18.17).

Reticular dermis forms the bulk of the dermis. It is composed of prominent broad bands of dense collagen with intervening long thick fibres of elastin, which usually run parallel to the skin surface. Within this tissue are the blood vessels, lymphatics and nerves of the skin.

The dermis contains two vascular plexuses

The main blood supply to the skin is located within the dermis and arises from larger vessels in the subcutaneous fat. Two distinct plexuses can be identified (see Fig. 18.1):
- A deep vascular plexus in the lower reticular dermis close to its border with the subcutis
- A superficial vascular plexus in the upper reticular dermis close to its junction with the papillary dermis.

Loops of small vessels from the superficial vascular plexus run up into the papillary dermis, with small capillaries lying close to the epidermal basement membrane. No blood vessels penetrate the epidermis.

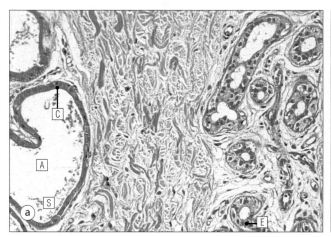
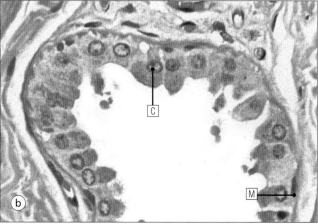

FIGURE 18.15 **Apocrine gland.** (a) Micrograph showing part of an actively secreting apocrine gland (A) from axillary skin, with part of an eccrine gland (E) for comparison. The apocrine gland has an inner layer of cuboidal epithelial cells (C) with markedly eosinophilic cytoplasm and an outer layer of discontinuous flat cells, which are thought to be myoepithelial. It is surrounded by a prominent eosinophilic basement membrane. The lumen is large, and a faintly pink homogeneous secretion (S) may be seen within it. (b) High-power view showing the roughly cuboidal eosinophilic lining cells (C) and the irregular luminal surface resulting from the secretory process, in which fragments of secretion-containing cytoplasm are 'pinched off' into the lumen. Flat myoepithelial cells (M) are present but inconspicuous.

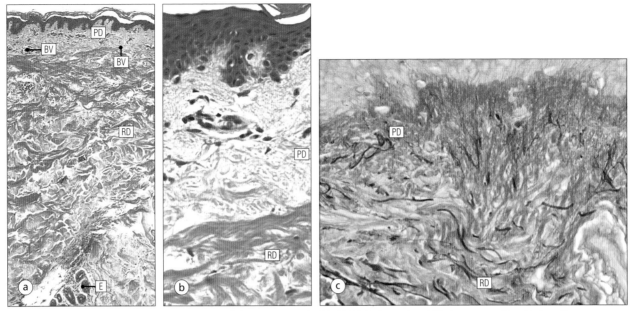

FIGURE 18.16 **Dermis.** (a) Low-power view of dermis stained with H&E. It is eosinophilic because of its high collagen content; the papillary dermis (PD), which contains less collagen, is paler. An eccrine unit (E) can be seen in the deeper part of the reticular dermis (RD). Note the concentration of small blood vessels (BV) at the junction between the papillary dermis and the densely collagenous reticular dermis. (b) High-power micrograph showing the different natures of the loose pale-staining papillary dermis (PD) and the more densely collagenous reticular dermis (RD). (c) Elastic van Gieson-stained section of upper dermis demonstrating elastic (black) and collagen (red) fibres, showing the difference between papillary dermis (PD) in which both collagen and elastin are fine and vertically orientated, and reticular dermis (RD) in which the collagen and elastin fibres are thicker and coarser and are mainly arranged longitudinally.

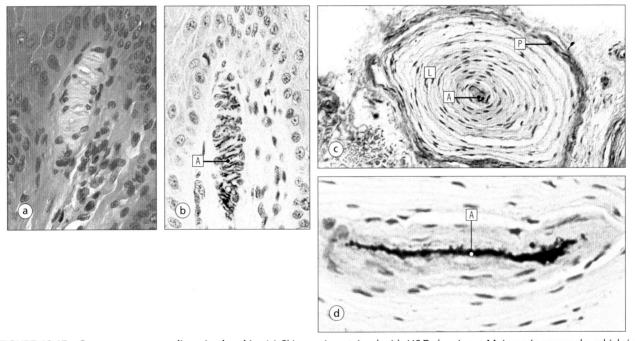

FIGURE 18.17 **Common nerve endings in the skin.** (a) Skin section stained with H&E showing a Meissner's corpuscle, which is an elongated oval body. Meissner's corpuscles are arranged vertically in the dermal papillae of hairless skin, particularly in fingers and toes, but also around lips and nipples. Internally, Meissner's corpuscles are composed of spirally arranged cells surrounded by a thin fibrocollagenous capsule. In H&E sections, the most commonly seen cells are flattened Schwann cells (see p. 99), the axons not being visible. (b) Meissner's corpuscle stained by an immunoperoxidase method for neurofilament protein (NFP) to demonstrate the spirally arranged axon (A). (c) Micrograph showing a Pacinian corpuscle in subcutaneous fat from the fingertip demonstrated by an immunoperoxidase method for NFP. It is a large, loosely laminated structure with a central core (axon, A) surrounded by concentrically arranged lamellae (L), which are modified Schwann cells separated from each other by fluid-filled spaces. The lamellae are more tightly packed peripherally and form a dense pseudocapsule (P). (d) A Pacinian corpuscle in longitudinal section stained by an immunoperoxidase method for NFP to show its longitudinally running central axon (A).

The dermis contains many arteriovenous anastomotic channels, including highly specialized shunts (**glomus bodies**), which are found mainly in the fingertips (see Fig. 18.22). Blood flow variation within the dermis is important to the skin's function as a thermoregulatory organ.

The skin appendages are supplied by branches from vessels connecting the deep and superficial vascular plexuses.

The dermis contains numerous nerves and nerve endings

The nerve supply of the skin is located in the dermis and comprises:

- A rich, non-myelinated supply derived from the sympathetic autonomic nervous system which controls the skin appendages and vascular flow
- An afferent myelinated and non-myelinated system, which detects cutaneous sensation.

Detection of cutaneous sensation is by variably specialized nerve endings (Fig. 18.17), the most important of which are:

- **Free nerve endings** (myelinated and unmyelinated), which detect pain (and its minor variant, itch) and temperature
- **Pacinian corpuscles** – encapsulated nerve endings with a characteristic structure – detect pressure and possibly vibration, and are usually found in the deep dermis or subcutaneous fat of the palms and soles
- **Meissner's corpuscles** – structured nerve endings confined to the dermal papillae – are most numerous on the feet and hands, and detect touch
- **Merkel cells** and their nerve attachments (see Fig. 18.10) are slowly adapting touch receptors.

Subcutaneous Tissue

Subcutaneous tissue is composed largely of adipose tissue

The adipose tissue in subcutaneous tissue is separated by fibrocollagenous septa and contains the main blood vessels and nerves from which the overlying dermis is supplied (Fig. 18.18). It acts as an effective heat insulator, food store and shock absorber.

Subcutaneous tissue may contain extensions of skin structures, for example:

- In the scalp it contains the lower parts of the long hair follicles
- Some apocrine and eccrine glands.

Features of Skin in Different Sites

The skin shows marked variation in structure at different sites

Most of the skin covering the body is protected by clothing and is not excessively traumatized; it is not particu-

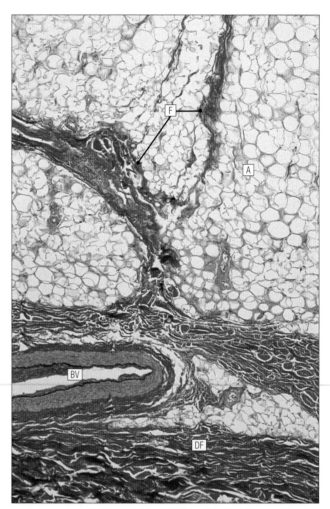

FIGURE 18.18 **Subcutaneous tissue.** Micrograph of subcutaneous tissue from the scalp. It is composed largely of adipose tissue (A) intersected by vertically running bands of fibrocollagenous tissue (F) that extend down from the deep dermis. In this example, the fibrous septa extend through the full thickness of subcutaneous tissues to join the dense fibrocollagenous layer (DF) covering the periosteum of the underlying skull. Subcutaneous tissue contains the major blood vessels (BV) from which the blood supply of the dermis arises.

larly specialized. Thus, skin on the back, abdomen, thighs and arms (Fig. 18.19) has:

- A thin epidermis producing only small amounts of loosely packed keratin
- A poorly-formed rete ridge system
- Small numbers of hair follicles producing fine hairs (large follicles and coarser hairs in men)
- Variable numbers of eccrine glands.

Sole. In contrast to the skin of the back, abdomen, thighs and arms, the skin of the sole (Fig. 18.20) is modified to withstand constant trauma. It has:

- A thick epidermis, which is covered by a thick layer of compact keratin
- A well-developed rete ridge system to prevent epidermal separation from shearing stress
- No hair follicles
- Abundant eccrine glands and ducts.

Scalp. The characteristic feature of the scalp is the presence of tightly packed hair follicles with their associated sebaceous glands (Fig. 18.21). In straight-haired people, the follicles are almost vertical, but in curly-haired people they are oblique, the degree of curliness depending on the degree of obliquity.

Fingertip. Fingertip skin shows two structural modifications: one to minimize damage from shearing stress, the other because of its role as a tactile sensory organ (Fig. 18.22). Thus, the skin in this region is characterized by:

- A thick epidermis with thick compact protective keratin
- A well-developed rete ridge system

- Numerous Meissner's corpuscles in the dermal papillae (see Fig. 18.17)
- Pacinian corpuscles in the dermis and subcutis (see Fig. 18.17)
- Specialized arteriovenous shunts (glomus bodies)
- Abundant eccrine sweat glands and ducts.

Axilla. The skin in the axilla and groin is similar, possibly because of our quadruped origins. Its most important features are:

- An abundance of highly active apocrine glands
- Numerous oblique hair follicles
- Numerous eccrine glands
- Thin epidermis (Fig. 18.23).

 PRACTICAL HISTOLOGY

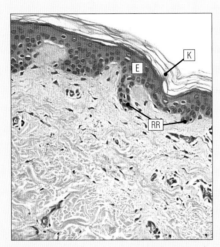

FIGURE 18.19 **Thin skin.** Micrograph showing the thin epidermal (E) and keratin (K) layers of thin skin, which is also characterized by a poorly-developed rete ridge system (RR), small numbers of hair follicles, and variable numbers of eccrine glands.

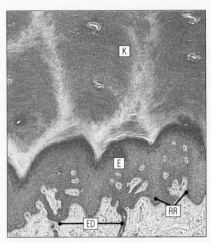

FIGURE 18.20 **Thick sole skin.** Micrograph showing the thick epidermal (E) and keratin (K) layers of thick skin, which is also characterized by a well-developed rete ridge system (RR) and numerous eccrine glands and ducts (ED).

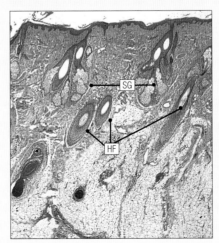

FIGURE 18.21 **Scalp skin.** Micrograph showing the tightly packed pilosebaceous units of scalp skin. Note the sebaceous glands (SG) and hair follicles (HF).

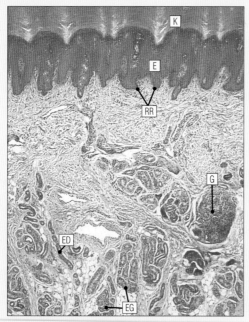

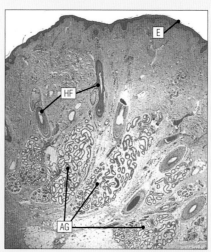

FIGURE 18.23 **Axillary skin.** Micrograph showing the abundant apocrine glands (AG), oblique hair follicles (HF) and thin epidermis (E) of axillary skin.

FIGURE 18.22 **Fingertip skin.** Micrograph showing the thick epidermis (E) and well-developed rete ridge system (RR) of fingertip skin, covered by thick compact protective keratin (K). Note the glomus body (G) and the abundant eccrine sweat glands (EG) and their ducts (ED).

Breast

Breasts develop as downgrowths from the epidermis along a line (milk line or streak) which runs obliquely from the axilla toward the groin on each side. In humans normally only one breast develops on each side, but occasionally an accessory breast develops, though only the nipple component persists after birth.

Nipple

> **Breast secretions emerge to the surface at the nipple**

At the tip of the nipple are the 12–20 small openings of the large nipple ducts (Fig. 18.24) arranged in a ring.

The nipple is a round, raised area of modified skin with a slightly convoluted epidermis, which shows increased melanin pigmentation after the first pregnancy.

The nipple is surrounded by the **areola**, which is modified skin containing large sebaceous units that form small nodular elevations (**Montgomery's tubercles**). The areola also shows increased melanin pigmentation after the first pregnancy.

Breast Development

> **Full development of the female breast occurs at puberty**

The nipple and its simple system of ducts is present at birth, but full development of the epithelial downgrowth does not occur until puberty, and then usually only in females.

At puberty, and under the influence of increasing oestrogen secretion:
- The breasts increase in bulk, due initially to an increase in adipose tissue
- The ductular system of the nipple becomes more complex, with branches extending into the adipose tissue (Fig. 18.25).

Normally, the male breast remains a rudimentary system of simple nipple ducts with a small amount of surrounding fibrocollagenous tissue. Occasionally, the male breast enlarges at puberty owing to an extension of the rudimentary duct system and an increase in periductal fibrous tissue. This is called **gynaecomastia** and is illustrated in Figure 18.26.

The growth and activity of the female breast are entirely hormone dependent. Continued oestrogen

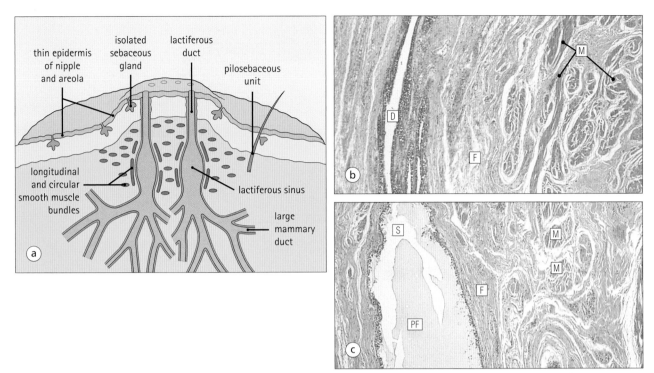

FIGURE 18.24 **Nipple.** (a) There are 12–20 openings arranged in a ring on the surface of the nipple, each being lined by keratinized stratified squamous epithelium. In the inactive, non-lactating breast they are normally plugged by keratin. Each opening is the site of emergence of a single lactiferous duct, which is lined by a two-layered epithelium, the basal layer being myoepithelial cells. Each lactiferous duct receives large mammary ducts, and there is a dilation, the lactiferous sinus, shortly afterwards. The support tissue consists of fibroadipose tissue containing numerous longitudinal and circular smooth muscle bundles. (b) Micrograph of a lactiferous duct (D) of the nipple, with surrounding fibrocollagenous stroma (F) and longitudinal and circular smooth muscle (M). (c) Micrograph of a part of a lactiferous sinus (S) just below the nipple. The sinus contains homogeneous proteinaceous fluid (PF) and is surrounded by fibrocollagenous stroma (F) and muscle (M).

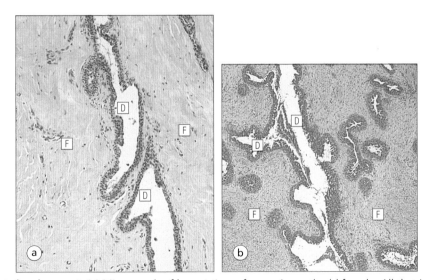

FIGURE 18.25 **Breast development.** (a) Micrograph of breast tissue from a 4-month-old female. All that is present is a system of scarcely branching nipple ducts (D) embedded in fibrocollagenous tissue (F). (b) Micrograph of breast tissue from an 11-year-old girl at the onset of puberty. The ductular system (D) is beginning to proliferate and produce branches, and the surrounding fibrocollagenous supporting tissue (F) is actively increasing in bulk.

CLINICAL EXAMPLE
GYNAECOMASTIA

Pronounced development of the male breast (Fig. 18.26) is called gynaecomastia. It occurs under the influence of excess oestrogen secretion, which may be either endogenous (e.g. at puberty) or exogenous (e.g. stilboestrol treatment for prostatic cancer).

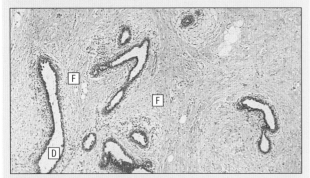

FIGURE 18.26 **Gynaecomastia.** Gynaecomastia is characterized by proliferation and branching of the mammary duct system, which often dilates (D), and by an increase in the periductal fibrocollagenous tissue (F).

secretion after the onset of puberty leads to progressive enlargement and complexity of the duct system.

The parenchyma of the breast is composed of 12–20 distinct lobes

Each lobe consists of a duct system, with its own separate opening in the nipple, embedded in adipose tissue containing fibrocollagenous septa. Particularly prominent septa separate the individual lobes and are attached to overlying skin by fibrocollagenous bands, which are sometimes called 'Cooper's suspensory ligaments'. On their deep surface the septa are attached to the fascia overlying the pectoralis muscle.

Mammary Duct and Lobule System

Each lobe of the breast is a system of ever-branching ducts that penetrate deep into the fibroadipose tissue of the breast.

Each duct is lined by columnar or cuboidal epithelium, with a continuous surface layer of epithelial cells with oval nuclei and an outer discontinuous layer of myoepithelial cells, which have clear cytoplasm.

Each duct is surrounded by loose fibrocollagenous support tissue containing a rich capillary network. Elastic fibres are present within this fibrous sheath in all but the smallest, most peripheral branches.

The duct system terminates in an ovoid mammary lobule

The branching duct system ends in a cluster of blind-ending terminal ductules, each cluster and its feeding duct comprising a **mammary lobule**.

KEY FACTS
BREAST

- The functional unit of the breast is a lobule surrounded by a specialized stroma
- Lobule epithelium is hormone sensitive and undergoes proliferation in pregnancy
- Myoepithelial cells surround each lobule and express secreted milk
- Milk is transported along duct systems to the nipple.

The terminal ducts and lobules are embedded in a loose fibrous support tissue, which is rich in capillaries and also contains a few lymphocytes, macrophages and mast cells. This tissue is surrounded by a more dense fibrocollagenous support tissue intermingled with adipose tissue (Fig. 18.27).

The structure of the mammary lobule undergoes minor transient structural change during the menstrual cycle

In the second half of the menstrual cycle, there is gradually increasing progesterone and oestrogen secretion by the corpus luteum produced in the ovary after ovulation (see p. 352). Progesterone stimulates proliferation of the epithelial cells in terminal ductules; they also become enlarged and begin to show evidence of early secretory activity. In addition, fluid and glycosaminoglycans accumulate in the loose intralobular fibrocollagenous stroma. These changes lead to a slight enlargement in the breasts, often accompanied by a feeling of discomfort. If fertilization occurs, the ovarian corpus luteum persists and enlarges, secreting ever-increasing amounts of progesterone, which stimulates the continued proliferation and secretory activity in the terminal ductules of the breast lobule. However, if fertilization does not occur, the progesterone levels fall dramatically at the end of the cycle and the structure of the breast lobule reverts to normal, with cessation of the early secretory activity.

Breast Changes in Pregnancy

Breast structure changes early in pregnancy

The vascularity and melanin pigmentation of the nipple and areola increase and the mammary lobules enlarge by hyperplastic proliferation of the terminal ductule epithelium, with some vacuolation appearing in the luminal epithelial cells.

By the second trimester, there is evidence of luminal cell secretion, which is copious by the third trimester and accumulates within the hyperplastic terminal ducts (Fig. 18.28).

With this expansion of the lobular units, there is an accompanying increase in the loose lobular support tissue and inflammatory cells. At term, and throughout lactation, the hyperplastic lobular units are distended by their lipid-rich proteinaceous secretion (milk).

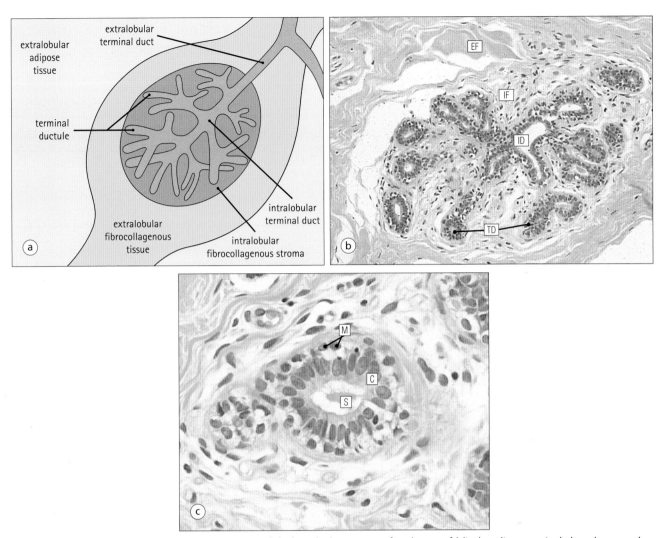

FIGURE 18.27 **Mammary lobule.** (a) A mammary lobule, which consists of a cluster of blind-ending terminal ductules together with the drainage duct system (extralobular and intralobular terminal ducts). Some lobules are located in the dense fibrocollagenous tissue of the breast, whereas others are in adipose tissue. (b) Micrograph of a typical mammary lobule embedded in fibrocollagenous tissue. Note the difference between the intralobular (IF) and extralobular (EF) fibrocollagenous tissue. In this inactive lobule, the epithelium of the terminal ductules (TD) is identical to that of the intralobular terminal duct (ID). The extralobular terminal duct is not visible. (c) High-power micrograph showing the epithelium of the intralobular terminal ductules. Essentially two-layered, the inner layer varies between a cuboidal and a low columnar pattern (C), whereas the outer layer consists of prominent myoepithelial cells (M). Note the minute amount of secretion (S) in the lumen of the duct resulting from menstrual cycle hormone secretion.

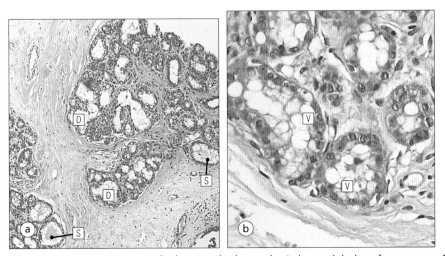

FIGURE 18.28 **Breast in pregnancy.** (a) Micrograph showing the hyperplastic breast lobules of pregnancy. The intralobular terminal ductules (D) are increased in size and complexity, and their lumina are distended by secretion (S) from the lining epithelium. (b) Micrograph showing clear vacuoles (V) containing lipid-rich secretion forming on the luminal aspect of terminal ductule lining epithelium.

Steroid hormones can only act on cells that bear receptors specific to the particular hormone; these receptors are binding proteins which link with the hormone and transmit the steroid signal to alter the activity of genes in the nucleus. The function of the breast is dependent on the steroid hormones oestrogen and progesterone, and receptors for both are present in mammary epithelium, particularly in the epithelium of the terminal ductules of the lobule (Fig. 18.29).

In breast cancer, the persistence of oestrogen and progesterone receptors in the tumour cells indicates the likely responsiveness of the tumour to some chemotherapeutic treatments, particularly antioestrogens.

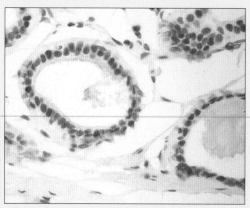

FIGURE 18.29 **Oestrogen receptors in lobule epithelium.** This photomicrograph demonstrates a brown positive immunocytochemical staining in the nuclei of lobular epithelium, indicating the presence of oestrogen receptor.

The breast only reaches its full functional activity during pregnancy and lactation

Functional maturation of the breast in pregnancy is under the influence of pituitary and ovarian hormones, which are secreted in high concentrations during pregnancy and throughout breastfeeding.

When breastfeeding ceases, the breast returns to its normal or resting state by gradual involution over a period of some months. The luminal cells return to their former size without cytoplasmic vacuolation and the lobular support tissue returns to its normal proportions.

Repeated exposure of the mammary lobules to varying oestrogen and progesterone secretions during numerous menstrual cycles can lead to disproportionate growth of various components and distortion of the normal architecture. Common changes are:

- Increased duct and ductular tissue (adenosis)
- Increased fibrocollagenous support tissues (fibrosis)
- Dilation of the larger mammary ducts.

Such changes when they occur are most severe in multigravid women and cause increased nodulation of the breast tissue, which is sometimes associated with cyst formation (Fig. 18.30). This is the most common disorder of the breast and is variably called 'fibroadenosis, cystic mammary dysplasia, benign mammary dysplasia or fibrocystic disease' of the breast.

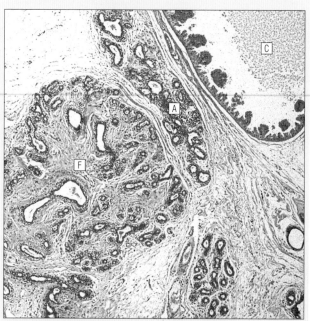

FIGURE 18.30 **Fibroadenosis.** Micrograph of section of breast showing the features of fibroadenosis: fibrosis (F), adenosis (A) and cyst formation (C).

Sometimes there is residual increased collagen in the involuting lobular support tissue, and this can lead to progressive distortion of the mammary lobules and persistent cystic dilation of some of the ducts.

CLINICAL EXAMPLE
CARCINOMA OF THE BREAST

The epithelial component of the extralobular mammary ducts, the intralobular mammary ducts and the terminal ductules may undergo cancerous change to produce one of the most important and common cancers in women, breast cancer. Cancers originating in the terminal ductules are called 'lobular carcinomas'; those from the ducts are called 'ductal carcinomas' (Fig. 18.31).

The breast is well equipped with small blood and lymphatic vessels, so spread of the cancer away from its site of origin in the breast is common and can lead to a poor outlook. Spread along lymphatics is usually to the axillary group of lymph nodes on the side of the affected breast, producing metastatic deposits in the nodes (see Fig. 8.14), whereas spread via the bloodstream usually occurs at a later stage, metastatic carcinoma being deposited in many organs, particularly the lungs and bones.

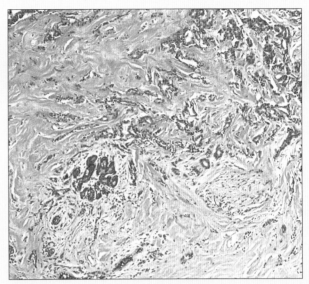

FIGURE 18.31 **Mammary carcinoma.** Micrograph showing the features of a typical carcinoma derived from mammary ducts. The cells have broken through into the surrounding fibroadipose tissue to produce an invasive carcinoma.

PRACTICAL HISTOLOGY

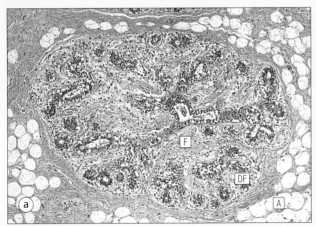
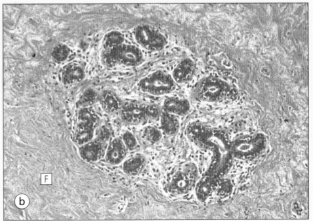

FIGURE 18.32 **Breast.** (a) Micrograph showing normal breast tissue from a 23-year-old woman. At the centre is a breast lobule in which the system of terminal ducts and ductules is embedded in loose intralobular fibrocollagenous stroma (F). There is a narrow surrounding zone of dense extralobular fibrocollagenous support tissue (DF), outside which is the soft adipose tissue (A) that forms the bulk of the breast. (b) Micrograph showing normal breast tissue from a 43-year-old woman. As women age, the amount of fibrocollagenous tissue (F) in the breast increases, replacing some of the adipose tissue. The mammary lobules become enclosed in dense collagen.

For online review questions, please visit
https://studentconsult.inkling.com.

? END OF CHAPTER REVIEW

True/False Answers to the MCQS, as Well as Case Answers, Can be Found in the Appendix in the Back of the Book.

1. **The basal layer of the epidermis**
   (a) Is responsible for the constant production of keratinocytes
   (b) Is composed of cuboidal or columnar keratinocytes
   (c) Is attached to the basement membrane by desmosomes
   (d) Contains scattered melanocytes
   (e) Contains keratinosomes

2. **Melanocytes**
   (a) Are pigmented because of the melanin they contain
   (b) Have long cytoplasmic processes which extend between keratinocytes
   (c) Are greatly increased in number in dark-skinned races
   (d) Contain characteristic spherical premelanosomes
   (e) Are neural derived and also act as mechanoreceptors

3. **In the skin appendages**
   (a) Sebaceous gland units usually open directly on to the skin surface
   (b) Apocrine glands secrete sweat
   (c) Eccrine glands are particularly frequent on the palms and soles
   (d) The internal root sheath of the hair follicle produces the hair shaft
   (e) Erector pili muscles control the position of the hair shafts

4. **The mammary lobule**
   (a) Is embedded in loose fibrous support tissue
   (b) Contains terminal ductules which are the main secretory component
   (c) Terminal ductule epithelium cells show vacuolation in the second half of the menstrual cycle
   (d) Contains myoepithelial cells which lie beneath the terminal ductule epithelium
   (e) Undergoes structural and functional atrophy after the menopause

CASE 18.1   A MAN WITH BLISTERS

A 62-year-old man is seen in the clinic because he has developed a tense blistering skin rash, most evident in the flexures of the arms. A skin biopsy is performed, which shows that the blistering is based at the epidermal–dermal junction, associated with an infiltrate of eosinophils.

Immunofluorescence staining shows a linear band of deposits of autoantibody IgG and C3 at the dermoepidermal junction. A blood sample from the patient shows circulating antibodies, which are shown to bind to the epidermal–dermal junction of a normal skin sample.

A diagnosis of bullous pemphigoid is made, an autoimmune condition in which autoantibodies are directed against a normal component of the hemidesmosome.

Q. Describe the structural and functional background to this case. Focus on the structural features of the epidermis that facilitate its anchorage to the dermis and how disruption of hemidesmosomes predisposes to blistering. Speculate which other structural defects may lead to blistering skin diseases.

CASE 18.2   A WOMAN WITH A LUMP IN THE BREAST

A 46-year-old woman presents to her doctor with an intermittently tender lump in the breast. Examination shows a firm, irregular mobile lump in the lower medial quadrant of the left breast approximately 2 cm in diameter. There is no attachment to other structures and no enlargement of local lymph nodes. Further investigation by imaging and histological sampling is planned.

Q. Describe the structural and histological background to this case. Concentrate on normal structures in the breast that may be the origin of neoplastic growth.

Chapter 19

Special Senses

Introduction

A vital function of the nervous system is the gathering of sensory information

Sensory information is derived from a variety of specialized sensory nerve endings. These include:
- Sensory endings in the skin to detect touch (fine touch, pressure), pain and temperature (see Chapter 18)
- Tendon endings and muscle spindles to detect movement and position of the limbs
- Chemoreceptive organs, such as the carotid body
- Sensory endings on the tongue to detect taste
- Sensory endings in the olfactory mucosa to detect smell.

In addition, information is obtained by the specialized sensory organs, the eye and the ear; the ear and the vestibular system detect sound, acceleration and position and the eye perceives light.

Ear

The ear is divided into the external ear, middle ear and inner ear

The external ear comprises the **pinna** and **external auditory canal**. The pinna is composed of elastic cartilage covered by hair-bearing skin. The external auditory canal is lined by hair-bearing skin. Within its subcutaneous tissues are wax-secreting **ceruminous glands**, which are modified sebaceous glands. The outer two-thirds of the canal is surrounded by elastic cartilage in continuity with the pinna; the inner third is surrounded by the temporal bone of the skull.

The middle ear is separated from the external ear by the tympanic membrane

The **tympanic membrane** marks the boundary between the external ear and the cavity of the middle ear, which is also termed the **tympanic cavity** (Fig. 19.1).

The tympanic membrane is a three-layered structure:
- The outer aspect is covered by stratified squamous epithelium
- The central portion is composed of fibrocollagenous support tissue containing numerous elastic fibres to provide mechanical strength

- The inner portion is lined by a low cuboidal epithelium which is continuous with that lining the rest of the middle ear.

The middle ear transmits sound vibrations to the inner ear

The middle ear cavity is lined by a low cuboidal epithelium and contains three auditory ossicles, the **incus**, **malleus** and **stapes**. These are:
- Composed of compact bone
- Articulated by synovial joints (see Chapter 13)
- Covered externally by the same low cuboidal epithelium that lines the inner ear.

Two small skeletal muscles, the stapedius and the tensor tympani, are associated with the ossicles and damp motion between the bones, which occurs in response to loud noise.

The middle ear cavity communicates directly with air-filled spaces in the mastoid bone (**mastoid sinuses**), which are lined by low cuboidal or flattened squamous epithelium.

The auditory (Eustachian) tube equalizes pressure in the middle ear cavity

The **auditory tube** extends from the middle ear cavity to the nasopharynx and is lined by ciliated epithelium similar to that of the respiratory tract. Its function is to equilibrate pressure between the middle ear cavity and the atmosphere.

Normally, the auditory tube is collapsed, but it is opened by movement of muscles in the nasopharynx, such as occurs with swallowing or yawning.

The inner ear is a series of fluid-filled sacs encased in bone

The inner ear consists of fluid-filled sacs (**membranous labyrinth**) that lie in cavities in the temporal bone of the skull (**bony or osseous labyrinth**).

The membranous labyrinth comprises the **cochlear duct**, the **saccule**, the **utricle** and **semicircular canals** and the **endolymphatic sac and duct**, the walls of which are composed of sheets of fibrocollagenous support tissue lined by a flat epithelium. These sacs are filled with a fluid called **endolymph** and have epithelial and sensory specializations to detect position and sound.

The osseous labyrinth is composed of three cavities: the vestibule, the semicircular canals and the cochlea,

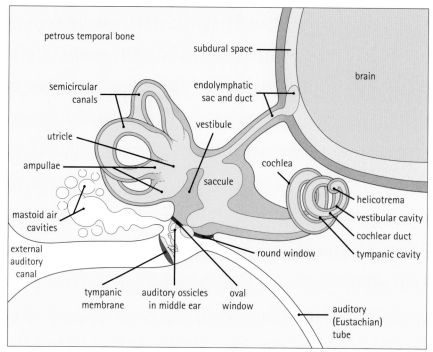

FIGURE 19.1 **Anatomy of the ear.** The ear consists of the external ear, middle ear and inner ear. The inner third of the external auditory canal of the external ear is surrounded by the temporal bone, and the middle ear and inner ear are contained within cavities in the temporal bone. The middle ear is an air-filled cavity containing the auditory ossicles. It is connected to the nasopharynx by the auditory (Eustachian) tube and is in direct continuity with the mastoid air cells. The inner ear is a fluid-filled cavity divided into three main spaces (semicircular canal space, vestibule and cochlea). Within the inner ear are a series of interconnecting fluid-filled sacs (semicircular canals, utricle, saccule and cochlear duct). The endolymphatic duct runs from the membranous sacs to the subdural space around the brain.

which are lined by periosteum and filled with fluid called **perilymph**.

Movement is detected in the inner ear by mechanoreceptors

Mechanoreceptors or **hair cells** are specialized epithelial cells bearing a highly organized system of microvilli (**stereocilia**) on their apical surface. Deflection of the microvilli causes electrical depolarization of the hair cell membrane, which is transmitted to the central nervous system by the connecting axons of sensory nerve cells (Fig. 19.2).

Patches of hair cells are located in three sites:
- Within the vestibular apparatus in the ampullae of the semicircular canals to detect acceleration
- Within the macula of the utricle and saccule to perceive the direction of gravity and static position
- Within the organ of Corti of the cochlea to detect sound vibration.

At each site, the hair cell microvilli are embedded in a gelatinous matrix, which moves according to the stimulus it is detecting. Movement of the microvilli towards the tallest row excites (depolarizes) the hair cell membrane, whereas movement towards the shortest row inhibits (hyperpolarizes) it.

Hair cells are arranged in different parts of the membranous labyrinth (Fig. 19.3) in order to sense movement generated by different causes.

Support cells surround the hair cells and are anchored to them at their apex by occluding junctions. These junctions maintain ionic gradients between the endolymph and the extracellular fluid around the cells, the gradients being reversed on depolarization.

Sound is detected in the inner ear by the organ of Corti in the cochlear duct

The **cochlear duct** is a blind-ended tubular diverticulum filled with endolymph. It makes two and three-quarter turns within the spiral-shaped bony cochlea in the temporal bone, and is compressed between two other tubular spaces, the **vestibular** and **tympanic cavities**, which are filled with perilymph (Fig. 19.4).

Within the cochlear duct is the **organ of Corti**, which is a special adaptation of the epithelial cells lining the cochlear duct and detects sound vibration (Fig. 19.5).

Gravity and static position are detected by hair cells in the macula of the utricle and the macula of the saccule

The macula of the utricle lies in the horizontal plane, whereas the macula of the saccule lies in the vertical plane at right-angles to the macula of the utricle (see Fig. 19.3).

Each macula is histologically identical and is composed of the following three cell types (Fig. 19.6):

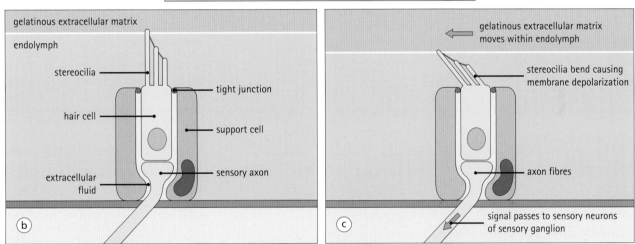

FIGURE 19.2 **Hair cell microvilli.** (a) The apical surface of each hair cell bears a highly organized system of microvilli (stereocilia), which are arranged as three parallel rows in a V- or W-shaped pattern. The height of the microvilli progressively decreases from the back to the front of the hair cell to form a so-called 'organ-pipe' arrangement. Fine filaments link individual microvilli from each row, with the tips of the shorter microvilli being coupled to the shafts of the taller microvilli behind. Whereas the hair cell is rigidly fixed in place by support cells, the tips of the tallest row of microvilli are embedded in a gelatinous extracellular matrix, which is free to move within the fluid cavities of the inner ear or vestibular system. (b) Hair cells are supported by adjacent cells and are in contact with the axon of a sensory nerve. The support cells are anchored to the hair cells by occluding junctions. The stereocilia are embedded in a gelatinous matrix. (c) Movement of the gelatinous matrix deflects the stereocilia, causing membrane depolarization of the hair cell, which is relayed to the central nervous system via the axon of a sensory nerve. Hair cells are arranged in different patterns in the cochlea and vestibular apparatus to detect acceleration (movement), gravity (position) or sound (hearing).

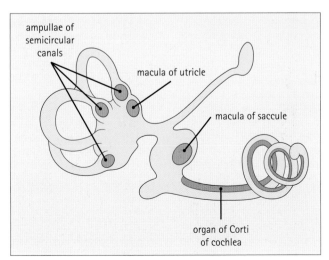

FIGURE 19.3 **Distribution of hair cells in the membranous labyrinth.** The hair cells are arranged in patches in the ampullae of the semicircular canals to detect acceleration, in the macula of the utricle and saccule to perceive gravity direction and static position, and in the organ of Corti of the cochlea to detect sound vibration.

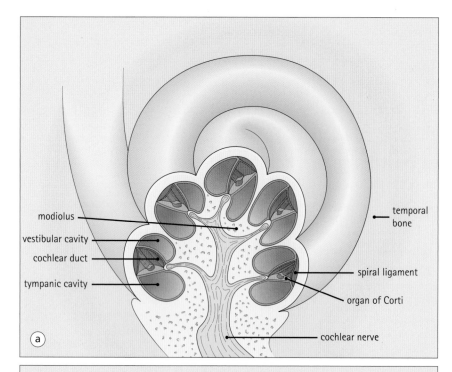

modiolus
vestibular cavity
cochlear duct
tympanic cavity

temporal bone
spiral ligament
organ of Corti
cochlear nerve

(a)

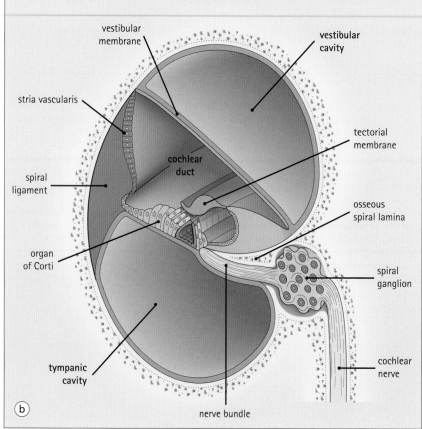

vestibular membrane
stria vascularis
spiral ligament
organ of Corti
tympanic cavity

vestibular cavity
tectorial membrane
cochlear duct
osseous spiral lamina
spiral ganglion
cochlear nerve
nerve bundle

(b)

FIGURE 19.4 **Cochlea.** (a) The cochlea of the osseous labyrinth contains three spaces, the vestibular cavity, the cochlear duct and the tympanic cavity. These spaces are wound in a spiral within the temporal bone. The central spiral of bone within the cochlea is called the 'modiolus'. The vestibular cavity and the tympanic cavity contain perilymph continuous with that in the vestibule (see Fig. 19.1), whereas the cochlear duct, which is continuous with and part of the membranous labyrinth, is filled with endolymph. At the apex of the cochlea, the vestibular and tympanic cavities connect at an opening termed the 'helicotrema'. The cochlear nerve emerges from the base of the cochlea and carries signals to the brain. (b) Shown here is a section through the cochlea. The vestibular membrane (Reissner's membrane) consists of two layers of flattened epithelium separated by a basement membrane, one cell layer being in continuity with the cells lining the vestibular cavity and the other in continuity with the cells lining the cochlear duct. The cells are held together by well-developed occluding junctions to maintain different electrolyte concentrations between the endolymph and the perilymph. The stria vascularis is a specialized area of epithelium with a rich vascular supply in the lateral wall of the cochlear duct. Many of the cells here have ultrastructural features indicating an ion transport function, and it is thought that they secrete endolymph. The basilar membrane is thicker than the vestibular membrane and consists of collagen fibres as well as a basement membrane. On one side it is covered by cells lining the tympanic cavity, and on the other by specialized cells lining the cochlear duct. Medially, the basilar membrane is continuous with the organ of Corti, which is a specialized area of support cells and sensory hair cells subserving hearing (see Fig. 19.5). The organ of Corti is supported by a spur of bone called the 'osseous spiral lamina'. Laterally, the basilar membrane is attached to the spiral ligament, which is a mass of tissue developed from the endosteum of the surrounding bone. Neurons of the spiral ganglion are present adjacent to the osseous spiral lamina.

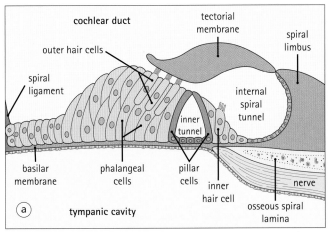

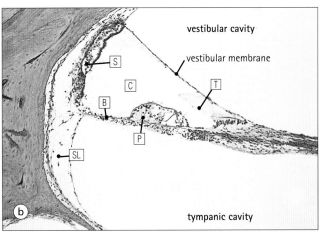

FIGURE 19.5 **Organ of Corti.** (a) The organ of Corti is composed of epithelial support cells and sensory hair cells. Medially, it rests on the rigid bony osseous spiral lamina; laterally it is located on the deformable basilar membrane. There are two groups of hair cells, an inner group and an outer group, which are separated by a small opening at the end of the osseous spiral lamina termed the inner tunnel (tunnel of Corti). The inner group are smaller and rounder than the outer group and arranged as a single row along the cochlea. The outer group are tall and thin and arranged in three to five parallel rows, depending on the position in the length of the cochlea. The hair cells are surrounded by epithelial support cells, the inner hair cells being completely surrounded, whereas the outer hair cells are enclosed only at their extreme apex and basal portions, leaving a bare mid-zone in contact with extracellular fluid. The microvilli of the outer hair cells are attached to a sheet of gelatinous extracellular matrix braced by filamentous proteins (tectorial membrane), but those of the inner hair cells are free. Axons make synaptic contact with the hair cells and run to the spiral ganglion. The tectorial membrane is secreted by epithelial cells (interdental cells). There are several classes of support cell in the organ of Corti. Pillar cells contain abundant scaffolding microtubules, and surround and support the triangular cavity (inner tunnel) at the level of the lip of the osseous spiral lamina. In contrast, phalangeal cells support the hair cells and are attached to them by occluding junctions at their apices, thus isolating the basal membrane of hair cells from the endolymph and maintaining electrochemical gradients. (b) Micrograph of the organ of Corti. Note the tectorial membrane (T), the mass of phalangeal cells bearing the hair cells (P), the basilar membrane (B), and the stria vascularis (S) on the spiral ligament (SL) within the cochlear duct (C).

ADVANCED CONCEPT
DETECTION OF SOUND IN THE INNER EAR

Sound waves cause vibration of the tympanic membrane, which is then transmitted to the oval window membrane via the auditory ossicles.

Pressure waves are thence transmitted to the perilymph of the vestibular cavity, causing the vestibular and basilar membranes to bow inward towards the tympanic cavity, and to the round window, which bows outward.

Because the tectorial membrane remains relatively rigid, bowing of the vestibular and basilar membranes causes relative movement of the hair cell stereocilia, which results in membrane depolarization.

The signal is transmitted to the sensory nerves of the spiral ganglion and then through the cochlear cranial nerve to the brain, where it is perceived as sound.

Low-frequency sound is detected by stereocilia towards the apex of the cochlea, whereas high-frequency sounds are detected at the base.

CLINICAL EXAMPLE
HEARING LOSS

Many diseases of the ear are associated with temporary or permanent hearing loss. Deafness can be divided into conductive and sensorineural types.

Conductive loss occurs when sound waves cannot be transmitted to the inner ear; common causes include blockage of the external auditory meatus (e.g. wax) or damage to the middle ear by infection ('otitis media').

Sensorineural loss is the result of damage to the inner ear, the nerves linking the cochlea with the brain, or in the brain itself. The most common type is called **presbycusis**, which occurs in elderly people; it results from reduction in hair cells, atrophy of the stria vascularis and neuron loss in the spiral ganglia.

Recently, it has been possible to place electronic implants into the cochlea to treat deafness. Sound is detected by an external device and this causes direct stimulation of the cochlear nerve, allowing hearing.

- Support cells (sustentacular cells), which are columnar cells with short apical microvilli
- Type I hair cells, which are polygonal in shape and surrounded by a network of afferent and efferent nerve endings
- Type II hair cells, which are cylindrical in shape, with basal synaptic afferent and efferent nerve endings.

In addition to an organ-pipe arrangement of tall microvilli stereocilia on their apical surface (see Fig. 19.2), these hair cells possess a single true cilium termed a **kinocilium**, which is located just behind the tallest row of stereocilia.

The stereocilia and kinocilium of each new hair cell are embedded in a gelatinous plaque of extracellular matrix called the **otolithic membrane**, which is

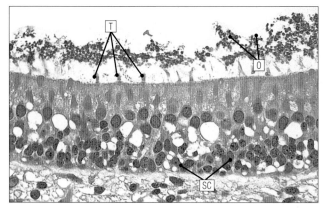

FIGURE 19.6 **Macula.** In this micrograph, the stereocilia of the hair cells of the macula are embedded in the otolithic membrane. The otoconia (O) are visible as numerous purple-stained particles. The stereocilia appear as pink tufts (T) arising from the cell surface, but neither individual microvilli nor type of hair cell can be identified at this magnification. The support cells (SC) appear as an epithelial sheet.

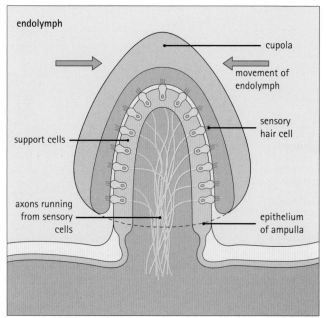

FIGURE 19.7 **Ampullary region of semicircular canal.** Within the ampullae of the semicircular canals, hair cells are arranged over a finger-like protrusion of the lining called the 'ampullary crista'. The hair cells are both type I and type II and are associated with adjacent support cells. The axons innervating the cells emerge from the base of the ampullary crista, being derived from sensory nerve cells in the ganglion of the vestibular nerve (Scarpa's ganglion), which connect with the vestibular nucleus in the brain stem. The hair cell stereocilia and kinocilium are embedded in the gelatinous matrix of the cupola which, unlike the tectorial membrane of the maculae, does not contain otoconia.

suspended in the endolymph. This membrane is covered by numerous small particles composed of protein and calcium carbonate, the **otoconia (otoliths)**.

The macula can detect the direction of gravity by sensing the direction of pull of the otolithic membrane and otoconia on the mass of hair cells that results from head movement either backwards and forwards (macula of utricle) or from side to side (macula of saccule).

Acceleration and motion are detected by hair cells in the ampullae at the end of the semicircular canals

There are three semicircular canals, which assume posterior, superior and horizontal positions.

Each ampulla is a 1 mm long dilated region of the membranous labyrinth and contains a patch of hair cells arranged in a tall finger-like structure (an **ampullary crista**). The stereocilia of the sensory hair cells are attached to a dome-shaped gelatinous matrix termed a 'cupola' (Fig. 19.7).

With rotary motion of the head, endolymph moves within the membranous labyrinth because of the static inertia of the fluid relative to the rest of the vestibular apparatus. Such movement causes displacement of the cupola, and the direction of this displacement is detected by the hair cells.

When integrated, perception from the three semicircular canals arranged in planes perpendicular to each other provides information on the direction and rate of acceleration of head movement.

Eye

The eye is designed to focus light on to specialized receptors that respond to light. It is composed of sclera, cornea, uvea and retina arranged around three chambers (Fig. 19.8).

The sclera proper is the outer fibrocollagenous coat of the globe of the eye

The sclera varies in thickness from 1 mm posteriorly to 0.5 mm anteriorly, and is composed of flat plates of collagen oriented in different directions, but parallel to the surface.

The sclera is composed of three layers:
- The episclera, an external layer of loose fibrocollagenous tissue running adjacent to the periorbital fat
- The stroma, the middle layer, which is composed of bundles of collagen thicker than those of the episclera
- The inner part of the sclera, adjacent to the choroid layer.

The collagen bundles of the stroma run in sweeping branching patterns, mainly looping from front to back, within the stroma. The lamina fusca contains small numbers of elastic fibres.

The blood vessels and nerves (including the optic nerve) running to and from the eye pass through the periscleral and scleral layers. The scleral stroma itself is avascular. Anteriorly, the sclera blends with the cornea in a transition zone (the limbus), which is 1 mm wide.

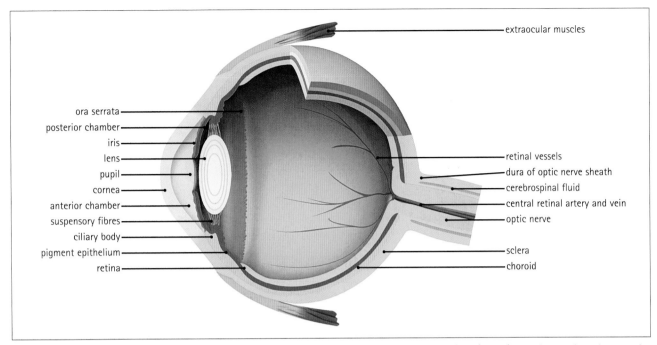

FIGURE 19.8 **Anatomy of the eye.** The eye is a spherical structure with a translucent disc-shaped area (cornea) on its anterior surface. This merges at its margins with a tough fibrocollagenous outer coat (sclera) at the limbus. The sclera surrounds the globe and is attached to a series of skeletal muscles (extraocular muscles) responsible for eye movement. The choroid is composed of blood vessels, support cells and melanocytes posteriorly and is continuous with the ciliary body and iris anteriorly, the iris being a disc-shaped membrane containing smooth muscle, with a central aperture (the pupil) to allow the passage of light. A special epithelial layer (retinal pigment epithelium) lies inside the choroid and inside this is the receptor and nerve cell layer of the eye (retina). The ora serrata marks the end of the specialized sensory layer of the retina anteriorly. Nerves from the retina emerge from the posterior aspect of the globe in the optic nerve, which is surrounded by a covering layer of fibrocollagenous tissue and cerebrospinal fluid, in continuity with that surrounding the brain. Blood is supplied to the retina by the central artery of the retina, which runs with the optic nerve. The transparent biconvex lens is suspended by a series of fine filaments from the ciliary body. The ciliary body contains smooth muscle and its contraction regulates the lens shape. The globe is divided into three chambers: the anterior chamber in front of the iris, the posterior chamber behind the iris, and the vitreous behind the lens. The anterior and posterior chambers contain a clear fluid called the aqueous. The vitreous is a gelatinous transparent extracellular matrix material.

The cornea is covered on both surfaces by epithelium

The cornea is the transparent disc-like anterior portion of the globe, and in the adult, typically measures 10.5 mm from top to bottom and 11.5 mm from side to side. It is more curved than the globe and protrudes anteriorly. The cornea has five layers (Fig. 19.9).

Corneal epithelium. The non-keratinizing squamous epithelium with a basal cell layer gives rise to five to six superficial layers with a total thickness of about 50 μm. Numerous free nerve endings terminate in this epithelium and are the afferent part of the blink (ciliary) reflex, which is mediated through the sensory part of the fifth cranial nerve.

Bowman's membrane. This is composed of fine collagen fibrils embedded in an extracellular matrix and is 8–10 μm thick. It is limited anteriorly by the basement membrane of the corneal epithelium, and blends posteriorly with the corneal stroma.

Corneal stroma. The main layer of the cornea is composed of 60–70 broad sheets of tightly bound, parallel collagen fibres (corneal lamellae) embedded in an extracellular matrix composed mainly of sulphated glycosaminoglycans. To provide maximum mechanical strength, the direction of the collagen fibres differs in each layer.

Between the lamellae are sparse inactive spindle-shaped fibrocytes (**keratocytes**).

As there are no blood vessels in the cornea, the regular parallel arrangement of the collagen and the paucity of cells render the cornea translucent and allow it to transmit light.

Descemet's membrane. This 7–10 μm thick hyaline layer on the posterior aspect of the corneal stroma is produced by the corneal endothelial cells and is a true basement membrane.

Corneal endothelium. This consists of a single layer of polygonal, plate-like cells that line the inner surface of the cornea. They are adapted for ion pumping and therefore possess numerous mitochondria, and are linked together by both desmosomal and occluding junctions.

The corneal endothelial cells pump fluid from the corneal stroma, thereby preventing excessive hydration of the extracellular matrix, which would result in opacification of the cornea.

The uvea is a specialized support tissue within the globe

The uvea is an intermediate layer in the eye between the dense support tissue of the sclera and the functional neural tissue of the retina. It contains blood vessels,

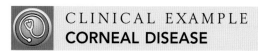

CLINICAL EXAMPLE
CORNEAL DISEASE

The cornea contributes to the refraction of light into the eye, and damage resulting in corneal opacity may impair vision.

Although loss of corneal epithelium (corneal abrasion) is exquisitely painful, it is soon repaired by regeneration of new cells. Damage to Bowman's membrane, however, results in the formation of an opaque corneal scar because repair is by the haphazard deposition of collagen. If such scarring occurs in the visual axis, it causes loss of visual acuity.

The corneal endothelial cells are not replaced during life, and in some instances, become depleted with age. They may also be damaged by disease processes in the anterior chamber of the eye. When the corneal endothelial cells are sufficiently depleted, fluid accumulates in the corneal stroma, which then becomes less transparent. Such waterlogging of the corneal stroma (corneal oedema) may cause the overlying epithelium to separate, and this is intensely painful.

Diseases of the cornea, including endothelial failure, may be treated by corneal transplantation.

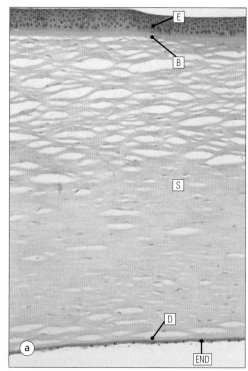

nerves, support cells, contractile cells and melanocytes, and is divided into three specialized areas: the choroid, ciliary body and iris.

The choroid has three layers and supports the retina

The choroid extends from the ora serrata to the optic nerve and contains the blood vessels and lymphatics supporting the retina (Fig. 19.10). It is a dark brown sheet and blends with the lamina fusca of the sclera in its outer portion, whereas in its inner portion it is attached to the retina. Next to the sclera is the **choroidal stroma**, which is a loose fibrocollagenous support tissue interspersed with melanocytes, lymphocytes and mast cells, and through which the main arteries and veins run. Inside this is the **choriocapillary layer**, which is a capillary layer supporting the deep layers of the retina and arises from the larger vessels in the stroma. Finally, at the interface between the choroid and the retinal pigment epithelium, is **Bruch's membrane**, which consists of:

- The basement membrane of the choriocapillary endothelial cells
- An outer collagen fibre layer 0.5 μm thick
- An elastic fibre layer 2 μm thick
- An inner collagen fibre layer
- The basement membrane of the retinal pigment epithelium (part of the retina).

The iris is part of the uvea and forms a diaphragm in front of the lens

The iris delineates the anterior and posterior chambers of the eye. It has a circular aperture (**pupil**) that can be opened and closed by the action of groups of smooth muscle. Contraction of the pupil reduces the amount of

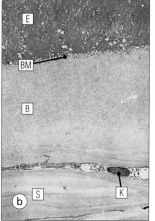

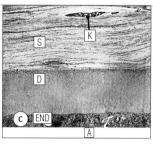

FIGURE 19.9 **Cornea.** (a) Micrograph of the five layers of the cornea showing epithelium (E), Bowman's membrane (B), stroma (S), Descemet's membrane (D) and endothelium (END). Bowman's membrane and Descemet's membrane appear as homogeneous hyaline layers that stain bright pink with H&E. In paraffin-processed material, as here, artifactual splitting of the collagen plates forming the corneal stroma is common and gives rise to small spaces. (b) Electron micrograph showing the base of a corneal epithelial basal cell (E) and its basement membrane (BM) resting on Bowman's membrane (B), in which a felt-like arrangement of fine collagen fibrils can just be discerned. Beneath this are the collagen lamellae of the corneal stroma (S) and a corneal fibrocyte (keratocyte, K). (c) Electron micrograph showing endothelium (END) resting on Descemet's membrane (D). Above are the collagen lamellae of the corneal stroma (S) and a corneal fibrocyte (keratocyte, K). Below is the anterior chamber (A).

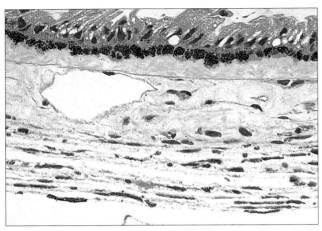

FIGURE 19.10 **Choroid.** Micrograph showing the vascular choroid layer posterior to the retinal pigment epithelium.

CLINICAL EXAMPLE
UVEAL DISEASE

The uvea is the site of several disease processes:

- Inflammation of the uvea is termed 'uveitis'. Anterior uveitis, affecting iris and ciliary body, presents as a painful red eye and reduced visual acuity. Uveitis may be a complication of several systemic inflammatory diseases and infections. Examples include ankylosing spondylitis, rheumatoid arthritis, Behçet's syndrome, syphilis, tuberculosis and inflammatory bowel disease. Uveitis affecting the back of the eye may be caused by direct infection
- The melanin-containing cells of the uvea give rise to the commonest tumour seen in the eye; a malignant melanoma. These tumours have the capacity to spread both locally and to distant organs by metastasis
- Albinism is a congenital condition characterised by absence of melanin from the uvea, either alone or from the whole body. Patients have poor vision and may have cerebellar ataxia.

CLINICAL EXAMPLE
RETINAL DETACHMENT

The term 'retinal detachment' is used to describe splitting of the retina through the photoreceptor layer to leave the attached pigment epithelium. Retinal detachment usually follows a tear in the retina caused either by retinal degeneration or by traction by the vitreous.

The vitreous is normally in contact with the whole of the retina and rotational shearing forces generated by pulling of the extraocular muscles are transmitted uniformly to the whole globe. If the vitreous becomes detached from the retina posteriorly, rotational shearing forces are focally concentrated and cause tearing of the retina.

If the retina does not reattach, the cell bodies of the rods and cones in the detached area degenerate, with loss of visual function.

light entering the eye and thereby reduces glare from light scattered from the periphery of the lens.

The iris contains pigmented cells and muscle and is composed of four layers: the **anterior limiting membrane**, the **stroma**, the **dilator muscle layer** and the **posterior epithelium** (Fig. 19.11).

The anterior limiting layer is an incomplete, fenestrated layer formed from stellate fibroblastic cells and stellate melanocytes.

The **stroma** is a loose fibrocollagenous support tissue associated with spindle-shaped fibroblasts (stromal cells), blood vessels, nerves and macrophages containing phagocytosed melanin pigment; at the pupil margin is the circumferentially arranged smooth muscle of the sphincter muscle of the pupil.

The blood vessels of the iris generally run in a radial direction, with frequent anastomotic channels forming circumferential vascular plexuses.

The dilator muscle layer is composed of the contractile processes of the myoepithelial cells of the inner layer of the posterior epithelium; it extends from the base of the iris to the sphincter muscle.

The **posterior epithelium** is composed of two layers of cells which are densely pigmented with melanin. The inner layer of cells are more correctly myoepithelial in type, with a basal zone around the nucleus containing melanin granules and an apical portion, which is melanin-free, constituting the dilator muscle layer. This inner layer is bound by desmosomal junctions to the outer layer cells, which contain numerous melanin granules and are continuous with the retinal pigment epithelial layer. The pigmented cells eliminate light from the eye and reduce glare.

Eye colour is determined by the relative number of melanocytes in the stroma. Few cells give a blue colour, whereas many melanin-containing cells produce a dark brown colour; grey and green are the intermediate colours.

The ciliary body contains the muscle that relaxes the lens

The **ciliary body** extends from the base of the iris to the ora serrata, where it is continuous with the choroid (see Fig. 19.8). In section (Fig. 19.12), the ciliary body is roughly triangular in shape and is composed of a vascular stroma, smooth muscle and covering epithelium; it has two anatomically recognizable regions: the **pars plica** and the **pars plana**.

The ciliary body contains the **ciliary muscle**, which is a form of smooth muscle. Contraction of the ciliary muscle lessens tension on the suspensory fibres of the lens and allows the lens to assume a more spherical shape.

The pars plica contains the ciliary processes, which are ridges or folds 2 mm long, each with a core of stroma and blood vessels and covered by two layers of columnar epithelium. The outer layer of epithelium is pigmented, but the inner layer, which is in contact with the aqueous, is not.

The non-pigmented epithelial cells in the grooves between the ciliary processes give rise to the suspensory

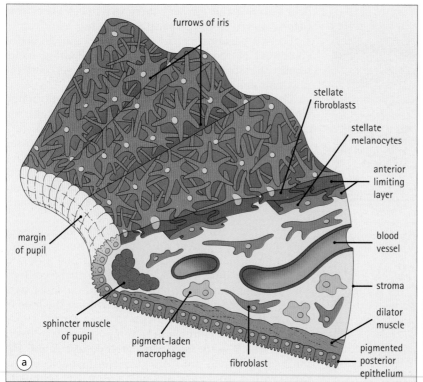

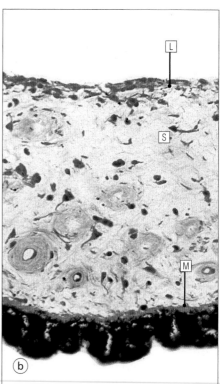

FIGURE 19.11 **Iris.** (a) The free margin of the iris at the pupil, showing its four constituent layers. An incomplete and fenestrated anterior limiting layer containing stellate fibroblasts and melanocytes lies on a loose fibrocollagenous stroma containing the sphincter muscle of the pupil, as well as radially orientated collagen fibres that give the iris its ribbed and trabeculated surface. Behind the stroma is the dilator muscle, which is backed posteriorly by two layers of melanin-pigmented cells. (b) Micrograph showing the histological appearance of the iris. The four layers are not well defined. The anterior limiting layer (L) merges with the stroma (S). The pigmented posterior epithelium cannot be resolved into two layers because of the density of melanin pigment. The dilator muscle (M) is visible as a pink band.

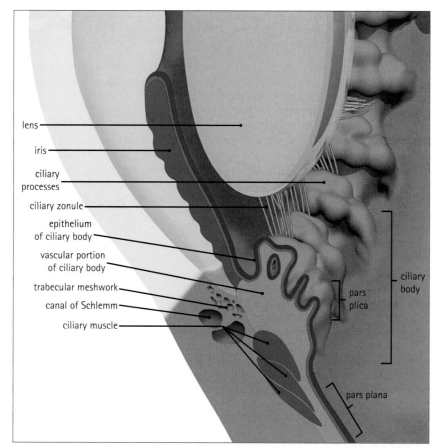

FIGURE 19.12 **Ciliary body.** The ciliary body is continuous with the base of the iris and is divided anatomically into the pars plica and pars plana. The ciliary processes give rise to the suspensory fibres of the lens (ciliary zonule) and the ciliary muscle controls the tension on the suspensory fibres, thereby controlling the shape of the lens. The epithelium of the pars plana secretes the aqueous.

fibres of the lens, which are composed mainly of the protein fibrillin. The ultrastructural features of these non-pigmented cells are those of ion-pumping cells; they secrete the aqueous.

The pars plana is a posterior flat area 4 mm long. Its stroma is continuous with the choroid, whereas the outer pigmented epithelium of the ciliary body is continuous with that of the retina at the ora serrata.

The retina contains photoreceptors along with support cells and nerve cells

The retina is the innermost layer of the eye and is derived embryonically from an outgrowth of the developing brain (the optic cup). It is composed of pigment epithelial cells, photoreceptor cells, retinal support cells and nerve cells.

Retinal pigment epithelial cells maintain and support photoreceptor cells

The retinal pigment epithelium is a single layer of melanin-containing polygonal cells extending from the optic nerve to the ora serrata. Internally, it lies adjacent to the photoreceptor layer of the retina; externally its basement membrane is a component of Bruch's membrane.

The apical surfaces of the pigmented epithelial cells are covered with large microvilli, which extend upward and surround the photoreceptors of the retina. Retinal pigment epithelial cells phagocytose worn-out components of the photoreceptor cells.

The two types of photoreceptor cell of the retina are termed rods and cones

The light-sensitive structures (**photoreceptor discs**) in the photoreceptor cell form huge stacks 600–1000 deep in the outer segment of the cell and originate as deep infolds of the cell membrane (Fig. 19.13).

In rods, photoreceptor discs are formed constantly and pinch off to form free discs, which are shed from the cell when old (Fig. 19.14). In cones, however, photoreceptor discs remain as deep infolds of cell membrane and do not form free discs. The turnover of cone photoreceptor discs is not clear, but it does not appear to be the same as that of rods.

Rods are about 2 μm thick and an average of 50 μm in length, possessing a roughly cylindrical outer segment. The tips of these cells are embedded in the microvilli of pigment epithelial cells, which phagocytose the old photoreceptor discs.

Cones are thicker and slightly shorter than rods, being 3–5 μm thick and about 40 μm long; their outer segment is conical in shape. Like rods, cones are also located close to the microvilli of the retinal pigment epithelial cells.

The distribution of rods and cones varies within the retina. Cones, which perceive colour, are concentrated in the optical centre of the retina in a small pit (the **fovea**). Rods, which perceive light intensity but not colour, are concentrated at the periphery of the retina.

Between the fovea and the periphery of the retina, there is a mixture of rods and cones (Fig. 19.15).

The retina contains two main types of support cell: Müller's cells and astrocytes

Müller's cells are tall, retinal support cells. They extend from the base of the inner segment of the photoreceptor cells, where they link to each other by adherent junctions (see Fig. 3.9) to form the structure known as the outer limiting membrane, up to the retinal surface, where they rest on the internal limiting membrane.

Astrocytes (see p. 92) act as support cells to the nerve cells throughout the retina and are characterized by long dendritic processes that form a scaffold for the delicate processes of nerve cells.

ADVANCED CONCEPT
MECHANISM OF LIGHT DETECTION

In the dark, the photoreceptor cell is strongly depolarized and this holds voltage-gated Ca^{2+} ion channels open in the synaptic region, resulting in the constant release of an inhibitory transmitter substance at the synaptic terminal. This inhibitor prevents firing of nerve cells connected to the photoreceptor.

When stimulated by light, the photoreceptor becomes hyperpolarized and release of the inhibitory transmitter substance at the synaptic terminal is reduced. This reduction allows the axons of nerve cells connected to the photoreceptors to fire.

Photoreceptor cells detect light through its interaction with rhodopsin molecules. These are membrane-associated glycoproteins in the photoreceptor discs, and are composed of a protein (opsin) and a light-sensitive group (cis-retinal).

When cis-retinal interacts with a photon it undergoes a conformational change to the transform, which causes a fall in the concentration of a secondary messenger (cyclic GMP) within the cytosol of the photoreceptor. This results in closure of sodium channels in the cell membrane and hence hyperpolarization.

Nerve cells of the retina interconnect to integrate the signals from photoreceptors

The retina contains several classes of nerve cell: bipolar cells, ganglion cells, horizontal cells, amacrine cells and interplexiform cells.

Bipolar cells connect with the synaptic end of the photoreceptor cells and transmit signals to ganglion cells. **Ganglion cells** send axons from the eye to the brain in the optic nerve.

Horizontal cells, amacrine cells and **interplexiform cells** are neurons that act as 'gates' to modulate the passage of impulses from the photoreceptors to the ganglion cells. Their processes interpose the connections between bipolar cells and photoreceptors, and between bipolar cells and ganglion cells. This group of gate cells allows the integration of signals from adjacent groups of photoreceptors.

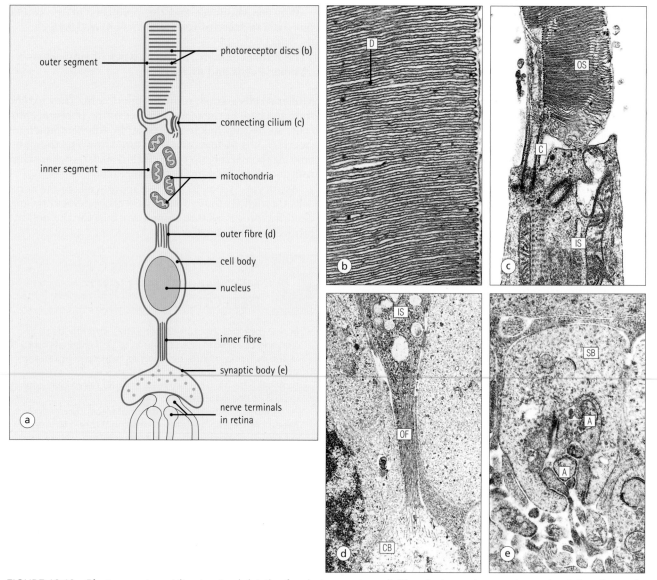

FIGURE 19.13 **Photoreceptors.** Ultrastructural details of a photoreceptor cell. The electron micrographs on the right refer to the areas labelled (b), (c), (d) and (e). Light is detected by its outer segment (OS), which contains flat plates of membrane (photoreceptor discs, D). The outer segment is connected to the inner segment (IS) by a connecting cilium (C). The inner segment contains numerous mitochondria. The cell body (CB) connects to the inner segment (IS) by a microtubule-rich outer fibre (OF). The synaptic body (SB) is cup-shaped and connects to axons (A) from other retinal neurons.

The sensory retina is composed of nine layers made up of different cell types

- The **photoreceptor layer** of rods and cones, which extends from the retinal pigment epithelium and consists of outer and inner segments of the photoreceptor cells (Fig. 19.16)
- The **external limiting membrane**, which is not a true membrane, but a line marking the zone of adherent junctions between Müller's cells
- The **outer nuclear layer**, consisting of the nuclei and cell bodies of the photoreceptor cells, which form eight to nine rows of nuclei
- The **outer plexiform layer**, which contains the cell processes and synaptic connections between the photoreceptor cells, bipolar neurons and horizontal cells

- The **inner nuclear layer**, which is composed of the nuclei and cell bodies of bipolar cells, horizontal cells, interplexiform cells and amacrine cells, as well as the nuclei of the Müller's cells
- The **inner plexiform layer**, containing the cell processes and synapses of bipolar cells, amacrine cells, interplexiform cells and ganglion cells
- The **ganglion cell layer**, consisting of a row of ganglion cells which have large nuclei with visible nucleoli, and prominent rough endoplasmic reticulum visible as Nissl substance
- The **nerve fibre layer**, composed of the axons of the ganglion cells en route to the central nervous system via the optic nerve with supporting astrocytic cells
- The **internal limiting membrane**, a barely visible basement membrane at the interface between the vitreous and the retina.

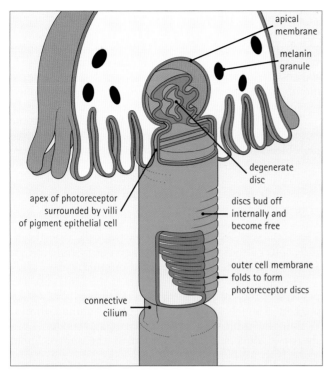

FIGURE 19.14 **Turnover of photoreceptor discs in rods.** In the rod photoreceptor cell, photoreceptor discs originate at the cilial pole of the outer segment as deep infoldings of the cell membrane. These migrate up through the cell and eventually bud off internally to form free discs within the outer segment. At the rod apex, effete and aged discs are eliminated and extruded into the extracellular space, where they are phagocytosed by the retinal pigment epithelial cell, into which the rod outer segment is buried. There is a constant flow of new photoreceptor discs along the rod outer segment.

The nuclei of rods are small and densely stained, whereas those of cones are larger and pale stained.

In the outer plexiform layer, the synaptic connections to rods are termed 'spherals', whereas those to cones are termed 'pedicles'. For both cell types, the terminal of a horizontal cell is interposed between the photoreceptor and the bipolar cell to form a structure termed a 'triad'. The horizontal cell can therefore modulate the impulse from the photoreceptors to the bipolar cells and allows integration of signals from adjacent photoreceptors.

The amacrine cells of the inner plexiform layer interpose processes between the processes of bipolar cells and ganglion cells and thereby modify the transmission of impulses from the bipolar cells. The interplexiform cells are similar to amacrine cells but also send a process to synapse in the outer plexiform layer. The ganglion cells of the ganglion layer are separated by the cytoplasm of Müller's cells.

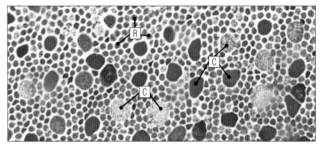

FIGURE 19.15 **Rods and cones.** Micrograph of a resin section taken tangentially through the retina at the level of the inner segment of the photoreceptors. Rods (R) are identified as thin circular profiles, and cones (C) are larger. There is a mosaic of rods and cones in this retinal area 6 mm temporal to the fovea.

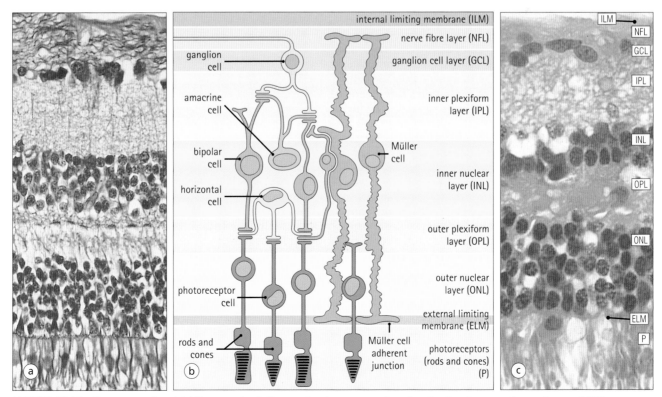

FIGURE 19.16 **Sensory retina.** (a) Micrograph of silver-stained sensory retina showing its nine constituent layers. (b) The sensory retina showing its nine layers. (c) Micrograph of H&E-stained sensory retina.

Ophthalmoscopic examination of the retina (funduscopy) is an important part of a general medical examination because it provides a direct view of blood vessels in a critical area of the circulation. Retinal blood vessels are frequently affected in disease, particularly diabetes mellitus.

In diabetes mellitus, the basement membrane of small blood vessels in the retina thickens and the vessels show dilatations termed microaneurysms.

The abnormal vessels become leaky and exude fluid into the retina, which is visible as white spots. Haemorrhages may also occur. This particularly affects the macula, leading to loss of visual acuity.

If these changes become severe, the blood supply to the retina is reduced (ischaemia) and this stimulates abnormal growth of new retinal blood vessels (proliferative retinopathy). The newly formed vessels may bleed and also result in retinal detachment.

The severity of diabetic retinopathy, which is the most common cause of blindness in the developed world, is greatly reduced by the careful control of blood sugar levels. Laser coagulation of leaking vessels delays or prevents the development of severe visual loss.

The retinal structure is modified in specialized areas

Optic disc. The axons of the nerve fibre layer converge at the optic disc, which is visible in the retina and gives rise to the optic nerve. This area is devoid of photoreceptors and therefore produces a blind spot in the visual field.

Macula. The macula is a small yellow area located 2.5 mm lateral (temporal) to the optic disc. At its centre, there is a thin zone of retina composed exclusively of cones (the fovea), each cone synapsing with a single bipolar cell and thence linking with a single ganglion cell, thus producing a high degree of resolution. This area is at the centre of the visual axis and provides highly detailed colour vision.

The yellow colour of the surrounding macula is due to the presence of yellow xanthophyll pigment in ganglion cells from the fovea, which are displaced laterally so that light can impinge on the cones of the fovea without being dispersed by an overlying neural layer.

Peripheral retina. In the peripheral retina, many photoreceptors are mapped on to one ganglion cell and form a receptive field with low visual resolution. Electrophysiology has shown that these receptive fields are triggered by different visual stimuli, for example some ganglion cells only fire in response to a bright light, whereas others only respond to a moving edge.

The retinal blood supply enters with the optic nerve at the back of the globe

The central artery and vein of the retina enter the back of the eye in the optic nerve and branch in the plane between the vitreous and the inner limiting membrane.

The capillaries, which form a dense plexus within the retina and supply all cells apart from the rods and cones, are characterized by tight junctions between their constituent endothelial cells to prevent diffusion of substances into the neural retina (i.e. they form a **blood–retinal barrier**). The rods and cones are supplied by choroidal vessels.

The retinal vessels are visible by ophthalmoscopic examination and may be damaged in disease, for example high blood pressure (hypertension) causes visible thickening of the arterial walls.

The optic nerve takes axons from the retina to the brain

The optic nerve contains the axons from the retinal ganglion cells en route to the central nervous system, as well as the central artery and vein of the retina.

The optic nerve leaves the retina at the optic disc and penetrates the collagen of the sclera through a sieve-like plate of channels in an area termed the **lamina cribrosa**. Within the orbit, the optic nerve is surrounded by a sheath of dura and an extension of the subarachnoid space (Fig. 19.17).

The optic nerve is invested in the pia arachnoid layers (see Chapter 6), and septa from this layer enter the optic nerve and divide the axons into fascicles.

If pressure of the cerebrospinal fluid (CSF) within the skull increases (raised intracranial pressure), pressure of the CSF around the optic nerve increases. Initially, this impairs cytoplasmic flow along the optic nerve axons, which swell and cause engorgement of the central artery and vein.

Ophthalmoscopic examination of a normal optic disc reveals that it is a cup-shaped depression, but in cases of raised intracranial pressure, the disc is swollen (papilloedema), with loss of the cup-shaped depression.

Papilloedema is an important physical sign and usually denotes abnormal brain swelling caused by disease.

The lens, a soft transparent biconvex structure composed of crystallins, is encased in a capsule

In the adult, the lens is 9 mm in diameter and 3.5 mm thick. It has:
- An outer capsule 10–20 μm thick of hyaline material containing type IV collagen
- A layer of large cuboidal epithelial cells (the lens epithelium) beneath the capsule
- A centre composed of tightly packed cells, which have lost their nuclei and become packed by special transparent proteins (crystallins) to form so-called 'lens fibres' (Fig. 19.18).

New lens cells are added to the margin of the lens throughout life from the lens epithelium, but the cells at the centre of the lens do not undergo turnover or

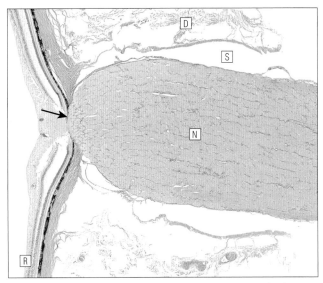

FIGURE 19.17 **Optic nerve and retina.** Micrograph showing the optic nerve (N) in longitudinal section. The central artery and vein of the retina run along its centre. The optic nerve leaves the retina (R) at the optic disc and penetrates the sclera through the lamina cribrosa (arrow). Around the optic nerve is the optic nerve sheath, which is composed of an extension of the dura (D) and subarachnoid space (S) and is filled with cerebrospinal fluid.

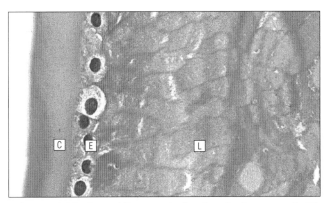

FIGURE 19.18 **Lens.** Micrograph showing the lens capsule (C) as a pink-staining hyaline layer, and the subcapsular lens epithelium (E). The centre of the lens (L) is composed of cells devoid of organelles (lens fibres) packed with crystalline proteins.

replacement and are therefore the oldest cells in the body of an adult.

The lens is avascular and is nourished by diffusion from the aqueous and vitreous.

The lens is suspended by suspensory fibres to the ciliary body, the radial arrangement of suspensory fibres being termed the **ciliary zonule**. These fibres are composed mainly of the fibrillar protein fibrillin (see Chapter 4).

The eye is divided into three chambers

The **vitreous body** is a transparent gelatinous structure located behind the lens and occupying the space bounded by the inner surface of the retina. The vitreous has a volume of 4 mL and is a specialized support tissue, being composed of a few scattered spindle-shaped cells (hyalocytes), fine, highly dispersed collagen fibres and an abundant extracellular matrix rich in hyaluronic acid.

The **anterior** and **posterior aqueous chambers** lie anterior to the lens, are delineated by the iris and communicate with each other via the aperture of the pupil (see Fig. 19.8).

The **aqueous humour** is a watery fluid resembling cerebrospinal fluid and is secreted at a rate of about 2 mL/min by the epithelial cells of the ciliary body in the posterior chamber. It provides nutrients to the structures it bathes, and flows from the posterior chamber through the pupil into the anterior chamber.

The aqueous then filters through a network of spaces lined by endothelium, the **trabecular meshwork** (see Fig. 19.12), which runs around the circumference of the root of the iris, at the periphery of the anterior chamber, and enters the **canal of Schlemm** (Fig. 19.19). This canal runs around the whole circumference of the limbus within the sclera. From the canal of Schlemm, the aqueous enters venous vessels.

The angle between the margin of the cornea and the iris root where the trabecular meshwork lies is the **iridocorneal drainage angle**.

KEY FACTS
THE EYE

- Aqueous humour is produced by the ciliary body, goes through the pupil and drains through the trabecular meshwork into the canal of Schlemm
- The cornea is kept translucent by the action of the ion-pumping endothelial cells on its inner surface
- The uvea contains melanocytes and comprises the choroid, ciliary body and iris
- The photoreceptor layer of the retina is maintained by its close contact with the retinal pigment epithelium
- The retina is supplied by a single artery that runs through the optic nerve
- The nerve fibres in the optic nerve originate from the retinal ganglion cells
- Cones are concentrated in an area of the macula termed the 'fovea', which is responsible for high-resolution colour vision.

There is a normal resistance to the flow of aqueous at the level of the trabecular meshwork, such that continued secretion and resorption of the aqueous results in a normal intrinsic resting pressure within the globe (intraocular pressure) of 10–22 mmHg.

Accessory Components of the Eye

The conjunctiva is composed of a mucin-secreting columnar epithelium

The normal conjunctiva is a translucent membrane that lines the inner surface of the eyelids (palpebral conjunctiva) and reflects on to the globe (bulbar conjunctiva) to

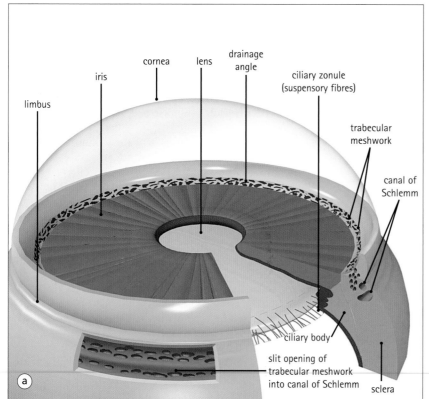

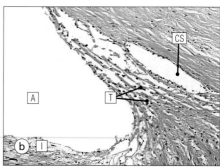

FIGURE 19.19 Canal of Schlemm and trabecular meshwork. (a) The canal of Schlemm runs around the circumference of the cornea at the limbus and communicates with the trabecular meshwork, which runs around the circumference of the root of the iris. The aqueous from the anterior chamber of the eye filters through the trabecular meshwork into the canal of Schlemm, and thence drains into venous vessels. (b) Micrograph showing the trabecular meshwork (T) as an area of slit-like spaces with the canal of Schlemm (CS) within the sclera. The aqueous filters from the anterior chamber (A) just above the iris (I).

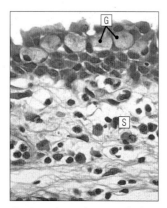

FIGURE 19.20 Conjunctiva. Micrograph showing conjunctival epithelium with goblet cells (G) containing mucin overlying the subepithelial support tissues (S), which contain vessels and lymphoid cells.

cover its anterior surface up to the margin of the cornea (limbus).

The conjunctiva is covered by two layers of stratified columnar epithelium, which give way to a flattened squamous epithelium towards the limbus. Goblet cells (see p. 49) are present in this epithelium but mainly in the medial portion, being scarce in the temporal bulbar conjunctiva (Fig. 19.20).

Beneath the epithelium, the conjunctival stroma is composed of loose fibrocollagenous support tissue with small blood vessels and lymphatics running through it. With ageing, there is loss of collagen in this tissue.

CLINICAL EXAMPLE
GLAUCOMA

Abnormalities in the drainage pathway of aqueous humour result in a rise in the intraocular pressure (glaucoma) which, if untreated, damages the nerve cells of the retina and causes blindness.

The eyelids contain many different secretory glands

The structure of both upper and lower eyelids is similar and comprises the following four layers:
- Skin
- Orbicularis muscle (a layer of skeletal muscle)
- Tarsal plate (a plate of dense fibroelastic tissue)
- Conjunctiva.

Within these layers are various types of gland (Fig. 19.21):

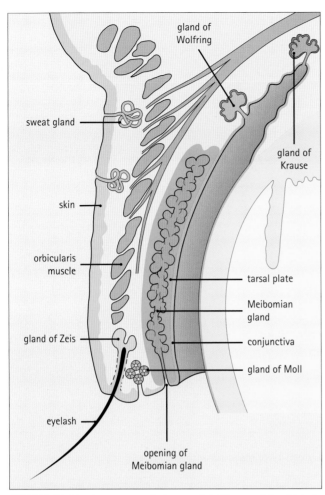

FIGURE 19.21 **Structure of the eyelid.** The eyelid, which is composed of skin, orbicularis muscle, tarsal plate and conjunctiva and contains various types of gland.

- Meibomian glands, sebaceous in type and secreting a lipid-rich substance that delays evaporation of the tear film that lubricates and protects the cornea
- Glands of Zeis, small sebaceous glands associated with the eyelashes
- Glands of Moll, apocrine sweat glands at the margin of the eyelid
- Glands of Krause, accessory lacrimal glands in the fornix of the conjunctiva
- Glands of Wolfring, accessory lacrimal glands just above the tarsal plate.

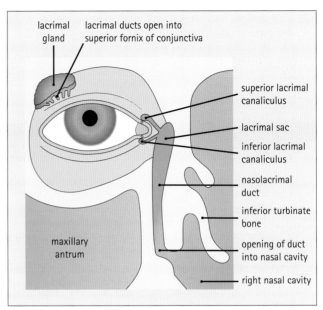

FIGURE 19.22 **Lacrimal apparatus.** The lacrimal gland discharges tear fluid onto the conjunctiva. Drainage from the conjunctival surfaces is via superior and inferior lacrimal puncta, located at the medial ends of the upper and lower eyelids. These open into small ducts (canaliculi) that unite to drain into the lacrimal sac. The lacrimal sac drains into the nasal space by the nasolacrimal duct, most of which runs within the bone.

The lacrimal glands produce tears, which drain via a duct system into the nose

Tears are produced by the main lacrimal gland, which is located beneath the conjunctiva on the upper lateral margin of the orbit, and by the accessory glands of Krause and Wolfring (see Fig. 19.21). The glands secrete a serous fluid and have a complex branched structure with secretory acini and ducts (see Fig. 3.25).

The main lacrimal gland drains into the upper fornix of the conjunctiva via a series of about 10 small ducts. Tears then wash over the surface of the eye and drain via two ducts located at the medial end of the eyelids. These ducts, the superior and inferior lacrimal ducts, merge into a common lacrimal duct and drain into the lacrimal sac; this empties, via the nasolacrimal duct, into the nasal cavity through an opening beneath the inferior turbinate bone (see Chapter 10 and Fig. 19.22).

The superior and inferior lacrimal ducts are lined by stratified squamous epithelium, whereas the lacrimal sac and nasolacrimal duct are lined by respiratory-type pseudostratified ciliated columnar epithelium.

For online review questions, please visit https://studentconsult.inkling.com.

END OF CHAPTER REVIEW

True/False Answers to the MCQS, as Well as Case Answers, Can be Found in the Appendix in the Back of the Book.

1. **Which of the following features are present in the ear?**
   (a) The pinna is composed of elastic cartilage
   (b) The ceruminous glands are modified apocrine glands
   (c) The tympanic membrane is lined on one side by cuboidal epithelium
   (d) The middle ear cavity is lined by ciliated pseudostratified epithelium
   (e) The auditory ossicles articulate by syndesmoses

2. **Which of the following features are seen in the inner ear?**
   (a) Hair cells have cilia on their surface to detect movement
   (b) The ampullae of the semicircular canals detect acceleration
   (c) The macula of the saccule detects sound
   (d) The vestibular and tympanic cavities contain perilymph
   (e) The basilar membrane is continuous with the organ of Corti

3. **Which of the following are present in the eye?**
   (a) The posterior chamber lies behind the lens
   (b) The lens is suspended from the ciliary body
   (c) The inner part of the cornea is lined by endothelium
   (d) The aqueous humour drains through the trabecular meshwork
   (e) Aqueous humour is produced by the epithelium of the ciliary body

4. **Which of the following features are true for the retina?**
   (a) Retinal pigment epithelial cells are responsible for phagocytosis of photoreceptor membranes
   (b) Cones are concentrated at the periphery of the retina
   (c) The photoreceptor layer is isolated from the rest of the retina by a belt of adherent junctions forming the external limiting membrane
   (d) The macula contains the fovea
   (e) The optic disc is devoid of photoreceptors

CASE 19.1   GRADUAL ONSET OF DEAFNESS

A 58-year-old man has been referred to a hearing assessment unit because he has experienced increasing difficulty with hearing. Physical examination of the tympanic membrane is normal and it is planned to perform audiography to determine the pattern of hearing loss.

Q. Describe the functional and structural background to this case. Concentrate on structural aspects of hearing that may be abnormal and lead to deafness.

CASE 19.2   A WOMAN WITH DETERIORATING VISION

A 63-year-old woman is seen in the clinic having been referred because of deterioration in her vision. Ophthalmoscopic examination shows some cupping of the optic disc and the intraocular pressure is elevated. A diagnosis of glaucoma is made.

Q. Describe the structural and functional background to this case. Focus on structural changes in the eye that might cause an increase in the intraocular pressure.

Appendix

Answers

Chapter 2 The Cell

1. (a) True, (b) False, (c) False, (d) False, (e) True
2. (a) True, (b) True, (c) False, (d) True, (e) True
3. (a) True, (b) False, (c) True, (d) True, (e) True
4. (a) True, (b) True, (c) False, (d) True, (e) True

Case 2.1 Answer

Lysosomes are membrane-bound intracellular organelles and are part of the acid vesicle system. These contain hydrolases that operate at the acidic pH found within the lysosome. In the acid vesicle system are more than 30 defined and specific acid hydrolases, which not only degrade abnormal large molecules but also recycle or process normal cell constituents. Lysosomes internalize material that is degraded by hydrolases. Among the many substances broken down within the lysosome is glycogen. The enzyme responsible for the breakdown of glycogen is acid maltase.

In this case, detectable acid maltase activity associated with the accumulation of glycogen within muscle is absent. This has led to muscle disease with clinical features of proximal muscle weakness.

This type of disease is called a **lysosomal storage disorder** and is caused by a genetic defect that leads to lack of activity of one of the enzymes normally found within lysosomes. The substance that would normally be broken down by the missing enzyme accumulates within the cells and causes damage. Clinical manifestations of lysosomal storage diseases are mostly related to damage to cells that are non-dividing permanent populations such as neurons, skeletal muscle and liver tissue.

The heart is abnormal because the cardiac muscle cells are also affected. Were an endomyocardial biopsy to be performed, this would also show abnormal accumulation of glycogen within cells.

Other causes of abnormal glycogen storage are also the result of genetic defects that lead to reduced activity of enzymes involved in glycogen metabolism.

This disease is defined as the following:

- A storage disorder – The disease is associated with abnormal accumulation and storage of a substance within cells
- A lysosomal storage disease – The disease is caused by absence of a lysosomal enzyme
- A glycogenosis – The disease is associated with the abnormal handling of glycogen.

Muscle diseases that are associated with abnormalities of skeletal muscle fibres are termed **myopathies**. In this case, the patient's condition would be classified as a metabolic myopathy.

Cardiac diseases that are caused by primary defects in myocardial muscle fibres are termed **cardiomyopathies**. This child would be classed as having a cardiomyopathy.

Case 2.2 Answer

When a tumour is encountered in a biopsy from a patient, optimal treatment depends on the type of tumour, which requires ascertaining its cell of origin. In most instances, this is not a diagnostic problem and routine histological examination is adequate. However, in some patients it is not clear from what organ or cell type a tumour has arisen. The case under discussion is a common clinical problem: metastatic disease (i.e. a malignant tumour that has spread from its organ or tissue of origin to another site such as a lymph node or the liver) is discovered in the absence of any known primary site.

In such cases, standard histological examination is supplemented by immunohistochemical assessment of the tumour to detect markers that might point to the cell of origin. It is common to apply to a tumour a panel of antibodies capable of detecting a wide range of possible tumours.

The intermediate filaments are composed of protein subunits and form part of the cytoskeleton. Different types of intermediate filaments characterize different cell types. The main types are as follows:

Cell type	Intermediate filament
Mesenchymal cells, as well as other cell types	Vimentin
Epithelial cells	Cytokeratins
Neurons	Neurofilament proteins
Glial cells	Glial fibrillary acidic protein (GFAP)
Muscle cells	Desmin

If immunostaining is performed using antibodies against specific intermediate filament proteins, it is possible to determine the cell of origin of a tumour.

In this case, expression of cytokeratins would lead to the conclusion that the tumour was of epithelial origin and was therefore some sort of carcinoma (**carcinoma** is the term used to refer to malignant tumour of an epithelial tissue).

Epithelial cells from different tissues can also express specific proteins useful in diagnosis. For example:

- Tumours derived from prostatic epithelium may be detected by immunostaining for prostate-specific antigen or prostate-specific acid phosphatase
- Tumours derived from the thyroid may be detected by immunostaining for thyroglobulin
- Tumours derived from the breast may express oestrogen receptor
- Tumours derived from the gastrointestinal tract may express carcinoembryonic antigen (CEA)
- Tumours of lymphoid tissues express markers of normal lymphoid cells
- Tumours of muscle often express desmin, the intermediate filament of muscle.

It would be very unusual for a tumour of the nervous system to spread to lymph nodes. However, tumours that arise in the nervous system can be characterized by immunostaining for GFAP and neurofilament proteins to determine their cell of origin.

Any tumour of neuroendocrine type can be characterized by detecting proteins expressed on neurosecretory granules, such as synaptophysin or chromogranin A.

Vimentin is expressed by so many cell types that it is not particularly helpful in diagnosis.

In some patients, a tumour becomes so poorly-differentiated that no specific pattern of expression of any protein is seen. Such anaplastic tumours generally carry a very poor prognosis.

Chapter 3 Epithelial Cells

1. (a) True, (b) True, (c) True, (d) False, (e) True
2. (a) True, (b) True, (c) False, (d) True, (e) True
3. (a) True, (b) True, (c) False, (d) False, (e) True
4. (a) False, (b) True, (c) False, (d) True, (e) False

Case 3.1 Answer

Normal cells and tissues are characterized by a uniformity of cytology and a coherence of tissue architecture.

Cell division is usually restricted to a specific part of a tissue, for example, the basal layer of the epidermis of the skin or the crypts in the intestinal mucosa. Cells are usually of uniform size within any given tissue and tend not to show much variation in size or shape. In normal cells, the nucleus staining is related to the activity of the cell.

Neoplastic cells from malignant tumours are often found to have nuclei that are more darkly staining than normal tissues (hyperchromatism). They also show variation in nuclear size and shape (pleomorphism), and evidence of cell proliferation exists in the form of mitoses.

In this case, the finding of cells with variable size and shape, mitoses and darkly-stained nuclei suggests a neoplastic process and raises the possibility that the lesions in the liver are tumours.

In any tissue, a malignant process can be caused by a tumour arising locally (primary tumour) or spreading to the tissue from another site (metastatic tumour).

Histological assessment of a tumour is an important part of diagnosis and may be the investigation that suggests the original site of origin. This is important because prognosis and therapy of tumours is related to the site of origin and histogenesis.

Differentiation of tissues can be detected by conventional stains, immunohistochemical staining, and electron microscopy. Stains such as Alcian blue or PAS can detect the presence of mucin. This would suggest that the tumour was epithelial in origin and also of glandular differentiation; therefore the tumour would be classified as an adenocarcinoma.

Immunohistochemistry can be used to detect proteins expressed by cells that are specific to different cell types.

Cell type	Intermediate filament
Mesenchymal cells, as well as other cell types	Vimentin
Epithelial cells	Cytokeratins
Neurons	Neurofilament proteins
Glial cells	Glial fibrillary acidic protein (GFAP)
Muscle cells	Desmin

In this case, expression of cytokeratins would lead to the conclusion that the tumour was of epithelial origin and was therefore some sort of carcinoma (**carcinoma** is the term used to refer to a malignant tumour of an epithelial tissue).

Epithelial cells from different tissues can also express specific proteins useful in diagnosis. For example:

- Tumours derived from prostatic epithelium may be detected by immunostaining for prostate-specific antigen or prostate-specific acid phosphatase
- Tumours derived from the thyroid may be detected by immunostaining for thyroglobulin
- Tumours derived from the breast may express oestrogen receptor
- Tumours derived from the gastrointestinal tract may express carcinoembryonic antigen (CEA)
- Tumours of lymphoid tissues express markers of normal lymphoid cells
- Tumours of muscle often express desmin, the intermediate filament of muscle.

It would be very unusual for a tumour of the nervous system to spread to the lymph nodes. However, tumours that arise in the nervous system can be characterized by immunostaining for GFAP and neurofilament proteins to determine their cell of origin.

Any tumour of neuroendocrine type can be characterized by detecting proteins expressed on neurosecretory granules, such as synaptophysin or chromogranin A.

Vimentin is expressed by so many cell types that it is not particularly helpful in diagnosis.

Case 3.2 Answer

The normal skin is a tough structure and is specifically designed to provide a resilient outer layer with important barrier functions. The toughness is provided by a variety of adhesion mechanisms that unite cells and extracellular matrix into a single structure.

In normal skin, epidermal cells are tightly held together by intercellular junctions called **desmosomes**.

The desmosomes are linked to the intermediate filament cytoskeleton of epidermal cells (called **keratins**). The basal layer of the epidermis is strongly linked to the basement membrane by hemidesmosomes, which also link into the cytokeratin intermediate filament cytoskeleton.

As the cells differentiate and move up the stratified epithelium, they remain tightly bound by desmosomal junctions but the cytokeratin proteins change to higher molecular weight forms. Cells in the upper part of the epithelium express genes coding for a variety of specialized proteins that interact with the cytokeratin filaments and the cell membrane to produce a resilient and mechanically robust compact mass (keratin). Small granules (keratohyaline granules) contain some of these specialized proteins.

Both desmosomes and hemidesmosomes are composed of multiple link proteins responsible for cell anchorage.

The basement membrane is anchored to the extracellular matrix of the dermis by several anchoring proteins and glycoprotein interactions.

In this case, one of the keratin intermediate filament proteins is abnormal because of a mutation in a coding gene. The consequence of this is to prevent complete anchoring of cells to one another. Although the desmosomes and hemidesmosomes bind cells together, within the cells there exists no cross-linking, which is normally mediated by keratin filaments. Trauma is associated with separation of cells that literally tear apart in the absence of a bracing network of keratin intermediate filaments. This leads to clinical blistering.

Chapter 4   Support Cells and the Extracellular Matrix

1. (a) True, (b) False, (c) True, (d) True, (e) True
2. (a) True, (b) False, (c) True, (d) False, (e) False
3. (a) False, (b) True, (c) True, (d) True, (e) True
4. (a) True, (b) True, (c) False, (d) False, (e) True

Case 4.1   Answer

The strength of bone is determined by its extracellular matrix proteins, as well as its mineralization. Osteoblasts elaborate the support matrix of bone, osteoid, which subsequently calcifies to form bone.

Osteoid is composed mainly of type I collagen, which is associated with the extracellular GAGs, chondroitin sulfate and keratin sulfate. Two glycoproteins, sialoprotein and osteocalcin, are mainly found in the bone matrix and bind calcium; therefore they may have a role in bone mineralization. In children, several types of so-called 'brittle bone disease' are recognized, properly called **osteogenesis imperfecta** (OI).

OI is a dominant inherited condition that leads to a disorder of type I collagen, which is the main extracellular matrix protein of bone. Four forms of OI have been described.

Type I

- Most common and mildest form
- Bones predisposed to fracture
- Most fractures occur before puberty

- Triangular face
- Sclerae have a blue or grey tint
- Patients may have spinal curvature
- Bone deformity absent or minimal
- Collagen structure is normal, but the amount is less than normal.

Type II

- Fractures are numerous and severe, resulting in bone deformity
- Most severe form
- Often lethal at or shortly after birth
- Small stature develops
- Collagen is improperly formed.

Type III

- Bones fracture easily
- Fractures are often present at birth
- Short stature develops with bone deformity
- Triangular face
- Sclerae have a blue or grey tint
- Patients may have spinal curvature
- Collagen is improperly formed.

Type IV

- Intermediate in severity between types I and III
- Bones fracture easily, most before puberty
- Triangular face
- Sclerae normal in colour
- Generally only moderate bone deformity
- Patients may have spinal curvature
- Collagen is improperly formed.

Chapter 5   Contractile Cells

1. (a) True, (b) False, (c) True, (d) True, (e) True
2. (a) True, (b) True, (c) False, (d) True, (e) True
3. (a) True, (b) True, (c) True, (d) True, (e) True
4. (a) True, (b) True, (c) True, (d) True, (e) True

Case 5.1   Answer

Cardiac muscle is a form of striated muscle. Individual cardiac muscle cells are joined end to end at intercalated discs to form long fibres. Nuclei are typically in the centre of each cardiac muscle cell.

The term **hypertrophic** refers to the fact that the mass of the heart is increased by an increase in the size of individual cardiac muscle cells. The term **cardiomyopathy** implies that heart disease has resulted from a primary defect in the cardiac muscle.

The main contractile proteins in cardiac striated muscle are actin and myosin. Myosin interacts with several other proteins to form a regular array of contractile proteins arranged in striations.

The proteins involved in muscle contraction may be abnormal because of a mutation in the coding gene. In some patients with mutation in a gene form of cardiac myosin, contraction of muscle fibres is inefficient, leading to cardiac hypertrophy (enlargement of individual muscle cells that causes an increase in total mass of the myocardium).

It is now recognized that mutation in the genes coding for several muscle proteins, each of which is part of the contractile mechanism, can lead to hypertrophic cardiomyopathy. Mutations in the genes for cardiac myosin-binding protein C (MYBPC3) and beta-myosin heavy chain (MYH7) account for about 80% of families with identified mutations.

Chapter 6   Nervous Tissue

1. (a) False, (b) False, (c) False, (d) False, (e) True
2. (a) False, (b) True, (c) False, (d) False, (e) True
3. (a) False, (b) False, (c) True, (d) False, (e) True
4. (a) False, (b) False, (c) False, (d) True, (e) True

Case 6.1   Answer

The main cell types in the brain are neurons, glial cells, astrocytes, oligodendrocytes, ependymal cells, and microglia. Outside the brain are epithelial cells associated with the meninges; such cells are called **meningothelial cells**. Tumours can arise from any of these cell types.

The most common tumours arise from glial cells (gliomas) in the form of astrocytic tumours. Less common are tumours of oligodendrocytes (oligodendrogliomas) and ependymal cells.

Tumours that contain neurons are not very common compared with those that are purely glial.

True tumours of the resting phagocytic cells of the brain, the microglia, are extremely rare. However, lymphoid cells that migrate through the brain can cause tumours – so-called **cerebral lymphomas**.

One of the most common tumours that affect the brain is derived from the epithelial cells of the meninges, which form meningiomas.

In childhood, tumours arise from small primitive cells that are believed to be related to the primitive neuroectoderm. Such tumours can have a variety of patterns of differentiation.

Case 6.2   Answer

A peripheral nerve is composed of the following:
- Axons
- Schwann cells, which make myelin
- Spindle-shaped fibroblast support cells, which produce fibrocollagenous tissue
- Blood vessels.

There are three types of support tissue in a nerve trunk: the endoneurium, the perineurium, and the epineurium.

Endoneurium is composed of longitudinally oriented collagen fibres, extracellular matrix material rich in glycosaminoglycans and sparse fibroblasts. It surrounds the individual axons and their associated Schwann cells, as well as capillary blood vessels.

Perineurium surrounds groups of axons and endoneurium to form small bundles (fascicles). It is composed of seven or eight concentric layers of epithelium-like flattened cells separated by layers of collagen. The cells are joined by junctional complexes, and each layer of cells is surrounded by an external lamina.

Epineurium is an outer sheath of loose fibrocollagenous tissue that binds individual nerve fascicles into a nerve trunk. The epineurium may also include adipose tissue, as well as a main muscular artery supplying the nerve trunk.

In a peripheral neuropathy, the structures most likely to be damaged are the axons or the myelin and Schwann cells. In some cases, disease is caused by abnormalities in blood vessels that lead to local ischaemia of a nerve.

The speed of conduction along nerves is limited by the electrical capacitance and resistance of the axon. Because wide axons have a lower capacitance than narrow ones, increasing the diameter of axons is a useful means of increasing the speed of nerve conduction. This is inefficient, however, because giant axons require high metabolic upkeep. The speed of conduction along axons is increased if leakage of current from the membrane is minimized by insulation by myelin. The reduction in conduction velocity in this patient suggests that the main problem is loss of myelin from nerves (demyelination).

Diabetic patients are especially prone to development of peripheral neuropathy.

Chapter 7   Blood Cells

1. (a) True, (b) True, (c) True, (d) False, (e) True
2. (a) False, (b) False, (c) True, (d) True, (e) True
3. (a) False, (b) True, (c) True, (d) True, (e) False
4. (a) True, (b) True, (c) False, (d) False, (e) False

Case 7.1   Answer

In aplastic anaemia the quantity of all cellular elements in the blood is reduced because of failure of the bone marrow to manufacture cells.

In normal bone marrow, stem cells divide and produce committed progenitor cells that produce the various cell lineages.

All cellular elements of the blood originate from a common pluripotential progenitor stem cell (haemopoietic stem cell, HSC). These pluripotential stem cells are present in very small numbers at sites of blood-cell formation, and even fewer of them can be found in the peripheral blood. Histologically, they resemble lymphocytes but can be identified by use of immunohistochemical techniques, because they have distinctive cell-surface antigens. The pluripotential cells divide and give rise to cells with a more restricted line of growth.

It is possible to divide blood-forming cells into four groups, depending on capacity for self-renewal, cell division and ability to form different cell types. Pluripotential stem cells are capable of forming any type of blood cell; multipotential progenitor cells are capable of forming a specific but wide range of blood cells; committed progenitor cells are capable of forming only one or two types of blood cells; and maturing cells are undergoing structural differentiation to form one cell type and so are incapable of division.

Growth control of blood stem cells is through secreted growth factors and local cell contacts.

The best understood mechanism of control of growth of the different types of haemopoietic stem cells is

through the action of growth factors. These substances are secreted systemically or locally and modulate three aspects of cell growth:
- Proliferation
- Differentiation
- Maturation.

Less well understood in the control of blood-cell formation is the role of local cell–cell contacts. Stromal cells in the bone marrow appear to be important in control of differentiation and maturation; however, the signals involved are at present uncertain.

Aplastic anaemia can be associated with a variety of conditions and can be encountered as a disease of unknown cause.
- Reduction in platelets leads to increased tendency to bleed
- Reduction in red cells leads to clinical features of anaemia
- Reduction in white cells leads to susceptibility to infection.

In this case, a bone marrow biopsy showed lack of precursor cells for all formed elements in the marrow. This indicates that the reduced cellularity of all elements in the blood is caused by a failure of marrow production rather than a process of increased peripheral consumption or loss of cells.

Chapter 8 Immune System

1. (a) True, (b) True, (c) False, (d) True, (e) True
2. (a) True, (b) True, (c) False, (d) True, (e) True
3. (a) False, (b) True, (c) False, (d) True, (e) True
4. (a) True, (b) True, (c) False, (d) True, (e) True

Case 8.1 Answer

This clinical case illustrates a common problem: an enlarged lymph node of uncertain cause. The lymph node is a bean-shaped organ with a fibrocollagenous capsule, from which fibrous trabeculae extend into the node to form a supporting framework.

Lymph nodes contain three functional compartments:
- A network of endothelial-lined lymphatic sinuses continuous with the lumina of the afferent and efferent lymphatic vessels
- A network of small blood vessels, where circulating lymphocytes enter the node
- A parenchymal compartment composed of superficial cortex, paracortex, and medulla.

The superficial cortex of the lymph node contains the densely staining spheroid aggregations of lymphocytes (lymphoid follicles). Some of the follicles (primary follicles) are of fairly uniform staining density; however, most of the follicles that respond to antigen have less densely staining germinal centres and are described as secondary follicles. The lymphocyte population of the follicles consists predominantly of B cells, but there are smaller populations of TH cells, macrophages and accessory cells.

The cell population of the paracortex consists of lymphocytes and accessory cells, which constantly move in and out of the region. T cells dominate the paracortex, entering the node from the blood via the HEVs and leaving via the efferent lymphatics. When activated, T cells enlarge to form lymphoblasts. These then proliferate to produce an expanded clone of activated T cells. In a T cell-dominated immunological response, the paracortex may expand into the medulla, producing a so-called 'paracortical reaction'. Activated T cells are then disseminated via the circulation to peripheral sites, where much of their activity occurs.

In this case, the lymph node is characterized by expansion of both cortex (B-cell) and paracortical (T-cell) areas. One aspect of the function of activated T-cells is the secretion of cytokines and the recruitment and activation of macrophages. This is the functional background to the formation of aggregates of histiocytic cells to form structures called **granulomas**.

When associated with necrosis, granulomatous inflammation in a lymph node is likely to have been caused by tuberculous infection.

Chapter 9 Blood and Lymphatic Circulatory Systems and Heart

1. (a) True, (b) True, (c) True, (d) False, (e) True
2. (a) False, (b) True, (c) False, (d) True, (e) True
3. (a) True, (b) False, (c) False, (d) True, (e) False
4. (a) True, (b) True, (c) True, (d) True, (e) True

Case 9.1 Answer

From this you can see the basis of the family practitioner's explanation to the widower. Anything solid that forms in the leg veins and breaks off will be carried in the venous flow into the right side of the heart, and from there into the pulmonary artery system. In detail, the route leads from the deep veins in the right calf into the right femoral vein, the right external iliac vein, the right common iliac vein and the inferior vena cava. The mass passes up the inferior vena cava and into the right atrium, through the tricuspid right atrioventricular valve into the right ventricle, and out of the heart through the pulmonary valve into the large common pulmonary artery trunk.

So far, the mass has passed through vessels that are increasingly large in bore. However, at the division of the common pulmonary trunk into right and left main pulmonary arteries, the vessels begin to have a smaller bore. Eventually, the solid mass meets a blood vessel that is too small in bore to permit further passage, and an impaction occurs, completely blocking off the blood vessel. The clinical effect on the patient depends on the size of vessel obstructed.

Another factor of importance in this case is the pathological process called **thrombosis**. You can refer to a pathology textbook for a thorough discussion of this topic; a brief introduction to it is presented in *Human Histology*, third edition. Thrombosis is the pathological process in which a solid thrombus forms within the blood circulatory system. A thrombus is composed of aggregated blood platelets meshed together with strands of fibrin, an insoluble polymeric protein molecule derived from the soluble blood protein fibrinogen. In simple terms, platelets aggregate on a damaged endothelial surface and release factors that, with other factors from the damaged vessel wall, initiate the so-called **coagulation cascade**, a sequence of stepwise chemical reactions that ultimately catalyses the conversion of soluble fibrinogen (a normal plasma protein) into insoluble fibrin. The fibrin meshes with the original aggregated platelets, and additional masses of platelets become adherent, stimulating yet more fibrin formation. Thus, in certain circumstances, a thrombus may grow relentlessly until it is big enough to completely block the lumen of a vessel (e.g. coronary artery thrombosis). Fragments of thrombus may break off from the original site of formation and pass to another site in the blood circulation. This is called **thromboembolism** and is the cause of death in this case.

Case 9.2 Answer

The diagnosis in this case is anteroseptal myocardial infarction of the left ventricle. The anatomy can be broken down as follows:

- Left ventricle – This is the most substantial and bulky component of the heart. The chamber receives oxygenated blood from the lungs via the left atrium and pumps it throughout the body at high pressure. Therefore it has a thick wall of contractile cardiac muscle lined by smooth endothelium and covered by the smooth pericardium. Because it has large work output, the muscle of the left ventricle has a high demand for oxygenated blood, supplied by coronary arteries
- Anteroseptal part of the left ventricle – This part of the left ventricle consists of the anterior wall of the left ventricle and the anterior half of the interventricular septum. This part of the heart is usually supplied by the anterior descending branch of the left coronary artery
- Myocardial infarction – This is the name given to the pathological process in which death of myocardium (cardiac muscle) results from an abrupt interference with its oxygenated blood supply. It usually follows sudden complete obstruction of a branch of a coronary artery.

In this case, complete obstruction of the anterior descending branch of the left coronary artery has led to necrosis of the myocardium in the anteroseptal part of the left ventricle.

The following symptoms, displayed by this man, are typical of myocardial infarction:

- Central crushing pain in the chest, which persists and does not improve with rest
- Breathlessness (see later)
- Distress.

The following physical signs, elicited on examination, are also typical:

- Shock (weak rapid pulse, low blood pressure)
- Cyanosis (see later)
- White froth on the lips (see later)
- Widespread crepitations over both lung fields (see later)
- Pericardial friction rub (see later).

The clinicopathological correlation of myocardial infarction can be briefly summarized as follows: the damaged left ventricle is unable to contract efficiently, so the left ventricular output is reduced; this produces the low blood pressure and a weak pulse, and the heart rate increases in an attempt to augment the cardiac output. The pulse rate is rapid.

Another manifestation of the failing function of the left ventricle is its inability to empty completely with each systole. With each diastole, the same amount of blood pours into the left ventricle from the left atrium, to be added to the blood remaining in the left ventricular chamber at the end of systole. A few heartbeats after the left ventricular wall failure, the left ventricle begins to dilate because of accumulated blood. The pressure rises in the left ventricle and is eventually transmitted backward into the left atrium and from there into pulmonary veins and back into the pulmonary capillaries. The increase in pulmonary capillary pressure has important clinical and pathological consequences.

High pressure in the extensive pulmonary capillary network leads to transudation of some of the fluid content of the blood in the capillaries into the alveolar air sacs. (The pulmonary capillaries are in intimate contact with the alveolar air sac wall.) The consequence of this is that the air sacs become filled with watery fluid, which displaces the air (i.e. pulmonary oedema), and this interferes with oxygenation of the blood, producing breathlessness and cyanosis, both of which (combined with the severe chest pain) produce distress. The white froth around the lips is mixed air and oedema fluid welling up from the millions of alveoli of the lungs, an indication of severe widespread pulmonary oedema. On auscultation of the lungs, the movement of inspired air trying to get into the alveoli full of watery fluid gives rise to the physical sign called **crepitation**.

Infarction of the full thickness of the left ventricular wall also leads to damage to the inner endocardium and the outer pericardium, both of which can produce major complications. An indication that the pericardium had been affected is the presence, on auscultation, of a pericardial friction rub, a high-pitched scratching noise that occurs in time with each systolic heartbeat.

Chapter 10   Respiratory System

1. (a) False, (b) False, (c) False, (d) True, (e) True
2. Answer: b, d, a, e, c
3. (a) False, (b) True, (c) False, (d) False, (e) False
4. (a) True, (b) False, (c) True, (d) False, (e) True

Case 10.1 Answer

This man's total loss of the sense of smell followed an episode of severe trauma to the skull, during which he sustained a crack fracture to the base of his skull in the anterior cranial fossa. The olfactory nerves and bulb lie on the floor of the anterior cranial fossa on either side of the midline, running in an anterior–posterior direction. They may be transected in a transverse fracture across the floor of the anterior cranial fossa, resulting in loss of the sense of smell.

Case 10.2   Answer

This man's loss of voice is the result of a structural abnormality in the laryngeal region, and the loss of voice means that the true cords are involved. Loss of voice has many causes, including bacterial or viral infection ('laryngitis'), but long-standing and progressive loss of voice means that a tumour must be excluded, particularly in elderly smokers. Phonation (voice production) is dependent on vibration of the freely moving true vocal cords under the control of the vocalis muscle and laryngeal nerves.

Even benign tumours can affect the structure of the true cord enough to produce symptoms such as hoarseness, but invasive malignant tumours so disrupt the anatomy of the true cord that progressive hoarseness eventually leads to complete loss of voice. This malignant tumour is derived from the stratified squamous epithelium that covers the outer surface of the true cord.

Malignant tumours can spread away from the site of origin by various mechanisms, including invasion into the lumen of a lymphatic vessel at the original tumour site, and clumps of tumour cells can break off and pass through the lymphatic vessels to regional lymph nodes. Spread to the lymph nodes in the side of the neck is common in carcinoma of the larynx. The true cords contain no lymphatic vessels except at the commissures, so spread to distant sites is common only when the primary tumour in the true cord extends to involve the commissures.

The other parts of the laryngeal apparatus, such as the false cords, are well supplied with lymphatic vessels, so tumours originating in these sites are much more likely to spread away from the primary site to regional lymph nodes than tumours confined to the true cord, with a correspondingly poor prognosis.

Case 10.3   Answer

Pneumonia has developed in both lungs, but it is confined to the basal parts of the lower lobes. **Pneumonia** is the old term (but still used) to describe a viral or bacterial infection of the lungs, although **pneumonitis** would be a better term. In bacterial pneumonia, bacteria gain access to the alveolar air sacs in two main ways: by being carried down in bronchial mucus from higher up the respiratory tree in situations in which the normal mucociliary ladder does not work, or by being inhaled directly into the air sacs.

In this patient, an elderly woman who has recently had an upper respiratory tract infection, the bacteria have initially colonized an upper respiratory tract that has been damaged by a preceding viral infection (influenza) that severely damaged the surface epithelium of the trachea and main and branch bronchi, destroying particularly the surface cilia normally responsible for sweeping the thin sheet of bronchial mucus upwards. In the absence of these defence mechanisms, the bronchial mucus slides down the bronchial tree under the influence of gravity and the bronchioles in the distal respiratory tree become blocked with mucus. As they pass downwards, the bacteria infect the trachea (tracheitis), the bronchi (bronchitis) and the bronchioles (bronchiolitis),

and when they reach the thin-walled terminal and respiratory bronchioles, the bacteria can pass out through the walls to infect the alveolar air sacs around the bronchioles. This pattern of spread of bacterial lung infection is called **bronchopneumonia**.

Chapter 11   Alimentary Tract

1. (a) True, (b) True, (c) False, (d) True, (e) True
2. (a) True, (b) True, (c) False, (d) True, (e) True
3. (a) False, (b) True, (c) True, (d) True, (e) False
4. (a) False, (b) True, (c) False, (d) False, (e) True

Case 11.1   Answer

This man is thought by his family practitioner to have gastroesophageal reflux disease (GERD) because of the history he gives, especially the fact that the pain is particularly frequent and severe at night when he lies down in bed. The basis of this disorder is that the acid secretions in the lumen of the stomach sometimes pass up into the lower oesophagus. Here, they damage and erode the stratified squamous epithelium of the lower oesophagus, which is not resistant to the effects of acid (unlike the tall, columnar epithelium lining the stomach, which has a thin protective layer of mucus secreted by the gastric mucous cells).

Reflux of gastric acid into the oesophagus is normally prevented by the gastroesophageal sphincter, which is partly structural (a ring of sphincteric smooth muscle in the wall at the gastroesophageal junction) and partly functional, with extrinsic pressure from the muscles of the diaphragm and the normal angulation at the gastroesophageal junction both playing a part. To understand the role of the diaphragm, read about hiatal hernia in your surgical textbook.

Case 11.2   Answer

The patient cites a very short history of severe uncontrollable diarrhoea, the stools being very watery and bloodstained. A biopsy shows loss of the mucosa with extensive superficial ulceration, and a diagnosis of acute ulcerative colitis is made.

The mucosa of the colon and rectum is lined by tall columnar epithelium arranged in straight tubular glands, and the majority of the epithelial cells are either absorptive or mucus secreting. The major function of the large intestine is to absorb water from the liquid small intestinal contents, which pass into it through the ileocaecal valve. Thus, the liquid small intestinal contents are converted into semisolid faeces by concentration through massive reabsorption of water, and the passage of the semi-solid faecal mass along the distal colon and rectum is eased by the mucus added to it from the colonic mucus-secreting goblet cells. At the bottom of the tubular glands are also neuroendocrine cells and stem cells; the latter are important in the healing process in this disease.

Extensive loss of mucosa of the large intestine in severe ulcerative colitis significantly interferes with the function of the large intestine; loss of so much absorptive epithelium means that the ileal contents pass through largely unchanged because the water is not absorbed, and no semisolid faeces is formed. Because the disease destroys and erodes much of the mucosa, the underlying submucosa, which contains abundant thin-walled blood vessels, is exposed and significant bleeding occurs, producing iron deficiency anaemia, as in this case. The sphincter mechanism in the anus (internal anal sphincter and external anal sphincter) has a very limited capacity to retain the liquid contents of the colon and rectum, and faecal incontinence is a problem.

Case 11.3   Answer

The mucosa and submucosa of the small bowel are thrown up into a large number of folds or plicae arranged circularly around the lumen. These are most prominent in the jejunum. The surface of the plicae is further arranged into villi, which protrude into the intestinal lumen. Tubular glands or crypts extend down from the base of the villi to the muscularis mucosae.

The small bowel mucosa is formed of enterocytes, which are tall columnar cells with round or oval nuclei in the lower third of the cell. The luminal surface of enterocytes is highly specialized; each cell bears 2–3000 tightly packed, tall microvilli, which are coated by a glycoprotein, the glycocalyx. This is composed of fine filamentous extensions of the microvillus cell membrane. The glycocalyx contains a number of enzymes (brush border enzymes, e.g. lactase, sucrase, peptidases, lipases and alkaline phosphatase), which are important in digestion and transport.

In coeliac disease, an immune response to ingested gluten found in wheatflour leads to death of cells in the small bowel epithelium. In response to cell death, there is increased production of epithelial cells by the crypts. The crypts become longer than normal. However, cell death of formed epithelial cells continues and the bowel mucosa does not form a villous pattern.

A consequence of losing the villous pattern is that the surface area of small bowel for absorption is reduced. This leads to small bowel malabsorption. Fat is especially not absorbed, so it remains in the stool making them greasy, pale and difficult to flush away (steatorrhoea). The absorption of iron, vitamin B_{12} and folate can also be affected, leading to anaemia.

Another consequence of having a rapid turnover of small bowel epithelial cells, is that they do not have time to achieve full differentiation. The expression of surface enzymes such as lactase and sucrase may not occur and so absorption of these sugars may not happen as they cannot be broken down into simple sugars.

In patients with coeliac disease, a diet free of gluten in wheatflour is advised. Immune-mediated damage ceases and the epithelial architecture of the small bowel returns to normal.

Chapter 12   Liver

1. (a) False, (b) True, (c) True, (d) True, (e) False
2. (a) False, (b) True, (c) True, (d) False, (e) True
3. (a) True, (b) True, (c) True, (d) True, (e) False
4. (a) True, (b) True, (c) True, (d) True, (e) True

Case 12.1   Answer

In this patient, collapse is likely to be related to a high blood ethanol level and also to the low blood glucose level. Alcohol is a recognized hepatotoxin and can interfere with normal liver function and cause liver cell damage. The main functions of the liver are as follows:

- Bile synthesis and secretion – The liver produces bile, which contains water, ions, phospholipids, bile pigments (mainly bilirubin glucuronide) and bile acids (glycocholic and taurocholic acids)
- Excretion of bilirubin – Bilirubin is produced in the spleen from the breakdown of the haem component of haemoglobin. In the liver, the bilirubin is conjugated with glucuronic acid, and the conjugate (bilirubin glucuronide) is excreted in the bile and thence the faeces
- Protein synthesis – The liver synthesizes many proteins, including albumin, and blood clotting factors, such as fibrinogen and prothrombin
- Gluconeogenesis – Lipids and amino acids are converted into glucose in the liver by gluconeogenesis
- Storage – Triglycerides, glycogen and some vitamins are stored in the liver
- Deamination of amino acids – In the liver, amino acids are deaminated to produce urea, which is excreted by the kidney
- Conjugation and chemical breakdown of toxins – The smooth endoplasmic reticulum of the liver possesses large numbers of enzymes that break down or conjugate toxic substances (e.g. alcohol, barbiturates) to convert them into other metabolites.

In this patient, the following three aspects of liver function have been found to be abnormal:

- Low blood sugar – possibly related to failure of gluconeogenesis
- Elevated bilirubin – possibly related to failure of bile synthesis and excretion
- Low serum albumen – related to failure of protein synthesis by the liver.

An additional clinical feature that is observed is ascites – the accumulation of fluid within the peritoneal cavity. The patient may be predisposed to this condition by a low serum albumen, with a corresponding low plasma oncotic pressure. Another factor that can cause ascites is a raised blood pressure in the portal venous system – portal hypertension. In the normal liver, blood from the portal vein runs through the liver in vessels in portal tracts, then into liver sinusoids. If a disturbance of liver structure occurs because of disease, then the flow of blood through the sinusoids may be impaired, leading to backpressure in the portal venous system and portal hypertension.

A disease that can result in all these features is cirrhosis, in which long-standing damage to liver cells leads to fibrosis (deposition of collagenous scar), death of liver cells and, through attempted regeneration, formation of nodules of liver cells. This disturbed architecture of the liver leads to disturbance of the vascular arrangement and portal hypertension. Reduction in liver cell mass and abnormal anatomy leads to failure of liver cell function, with elevated bilirubin, impaired gluconeogenesis and failure of secretion of serum proteins. This pattern of disease is termed **chronic liver disease**, as it results from long-standing damage.

In this instance, it is most likely that chronic alcohol abuse has led to liver cell damage and eventual development of cirrhosis.

Chapter 13   Musculoskeletal System

1. (a) False, (b) True, (c) True, (d) True, (e) False
2. (a) False, (b) True, (c) True, (d) False, (e) False
3. (a) True, (b) False, (c) False, (d) True, (e) True
4. (a) True, (b) True, (c) True, (d) False, (e) True

Case 13.1   Answer

When bones are so severely fractured that displacement occurs, normal bone fracture repair cannot take place because the fractured bone ends are too far apart. The aim of surgical treatment is to put the ends of the fractured bone together ('fracture reduction') and hold them in close apposition ('fracture fixation'), so that speedy healing can occur. Given that this fracture required fixation with metal pins and plates, one can assume that considerable displacement was present.

Even when the fracture is reduced and fixed in this way, it takes at least 8 weeks for the fracture to repair, during which time the movement of the limb is limited, and the patient is unable to bear weight on it for some weeks. During this time, the muscles of the limb are grossly underused, and they can undergo significant atrophy as a result of disuse, leading to reduction in the muscle mass and weakness in the limb, when it is eventually fully mobilized. These changes can be minimized by a programme of physiotherapy to keep the muscles in use, even if they are not used for walking.

Physiotherapy to the thigh and calf muscles is essential from the outset for the following two reasons:
- It is essential for prevention of disuse atrophy of the muscle, which develops because of physical inactivity during the period of fracture healing
- It minimizes the risk for leg vein thrombosis (see Case 9.1).

Case 13.2   Answer

Dystrophin is a protein that is associated with the cell membrane of skeletal muscle fibres and is responsible for providing a link between the intracellular proteins that mediate contraction and the extracellular proteins in the external membrane surrounding each muscle fibre.

If dystrophin is not expressed, then forces generated by contraction of muscle fibres are not transmitted efficiently to the extracellular matrix. In normal muscle, contraction forces are coordinated and transmitted uniformly through the extracellular matrix to allow the muscle to behave as a single mass.

In patients without expression of dystrophin, contraction causes tearing of the cell membrane, leading to death of muscle fibres. Although some regeneration of muscle fibres can occur, over time, fibres are lost and

fibrosis develops in muscle, manifest in permanent muscle weakness.

It is now realized that mutation in genes coding for other membrane linking proteins can also result in muscular dystrophy.

Case 13.3   Answer

The hip joint is a typical synovial joint between the head of the femur and the cup-like acetabulum of the pelvis, into which the femoral head fits in the form of a ball and socket joint. Because it is a synovial joint, both articular surfaces are normally coated by a layer of articular cartilage, and the smooth and virtually friction-free movement of the two articular surfaces is assisted by the presence between them of a thin film of slippery lubricating synovial fluid produced by the synovial lining of the internal surface of the joint capsule.

In the normal structure of the femoral head, a thick coat of smooth articular cartilage on the articular surface rests on the dense compact cortical bone, from which the complex interfacing network of trabecular bone struts run to occupy the medullary cavity of the bone.

In the disease suffered by this patient (osteoarthritis, or osteoarthrosis), constant frictional damage occurs over very many years, leading to progressive erosion and thinning of the articular cartilage on the two opposing surfaces of the two bones participating in the joint. Eventually, all the articular cartilage is eroded away, and the cortical bone of the head of the femur is in constant contact with the cortical bone of the acetabular cup. The cortical plates of the two bones undergo thickening to withstand the extra forces they must resist once the cushioning effect of the cartilage has gone. The cortical bone not only becomes thickened, but it becomes even more compact as a result of the severe compressive forces to which it is subjected, and the constant friction of the two hard cortical bone surfaces leads to the bone surfaces becoming very compact and highly 'polished' (a process called **eburnation**). The vertical compressive forces on the femoral head lead to variable degrees of flattening of the usually round head, because some of the bone trabeculae under the reinforced cortical plate may buckle.

A further structural change that occurs in the femoral head is the formation of protuberant bony 'osteophytes' at the periphery of the head. This occurs because of reactive new bone formation as a result of abnormal transmission of the compressive and frictional forces operating as the structure of the femoral head changes with the progression of the disease.

Production of osteoarthritic changes. As described previously, the main changes that occur are the result of progressive excessive wear and tear, and most can be explained purely by the physical forces involved. Osteoarthritis is very common in the hip in the elderly but also occurs in joints that are heavily used, for example, in the fingers of keyboard operators and the knees of athletes such as soccer players. However, development of the disease is not inevitable, and evidence suggests that genetic factors may have an influence, particularly on the function and response of the chondrocytes in the articular cartilage to trauma.

Case 13.4   Answer

This patient gives a clinical history of an intervertebral disc protrusion, causing symptoms of back pain ('lumbago') and pain in the buttock and down the back of the leg with neurological symptoms ('sciatica').

The bony vertebral bodies are separated from one another by intervertebral discs, which act as both shock absorbers and as non-synovial joints, allowing limited anteroposterior and lateral flexion and extension of the spine.

Each intervertebral disc is composed of fibrocartilage with a central area of soft gelatinous fibromyxoid tissue called the **nucleus pulposus**, around which the denser fibrocartilage is arranged as a surrounding shell, called the **annulus fibrosus**. In disc protrusion, the central nucleus pulposus material bulges out through the lateral wall, barely restrained by the thin annulus fibrosus. The cause of this is not certain, but extruded disc material removed at surgery for the treatment of disc protrusion shows the annulus fibrosus to be thinned and partly disrupted by rather pale, disorganized nucleus pulposus material that looks waterlogged.

The bulging disc material presses on spinal nerves as they emerge from the spinal cord on their way to the pelvis and lower limbs. This physical pressure on the nerves produces the neurological symptoms and signs of sciatica.

Chapter 14   Endocrine System

1. (a) False, (b) True, (c) True, (d) False, (e) True
2. (a) False, (b) False, (c) True, (d) True, (e) True
3. (a) iii, (b) iv, (c) i, (d) ii
4. (a) False, (b) True, (c) False, (d) True, (e) True

Case 14.1   Answer

To understand the answer to this question, you need to be familiar with the normal histology of the thyroid gland, the structural and functional relationships of the thyroid acinar cells and the feedback control of thyroid hormone secretion.

The surgeon was particularly interested in the palpation of the front of the neck because he suspected the thyroid gland was the source of the problem, and there was a good chance that the entire gland or part of it would be sufficiently enlarged that it would be easily palpable. Sometimes, the gland is so enlarged that it is easily visible (goitre).

This patient has thyroid hyperplasia, in which the thyroid acini contain increased numbers of thyroid epithelial cells. Normally, a high proportion of the epithelial cells lining the thyroid acini are small and in an inactive phase; only a few cells at any one time are actively involved in synthesizing thyroid hormone or reprocessing formed thyroglobulin from the stored thyroid colloid to produce active thyroid hormone. The proportion of active to inactive thyroid cells varies according to the body's requirement for thyroid hormone, controlled by a feedback mechanism involving thyroid-stimulating hormone (TSH) secreted by the anterior pituitary gland. In thyroid hyperplasia, this feedback mechanism is circumvented; the thyroid epithelial cells increase in number, and a much higher proportion becomes actively involved in synthesizing and mobilizing thyroid hormone, irrespective of the body's needs. This leads to the clinical syndrome of thyrotoxicosis, in which constant excessive output of active thyroid hormone increases the body's metabolic rate, leading to increased appetite, weight loss, irritability, restlessness, sleeplessness, clumsiness, physical hyperactivity, palpitations, diarrhoea and heat intolerance.

This patient suffers from many of the listed symptoms as a result of the continuous high output of active thyroid hormone by her histologically abnormal thyroid gland.

Case 14.2   Answer

This patient was thought to have Cushing's disease. Most patients have upper body obesity with a rounded face and increased fat deposition around the neck and shoulders. Abdominal striae are purple-red stretch marks that can appear on the abdomen, arms, breasts, buttocks and thighs. High blood pressure is common. Many patients also complain of fatigue and have muscle weakness. Impaired glucose tolerance may result in diabetes mellitus.

The disease is caused by excessive levels of the hormone cortisol. Cortisol is produced by the cells of the adrenal cortex. This is regulated by secretion of adrenocorticotropic hormone (ACTH) by the adenohypophysis of the pituitary gland, which stimulates production. The release of ACTH is in turn, regulated by influences from the hypothalamic region of the brain and the secretion of corticotropin-releasing factor (CRF), which stimulates secretion.

When levels of cortisol in the blood reach appropriate levels, the hypothalamus and pituitary release less CRF and ACTH. This feedback system regulates the amount of cortisol released by the adrenal glands.

The theoretic causes of excess secretion of cortisol could reside in the hypothalamus, the pituitary gland or the adrenal gland.

Excessive CRF secretion may lead to overproduction of cortisol. In practice, this does not commonly explain cases of Cushing's disease; when it does happen, its origin is not the hypothalamus, but rather it has an ectopic cause, usually a lung tumour.

Excessive secretion of ACTH may happen in the presence of a tumour of the pituitary gland (pituitary adenoma). In this situation, the tumour continues to secrete ACTH independently of any regulation by levels of CRF.

In some patients, ACTH can be secreted from an ectopic site, for example a lung tumour.

Excessive cortisol may be the result of autonomous secretion by an abnormality in the adrenal gland. The usual cause is a tumour of the adrenal cortex. In most cases, this is an adenoma (benign), but in some patients, it can be an adrenal cortical carcinoma (malignant).

Chapter 15   Urinary System

1. (a) True, (b) True, (c) False, (d) True, (e) True
2. (a) True, (b) True, (c) True, (d) False, (e) False

3. (a) False, (b) True, (c) False, (d) True, (e) True
4. (a) True, (b) True, (c) False, (d) False, (e) True

Case 15.1 Answer

This child shows the features of the nephritic syndrome (acute glomerulonephritis), which is composed of the following:

- Haematuria and passage of reduced amounts of urine (oliguria)
- Transient rise in blood pressure
- Transient rise in blood urea
- Oedema, particularly periorbital.

The features are the result of structural abnormalities in all the glomeruli in both kidneys. The normal thin layer of endothelial cells lining the glomerular capillaries proliferates so that the lumina of the capillaries are completely blocked and prevent the passage of blood through them. This leads to an increase in vascular peripheral resistance, leading to a rise in blood pressure. Because little blood passes through the glomeruli, little ultrafiltration occurs across the glomerular filtration barrier; the volume of urine passed is greatly reduced (oliguria), and the blood urea rises.

The pathogenesis of the nephritic syndrome is complex, but the basic abnormality is an immunological injury to the glomerulus, with the deposition of immune complexes in the membrane, the presence of which stimulates the proliferation of the endothelial cells.

Fortunately, in most cases, the nephritic syndrome in children is short-lived. The immune complexes in the glomerular basement membrane disappear and the proliferated endothelial cells regress until the capillaries are again lined by a thin layer of flat endothelial cells. As the capillaries regain their lumen, blood flows through them once more; the blood pressure falls and ultrafiltration resumes, so that urine output increases and the blood urea level falls.

Case 15.2 Answer

This man has the combination of symptoms, signs and laboratory findings that constitute the nephrotic syndrome:

- Excessive protein loss in the urine (proteinuria)
- Low serum albumen levels (hypoalbuminaemia)
- Oedema, particularly of the hands and feet.

Because of an abnormality in the glomerular filtration barrier, large amounts of protein pass out from the blood plasma in the glomerular capillary lumen into the urinary space. The normally functioning glomerular filtration barrier holds back most of the plasma protein. The protein (particularly the smaller protein molecules such as albumen) passes down the tubular system in the glomerular filtrate. Normally, any small amounts of protein that pass through the normally functioning glomerular filtration barrier are reabsorbed in the proximal convoluted tubule, so that the urine eventually contains no protein at all. However, in the nephrotic syndrome, the amount of protein in the glomerular filtrate far exceeds the tubule's capacity to reabsorb it, so protein is present in the final concentrated urine. This is called **proteinuria**.

When protein loss (particularly albumen) in the urine has been severe and prolonged, the amount of protein loss exceeds the capacity of the liver to synthesize new albumen. When the blood is tested for protein content, it is found that the level of albumen is low. This is called **hypoalbuminaemia**.

With a low serum albumen, the forces that control the balance of fluid between the intravascular and extravascular (tissue) fluid are disturbed. One of the important factors that draws fluid into the intravascular space (at capillary level) from the interstitium of the tissues is the osmotic (oncotic) pressure exerted by the high levels of protein in the plasma within the capillaries; this sucks in fluid from the extravascular space. When the plasma protein levels are low, this oncotic pressure is reduced, and less interstitial fluid is drawn into the capillary lumina. Therefore, fluid accumulates in the tissue interstitium, leading to tissue oedema.

Case 15.3 Answer

The component of the nephron damaged in this case is the tubule system, particularly the metabolically active proximal and distal tubules, which are so important in fluid and ion exchange and therefore in maintaining homeostasis.

The capillaries that supply the tubules (peritubular capillaries) are at the end of a long and complicated vascular supply to the kidney: renal artery, main renal artery branch, segmental artery, interlobular artery, arcuate artery, interlobular artery, afferent arteriole, glomerular capillary network, efferent arteriole and peritubular capillary network. Perfusion of blood through this very distal capillary system is always likely to be compromised if any central loss of perfusion pressure occurs, and the cells that they supply, i.e. the epithelial cells of the tubules, are likely to suffer from hypoxia. Unfortunately, these cells have a very high oxygen requirement, as they are so rich in mitochondria because of their high metabolic activity.

In this case, the patient suffered multiple injuries involving severe loss of blood (from a ruptured spleen and bone fractures) and was hypotensive and hypovolaemic for a long period. During such a time, perfusion through the most peripheral blood vessels such as the peritubular capillaries is greatly reduced and oxygenation of tissues (including the tubular epithelial cells) becomes inadequate for normal cell function. The ion-pumping activities cease, and many of the tubular epithelial cells therefore die (acute tubular necrosis). The failure of their function leads to severe disorders of electrolyte balance, metabolic acidosis and hyperkalaemia being the first to be manifest on blood testing. Reduced blood perfusion through the glomerular capillaries leads to reduced ultrafiltration, with consequent reduction in the production of glomerular filtrate, and therefore urine. In this case, perfusion of blood through the kidney vessels was so greatly reduced that no urine was produced at all (anuria).

This man has an excellent chance of recovery once his blood loss is stopped. He will then cease to be hypovolaemic and hypotensive, and the blood flow through his peripheral blood vessels will return to normal. Normal perfusion through the glomerular capillaries will allow ultrafiltration to occur, and urine will be produced again.

Normal perfusion in the peritubular capillaries will allow adequate oxygenation of any tubular epithelial cells that have survived, and they will begin to pump ions again in a small way. However, the tubular epithelial cells have a great capacity to regenerate; the tubules soon become completely repopulated by functional epithelial cells, and normal homeostatic mechanisms return.

Chapter 16 Male Reproductive System

1. (a) False, (b) True, (c) True, (d) True, (e) True
2. (a) True, (b) True, (c) False, (d) True, (e) False
3. (a) False, (b) True, (c) True, (d) False, (e) True
4. (a) False, (b) True, (c) True, (d) True, (e) True

Case 16.1 Answer

After leaving the bladder, the male urethra passes through the prostate gland before running through the penis. As it passes through the prostate, the urethra can become compressed if the prostate gland becomes enlarged. Enlargement of the prostate gland is common in men older than 60 years and results from hyperplasia of the glands in the mucosal (inner periurethral) and submucosal (outer periurethral) groups. This proliferation of glands leads to enlargement of the entire gland, and the normally tubular prostatic urethra is squashed into a narrow slit-like shape, producing partial obstruction. This leads to difficulty in emptying the bladder during micturition. The symptoms experienced by this man (urinary frequency, poor stream, difficulty in starting and stopping) are typical of those resulting from prostatic obstruction of the urethra.

As a result of this obstruction of the urethra, some urine is always left behind in the bladder at the end of micturition (residual urine); the amount retained increases with the severity of the obstruction, and the bladder may become permanently distended. The bladder has to work harder than normal to empty against the obstruction, and as a result, the smooth muscle in the wall of the bladder undergoes work hypertrophy. The bladder wall becomes thicker as the three muscle layers undergo hypertrophy, and the enlarged muscle bands can be seen through the mucosa (trabeculations).

Case 16.2 Answer

The testes develop high on the posterior abdominal wall during early embryological development and migrate down into the scrotal sac before birth. It is believed that the lower temperature in the scrotum is essential for normal development of the germ cells and their subsequent maturation into spermatozoa in the process called **spermatogenesis**. The normal mature testis is composed of seminiferous tubules lined internally by germ cells (spermatogonia), which, under the influence of testosterone secreted by the Leydig cells lying in the interstices between seminiferous tubules, undergo the division and maturational processes known as **spermatocytogenesis** and **spermatogenesis** to produce motile spermatozoa. This process begins with the onset of puberty. Formed

spermatozoa pass into the rete testis, then into efferent ductules and into the epididymis. From there, they pass into the long tubular vas deferens (ductus deferens), which runs in the spermatic cord from epididymis into the ejaculatory ducts, which run through the prostate gland and open into the prostatic urethra at the utricle. At the beginning of the ejaculatory ducts, the vas deferens is joined by short ducts from the seminal vesicles, the secretions of which provide nutrients for the spermatozoa.

Absence of spermatozoa in the ejaculate means that either the testes are not making spermatozoa or the passage of spermatozoa from the testes to the urethra is completely obstructed on both sides. In this case, the most likely cause is that the testes are not making spermatozoa as a result of failure of the testes to descend into the scrotum during intrauterine life (cryptorchid testes). In such circumstances, the germinal epithelium does not develop, even though the testes are often drawn down into the scrotal sac surgically in childhood. Once all the germ cells have died, there does not seem to be any capacity for regeneration once conditions improve. Without germinal epithelium to form the internal lining of the seminiferous tubules, the only cells present are the Sertoli cells. The tubules remain small, with thick basement membranes, and the testis as a whole remains small, showing little of the enlargement that normally occurs at puberty. The testosterone-secreting Leydig (interstitial) cells are not damaged in undescended testes and continue to secrete hormone, so secondary sexual characteristics develop normally.

Other causes of germ cell destruction in the testes exist, including viral infection in mumps. If the cause of absence of spermatozoa in the ejaculate is not apparent, a needle biopsy of the testis can be performed.

Chapter 17 Female Reproductive System

1. (a) False, (b) True, (c) True, (d) True, (e) False
2. (a) True, (b) False, (c) True, (d) True, (e) True
3. (a) True, (b) False, (c) True, (d) False, (e) True
4. (a) True, (b) True, (c) False, (d) True, (e) True

Case 17.1 Answer

In order for an ovum to be fertilized and become implanted after its release from the ovary, it must pass down the uterine (fallopian) tube. The fertilized ovum then must implant itself in the endometrium of the uterus at the correct phase.

Ovarian factors are a common cause of female infertility. It is possible that endocrine factors prevent maturation of the follicle and release of an ovum; however, this appears to be excluded in this case on investigation.

The next most common group of disorders relates to problems in the uterine tubes. The uterine tubes convey ova from the ovary to the lumen of the body of the uterus (endometrial cavity). They are also the usual sites of fertilization of the ovum by spermatozoa. After fertilization, the tube transmits the fertilized ovum to the endometrial cavity, where implantation can take place. Each uterine tube is 10–12 cm long and extends from a dilated open end close to the ovary to a narrow portion that passes through the myometrial wall of the uterus before opening into the uterine cavity.

The infundibulum of the uterine tube is surrounded by a fringe of epithelial-coated fimbriae. In some diseases, the fimbriae become densely adherent to the surface of the ovary, such that it is not possible for a released ovum to enter the tube. The uterine tube is a muscular tube lined by specialized epithelium that is variably folded and plicate, differing in appearance at different sites. In the presence of disease of the tube, such as that causing narrowing, or disease of the lining epithelium, the ovum may be impeded in its passage down the tube. Two types of epithelial cell line the uterine tube: ciliated cells and secretory cells. The ciliated cells may be responsible for movement of the ovum through the infundibulum and ampulla, although tubal peristalsis probably plays a greater role. Ciliated cells may also have a role in propelling the spermatozoa in the opposite direction. Rare genetic conditions in which cilial motility is impaired may be associated with impaired fertility.

Endometrial or uterine factors may also lead to infertility. Implantation has to take place in an endometrium in the secretory phase. If endocrine factors are such that the endometrium is not in a secretory phase, then implantation may not occur. Inflammatory conditions and anatomical abnormalities of the endometrium, such as polyps, may also interfere with implantation. In some women, scarring and narrowing of the endometrial cavity may prevent implantation.

Chapter 18   Skin and Breast

1. (a) True, (b) True, (c) False, (d) True, (e) False
2. (a) False, (b) True, (c) False, (d) False, (e) False
3. (a) False, (b) False, (c) True, (d) True, (e) True
4. (a) True, (b) True, (c) True, (d) True, (e) True

Case 18.1   Answer

This disease (bullous pemphigoid) is caused by an abnormality at the epidermal basement membrane, so it is important to know its structure.

The basement membrane between epidermis and dermis has three main layers: an electron-lucent lamina lucida on the epithelial side; an electron-dense lamina densa beneath it; and, on the dermal side of the lamina densa, an ill-defined layer called the fibroreticular lamina, through which various anchoring fibrils (type VII collagen) and microfibrils (fibrillin) pass and connect to collagen and elastin fibres in the dermis. These firmly tether the basement membrane to the underlying dermis. On the other (epidermal) side of the basement membrane, the basal cells of the epidermis are firmly bound to the basement membrane through specialized structures called **hemidesmosomes,** which connect to the lamina densa by anchoring filaments that pass from the hemidesmosome to the lamina densa through the lamina lucida.

At least 17 different antigens have been identified in the various layers of the basement membrane, two of which are known as the **bullous pemphigoid antigens** (BPAG-1 and BPAG-2). One of these resides in the hemidesmosome, and the other is located in the lamina lucida. In the disease bullous pemphigoid, autoantibodies develop against these two antigens, and an antigen-antibody reaction occurs at the site of the antigens, that is, in the hemidesmosomes and lamina lucida. The damage to the antigen molecules by this autoimmune process leads to weakness of the epidermal basement membrane, and separation of the epidermis from the dermis occurs in the plane of the lamina lucida. Fluid accumulation in this separation space leads to the lifting of the epidermis to form a fluid-filled blister. Electron microscopy of an early blister shows that the separation occurs in the lamina lucida, the lamina densa being left behind on the surface of the dermis at the base of the blister.

The blood test demonstrates the presence of antibodies against the bullous pemphigoid antigens (BPAG-1 and BPAG-2) circulating in the bloodstream, and the immunofluorescence staining of the skin biopsy shows the presence of antibodies confined to the basement membrane.

Other blistering diseases are associated with different abnormalities in the way in which epidermal cells adhere to each other and the methods by which the basement membrane is stuck firmly down onto the dermis.

Case 18.2   Answer

The functional unit of the female breast is the **mammary lobule**, composed of a series of blind-ending terminal ductules that open into an intralobular terminal duct. The intralobular terminal duct can carry secretions to a larger duct that lies outside the lobule – the extralobular terminal duct; this then connects with extralobular terminal ducts from adjacent lobules before opening into a series of increasingly larger ducts, the largest of which open to the exterior at the nipple. The terminal ductules and the intralobular terminal duct are embedded in a loose fibrous support tissue, the intralobular fibrocollagenous stroma, and all lobules have a supporting packing of adipose tissue and some denser fibrous tissue around them. The epithelium of the blind-ending terminal ductules is hormone sensitive, responding to hormone secretion (by ovary and pituitary) by synthesizing a lipid- and protein-rich fluid (mild). This reaches maximum effectiveness during late pregnancy and lactation, when the lobules increase enormously in size as a result of hyperplasia of the terminal ductule epithelium, as they increase the amount of milk synthesized under the influence of continued secretion of lactation-stimulating hormones by the ovary and the pituitary gland. The glandular component of the lobules undergoes hyperplasia, and the breast enlarges as a whole. When lactation ceases, the lobules slowly return to their normal size. The lobules also alter slightly in the second half of each menstrual cycle, because the terminal ductule epithelial cells begin the process of synthesizing milk under the influence of progesterone from the corpus luteum in the ovary; however, this stops as soon as menstruation occurs and the hormone level drops. This is the reason for the slight breast enlargement and tenderness experienced by some women just before menstruation.

Over a period of many years, the cyclical changes of enlargement and shrinkage during menstruation, pregnancies and lactation can lead to distortion of the normal architectural arrangements of the lobules and ducts. In particular, the fibrous tissue (both the dense extralobular and the loose intralobular) increases in amount, and bands of fibrous tissue split up some lobules and constrict and obstruct some of the ducts so that they become blocked and distended. Fibroadenosis is an extreme example of this change and is composed of irregular fibrosis, distortion of the lobular glandular tissue (adenosis) and marked dilatation of the obstructed ducts (cystic change). On palpation, such an area in the breast is irregular in outline, rubbery, not adherent to overlying skin or underlying muscle and may be tender. When cyst formation is prominent, part of the lump may be fluctuant.

Chapter 19 Special Senses

1. (a) True, (b) True,   (c) True,   (d) False, (e) False
2. (a) False, (b) True,   (c) False, (d) True,   (e) True
3. (a) False, (b) True,   (c) True,   (d) True,   (e) True
4. (a) True,   (b) False, (c) True,   (d) True,   (e) True

Case 19.1 Answer

There are three main groups of causes of deafness, categorized as conductive, sensorineural and mixed.

Conductive hearing loss occurs when sound vibrations are impeded in transmission from the outer ear through to the middle ear structures, affecting hearing before the sound reaches the cochlea and the nerve receptors of the inner ear. Causes include blockage in the auditory canal, accumulation of secretions in the middle ear and abnormalities in the arrangement or mobility of the auditory ossicles.

Sensorineural hearing loss results from damage to the neural receptors of the inner ear (the hair cells in the organ of Corti of the cochlea), the nerve pathways to the brain (auditory nerve) or the areas of the brain that process sound information.

Some causes of sensorineural deafness are birth-related or involve diseases in early childhood, for example, Rh incompatibility or birth anoxia. Feto-maternal infections, such as rubella, measles and cytomegalovirus infection may be associated with deafness.

In many conditions that lead to sensorineural deafness, the root of disease is genetic. In many instances, the genes for these conditions have been discovered and the gene products linked to abnormal function of cochlea hair cells.

In adult life, toxic substances including some medicines, may lead to sensorineural deafness. Continued exposure to loud noise, as in certain industries, can result in damage to the inner ear and lead to permanent hearing loss. An uncommon cause of sensorineural deafness is a tumour of the acoustic nerve, derived from support cells of the nerve, called an **acoustic neuroma**. Trauma to the skull base involving the inner ear can also result in deafness.

Mixed hearing loss is a combination of conductive and sensorineural hearing losses.

Case 19.2 Answer

The intraocular pressure is determined by the secretion and drainage of the aqueous humour. The anterior and posterior aqueous chambers lie anterior to the lens, on each side of the iris, and communicate with each other via the aperture of the pupil.

The aqueous humour is a watery fluid resembling cerebrospinal fluid and is secreted at a rate of approximately 2 mL per minute by the epithelial cells of the ciliary body in the posterior chamber. The aqueous filters through a network of spaces lined by endothelium, the trabecular meshwork, which runs around the circumference of the root of the iris and at the periphery of the anterior chamber and enters the canal of Schlemm. This canal runs around the whole circumference of the limbus within the sclera. From the canal of Schlemm, the aqueous enters venous vessels. The angle between the margin of the cornea and the iris root where the trabecular meshwork lies is the 'iridocorneal drainage angle'.

There is a normal resistance to the flow of aqueous at the level of the trabecular meshwork, such that continued secretion and resorption of the aqueous results in a normal intrinsic resting pressure within the globe (intraocular pressure) of 10–22 mmHg.

If the structures involved in the drainage of aqueous are abnormal, then drainage may be impaired, leading to an increase in the intraocular pressure, called **glaucoma**.

Conditions that lead to glaucoma include the following:
- Physical blockage of the drainage angle by particulate matter in the anterior chamber, proliferating blood vessels or trauma that literally blocks the trabecular meshwork
- Blocking of the drainage angle and entrance to the trabecular meshwork by close apposition of the iris to the back of the cornea.

In many cases, no physical blockage of the drainage angle can be demonstrated, and there is a functional blockage of drainage of the aqueous. Some causes of glaucoma have a familial basis. Some forms of glaucoma are congenital and are present in early childhood.

Index

Page numbers followed by 'f' indicate figures and 'b' indicate boxes.